Phillips' Science *of* DENTAL MATERIALS

Phillips' Science of

DENTAL MATERIALS

KENNETH J. ANUSAVICE, PhD, DMD

Associate Dean for Research
Chair, Department of Dental Biomaterials
Director, Center for Dental Biomaterials
College of Dentistry
University of Florida
Gainesville, Florida

ELEVENTH EDITION

with 572 illustrations

Selected artwork by:
José dos Santos, Jr.

Graphical illustrations by:
Chiayi Shen

SAUNDERS
An Imprint of Elsevier

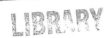
PHILLIPS' SCIENCE OF DENTAL MATERIALS   ISBN 0-7216-9387-3

NOTICE

Dentistry is an ever-changing field. Standard safety precautions must be followed, but as new research and clinical experience broaden our knowledge, changes in treatment and drug therapy may become necessary or appropriate. Readers are advised to check the most current product information provided by the manufacturer of each drug to be administered to verify the recommended dose, the method and duration of administration, and contraindications. It is the responsibility of the licensed prescriber, relying on experience and knowledge of the patient, to determine dosages and the best treatment for each individual patient. Neither the publisher nor the editor assumes any liability for any injury and/or damage to persons or property arising from this publication.

Previous editions copyrighted 1996, 1991, 1982, 1973, 1967, 1960, 1954, 1946, 1940, 1936 by W.B. Saunders Company

Library of Congress Cataloging-in-Publication Data

Phillips' science of dental materials / [edited by] Kenneth J. Anusavice; selected artwork by José dos Santos Jr. — 11th ed.
  p. ; cm.
    Includes bibliographical references and index.
    ISBN 0-7216-9387-3
    1. Dental materials. I. Title: Science of dental materials. II. Anusavice, Kenneth J. III. Phillips, Ralph W.
    [DNLM: 1. Dental Materials. WU 190 P5625 2003]
    RK652.5.P495 2003
    617.6'95—dc21   2003045747

Publishing Director: Linda L. Duncan
Executive Editor: Penny Rudolph
Senior Developmental Editor: Kimberly Alvis
Publishing Services Manager: Patricia Tannian
Project Manager: Sharon Corell
Designer: Gail Morey Hudson
Cover Design: Julia Dummitt

Printed in the United States of America

Last digit is the print number: 9   8   7   6   5   4   3   2   1

Contributors

Sibel A. Antonson, DDS, PhD
Assistant Professor and Director of Dental
　Biomaterials
Department of Restorative Dentistry
NOVA Southeastern University
College of Dental Medicine
Fort Lauderdale, Florida

William A. Brantley, PhD
Professor and Director, Graduate Program in Dental
　Materials Science
Section of Restorative Dentistry, and Prosthetic
　Dentistry
College of Dentistry
The Ohio State University
Columbus, Ohio

Paul Cascone, PhD
Senior Vice President, Technology
The Argen Corporation
San Diego, California

Josephine F. Esquivel-Upshaw, DMD, MS
Assistant Professor
Department of General Dentistry
University of Texas Health Science Center at San
　Antonio
San Antonio, Texas

Grayson W. Marshall, Jr., DDS, MPH, PhD
Professor and Chair, Division of Biomaterials and
　Bioengineering
Department of Preventive and Restorative Dental
　Sciences
University of California, San Francisco
San Francisco, California

Sally J. Marshall, PhD
Professor and Vice Chair for Research
Department of Preventive and Restorative Dental
　Sciences
University of California, San Francisco
San Francisco, California

Barry K. Norling, BSChE, MSChE, PhD
Associate Professor
Department of Restorative Dentistry
University of Texas Health Science Center at San
　Antonio
San Antonio, Texas

Rodney D. Phoenix, DDS, MS
Associate Professor and Head, Removable Partial
　Denture Division
Department of Prosthodontics
The University of Texas Health Science Center at
　San Antonio
San Antonio, Texas

H. Ralph Rawls, PhD
Professor and Head, Division of Biomaterials
Department of Restorative Dentistry
University of Texas Health Science Center at San
　Antonio
San Antonio, Texas

Chiayi Shen, PhD
Associate Professor
Department of Dental Biomaterials
University of Florida
Gainesville, Florida

John C. Wataha, DMD, PhD
Professor
Department of Oral Rehabilitation
Medical College of Georgia
Augusta, Georgia

The eleventh edition of
Phillips' Science of Dental Materials
is dedicated to the memory of
Dr. Harold Stanley
who passed away in 2001.

Stan's remarkable contributions to the field of
dental materials will benefit the dental profession and
our dental patient population well into the future.
He has served dentistry with the highest level of
moral and ethical standards, and he has set the standard for
excellence in scholarship for all future dental materials scientists.

Preface

This book represents a comprehensive overview of the composition, biocompatibility, physical properties, mechanical properties, manipulative variables, and performance of direct and indirect restorative materials and auxiliary materials used in dentistry. The book is intended as a textbook for dental students, dental hygiene students and practicing hygienists, laboratory technicians, and dental materials scientists. It is also designed as an authoritative reference book for dentists, dental assistants, and corporate marketing staff. Although the scientific concepts presented in some chapters are somewhat advanced, the text information in most chapters can be readily understood by individuals with a general college education.

The eleventh edition of *Phillips' Science of Dental Materials* is divided into four sections to reflect the focus of the chapters contained in each part. *Part I, General Classes and Properties of Dental Materials,* consists of eight chapters that cover the structure, physical properties, mechanical properties, and biocompatibility of restorative and auxiliary materials used in dentistry. *Part II: Auxiliary Dental Materials,* contains five chapters on impression materials, gypsum products, dental waxes, casting investments and procedures, and finishing and polishing abrasives and procedures. *Part III: Direct Restorative Materials,* is focused on five areas, bonding, restorative resins, dental cements, dental amalgams, and direct-filling gold. *Part IV: Indirect Restorative Materials,* consists of five chapters including dental casting and soldering alloys, wrought metals, dental ceramics, denture base resins, and dental implants. Direct and indirect materials are used to restore function and/or aesthetics in mouths containing damaged, decayed, or missing teeth by producing the restoration *directly* within the prepared tooth or a prosthesis *indirectly* in a dental laboratory before placement in the oral cavity, respectively.

The previous 30 chapters have been condensed into the 23 chapters of the eleventh edition by combining Chapters 3 and 16 into the new Chapter 3, *Physical Properties of Dental Materials;* Chapters 6, 7, and 8 into the new Chapter 9, *Impression Materials;* Chapters 22 and 23 into the new Chapter 12, *Casting Investments and Procedures;* Chapters 24 and 25 into the new Chapter 16, *Dental Cements;* Chapters 17 and 18 into the new Chapter 17, *Dental Amalgams;* and Chapters 20 and 27 into the new Chapter 19, *Dental Casting and Soldering Alloys.* This condensed format places similar topics into one chapter, making it easier to find information on any given topic.

Each of the chapters contains an introductory *terminology* section that is designed to familiarize the reader with key words and definitions and a number of *critical thinking questions,* which are intended to stimulate thinking and to emphasize important concepts. The answers to these questions are generally found in the section or sections immediately after each question. Although the terminology is associated with generally accepted scientific and dental definitions, it is not intended to be a comprehensive dictionary of all terms used in dental biomaterials science.

Several of the chapters represent totally new approaches to the specific subject. Chapter 1 has been revised to provide an introductory overview of the use of dental materials, the historical evolution of biomaterials, and standards for safety and quality assurance. Chapters 5, 6, 19, and 20 have been restructured to reflect an updated review of casting and wrought metals. Chapter 7 reflects a new approach on the science of dental polymers. Chapter 8 is a totally new summary of the basic principles and clinical implications of biocompatibility evaluation. Chapter 9 represents an integration of the three previous chapters on impression materials. Chapter 14 is a new overview of the systems and principles for use of dental adhesives. Chapter 15 reflects a more applied review of restorative resins. Chapter 16 on dental cements is an expanded description of cement composition, manipulative characteristics, and clinical performance based on the integration of the previous Chapters 24 and 25. Chapter 21 represents an updated summary of ceramics used for metal-ceramic and all-ceramic prostheses. Finally, Chapter 23 is a new overview of dental implants with an emphasis on implant material and design considerations relative to clinical performance.

Aims and Need for This Book

The aims of this textbook are: (1) to introduce dental materials science to students with little or no dental background and facilitate their study of physical and chemical properties that are related to selection of these products by the dentist, (2) to describe the basic properties of dental materials that are related either to clinical manipulation by dentists and/or dental laboratory technicians, (3) to characterize the durability and aesthetics of dental restorations and prostheses made from the restorative materials, and (4) to identify characteristics of materials that affect their biological safety. It is assumed that the reader possesses an introductory knowledge of physics as well as inorganic and/or organic chemistry.

The information in this book is intended to bridge the gap between the knowledge obtained in basic courses in materials science, chemistry, physics, and the dental clinic. As previously noted, a dental technique does not need to be an empirical process, but rather it can be based on sound scientific principles as more information is available from further research. In any basic science, principles should be emphasized. The chapters that follow focus more on why the materials react as they do and how the manipulation variables affect their performance in a dental laboratory or dental clinic.

One of the differences between a professional and a tradesman is that the former possesses basic knowledge with which he or she can establish conditions for a situation such that a prediction of eventual success of a project is reasonably ensured. A riveter must be responsible for the joined beams in a bridge, but the engineer is responsible for the design of the bridge, especially where the rivets and every truss and beam are to be placed and joined, and for the selection of the materials with which the structure is constructed. If the engineer knew nothing about the physical and chemical properties of the steels and other metals with which the bridge is made, the structure would be more likely to fail.

The dentist and the engineer have much in common. Dentists must estimate the stresses present in a dental prosthesis that they will build and be guided by such analyses in the design of the structure. They should possess a sufficient knowledge of the physical properties of the different types of materials that they use so that they can exercise the best judgment possible in their selection. For example, they must know whether the clinical situation requires the use of an amalgam, a resin-based composite, a cement, a casting alloy, a ceramic, or a metal-ceramic. Only if they know the physical and chemical properties of each of these materials are they in a position to make such a judgment. In addition to the mechanical requirements of the materials, there are also certain aesthetic and physiologic requirements that often complicate the situation beyond the difficulties usually experienced by the engineer.

Once the dentist has selected the type of material to be used, a commercial product must be chosen. It is the intention of major dental manufacturers to cooperate with dentists in supplying them with materials of the highest quality. The competition is keen, however, and the dentist should be able to evaluate the claims of the respective manufacturers from an informed, intelligent perspective. It is unfortunate that there are a few unprincipled dental manufacturers who make preposterous claims and who exploit the dentist for their own profit. For the dentists' protection and for the protection of their patients, they must be able to recognize spurious practices of this sort. Courses or lectures in dental materials attempt to provide dentists with certain criteria of selection so as to enable them to discriminate between fact and unproven claims.

Furthermore, it is hoped that students of dental materials are given an appreciation of the broad scientific scope of their chosen profession. Because a great deal of the daily practice of dentistry involves the selection and use of dental materials for patient treatment procedures, it is obvious that the science of dental materials is critically important.

The advances being made in dental materials science suggest that intriguing changes will continue to occur in the practice of dentistry. Based on your knowledge of materials science principles, you should be prepared to analyze the benefits and limitations of these dental materials to make rational decisions on their selection and use in a clinical practice.

Not all the materials used in dentistry are included in this book. For example, anesthetics, medicaments, and therapeutic agents such as fluoride varnish, xylitol, and chlorhexidine are not within the scope of this book. The science of dental materials generally encompasses some of the properties of natural oral tissues (enamel, dentin, cementum, pulp tissue, periodontal ligament, and bone) and the synthetic materials that are used for prevention and arrest of dental caries, for periodontal therapy, and for reconstruction of missing, damaged, or unaesthetic oral structures. These categories include materials employed in dental disciplines such as preventive dentistry, public health dentistry, operative dentistry, oral and maxillofacial surgery, orthodontics, periodontology, pediatric dentistry, and prosthodontics.

Organization

The engineering curriculum of most major universities includes the discipline of materials science. This is concerned with the microstructural features of materials and with the dependence of properties on these internal structures. The sequence of instruction generally progresses from atomic to macroscopic structures, from the simple to the more complex. Knowledge in this field is derived from various disciplines, such as physical chemistry, solid-state physics, polymer science, ceramics, engineering mechanics, and metallurgy. Because fundamental principles of the physical sciences and engineering and microstructure govern the properties of all materials, it is logical to study the microstructural characteristics before proceeding to the macrostructural features.

Following the overview of dental materials (Chapter 1), *Part I* focuses on the structure and properties of materials. This importance of relating properties of a material to its atomic or crystalline structure is emphasized in Chapter 2, which deals with the structure of matter and certain principles of materials science that are not usually included in a college physics course. These principles are in turn related to the properties of dental materials, as discussed in Chapters 3 and 4. The requirements placed on dental structures and materials are demanding and unique. To design prostheses appropriately, the dentist must be aware of the limitations of restorative materials and the demanding conditions that exist in the oral cavity. These factors are also discussed in Chapters 3 and 4. One should be increasingly aware of the difficulties involved in selecting a material that is technique insensitive, biocompatible, and durable. These characteristics are emphasized in the discussions that follow on specific materials.

Following the chapters on the structure of matter and the physical and mechanical properties of dental materials are overview chapters dealing with metals and alloys, polymers, and ceramics, and the biocompatibility of dental materials.

The basic science of physical metallurgy is concerned with the properties of metals and alloys, whereas the study of metallography involves the microstructure of metals that result from their solidification (Chapter 5). The constitution of alloys represents the equilibrium phases that result in an alloy system as a function of temperature and composition (Chapter 6). Chapter 7 focuses on dental polymers.

It is obvious from the earlier discussion of the regulatory agencies in dentistry, such as the ADA Council on Scientific Affairs, the FDA, the ISO and the FDI that the precursor to the marketing or selection of a dental material is its biocompatibility with oral tissues. These biological considerations are covered in Chapter 8 and are noted thereafter throughout the book.

Chapters 9 through 13 in *Part II* describe auxiliary materials and techniques that are used to fabricate and finish the surfaces of dental restorations and prostheses. These materials include impression materials (Chapter 9), gypsum products (Chapter 10), dental waxes (Chapter 11), casting investments and procedures (Chapter 12), and finishing and polishing materials (Chapter 13).

The chapters in *Part III* for direct restorative materials include bonding (Chapter 14), restorative resins (Chapter 15), dental cements (Chapter 16), dental amalgams (Chapter 17), and direct filling gold (Chapter 18).

Chapters in *Part IV* on indirect restorative materials include dental casting and soldering alloys (Chapter 19), wrought metals (Chapter 20), dental ceramics (Chapter 21), denture base resins (Chapter 22), and dental implants (Chapter 23).

Many branches of science are incorporated in the information presented and various specialized branches of chemistry are applied. Practically all of the engineering applied sciences have contributed to the subject. There is also an increasing awareness by the dentist that the biological properties of dental materials cannot be divorced from their mechanical and physical properties. Thus, interwoven throughout the book are discussions of the pertinent biological characteristics to be considered in the selection and use of dental materials.

Kenneth J. Anusavice, PhD, DMD

ACKNOWLEDGMENTS

The eleventh edition of *Phillips' Science of Dental Materials*, previously named *Skinner's Science of Dental Materials* in the ninth and earlier editions, has undergone significant changes that are consistent with the rapidly changing trends in the field of dental materials science and the practice of dentistry. Increased emphasis has been placed on biocompatibility, adhesion, dentin bonding principles, fluoride-releasing materials, resin-based composites, ceramic-based prostheses, dental polymers, and dental implants.

Many individuals should be recognized both for their contributions to the fields of dental materials science and to the revision of this textbook. Foremost is Chiayi Shen of our Department of Dental Biomaterials at the University of Florida. Dr. Shen has made significant recommendations for modifying the format of the eleventh edition by consolidating the 23 chapters into four main sections. He is also one of the main contributors to Chapters 9 and 16. William Brantley also made significant contributions to the revision of Chapters 3, 5, 6, 19, and 20. New chapters were written by Ralph Rawls, John C. Wataha, Barry Norling, and Josephine Esquivel-Upshaw. Much of the new artwork was created by José dos Santos, Jr. Other individuals who provided significant input include Michael Bagby, Wulf Brämer, Paul Cascone, Ivar Mjör, and Sam Sarma.

I express my appreciation to those who contributed to the tenth edition of this textbook, but who were not contributors to the eleventh edition. Several of the revised chapters may contain portions of the sections they created in the last edition. They include Charles F. DeFreest, Jack Ferracane, J. Rodway Mackert, Jr., Miroslav Marek, Victoria A. Marker, Robert Neiman, Karl-Johan Söderholm, and Harold R. Stanley. These individuals provided significant input to the tenth edition in which several significant changes had been introduced to enhance readability and the clinical perspectives of dental biomaterials. In their quest to promote evidence-based dentistry, they blended basic science and applied research findings with manipulative variables to provide improved balance between science and clinical practice.

Proofreading assistance was provided by my wife, Sandi, who has supported my academic pursuits in many ways. Her patience and understanding during the preparation of the eleventh edition were critically important to its timely completion.

I also express my gratitude to those who helped to shape my professional career. These individuals include Robert T. DeHoff, Professor of Materials Science and Engineering at the University of Florida, who guided my PhD training and enhanced my technical writing skills, Robert Kinzer, a former Chairman of

Restorative Dentistry at the Medical College of Georgia, who encouraged me to pursue dental school training and who supported the development of my didactic and clinical teaching skills, and Carl W. Fairhurst, former Professor of Restorative Dentistry at the Medical College of Georgia, who provided opportunities to advance my research skills. My research career has advanced more rapidly because of their guidance and support. In addition, financial support during my dental career has been provided by the National Institute of Dental and Craniofacial Research of the National Institutes of Health. This support is greatly appreciated.

Finally, I would like to thank the staff at Elsevier Inc. for their assistance in organizing and expediting the activities related to publishing the eleventh edition. These individuals include Penny Rudolph, Kimberly Alvis, and Courtney Sprehe.

Kenneth J. Anusavice, PhD, DMD

Contents

I

GENERAL CLASSES AND PROPERTIES OF DENTAL MATERIALS

1

Overview of Materials for Dental Applications

Kenneth J. Anusavice

OUTLINE

What Are Dental Materials?

Historical Use of Restorative Materials

Standards for Dental Materials

ADA Acceptance Program

General Provisions for ADA Acceptance

U.S. Food and Drug Administration Regulations

International Standards

ISO Standards, Subcommittees, and Working Groups

Other Dental Standards Organizations

How Safe Are Dental Restorative Materials?

KEY TERMS

Auxiliary dental—Substance that is used in the construction of a dental prosthesis but that does not become a part of the structure.

Direct restorative material—A cement, metal, or resin-based composite that is placed and formed intraorally to restore teeth or enhance aesthetics.

Indirect restorative material—A ceramic, metal, metal-ceramic, or resin-based composite used extraorally to produce prostheses, which replace missing teeth, enhance aesthetics, and/or restore damaged teeth.

Preventive dental material—Cement, coating, or restorative material that either seals pits and fissures or that releases a therapeutic agent such as fluoride or chlorhexidine to prevent or arrest the demineralization of tooth structure.

Restorative dental—Metallic, ceramic, metal-ceramic, or resin-based substance used to replace, repair, or rebuild teeth, and/or to enhance aesthetics.

Temporary restorative material—Cement or resin-based composite used for a period of a few days to several months to restore or replace missing teeth or tooth structure until a more long-lasting prosthesis or restoration can be placed.

CRITICAL QUESTION

What are the differences among preventive, restorative, preventive/restorative, and auxiliary dental materials used for the construction of a fixed partial denture (bridge)?

WHAT ARE DENTAL MATERIALS?

The overriding goal of dentistry is to maintain or improve the quality of life of the dental patient. This goal can be accomplished by preventing disease, relieving pain, improving mastication efficiency, enhancing speech, and improving appearance. Because many of these objectives require the replacement or alteration of tooth structure, the main challenges for centuries have been the development and selection of biocompatible, long-lasting, direct-filling tooth restoratives and indirectly processed prosthetic materials that can withstand the adverse conditions of the oral environment. Figure 1-1 is a schematic cross-section of a natural tooth and supporting bone and soft tissue. Under healthy conditions, the part of the tooth that extends out of adjacent gingiva tissue is called the *clinical crown,* and that below the gingiva is called the *tooth root.* The crown of a tooth is covered by enamel. The root is covered by cementum, and it consists of dentin and tissue within one or more root canals.

Historically, a wide variety of materials have been used as tooth crown and root replacements, including animal teeth, bone, human teeth, ivory, seashells, ceramics, and metals. Restorative materials for the replacement of missing portions of tooth structure have evolved more slowly over the past several centuries.

The four groups of materials used in dentistry today are metals, ceramics, polymers, and composites. Despite recent improvements in the physical properties of these materials, none of these are permanent. Dentists and materials scientists will continue the search in the 21st century for the ideal restorative material. An ideal restorative material would (1) be biocompatible, (2) bond permanently to tooth structure or bone, (3) match the natural appearance of tooth structure and other visible tissues, (4) exhibit properties similar to those of tooth enamel, dentin, and other tissues, and (5) be capable of initiating tissue repair or regeneration of missing or damaged tissues.

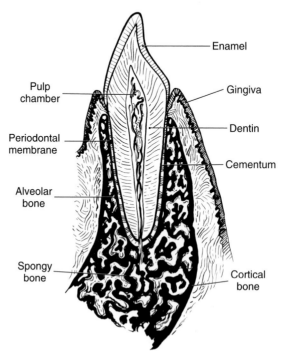

Fig. 1-1 Schematic illustration of a cross-sectional view of a natural anterior tooth and supporting tissues.

Dental materials may be classified as *preventive materials, restorative materials,* or *auxiliary materials.* **Preventive dental materials** include pit and fissure sealants; sealing agents that prevent leakage; materials that are used primarily for their antibacterial effects; and liners, bases, cements and restorative materials that are used primarily because they release fluoride (compomer, hybrid ionomer, glass ionomer cement, zinc silicophosphate cement), chlorhexidine, or other therapeutic agents used to prevent or inhibit the progression of tooth decay (*dental caries*). Table 1-1 summarizes the types of preventive and restorative materials, their applications, and their potential durability. In some cases a preventive material may also serve as a restorative material that may be used for a short-term application (up to several months), for moderately long time periods (1 to 4 years), or for longer periods (5 years or more). Dental restoratives that have little or no therapeutic benefit may also be used for short-term (temporary) use, or they may be indicated for applications requiring moderate durability or long-term durability. For example, restorative materials that do not contain fluoride can be used for patients who are at a low risk for caries.

Restorative dental materials consist of all synthetic components that can be used to repair or replace tooth structure, including primers, bonding agents, liners, cement bases, amalgams, resin-based composites, compomers, hybrid ionomers, cast metals, metal-ceramics, ceramics, and denture polymers. These materials can also be

Table 1-1   Comparative Applications and Durability of Preventive and Restorative Dental Materials

Material type	Applications of products	Potential preventive benefit	Durability
Resin adhesive	A	F (certain products)	M
Resin sealant	S	S	M
Resin cement	L	F (certain products)	M
Compomer	B, L, R	F	M
Hybrid ionomer	B, L, R	F	M
Glass ionomer (GI)	A, B, L, R, S	F, S	L, M
Metal-modified GI	R	F	L, M
Zinc oxide–eugenol	B, L, T		L, M
Zinc phosphate	B, L		M
Zinc polycarboxylate	B, L		M
Zinc silicophosphate	B, L	F	M
Resin composite	R	F (certain products)	H
Dental amalgam	R		H
Ceramic	R		H
Metal/ceramic	R		H
Metal/resin	R		M, H
Acrylic resin (temporary use)	T		L
Denture acrylic	R		H
Cast metal	R		H
Wrought metal	R		H

Applications: **A,** Adhesive; **B,** base; **L,** luting agent; **S,** pit/fissure sealant; **R,** restorative; **T,** temporary restorative.
Potential preventive benefit: F, Fluoride-releasing material; **S,** sealing agent.
Durability: L, Low; **M,** moderate; **H,** high.

designed as controlled-delivery devices for release of therapeutic or diagnostic agents. Restorative materials may be used for temporary, short-term purposes (such as temporary cements and temporary crown and bridge resins), or for longer-term applications (dentin bonding agents, inlays, onlays, crowns, removable dentures, fixed dentures, and orthodontic appliances). Restorative materials may further be classified as **direct restorative materials** or **indirect restorative materials,** depending on whether they are used (1) intraorally to fabricate restorations or prosthetic devices directly on the teeth or tissues or (2) extraorally, in which the materials are formed indirectly on casts or other replicas of the teeth and other tissues. **Auxiliary dental materials** are substances that are used in the process of fabricating dental prostheses and appliances but that do not become part of these devices. These include acid-etching solutions, impression materials, casting investments, gypsum cast and model materials, dental waxes, acrylic resins for impression and bleaching trays, acrylic resins for mouth guards and occlusion aids, and finishing and polishing abrasives.

Temporary restorative materials are a subcategory of restorative materials and include products used for dental restorations and appliances that are not intended for moderate-term or long-term applications. Examples include temporary cements used for luting, temporary cements, or other restoratives used for fillings, orthodontic wires, and acrylic resins used for temporary inlays, onlays, crowns, and fixed partial dentures.

CRITICAL QUESTION

What technological advances led to the development of a more precise fit of indirectly made prostheses?

HISTORICAL USE OF RESTORATIVE MATERIALS

Dentistry as a specialty is believed to have begun about 3000 B.C. Gold bands and wires were used by the Phoenicians (after 2500 B.C.). Around 700 B.C. the Etruscans carved ivory or bone for the construction of partial denture teeth that were fastened to natural teeth by means of gold wires or bands. The gold bands were used to position extracted teeth in place of missing teeth.

Although inscriptions on Egyptian tombstones indicate that tooth doctors were considered to be medical specialists, they are not known to have performed restorative dentistry. However, some teeth found in Egyptian mummies were either transplanted human teeth or tooth forms made of ivory. The earliest documented evidence of tooth implant materials is attributed to the Etruscans as early as 700 B.C. Around 600 A.D. the Mayans used implants consisting of seashell segments that were placed in anterior tooth sockets. Hammered gold inlays and stone or mineral inlays were placed for aesthetic purposes or traditional ornamentation by the Mayans and later by the Aztecs. The Incas performed tooth mutilations using hammered gold, but the material was not placed for decorative purposes.

Cavities in teeth have been replaced or restored since ancient times to the eighteenth century with a variety of materials including stone chips, ivory, human teeth, turpentine resin, cork, gums, and metal foils (lead and tin). More recently, gutta percha, cements, metal-modified cements, unfilled synthetic resin, composites, other metals (gold leaf, amalgam, and a variety of cast metals and alloys), ceramics, and metal-ceramics have been used for tooth restoration. Paré (1509–1590), surgeon to four kings, used lead or cork for tooth fillings. Queen Elizabeth I (1533–1603) used cloth fragments to fill the cavities in her teeth. Fauchard (1678–1761), the father of modern dentistry, used tin foil or lead cylinders for filling tooth cavities. Wealthy patients preferred to have teeth that were made of agate, mother of pearl, silver, or gold. Modern dentistry began in 1728, when Fauchard published a treatise describing many types of dental restorations, including a method for the construction of artificial dentures made from ivory.

Gold foil has also been employed for dental restorative purposes. Pfaff (1715–1767), the dentist of Frederick the Great of Prussia, used gold foil to cap the pulp chamber. Bull began producing beaten gold in Connecticut for dental applications in 1812. Arculanus recommended gold-leaf dental fillings in 1848. Sponge gold was introduced in 1853 in the United States and England to replace gold leaf. In 1855 Arthur promoted the use of cohesive gold in the United States. In 1897 Philbrook described the use of metal fillings made from wax patterns of the tooth cavity.

Using filings from silver coins mixed with mercury, Taveau (1816) developed in France what is likely the first dental amalgam. The Crawcour brothers, who emigrated from France to the United States, introduced Taveau's amalgam fillings in 1833; however, graduates of the Baltimore Dental College subsequently took an oath not to use amalgams in their practices. Many dentists criticized the poor quality of the early amalgam restorations. This controversy led to the "amalgam war" from 1840 to 1850, during which time heated debates occurred over the benefits and drawbacks of dental amalgam. Research on amalgam formulations from the 1860s through the 1890s greatly improved the handling properties and the clinical performance of amalgam filling materials. In 1895 Black proposed standardized cavity preparations and manufacturing processes for dental amalgam products.

Gold shell crowns were described by Mouton in 1746, but they were not patented until 1873 by Beers. In 1885 Logan patented a porcelain fused to a platinum post, replacing the unsatisfactory wooden posts previously used to build up intraradicular (within the tooth root) areas of teeth. In 1907 the detached-post crown was introduced, which was more easily adjustable.

In 1756 Pfaff described a method for making impressions of the mouth in wax, from which he constructed a model with plaster of Paris. Pfaff's use of plaster of Paris allowed dentists to make impressions of the patient's edentulous jaws in the mouth. Duchateau, a French pharmacist, and de Chemant, a dentist, designed a process in 1774 for producing hard, decay-proof porcelain dentures. In 1789 de Chemant patented an improved version of these "mineral paste" porcelain teeth. The porcelain inlay was introduced soon thereafter in the early 1800s. However, porcelain bonding to metals was not fully refined for metal-ceramic crowns until the mid 1900s.

The dentures of George Washington (1732–1799) fit poorly, and he suffered terribly throughout his presidency (1789–1797). Washington never wore wooden teeth as has been erroneously reported; he wore dentures made of some of his own teeth, cows' teeth or hippopotamus' teeth, ivory, or lead. Prior to his first term as president, he had worn partial dentures that were fastened to his remaining teeth. During the inauguration for his first term as president in 1789, Washington had only one natural tooth remaining and he wore his first full set of dentures made by John Greenwood. The base of these dentures was made of hippopotamus ivory carved to fit the jaw ridges. The upper denture contained ivory teeth, and the lower denture consisted of eight human teeth fastened by gold rivets that screwed into the denture base. The two dentures were secured in his mouth by spiral springs.

In 1808 Fonzi, an Italian dentist, developed an individual porcelain tooth form that was held in place with an embedded platinum pin. Planteau, a French dentist, first introduced porcelain teeth in the United States in 1817. In 1822 Charles Peale, an artist, fired mineral teeth in Philadelphia, and Samuel Stockton began the commercial production of porcelain teeth soon thereafter in 1825. Ash further developed an improved porcelain tooth in England around 1837.

Evans (1836) refined the method of making accurate measurements in the mouth. However, it was not until 1839 that Charles Goodyear's invention of a low-cost vulcanized rubber allowed dentures to be molded accurately and to fit the mouth. Vulcanized rubber denture bases that held denture teeth accelerated the demand for accurately fitting dentures at a reasonably low cost. Since 1839 denture bases have advanced in quality through the use of acrylic resins and cast metals. In 1935 polymerized acrylic resin was introduced as a denture base material to support artificial teeth.

Up to this point, we have focused primarily on the historical evolution of direct filling materials and some rather crude indirect materials. Prior to the 20th century, because of inadequate technology and lack of electricity, fillings were of rather poor quality and did not fit well within the teeth. However, in 1907 Taggert developed a more refined method for producing cast inlays. Cast alloys were introduced later in the 20th century, further developing this technology. Commercially pure titanium (CP Ti), noble alloys, and base metal alloys of nickel-chromium, cobalt-chromium, or cobalt-nickel-chromium are now available for use in the production of cast inlays, onlays, crowns, and frameworks for fixed all-metal or metal-ceramic dentures and for removable dentures. Few major improvements in the construction of fixed partial dentures (bridges) occurred until the early 1900s. Mason developed a detachable facing to a crown to hold an artificial tooth in place for an adjacent missing tooth. Thomas Steele (1904), a colleague of Mason, introduced interchangeable facings that solved the problem of fractured facings.

Even though the practice of dentistry antedates the Christian era, comparatively little historical data exist on the science of dental materials. The use of fluoride to prevent tooth demineralization originated from observations in 1915 of low decay rates of people in areas of Colorado whose water supplies contained significant fluoride concentrations. Controlled water fluoridation (1 ppm) to reduce tooth decay (demineralization) began in 1944, and the incidence of tooth decay in children who have had access to fluoridated water has decreased by 50% since then. The use of pit and fissure sealants and fluoride-releasing varnishes and restorative materials has reduced the caries incidence even further.

Little scientific information about dental restorative materials has been available until recently. Prior to this knowledge, the use of these materials was entirely an art, and the only testing laboratory was the mouth of the patient. Today, despite the availability of sophisticated technical equipment and the development of standardized testing methods for evaluating the biocompatibility of preventive and restorative materials, this testing sometimes still occurs in the mouths of our patients. The reasons for this situation are diverse. In some instances, products are approved for human use without being tested in animal or human subjects. In other instances, dentists use materials for purposes that were not indicated by the manufacturer; for example, a ceramic product may be used for posterior fixed partial dentures (FPDs) when the product has been recommended only for inlays, onlays, crowns, and anterior three-unit FPDs.

The first important awakening of scientific interest occurred during the middle of the 19th century, when research studies on amalgam began. At about the same time, some reports appeared in the literature of studies on porcelain and gold foil. These sporadic advances in knowledge finally culminated in the investigations of G.V. Black, who began his research studies in 1895. Hardly a phase of dentistry exists that was not explored and advanced by this pioneer in restorative dentistry.

STANDARDS FOR DENTAL MATERIALS

The next great advance in the knowledge of dental materials and their manipulation began in 1919. During that year the U.S. Army requested the National Bureau of Standards (now known as the *National Institute of Standards and Technology [NIST]*) to set up specifications for the evaluation and selection of dental amalgams for use in federal service. This research was done under the leadership of Wilmer Souder, and an excellent report on this study was published in 1920.

The information contained in the Souder report was received enthusiastically by the dental profession, and similar testing data were then requested for other dental materials. At that time, the U.S. government could not allocate sufficient funds to continue the work, so a fellowship was created and supported by the Weinstein Research Laboratories. Under such an arrangement, the sponsor provided money for the salaries of research associates and a certain amount of equipment and supplies. The associates then worked in the National Bureau of Standards under the direction of the staff members. For all practical purposes, these associates were members of the staff supported by private interests. All findings were published and became common property under this particular arrangement. Working under Dr. Souder's direction, several research associates investigated the properties of dental wrought gold materials, casting gold alloys, and accessory casting materials. This phase of the work resulted in the publication of an extensive and valuable research report.

In 1928, the Dental Research Fellowship at the National Bureau of Standards was assumed by the American Dental Association (ADA). The research carried out by the ADA research associates in conjunction with the staff members of NIST has been of inestimable value to the dental profession, and it has earned for this group an international reputation. Researchers such as Wilmer Souder, George C. Paffenbarger, and William T. Sweeney will undoubtedly be remembered historically as the pioneers whose work began a new era of intense research in the field of dental materials. It was the enthusiasm of these men that prompted the organization of the first academic courses in dental materials to be taught in U.S. dental schools and abroad.

CRITICAL QUESTION

What is the primary purpose of specifications and standards for dental materials?

ADA ACCEPTANCE PROGRAM

The work at the American Dental Association (ADA) is divided into a number of categories, including the measurement of the clinically significant physical and chemical properties of dental materials and the development of new materials, instruments, and test methods. Until 1965, one of the primary objectives of the facility at NIST was to formulate standards or specifications for dental materials. However, when the ADA Council on Dental Materials and Devices (now known as the *Council on Scientific Affairs*) was established in 1966, it assumed responsibility for standards development and initiated the certification of products that meet the requirements of these specifications.

Such specifications are standards by which the quality and properties of particular dental materials can be gauged. These standards identify the requirements for the physical and chemical properties of a material that ensure satisfactory performance if the material is properly manipulated and used by the dental laboratory technician and the dentist. The Acceptance Program of the Council on Scientific Affairs incorporates these specifications in the evaluation of dental products, and the products are tested for compliance with specification requirements. When a product is classified as *Accepted*, the manufacturer is permitted to signify on the label of the product the notation "ADA Accepted."

The ADA, accredited by the American National Standards Institute (ANSI), is also the administrative sponsor of two standards-formulating committees operating under the direction of ANSI. The ADA Standards Committee for Dental Products (SCDP) develops specifications for all dental materials, instruments, and equipment, with the exception of drugs and x-ray films. The Council on Scientific Affairs (CSA) is also responsible for the evaluation of drugs, tooth-cleaning and tooth-whitening agents, therapeutic agents used in dentistry, dental equipment, and dental x-ray film.

Working groups of ADA SCDP formulate the specifications. When a specification has been approved by the ADA SCDP and the ADA CSA, it is submitted to the American National Standards Institute. On acceptance by that body, it becomes an American National Standard. Thus the Council on Scientific Affairs also has the opportunity of accepting it as an ADA specification.

New specifications are continually being developed to apply to new program areas. Likewise, existing specifications are periodically revised to reflect changes in product formulations and new knowledge about the behavior of materials in the oral cavity, for example, the ANSI/ADA Specification No. 1 for dental amalgam, which was revised in January 2003.

The ADA Seal of Acceptance

Dentists and consumers of dental products have long recognized the ADA Seal of Acceptance as an important symbol of a dental product's safety and effectiveness. For more than 125 years, the ADA has sought to promote the safety and effectiveness of dental products. The first Seal of Acceptance was awarded in 1931. Although this program is strictly voluntary, over 400 companies participate in the Seal program. Manufacturers commit significant resources to evaluate, test, and market products in the Seal program. Approximately 1250 dental products carry the Seal of Acceptance. Of these, about 60% are products prescribed or used by dentists, such as antibiotics or dental restorative materials. The remaining 40% are dental products sold to consumers, such as toothpaste, dental floss, manual and electric toothbrushes, and mouth rinses.

Classification of Products Evaluated by the ADA Council on Scientific Affairs

Products that meet the standards of acceptance with respect to safety, efficacy, composition and labeling, package inserts, advertising, and other promotional material are accepted. Once accepted, the products are listed and may be described in suitable reports and advertisements in *The Journal of the American Dental Association*. The manufacturer may then use the Council's Seal of Acceptance and may be required to use an authorized statement if the ADA Seal is used in the advertisement. Products are usually accepted for a period of up to 5 years. Acceptance is renewable and may be reconsidered at any time. If there is a change in the manufacturer or distributor of a product, the period of acceptance expires automatically. *Provisionally accepted* products consist of those that lack sufficient evidence to justify classification as *accepted*, but for which there is reasonable evidence of safety and usefulness, including clinical feasibility. These products meet the other qualifications established by the Council.

The Council may authorize the use of a suitable statement to define specifically the area of usefulness of products classified as *provisionally accepted*. Classification in this category is reviewed each year and is not ordinarily continued for more than 3 years. Products that are obsolete, markedly inferior, ineffective, or dangerous to the health of the user are declared *unaccepted*. When it is in the best interest of the public or the profession, the Council may submit reports on unaccepted products to the editor for publication in *The Journal of the American Dental Association*. Decisions of the Council are based on available scientific evidence and are subject to reconsideration at any time that a significant amount of new evidence becomes available.

CRITICAL QUESTION

Can a manufacturer alter the composition of an ADA-accepted product and maintain the ADA Seal of Acceptance?

GENERAL PROVISIONS FOR ADA ACCEPTANCE
Composition, Nature, and Function

A quantitative statement of composition and adequate information on the properties of all ingredients must be provided to the Council. For instruments and equipment, a description of the materials used in the construction and the method of operation must be provided. Any change in the composition, nature, or function of an accepted product must be submitted to the Council for review and approval before a modified product is marketed.

The company that seeks ADA acceptance should provide evidence that manufacturing and laboratory control facilities are under the supervision of qualified personnel, that these facilities are adequate to ensure purity and uniformity of products, and that products are produced in compliance with the Good Manufacturing Practice Code. The company must permit representatives of the Council to visit laboratories and factories on request. For products whose guidelines include an official American Dental Association Specification, the manufacturer must conduct testing on a regular basis to determine continued compliance with the specification; these test records must be made available to the Council on request. In addition the manufacturer must make available to the Council on request test records and data for any batch of an accepted product.

Required Information

The product must conform to appropriate standards or specifications. For products that fall under the scope of official American Dental Association Specifications, the following information should be submitted: (1) the serial or lot number; (2) the composition; (3) the physical properties, as obtained by standard test methods; and (4) data covering every provision of the official specification. Responsibility for guaranteeing that the product complies with an official specification lies solely with the manufacturer and not with the American Dental Association.

The Council, at any time and without notice to the manufacturer, may authorize the testing of any or all such products. In the event that a sample fails the testing, the product will be removed from the List of Accepted Products. Test samples are procured at the expense of the manufacturer. If a product is removed from the List of Accepted Products, it may subsequently be resubmitted provided that the product that failed the testing has been removed from the market.

Names that are misleading or that suggest diseases or symptoms are not acceptable. This provision may not apply to certain biological products such as serums or vaccines. Because the uses of a product may change, the product name should indicate the generic type of material or its composition rather than a proposed use for the product. However, under certain circumstances the Council may accept a name that denotes a long-established physiological action or use, particularly for a mixture.

Evidence pertaining to mechanical and physical properties, operating characteristics (when applicable), actions, dosage, safety, and efficacy must be submitted by the company. Information on acceptable standard test methods for physical properties may be secured by request to the Council on Scientific Affairs. In general, the data required on physical tests must include a brief description of the apparatus used in performing the tests, a complete statement of the results obtained, the names of the observers, and the date of the test.

The company must provide objective data from properly designed clinical and laboratory studies. Extended clinical experience may be used, in part, as a basis for evaluation of a product. Products that fall under the scope of an official American Dental Association Specification will be tested for compliance with the specification by the American Dental Association. Test samples, unless otherwise indicated in the appropriate specification, may be procured on the open market at the expense of the manufacturer.

The company must disclose any past, present, or anticipated financial arrangements between the clinical investigator and the company, its affiliates, or subsidiaries, including, but not limited to, consulting agreements, speakers' fees, grants or contracts to conduct research, or membership on the company's advisory committees. If the Council determines that the financial interests raise a question about the integrity of the data, the Council may take any action it deems necessary to ensure the reliability of the data, including, but not limited to the following:

■ Requesting that the company submit further analyses of the data
■ Requesting that the company conduct additional independent studies
■ Rejecting the data

Information Required for Renewal of Acceptance

For renewal of acceptance the manufacturer may be required to submit evidence demonstrating continued acceptable clinical performance of the product. This evidence may be in the form of new clinical studies, reports of adverse reactions or follow-up investigations of previously submitted clinical studies.

The Council may occasionally find it necessary to review the status of a product's acceptance. Decisions of the Council are based on available scientific evidence and are subject to reconsideration at any time. If a significant amount of new scientific evidence demonstrates that a product is no longer safe or effective, or if a product is deemed obsolete, markedly inferior, or dangerous to the health of the user, Council acceptance will be withdrawn.

CRITICAL QUESTIONS

What are the differences among FDA Class I, Class II, and Class III devices? Which class of regulations does a dental implant need to satisfy?

U.S. FOOD AND DRUG ADMINISTRATION REGULATIONS

On May 28, 1976, legislation was signed into law that gave the U.S. Food and Drug Administration (FDA) the regulatory authority to protect the public from hazardous or ineffective medical (and dental) devices. This legislation was the culmination of a series of attempts to provide safe and effective products, beginning with the passage of the Food and Drug Act of 1906, which did not include any provision to regulate medical device safety or the claims made for devices.

The newer legislation, named the Medical Device Amendments of 1976, requires the classification and regulation of all noncustomized medical devices that are intended for human use. According to the Federal Register, the term *device* includes any instrument, apparatus, implement, machine, contrivance, implant, or in vitro reagent that is used in the diagnosis, cure, mitigation, treatment, or prevention of disease in man and that does not achieve any of its principal intended purposes through chemical action within or on the body of humans or animals and that is not dependent on being metabolized for the achievement of any of its principal intended purposes.

Some dental products, such as those containing fluoride, are considered drugs, but most products used in the dental clinic are considered to be devices, and thus they are subject to control by the FDA Center for Devices and Radiological Health. Also subject to this control are over-the-counter products sold to the public, such as toothbrushes, dental floss, and denture adhesives.

The classification of all medical and dental items is developed by panels composed of nongovernmental dental experts, as well as representatives from industry and consumer groups. The Dental Products Panel identifies any known hazards or problems associated with a device and then categorizes the item into one of three classification groups based on relative risk factors. *Class I devices* are considered to be of low risk, and they are subject to general controls, including the registration of the manufacturer's products, adherence to *good manufacturing practices*, and certain record-keeping requirements. If it is deemed that such general controls are not in themselves adequate to ensure safety and effectiveness as claimed by the manufacturer, the item is placed into the category of *Class II devices*. Products in this class are required to meet performance standards established by the FDA or appropriate standards from other authoritative bodies, such as those of the ADA. These performance standards may relate to components, construction, and properties of a device, and they may also indicate specific testing requirements to ensure that lots or individual products conform to the regulatory requirement.

Class III, the most stringent category, requires that devices be approved for safety and effectiveness before they are marketed. All implanted or life-supporting devices are placed in this premarket clearance category. Specific data must be provided to demonstrate safety and efficacy before marketing. In certain instances, the product or device may be substantially equivalent to other approved products, and under these circumstances, only the demonstration of equivalence is necessary. Any item that does not have adequate clinical or scientific information available to permit the formulation of a performance standard is placed in the premarket approval category. For example, one of these devices, the endosseous implant for prosthetic attachment, is considered a high priority relative to the need for adequate data to demonstrate safety and effectiveness. Manufacturers of this device need to submit premarket approval applications for their implants. These are then evaluated by the Dental Products Panel to determine whether new implants can be marketed. Guidelines that have been developed by the FDA are available to all interested parties to provide the preclinical and clinical requirements for the preparation of a premarket approval application.

Several hundred dental items have been classified into one of these three categories. The FDA program, in conjunction with the ADA Acceptance Program for dental products, provides a crucial framework for standards development and provides initial evidence that the product will be safe and effective as claimed. Other countries have national government agencies comparable to the FDA that also include dental materials and devices within the jurisdiction of their regulatory authority.

INTERNATIONAL STANDARDS

Two organizations, the Fédération Dentaire Internationale (FDI) and the International Organization for Standardization (ISO), are working toward the establishment of specifications for dental materials on an international level. Originally, the FDI initiated and actively supported a program for the formulation of international specifications for dental materials. As a result of that activity, several specifications for dental materials and devices have been adopted.

The ISO is an international, nongovernmental organization whose objective is the development of international standards. This body is composed of national standards organizations from more than 80 countries. The American National Standards Institute is the U.S. member. A request by the FDI to the ISO that they consider FDI specifications for dental materials as ISO standards led to the formation of an ISO technical committee (TC), TC 106–Dentistry. The responsibility of this committee is to standardize terminology and test methods and to develop standards (specifications) for dental materials, instruments, appliances, and equipment. Additional information on ISO standards is provided in the following section.

Several FDI specifications have now been adopted as ISO standards. Since 1963, more than 100 new standards have been developed or are currently under development in ISO TC 106 through cooperative programs with the FDI. Thus considerable progress has already been realized in achieving the ultimate goal of a broad range of international specifications for dental materials and devices.

The benefit of such specifications to the dental profession has been invaluable, considering the worldwide supply and demand for dental materials, instruments, and devices. Dentists are provided with criteria for selection that are impartial and reliable. In other words, if dentists use primarily those materials that meet the appropriate specifications, they can be confident that the materials will be satisfactory. Probably no other single factor has contributed as much to the high level of dental practice as has this specification program. Awareness by dental laboratory technicians and dentists of the requirements of these specifications is essential in recognizing the limitations of the dental materials with which they are working. As is discussed frequently in the chapters to follow, no dental material is perfect in its restorative role, just as no artificial arm or leg can serve as well as the original body member that it replaces.

Research on dental materials supervised by the ADA Council on Scientific Affairs or other national standard organizations is of vital concern in this textbook on dental materials. The ADA specifications for dental materials are referred to throughout the following chapters, although specific details regarding the test methods employed are omitted. For those products sold in other countries, the counterpart ISO standards, if applicable, should be used as a reference source. It is assumed for the discussions in this textbook that the student has access to a collection of specifications and Acceptance Program guidelines of the ADA or other national or international standards.

CRITICAL QUESTION

 Of the seven ISO TC 106 subcommittees and 52 working groups, which ones are responsible for direct and indirect restorative materials?

ISO STANDARDS, SUBCOMMITTEES, AND WORKING GROUPS
ISO Technical Committee 106

In 2002 the Internal Organization for Standardization had 224 TCs to develop standards for testing the safety and efficacy of dental products. Of these TCs, TC 106 is the committee responsible for dental standards, terminology used in standards, methods of testing, and specifications applicable to materials, instruments, appliances and equipment used in all branches of dentistry. A total number of 134 ISO dental standards have been published related to the TC and its subcommittees (SCs) and working groups (WGs). In 2002 representatives from 25 member countries and 20 observer countries were involved. There are seven subcommittees for ISO standards involving dental products. The following subcommittees cover all the dental products included in the ISO standards program under the direction of TC 106.

TC 106/SC1: Filling and Restorative Materials. The following 10 working groups are included: *WG1*—Zinc oxide–eugenol cements and noneugenol cements; *WG2*—Endodontic materials; *WG5*—Pit and fissure sealants; *WG7*—Amalgam/mercury; *WG9*—Resin-based filling materials; *WG10*—Dental luting cements, bases, and liners; *WG11*—Adhesion test methods; *WG12*—Resin-based cements; *WG13*—Orthodontic products; and *WG14*—Orthodontic elastics.

TC 106/SC2: Prosthodontic Materials. The following 17 working groups develop standards for prosthodontic materials: *WG1*—Dental ceramics; *WG2*—Dental base metal alloys; *WG6*—Color stability test methods; *WG7*—Impression materials; *WG8*—Noble metal casting alloys; *WG9*—Synthetic polymer teeth; *WG10*—Resilient lining materials; *WG11*—Denture base polymers; *WG12*—Corrosion test methods; *WG13*—Investments; *WG14*—Dental brazing materials; *WG16*—Polymer veneering and die materials; *WG17*—Ceramic denture teeth; *WG18*—Dental waxes and baseplate waxes; *WG19*—Wear test methods; *WG20*—Artificial teeth; and *WG21*—Metallic materials.

TC 106/SC3: Terminology. There are four working groups in SC3: *WG1*—Harmonization of dental codes and abbreviations; *WG2*—Dental vocabulary (Revision of ISO 1942 and thematic coding of its terms); *WG3*—Communication and communications; and *WG4*—Definition of new terms related to the needs of dental standards.

TC 106/SC4: Dental Instruments. The following six working groups are included in SC4: *WG1*—Dimensions of rotary instruments; *WG5*—Numbering system; *WG7*—Dental handpieces; *WG8*—Dental hand instruments; *WG9*—Root-canal instruments; and *WG10*—Dental injection systems.

TC 106/SC6: Dental Equipment. There are six working groups in SC6: *WG1*—Dental operating light; *WG2*—Dental patient chair and dental unit; *WG3*—Dental operator's stool; *WG5*—Amalgamators, dispensers and capsules; *WG7*—Powered polymerization activators; and *WG8*—Suction equipment.

TC 106/SC7: Oral Hygiene Products. The following four working groups are included in SC7: *WG1*—Manual toothbrushes; *WG2*—Powered oral hygiene devices; *WG3*—Auxiliary oral hygiene products; and *WG4*—Toothpastes.

TC 106/SC8: Dental Implants. The five working groups in SC8 are as follows: *WG1*—Implantable materials; *WG2*—Preclinical biological evaluation and testing; *WG3*—Content of technical files; *WG4*—Mechanical testing; and *WG5*—Dental implants—Terminology.

How Are ISO Standards Developed?

Manufacturers, dental vendors, users, consumer groups, testing laboratories, governments, the dental profession, and research organizations provide input information and requirements for the development of standards. International standardization is market-driven and is based on voluntary involvement of all interests in the marketplace.

The need for a standard is usually expressed by an industry sector, which communicates this need to a national member body. The latter proposes the new work item to the ISO as a whole. Once the need for an International Standard has been established, the first phase involves definition of the technical scope of the future standard. This phase is usually carried out by working groups, which comprise technical experts from countries interested in the subject. Once agreement has been reached on which technical aspects are to be covered in the standard, a second phase is entered, during which countries determine the detailed specifications within the standard. The final phase constitutes the formal approval of the resulting draft International Standard, by 75% of all voting members, following which the agreed text is published as an ISO International Standard.

Most standards require periodic revision because of technological evolution, new methods and materials, new quality tests, and new safety requirements. To account for these factors, all ISO standards should be reviewed at intervals of not more than 5 years. On occasion, it is necessary to revise a standard earlier.

OTHER DENTAL STANDARDS ORGANIZATIONS

The work at the National Institute of Standards and Technology in Gaithersburg, Maryland, has stimulated comparable programs in other countries. The Australian Dental Standards Laboratory was established in 1936 (until 1973 this facility was known as the *Commonwealth Bureau of Dental Standards*). H.K. Worner and A.R. Docking, the first two directors, are recognized for their leadership in the development of the Australian specifications for dental materials. Other countries that have comparable organizations for developing standards and certifying products are Canada, Japan, France, Czech Republic, Germany, Hungary, Israel, India, Poland, and South Africa. Also, by agreement among the governments of Denmark, Finland, Iceland, Norway, and Sweden, the Scandinavian Institute of Dental Materials, better known as NIOM (Nordisk Institutt for Odontologisk Materialprøvning), was established in 1969 for testing, certification, and research regarding dental materials and equipment to be used in the five countries. NIOM became operational in 1973.

Also in Europe, the Comité Européen de Normalisation (CEN) established Task Group 55 to develop European standards. After the establishment of the European Economic Community, the CEN was given the charge to outline recommendations of standards for medical devices, including dental materials. In fact, the proper term to describe *dental materials, dental implants, dental instruments,* and *dental equipment* in Europe is *medical devices used in dentistry*. The CE marking on product labels denotes the European mark of conformity with the Essential Requirements in the Medical Device Directive that became effective on January 1, 1995. All medical devices marketed in the European Union countries must have the CE mark of conformity. For certain products, some countries may enforce their own standards when other countries or the international community have not developed mutually acceptable requirements. For example, Sweden restricts the use of nickel in cast dental alloys because of biocompatibility concerns, whereas no such restriction applies to those alloys in the United States. Iceland, Liechtenstein, and Norway are also signatories of the European Economic Area Agreement and require the CE marking and NIOM's Notified Body registration number on medical device packaging.

An increasing number of universities in the United States and abroad have established laboratories for research in dental materials. In the past few years, this source of basic information on the subject has exceeded that of all other sources combined. Until recently, dental research activities in universities were centered solely in dental schools, with most of the investigations being conducted by the dental faculty. Now, however, research in dental materials is also being conducted in some universities that do not have dental schools. This dental-oriented research in areas such as metallurgy, polymer science, materials science, engineering, and ceramics is being conducted in basic science departments. These expanding fields of research in dental materials illustrate the interdisciplinary aspects of the science. Since the final criterion for the success of any material or technique is its service in the mouth of the patient, countless contributions to this field have been made by dental clinicians. The observant clinician contributes invaluable information by his or her keen observations and analyses of failures and successes. Accurate record keeping and well-controlled practice procedures form an excellent basis for valuable clinical research.

The importance of clinical documentation for claims made relative to the in vivo performance of dental materials is now readily apparent. For example, the Acceptance Program of the Council on Scientific Affairs requires clinical data, whenever appropriate, to support the laboratory tests for physical properties. During the past two decades there has been an escalation in the number of clinical investigations designed to correlate specific properties with clinical performance criteria. These studies are designed to establish the precise behavior of a given material or system. In the chapters that follow, frequent reference is made to such investigations.

Another source of information is derived from manufacturers' research laboratories. The far-sighted manufacturer recognizes the value of a research laboratory relative to the development and production control of products, and unbiased information from such groups is particularly valuable. During the writing of this textbook, as with the previous edition, the counsel of scientists from dental and nondental industries was called upon. In this way the product formulations described in the succeeding chapters reflect with greater accuracy the commercial materials used by the dentist.

This diversity of research activity is resulting in an accelerating growth in the body of knowledge related to dental materials. For example, in 1978 approximately 10% of all U.S. support for dental research was focused on restorative dental materials. The percentage would no doubt be considerably higher if the money spent by industry for the development of new materials, instruments, and appliances were included. This growing investigative effort is resulting in a marked increase in the number of new materials, instruments, and techniques being introduced to the profession. For these and other reasons, an intimate knowledge of the properties and behavior of dental materials is imperative if the modern dental practice is to remain abreast of changing developments.

How is it possible for dental materials that have not been accepted by the American Dental Association to be sold to dentists and consumers?

HOW SAFE ARE DENTAL RESTORATIVE MATERIALS?

Specifications and standards have been developed to aid producers, users, and consumers in the evaluation of the safety and effectiveness of dental products. However, the decision of producers to test their materials according to national and international standards is purely voluntary. The existence of materials evaluation standards does not preclude anyone from manufacturing, marketing, buying, or using dental or medical devices that do not meet these standards. However, producers or marketers of products and devices are expected to meet the safety standards established for those products in the countries in which they are sold. Thus it is possible for a producer to be given premarket approval by the FDA to sell a dental device such as a dental restorative material without the device being approved by the ADA in accordance with the specification or Acceptance Program requirements. Nevertheless, these agencies are becoming increasingly dependent on one another to ensure that all products marketed world-wide are safe and effective.

No dental device (including restorative materials) is absolutely safe. Safety is relative, and the selection and use of dental devices or materials are based on the assumption that the benefits of such use far outweigh the known biological risks. However, there is always uncertainty over the probability that a patient will experience adverse effects from dental treatment. The two main biological effects are allergic and toxic reactions. Paracelsus (1493–1541), a Swiss physician and alchemist, formulated revolutionary principles that have remained an integral part of the current field of toxicology. He stated that "all substances are poisons; there is none which is not a poison. The right dose differentiates a poison from a remedy." (Gallo and Doull, 1991.)

The major routes by which toxic agents enter the body are through the gastrointestinal tract (ingestion), lungs (inhalation), skin (topical, percutaneous, or dermal) and parenteral routes (Klaassen and Eaton, 1991). Exposure to toxic agents can be subdivided into acute (less than 24 hr), subacute (repeated, 1 month or less), subchronic (1 to 3 months), and chronic (longer than 3 months). For many toxic agents, the effects of a single exposure are different from those associated with repeated exposures.

Like toxicity, chemical allergy may also be dose-dependent, but it often results from low doses of chemical agents once sensitization has occurred. For a dental restorative material to produce an allergic reaction, most chemical agents or their metabolic products function immunologically as haptens and combine with endogenous proteins to form an antigen. The synthesis of sufficient numbers of antibodies takes 1 to 2 weeks. A later exposure to the chemical agent can induce an antigen-antibody reaction and clinical signs and symptoms of an allergy. Munksgaard (1992) concluded that occupational risks in dentistry are low and that patient risk for side effects of dental treatment is extremely low. Adverse reactions to dental materials have been reported to occur in only 0.14% of a general patient population (Kallus and Mjör, 1991) and in 0.33% of a prosthetic patient population (Hensten-Pettersen and Jacobsen, 1991).

Acknowledgment

The author expresses appreciation to Dr. Wayne Wozniak and Dr. Sharon Stanford of the American Dental Association for their helpful suggestions.

SELECTED READINGS

American Dental Association Seal Program, ADA website: *http://www.ada.org/public/topics/seal.html*

Coleman RL: Physical Properties of Dental Materials. National Bureau of Standards Research Paper No. 32. Washington, DC, US Government Printing Office, 1928.
This publication is the first major effort to relate physical properties of dental materials to the clinical situation. The American Dental Association specification program was established based on this historical review of the philosophy and the content of the facility created at the National Bureau of Standards.

Federal Register: Medical Devices; Dental Device Classification; Final Rule and Withdrawal of Proposed Rules. August 12, 1987, p 30082.
A listing of the dental materials and devices classified in Category III by the Food and Drug Administration as of that date.

Food and Drug Administration (FDA) website: *http://www.fda.gov*

FDA Center for Devices and Radiological Health, website: *http://www.fda.gov/cdrh/consumer/c-products.shtml*

Gallo MA, and Doull J: History and scope of toxicology. In: Casarett and Doull's Toxicology. New York, Pergamon Press, 1991, pp 3–11.

Hensten-Pettersen A, and Jacobsen N: Perceived side effects of biomaterials in prosthetic dentistry. J Prosthet Dent 65:138, 1991.

International Organization for Standardization (ISO) website: *http://www.iso.org*

International Organization for Standardization (ISO) TC 106–Dentistry website: *http://www.iso.org/iso/en/stdsdevelopment/techprog/workprog/TechnicalProgrammeTCDetailPage.TechnicalProgrammeTCDetail?COMMID=2916*

Kallus T, and Mjör IA: Incidence of adverse effects of dental materials. Scand J Dent Res 99:236, 1991.

Klaassen CD, and Eaton DL: Principles of toxicology. In: Casarett and Doull's Toxicology. New York, Pergamon Press, 1991, pp 12–49.

Munksgaard EC: Toxicology versus allergy in restorative dentistry. In: Advances in Dental Research. Bethesda, International Association for Dental Research, Sept 1992, pp 17–21.

Phillips RW: Changing trends of dental restorative materials. Dent Clin North Am 33(2):285, 1989.
A review of the trends in biomaterials that are influencing dental restorative procedures, particularly in aesthetic dentistry. Emphasis is on bonding technology and its application.

ADDITIONAL READINGS ON DENTAL HISTORY

American Dental Association: 125th anniversary commemoration. J Am Dent Assoc 108(4):473-586, 1984.

Asbell MB: Dentistry, a Historical Perspective. Bryn Mawr, PA, Torrence & Co, 1988.
An historical account of the history of dentistry from ancient times, with emphasis on the United States from the colonial to the present period.

Bennion E: Antique Dental Instruments. New York, Sotheby's Publishing, 1986.

Black CE, and Black BM: From Pioneer to Scientist. St. Paul, MN, Bruce Publishing, 1940.
The life story of Greene Vardiman Black, "Father of Modern Dentistry," and his son Arthur Davenport Black, late Dean of Northwestern University Dental School.

Carter WJ, and Graham-Carter J. Dental Collectibles and Antiques. 2nd ed. Bethany, OK, Dental Folklore Books, 1992.

Gardner PH: Foley's Footnotes: A Treasury of Dentistry. Wallingford, PA, Washington Square East Publishing, 1972.

Glenner RA, Davis AB, and Burns SB: The American Dentist. Missoula, MT, Pictorial Histories Publishing, 1990.
A pictorial history with a presentation of early dental photography in America.

Guerini V: A History of Dentistry, from the Most Ancient Times Until the End of the Eighteenth Century. Pound Ridge, NY, Milford House, 1909.

Hoffmann-Axthelm W: History of Dentistry. Chicago, Quintessence Publishing, 1981.

Koch, CRE: History of Dental Surgery. Chicago, National Art Publishing, 1909.

Lufkin AW: A History of Dentistry. Philadelphia, Lea & Febiger, 1948.

McCluggage RW: A History of the American Dental Association, A Century of Health Service. Chicago, American Dental Association, 1959.

Ring ME: Dentistry: An Illustrated History. New York, Harry N Abrams Inc, 1985.

Weinberger BW: An Introduction to the History of Dentistry. St Louis, Mosby, 1948.
Includes medical and dental chronology and bibliographic data (2 volumes).

Weinberger BW: Pierre Fauchard, Surgeon-Dentist. Minneapolis, MN, Pierre Fauchard Academy, 1941.
A brief account of the beginning of modern dentistry, the first dental textbook, and professional life 200 years ago.

Wynbrandt J: The Excruciating History of Dentistry: Toothsome Tales and Oral Oddities from Babylon to Braces. New York, St Martin's Press, 1998.

2

Structure of Matter and Principles of Adhesion

Kenneth J. Anusavice

OUTLINE

Change of State

Interatomic Primary Bonds

Interatomic Secondary Bonds

Interatomic Bond Distance and Bonding Energy

Thermal Energy

Crystalline Structure

Noncrystalline Solids and Their Structures

Diffusion

Adhesion and Bonding

Adhesion to Tooth Structure

KEY TERMS

Acid-etching technique—Process of roughening a solid surface by exposing it to an acid and thoroughly rinsing the residue to promote micromechanical bonding of an adhesive to the surface.

Adherend—A material substrate that is bonded to another material by means of an adhesive.

Adhesion—A molecular or atomic attraction between two contacting surfaces promoted by the interfacial force of attraction between the molecules or atoms of two different species; adhesion may occur as chemical adhesion, mechanical adhesion (structural interlocking), or a combination of both types.

Adhesive—Substance that promotes adhesion of one substance or material to another.

Adhesive bonding—Process of joining two materials by means of an adhesive agent that solidifies during the bonding process.

Cohesion—Force of molecular attraction between molecules or atoms of the same species.

Contact angle—Angle of intersection between a liquid and a surface of a solid that is measured from the solid surface through the liquid to the liquid/vapor tangent line originating at the terminus of the liquid/solid interface; used as a measure of wettability, whereby no wetting occurs at a contact angle of 180° and complete wetting occurs at an angle of 0°.

Diffusion coefficient—Proportionality constant representing the amount of a substance diffusing through a unit area and a unit thickness under the influence of a unit concentration gradient at a given temperature.

Glass transition temperature—Temperature at which a sharp increase in the thermal expansion coefficient occurs, indicating increased molecular mobility.

Heat of vaporization—Thermal energy required to convert a solid to a vapor.

Latent heat of fusion—Thermal energy required to convert a solid to a liquid.

Linear coefficient of expansion—Relative linear change in length per unit of initial length during heating of a solid per °K within a specified temperature range.

KEY TERMS—cont'd

Melting temperature (melting point)—Equilibrium temperature at which heating of a pure metal, compound, or eutectic alloy produces a change from a solid to liquid.

Metallic bond—Primary bond between metal atoms.

Micromechanical bonding—Mechanical adhesion associated with bonding of an adhesive to a roughened adherend surface.

Self-diffusion—Thermally driven transfer of an atom to an adjacent lattice site in a crystal composed of the same atomic species.

Smear layer—Tenacious deposit of microscopic debris that covers enamel and dentin surfaces that have been prepared for a restoration.

Stress concentration—State of elevated stress in a solid caused by surface or internal defects or by marked changes in contour.

Supercooled liquid—A liquid that has been cooled at a sufficiently rapid rate to a point below the temperature at which an equilibrium phase change can occur.

Surface tension—Interfacial tension, usually between a liquid and a solid surface, which occurs because of unbalanced intermolecular forces.

Wettability—Relative affinity of a liquid for the surface of a solid.

Wetting—Relative interfacial tension between a liquid and a solid substrate that results in a contact angle of less than 90°.

Wetting agent—A surface-active substance that reduces the surface tension of a liquid to promote wetting or adhesion.

Vacancy—Unoccupied atom lattice site in a crystalline solid.

van der Waals forces—Short-range force of physical attraction that promotes adhesion between molecules of liquids or molecular crystals.

CHANGE OF STATE

To gain an understanding of dental materials, we must begin with a basic knowledge of their atomic or molecular structure and their behavior during handling and use in the oral environment. Our scientific understanding of this behavior is limited. Because environmental factors are critically important for clinical success, extrapolation of in vitro information to the clinical (in vivo) situation should be approached with extreme caution.

The performance of all dental materials, whether ceramic, polymeric, or metallic, is based on their atomic structure. The collective physical and chemical reactions of the atoms determine the properties of the material. Therefore a short review of matter is justified to lay a foundation for a basic understanding of dental materials.

Atoms and molecules are held together by atomic interactions. When water boils, energy is needed to transform the liquid to vapor; this quantity of energy is known as the **heat of vaporization**. During condensation of water vapor, the same amount of heat is released to the environment, thus satisfying the conservation of energy. The heat of vaporization is defined as the amount of heat needed to evaporate 1 g of liquid to the vapor state at a given temperature and pressure. For example, 540 cal of heat is required to vaporize 1 g of water at 100° C at a pressure of 1 atm. Thus we can conclude that the gaseous state possesses more kinetic energy than does the liquid state.

Although molecules in the gaseous state exert a certain amount of mutual attraction, they can move readily because of their high kinetic energy. This also explains why gaseous molecules need to be confined to avoid dispersion. Atoms present in a liquid can also diffuse, but because their mutual attractions are greater in the liquid state than in the gaseous state, kinetic energy of the liquid must be increased to achieve separation. If the kinetic energy of a liquid decreases sufficiently when its temperature is decreased, a second transformation in state may occur and the liquid may change to a solid. Kinetic energy is released in the form of heat when the liquid freezes. In this instance, the energy released is known as the **latent heat of fusion**. For example, when 1 g of water freezes, 80 cal of heat are released. If 1 g of a solid is changed to a liquid, the reverse is true and an input of energy is required. For pure metals and some other solids, the temperature at which this change occurs is known as the **melting temperature**.

Because energy is required for the transformation from a solid to a liquid state, the attraction between atoms (or molecules) in the solid state must be greater than that in either the liquid or the gaseous state. If this were not true, atoms would separate easily. In addition, metals would deform readily, and they could exist in the vapor phase at low temperatures.

The temperature at which a liquid boils or solidifies depends partly on environmental pressure. A liquid can vaporize (or evaporate) at any temperature between its freezing and boiling points, provided that the space above the liquid is not already saturated or supersaturated with the vapor. Within a closed container, as the vapor density above the liquid increases, the vapor pressure produced by the molecules in the gaseous state also increases. This vapor density, as well as the resulting vapor pressure, attains a constant value in equilibrium, because the molecules enter and leave the liquid phase at an equal rate. It is possible for some solids to transform directly to a gas phase through the process of sublimation. However, this phenomenon is of little practical importance with respect to dental materials.

CRITICAL QUESTION

Which types of primary bonds control the properties of dental resins and cast alloys?

INTERATOMIC PRIMARY BONDS

The forces that hold atoms together are called cohesive forces. These interatomic bonds may be classified as primary or secondary. The strength of these bonds and their ability to reform after breakage determine the physical properties of a material. Primary atomic bonds (Fig. 2-1) may be of three different types: (1) ionic, (2) covalent, and (3) metallic.

Ionic Bonds

Ionic bonds (Fig. 2-1, *A*) result from the mutual attraction of positive and negative charges. The classic example is sodium chloride (Na^+Cl^-). Because the sodium atom contains one valence electron in its outer shell and the chlorine atom has seven electrons in its outer shell, the transfer of the sodium valence electron to the chlorine atom results in the stable compound NaCl. Ionic bonds result in crystals whose atomic configuration is based on a charge and size balance. In dentistry, ionic bonding exists in certain crystalline phases of some dental materials, such as gypsum and phosphate-based cements.

Covalent Bonds

In many chemical compounds, two valence electrons are shared by adjacent atoms (Fig. 2-1, *B*). The hydrogen molecule, H_2, is an example of covalent bonding. The single valence electron in each hydrogen atom is shared with that of the other

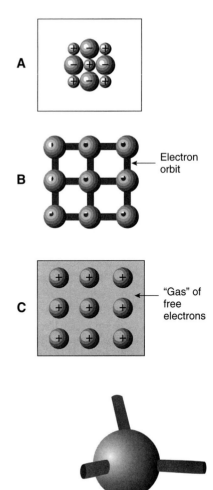

Electron
orbit

"Gas" of
free
electrons

Fig. 2-1 **A,** Ionic bond formation—characterized by electron transfer from one element (positive) to another (negative). **B,** Covalent bond formation—characterized by electron sharing and very precise bond orientations. **C,** Metallic bond formation—characterized by electron sharing and formation of a "gas" or "cloud" of electrons that bonds the atoms (which become positively charged because of the electron gas formation) together in a lattice. (Courtesy of K-J. Söderholm.)

Fig. 2-2 Carbon atom with an sp[3] orbit formation. This type of hybrid configuration is also common for silicon. (Courtesy of K-J. Söderholm.)

combining atom, and the valence shells become stable. Covalent bonding occurs in many organic compounds, such as dental resins, in which the compounds link to form the backbone structure of hydrocarbon chains. The carbon atom has four valence electrons forming an sp[3] hybrid configuration (Fig. 2-2) and can be stabilized by combining with hydrogen. A typical characteristic of covalent bonds is their directional orientation.

Metallic Bonds

The third type of primary atomic interaction is the **metallic bond** (Fig. 2-1, *C*), which results from the increased spatial extension of valence-electron wave functions when an aggregate of metal atoms is brought close together. This type of bonding can be understood best by studying a metallic crystal such as pure gold. Such a crystal consists only of gold atoms. Like all other metals, gold atoms can easily donate electrons from their outer shell and form a "cloud" of free electrons. The contribution of free electrons to this cloud results in the formation of positive ions that can be neutralized by acquiring new valence electrons from adjacent atoms.

Because of their ability to donate and recover electrons, atoms in a metal crystal exist as clusters of positive metal ions surrounded by a cloud of electrons. This structure is responsible for the excellent electrical and thermal conductivity of metals and also for their ability to deform plastically. The electrical and thermal conductivities of metals are controlled by the ease with which the free electrons can move through the crystal, whereas their deformability is associated with the slip of atoms along crystal planes. During slip deformation, electrons easily regroup to retain the cohesive nature of the metal.

INTERATOMIC SECONDARY BONDS

In contrast with primary bonds, secondary bonds (Fig. 2-3) do not share electrons. Instead, charge variations among molecules or atomic groups induce polar forces that attract the molecules. Since there are no primary bonds between water and glass, it is initially difficult to understand how water drops can bond to an automobile windshield when they freeze to ice crystals. However, the concepts of hydrogen bonding and secondary bonding—two types of bonds that exist between water and glass—allow us to explain this adhesion phenomenon.

Hydrogen Bonding

Hydrogen bonding can be understood by studying a water molecule (Fig 2-4). Attached to the oxygen atom are two hydrogen atoms. These bonds are covalent because the oxygen and hydrogen atoms share electrons. As a consequence, the protons of the hydrogen atoms pointing away from the oxygen atom are not shielded

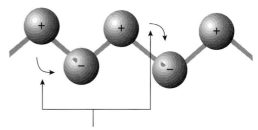

Fig. 2-3 Secondary bond formation. Charge variations along molecules induce polar forces that attract other molecules. (Courtesy of K-J. Söderholm.)

Differences in electron densities result in charge variations along the molecule

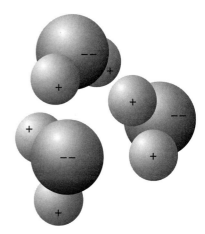

Fig. 2-4 Hydrogen bond formation between water molecules. The polar water molecule ties up adjacent water molecules via an H●●●O interaction between molecules. (Courtesy of K-J. Söderholm.)

efficiently by the electrons, and the proton side of the water molecule is positively charged. On the opposite side of the water molecule, the electrons that fill the outer orbit of the oxygen atom provide a negative charge. Thus a permanent dipole exists that represents an asymmetric molecule. The hydrogen bond, which is associated with the positive charge of hydrogen caused by polarization, is an important example of this type of secondary bonding.

When a water molecule intermingles with other water molecules, the hydrogen (positive) portion of one molecule is attracted to the oxygen (negative) portion of its neighboring molecule and hydrogen bridges are formed. Polarity of this nature is important in accounting for the intermolecular reactions in many organic compounds, such as the sorption of water by synthetic dental resins.

Van der Waals Forces

Van der Waals forces form the basis of a dipole attraction (Fig. 2-5). For example, in a symmetric molecule, such as an inert gas, the electron field constantly fluctuates. Normally, the electrons of the atoms are distributed equally around the nucleus and produce an electrostatic field around the atom. However, this field may fluctuate so that its charge becomes momentarily positive and negative, as shown in Figure 2-5. A fluctuating dipole is thus created that will attract other similar dipoles. Such interatomic forces are quite weak.

INTERATOMIC BOND DISTANCE AND BONDING ENERGY
Bond Distance

Regardless of the type of matter, there is a limiting factor that prevents the atoms or molecules from approaching each other too closely. This factor is the distance between the center of an atom and that of its neighbor, which is limited by the diameter of the atoms involved. Although the atom is treated as a discrete particle with boundaries and volume, its boundaries are established by the electrostatic fields of the electrons. If the atoms approach too closely, they are repelled from each other by their electron charges. On the other hand, forces of attraction tend to draw the atoms together. The position at which these forces of repulsion and attraction become equal in magnitude (but opposite in direction) is the equilibrium position of the atoms shown in Figure 2-6. In this position, the repelling forces are equal in magnitude to the attracting forces. Atom **B** can be displaced to position **B'** by a disturbing mechanical, thermal, or electrical force. A force may also cause the atoms to move more closely together (position **B″** in Fig. 2-6). As the forces of attraction

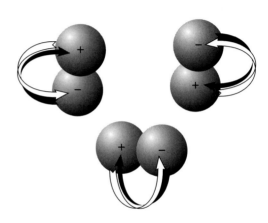

Fig. 2-5 Fluctuating dipole that binds inert gas molecules together. The **arrows** show how the fields may fluctuate so that the charges become momentarily positive and negative. (Courtesy of K-J. Söderholm.)

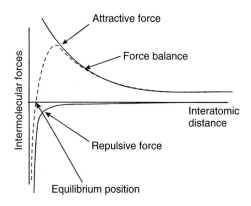

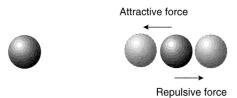

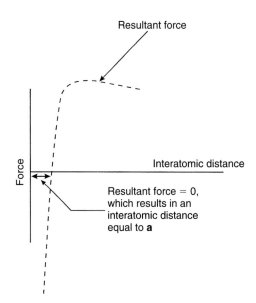

Fig. 2-6 Attractive and repulsive forces balance each other, and atom B attains its equilibrium position. (Courtesy of K-J. Söderholm.)

increase, the interatomic space decreases. On the other hand, the forces of repulsion remain relatively inactive until the atoms are sufficiently close to each other. The sum or resultant of the two forces is indicated by the broken line in Figures 2-6 and 2-7. The resultant force in Figure 2-6 becomes zero; that is, the magnitudes of the two forces are equal at the intersection of the broken line with the horizontal axis. At equilibrium, the interatomic distance represents the distance between the centers of the atoms involved (distance **a** in Fig. 2-7).

Fig. 2-7 When the equilibrium position is reached, the interatomic distance is **a**. If the atom is moved from this position, either a negative (repulsive) or a positive (attractive) force is required to move the atom back to its equilibrium position as shown in Fig. 2-6. (Courtesy of K-J. Söderholm.)

Bonding Energy

Because conditions of equilibrium are usually described in terms of energy rather than interatomic forces, the relationships in Figure 2-7 can be more logically explained in terms of interatomic energy. According to the laws of physics, energy can be defined as a force integrated over a distance. If the resultant force (F), represented by the dashed line in Figure 2-7, is integrated over the interatomic spacing (a), the graph shown in Figure 2-8 will result. The horizontal axis in Figure 2-8 represents the interatomic distance, and the interatomic or bonding energy is plotted on the vertical axis. In contrast with the resultant force plotted in Figure 2-6, the energy does not change a great deal initially as two atoms come closer together. As the resultant force approaches zero (see Fig. 2-7), the energy decreases (see Fig. 2-8). The energy finally reaches a minimum when the resultant force becomes zero. Thereafter the energy increases rapidly (see Fig. 2-8), because the resultant repulsive force (see Fig. 2-7) increases rapidly with little change in interatomic distance. The minimal energy corresponds to the condition of equilibrium and defines the equilibrium interatomic distance.

THERMAL ENERGY

Thermal energy is accounted for by the kinetic energy of the atoms or molecules at a given temperature. The atoms in a crystal at temperatures above absolute zero are in a constant state of vibration, and the average amplitude is dependent on the temperature. The higher the temperature, the greater the amplitude and, consequently, the greater the kinetic or internal energy. Further consideration of Figures 2-7 and 2-8 can provide additional interpretations of these phenomena.

For a certain temperature, the minimal energy occurs at equilibrium and is denoted by the lowest point of the curve in Figure 2-8. As the temperature increases, the amplitude of the atomic (or molecular) vibration increases. It follows also that the mean interatomic spacing increases (see Figs. 2-8 and 2-9), as well as the internal energy. The overall effect represents the phenomenon known as thermal expansion (Fig. 2-9).

If the temperature continues to increase, the interatomic spacing will increase and eventually a change of state will occur. A solid changes to a liquid, and the liquid subsequently changes to a vapor. It follows from Figure 2-9, *A* and *B*, that the deeper the lowest point of the curve, the greater the amount of energy required to

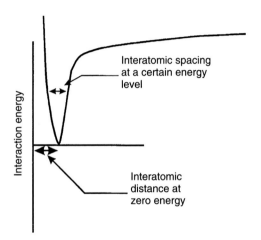

Fig. 2-8 By multiplying the force shown in Fig. 2-7 by the atomic displacement from its equilibrium position, the energy change can be plotted as a function of displacement in either direction. (Courtesy of K-J. Söderholm.)

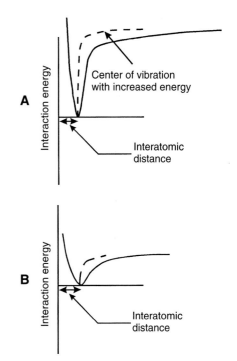

Fig. 2-9 The depth of the energy curve is determined by the magnitude of the attractive-repulsive forces. Thus for a shallower curve **B**, less energy is needed to separate the atoms than for deeper curve **A**. (Courtesy of K-J. Söderholm.)

achieve melting and boiling and, consequently, the higher the melting and boiling temperatures. By the same reasoning, it can be argued that the lower the minimum value of the energy curve is, the lower the thermal expansion per degree of temperature increase, because the interatomic spacing does not necessarily increase as the depth of the trough increases. In other words, the **linear coefficient of thermal expansion** (α) of materials with similar atomic or molecular structures tends to be inversely proportional to the melting temperature.

Figures 2-7 and 2-8 illustrate another interesting relationship between melting temperature and the force required to move atoms away from their equilibrium spacing. As shown in Figure 2-7, the net force on the atoms at the equilibrium spacing is zero, but small displacements result in rapidly increasing forces that maintain the equilibrium spacing. The stiffness of the material is proportional to the rate of change of the force, with a change in displacement measured by the slope of the net force curve near at interatomic distance equal to **a.** A greater slope of the force curve versus distance implies a narrower, deeper trough in the energy versus distance curve (see Fig. 2-8). Hence a high melting point is usually accompanied by a greater stiffness.

Thermal conductivity is related to interatomic spacing only to the extent that the heat is conducted from one atom or molecule to the next as adjacent basic structural units are affected by the kinetic energy of their neighbors. However, the number of "free" electrons in the material influences its thermal conductivity. As discussed previously, metallic structures such as dental casting alloys and dental amalgams contain many free electrons, and most metals are effective conductors of heat as well as electricity. On the other hand, nonmetallic materials, such as resin-based composites and denture acrylics, do not contain many free electrons, and consequently, they are generally poor thermal and electrical conductors.

The preceding principles represent generalities, and exceptions do occur. Nevertheless, they allow us to estimate the influence of temperature on the properties of most of the dental materials to be discussed in subsequent chapters.

Which dental substances are examples of crystalline materials? Which are noncrystalline materials? Which are combinations of crystalline and noncrystalline materials?

CRYSTALLINE STRUCTURE

Thus far, for the purpose of explaining specific concepts, we have generally assumed the presence of only two atoms or molecules. Dental materials consist of many millions of such units. But how are the structural units arranged in a solid, and how are they held together? In 1665, Robert Hooke (1635–1703) simulated the characteristic shapes of crystals by stacking musket balls in piles. It was 250 years later before anyone knew that he had created an exact model of the crystal structure of many familiar metals, with each ball representing an atom.

Atoms are bonded to each other by either primary or secondary forces. In the solid state, they combine in a manner that ensures minimal internal energy. For example, sodium and chlorine share one electron, as previously described. In the solid state, however, the atoms do not simply form only pairs; in fact, all of the positively charged sodium ions attract all of the negatively charged chlorine ions. The result is that they form a regularly spaced configuration known as a space lattice or crystal. A space lattice can be defined as any arrangement of atoms in space in which every atom is situated similarly to every other atom. Space lattices may be the result of primary or secondary bonds.

There are 14 possible lattice types or forms, but many of the metals used in dentistry belong to the cubic system; that is, the atoms crystallize in cubic arrangements. The simplest cubic space lattice is shown in Figure 2-10, with the spheres representing the positions of the atoms. Their positions are located at the points of intersection of three sets of parallel planes, each set being perpendicular to the other two sets of planes. These planes are often referred to as crystal planes. All dental amalgams, cast alloys, wrought metals, gold foil, and dental amalgam are crystalline. Some pure ceramics, such as alumina and zirconia core ceramics, are entirely crystalline. Other ceramics, such as dental porcelains, consist of noncrystalline glass matrix and crystalline inclusions that provide desired properties, including color, opacity, and increases in thermal expansion coefficients, radiopacity, strength, and fracture toughness.

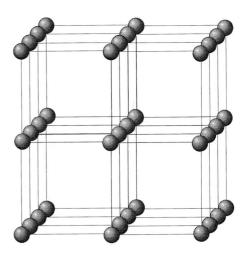

Fig. 2-10 Simple cubic space lattice. (Courtesy of K-J. Söderholm.)

Shown in Figure 2-11, *A*, is one unit cell of the simple cubic space lattice. The cells are repeated in three-dimensional space, as indicated in Figure 2-10. The simple cubic arrangements are shown in Figures 2-10 and 2-11, *A*. The arrangements shown in Figure 2-11, *B* and *C*, represent the cubic space lattices of practical importance. Also, Figures 2-10 and 2-11 are diagrammatic only. The atoms are actually closely packed so that the interatomic spacing is equal to the sum of their radii. The closer packing arrangement for a model of a body-centered cubic structure is shown in Figure 2-12, and a similar model for a face-centered cubic lattice is pictured in Figure 2-13.

The type of space lattice is defined by the length of each of three unit cell edges (called the *axes*) and the angles between the edges. For example, the cubic space

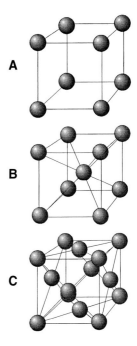

Fig. 2-11   Single cells of cubic space lattices. **A**, Simple cubic. **B**, Body-centered cubic. **C**, Face-centered cubic. (Courtesy of K-J. Söderholm.)

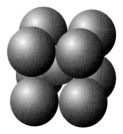

Fig. 2-12   Model of a body-centered cubic crystal. (Courtesy of K-J. Söderholm.)

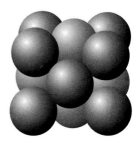

Fig. 2-13   Model of a face-centered cubic crystal. (Courtesy of K-J. Söderholm.)

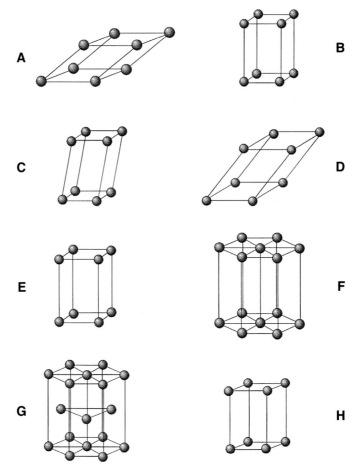

Fig. 2-14   Other simple lattice types of dental interest. **A**, Rhombohedral. **B**, Orthorhombic. **C**, Monoclinic. **D**, Triclinic. **E**, Tetragonal. **F**, Simple hexagonal. **G**, Close-packed hexagonal. **H**, Rhombic. (Courtesy of K-J. Söderholm.)

lattice (see Fig. 2-11, *A*) is characterized by axes that are all of equal length and meet at 90-degree angles. Other types of space lattices are diagrammed in Figure 2-14.

NONCRYSTALLINE SOLIDS AND THEIR STRUCTURES

Structures other than crystalline forms can occur in the solid state. For example, some of the waxes used by a dentist or laboratory technician may solidify as amorphous materials so that the molecules are distributed at random. Even in this case, there is a tendency for the arrangement to be regular.

Glass is also considered to be a noncrystalline solid, because its atoms tend to develop a short-range order instead of the long-range order characteristic of crystalline solids. The ordered arrangement of the glass is more or less locally interspersed with a considerable number of disordered units. Because this arrangement is also typical of liquids, such solids are sometimes called **supercooled liquids.**

A resin-based composite consists of a resin matrix, filler particles, and an organic coupling agent that bonds the filler particles to the resin matrix. In some cases, the filler particles are made from radiopaque glasses that are noncrystalline. Composites have a noncrystalline matrix and may or may not contain crystalline filler particles.

The structural arrangements of the noncrystalline solids do not represent such low internal energies as do crystalline arrangements of the same atoms and molecules. Noncrystalline solids do not have a definite melting temperature, but rather they gradually soften as the temperature is raised. The temperature at which there is an abrupt increase in the thermal expansion coefficient, indicating increased molecular mobility, is called the **glass transition temperature (T_g)** and it is characteristic of the particular glassy structure. Occasionally, the term is shortened to glass temperature. Below T_g, the glassy structure loses its fluid characteristics and has significant resistance to shear deformation. Synthetic dental resins are examples of materials that often have glassy structures.

CRITICAL QUESTION

Why are mercury and gallium of interest as components of direct restorative materials?

DIFFUSION

Diffusion of molecules in gases and liquids is well known. However, molecules or atoms diffuse in the solid state as well. As previously described, the atoms in a space lattice are constantly in vibration about their centers. The average kinetic energy of vibration over the entire crystal is related to the temperature. At absolute zero the vibration ceases, the energy becomes zero, and the atom occupies the center of vibration (see Fig. 2-9). At any temperature above the absolute zero temperature ($-273°$ C), atoms (or molecules) of a solid possess some kinetic energy. An understanding of diffusion in a solid requires two new concepts.

The first concept pertaining to diffusion in a solid is that all the atoms do not possess the same amount of energy. Rather, there is a distribution of atoms with a particular energy that varies from very low to high, with the average energy related to the absolute zero temperature. Even at very low temperatures, some atoms have high energies.

If the energy of a particular atom exceeds the bonding energy, it can move to another position in the lattice. In a noncrystalline solid with only short-range order, there is a strong probability that a high-energy atom will be located adjacent to a vacant position.

The second concept required to describe solid-state diffusion in crystalline solids is the fact that at any temperature above the absolute zero temperature, there are a finite number of missing atoms (called **vacancies**), representing open areas through which diffusion can occur. Atoms change position in pure, single-element solids even under equilibrium conditions; this process is known as **self-diffusion**. However, self-diffusion is generally not of practical importance, because no visible or measurable dimensional changes occur. As with any diffusion process, the atoms or molecules diffuse in the solid and liquid states in an attempt to reach an equilibrium state. For example, sugar molecules in solution tend to diffuse to achieve a uniform concentration. As discussed later, a concentration of atoms in a metal can also be redistributed through the diffusion process.

Diffusion may also occur in the other direction to produce a concentration of atoms in a solution. For example, if the sugar in the water becomes supersaturated, the molecules of sugar diffuse toward each other, and the sugar crystallizes out of solution. In the same manner, too many copper atoms in a solid alloy of copper and silver may cause supersaturation and diffusion of the copper atoms to increase the concentration of copper locally, causing them to precipitate out of solution.

Diffusion rates for a given substance depend mainly on temperature and the chemical potential gradient or concentration gradient. The higher the temperature or the higher the chemical potential gradient, the greater the rate of diffusion. The diffusion rate varies with the concentration gradients, atom size, interatomic or intermolecular bonding, and lattice imperfections. Thus different dental materials exhibit a range of characteristic diffusion rates. The diffusion constant that is uniquely characteristic of a given element in a compound, crystal, or alloy is known as the **diffusion coefficient**, usually designated as D. The diffusion coefficient is defined as the amount of a substance that diffuses across a given unit area (e.g., 1 cm^2), through a unit thickness of the substance (e.g., 1 cm), in one unit of time (e.g., 1 sec). In general, the diffusion coefficient of a pure metal is related to its melting temperature; that is, the lower its melting point, the greater its diffusion coefficient.

The diffusion coefficients of elements in most crystalline solids at room temperature are very low. Diffusion in dental alloys is so slow at room temperature that it cannot be detected in a practical sense; however, at temperatures only a few hundred degrees higher, the properties of the metal change markedly by atomic diffusion. Diffusion in a noncrystalline material may occur at a more rapid rate, and often may be evident at room or body temperature. The disordered structure enables the molecules to diffuse more rapidly with less activation energy. Some metals melt at temperatures below mouth temperature. For example, the melting points of mercury and gallium are $-38.36°$ C ($-37.05°$ F) and $29.78°$ C ($85.60°$ F) respectively. Thus, because the diffusion rate of these atoms into solid alloy particles may be fairly rapid at intraoral temperature, new metal compounds can be formed that may be useful as direct restorative materials.

ADHESION AND BONDING

The phenomenon of adhesion applies to many situations in dentistry. For example, leakage adjacent to dental restorative materials results from an insufficient or incomplete adhesion. The retention of artificial dentures is probably dependent, to some extent, on adhesion between the denture and saliva and between the saliva and soft tissue. Certainly, the attachment of plaque or calculus to tooth structure can be partially explained by an adhesion mechanism. Therefore, an understanding of the fundamental principles associated with the phenomenon is essential to the dentist.

When two substances are brought into intimate contact with each other, the molecules of one substance adhere, or are attracted to, molecules of the other substance. This force is called **adhesion** when unlike molecules are attracted and **cohesion** when molecules of the same kind are attracted. The material or film used to cause adhesion is known as the **adhesive**; the material to which it is applied is called the **adherend**.

In a broad sense, adhesion is simply a surface attachment process. The term adhesion is usually qualified by specification of the type of intermolecular attraction that may exist between the adhesive and the adherend.

Mechanical Bonding

Strong attachment of one substance to another can also be accomplished by mechanical bonding or retention rather than by molecular attraction. Such structural retention may be gross in nature, as seen by applications involving the use of screws, bolts, or undercuts. Mechanical bonding may also involve more subtle mechanisms such as the penetration of the adhesive into microscopic or submicroscopic irregularities (e.g., crevices and pores) in the surface of the substrate. A fluid or slightly viscous liquid adhesive is best suited for such a procedure, because it readily penetrates into these surface defects. On hardening, the numerous adhesive projections embedded in the adherend surface provide the anchorage for mechanical attachment (retention).

This **micromechanical bonding** mechanism has been commonly used in dentistry because of the absence of truly adhesive cements or restorative materials. For example, retention of cast restorations, such as a cast gold alloy crown or a base metal endodontic post and core, is enhanced by mechanical attachment of the cementing agent into irregularities that exist on the internal surface of the casting and those that are present in the adjoining tooth structure.

A more recent example of mechanical bonding is that of resin (plastic) restorative materials. Because these resins do not have the capability of truly adhering to tooth structure, leakage adjacent to the restoration may occur. Such leakage patterns contribute to marginal stain, secondary caries, and irritation of the pulp. A specific technique must be used to minimize the risks associated with deleterious agents that may migrate toward the pulp. Before insertion of the resin, the enamel of the adjoining tooth structure is exposed to phosphoric acid for a short period. This is referred to as the **acid-etching technique**. The acid produces minute pores and other irregularities in the enamel surface into which the resin subsequently flows when it is placed into the preparation. On hardening, these resin projections provide improved mechanical retention of the restoration, thereby reducing the possibility of interfacial leakage.

The acid-etching technique is an example of how bonding between a dental material and tooth structure can be achieved through mechanical mechanisms, rather than through molecular adhesion. This process is sometimes referred to as "micromechanical bonding." The principles of adhesion and the factors associated with this phenomenon are discussed further in the following sections.

Surface Energy

For adhesion to exist, the surfaces must be attracted to one another at their interface. Such a condition may exist regardless of the phases (solid, liquid, or gas) comprising the two surfaces, with the exception that adhesion between two gases is not expected, because they lack an interface.

The energy at the surface of a solid is greater than that of its interior. For example, consider the space lattice shown in Figure 2-15. Inside the lattice, all the atoms are equally attracted to one another. The interatomic distances are equal, and the energy

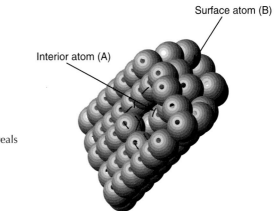

Surface atom (B)

Interior atom (A)

Fig. 2-15 Comparing an atom under the surface **(A)** with one on the surface **(B)** reveals that a bond balance exists around interior atom **A,** while surface atom **B** is free to develop bonds to atoms or molecules approaching the surface. (Courtesy of K-J. Söderholm.)

is minimal. At the surface of the lattice, the energy is greater because the outermost atoms are not equally attracted in all directions, as diagrammed in Figure 2-15. The interior atom A has a balanced array of nearest neighbors surrounding it, whereas surface atom B has an unbalanced number of adjacent atoms.

The increase in energy per unit area of surface is referred to as the surface energy or **surface tension**. A soap film contracts, and drops of a liquid form spherical shapes by minimizing surface area because this surface tension condition represents the state of lowest energy.

The surface atoms of a solid tend to form bonds to other atoms in close proximity to the surface and reduce the surface energy of the solid. This attraction across the interface between unlike molecules is called **adhesion**. For example, molecules in the air may be attracted to the surface and become adsorbed on the material surface. Silver, platinum, and gold adsorb oxygen readily. For gold, the bonding forces are of the secondary type; but in the case of silver, the attraction may be controlled by chemical or primary bonding, and silver oxide may form.

When primary bonding is involved, the adhesion is termed *chemisorption,* as compared with physical bonding by van der Waals forces. In chemisorption, a chemical bond is formed between the adhesive and the adherend. An example of this type of adhesion is an oxide film formed on the surface of a metal or a layer of solder bonded to a metallic substrate. Thus, van der Waals forces are weaker than primary bonding because they are intermolecular rather than intramolecular.

The development of van der Waals forces invariably precedes chemisorption. As the distance between the adhesive and the adherend diminishes, primary bonding may become effective. However, chemisorption is limited to the monolayer of adhesive present on the adherend. The surface energy and the adhesive qualities of a given solid can be reduced by any surface impurity, such as adsorbed gas, an oxide, or human secretions. The functional chemical groups available or the type of crystal plane of a space lattice present at the surface may affect the surface energy. In summary, the greater the surface energy, the greater the capacity for adhesion.

CRITICAL QUESTION

What conditions are necessary to achieve the strongest level of bonding?

Wetting

It is difficult to force two solid surfaces to adhere. Regardless of how smooth these surfaces may appear, they are likely to be extremely rough when viewed on an atomic or molecular scale. Consequently, when they are placed in apposition, only the "peaks" or asperities are in contact. Because these areas usually constitute only a small percentage of the total surface area, no perceptible adhesion takes place. The attraction is generally negligible when the surface molecules of the attracting substances are separated by distances greater than 0.7 nm (0.0007 µm).

One method of overcoming this difficulty is to use a fluid that flows into these irregularities to provide contact over a greater part of the surface of the solid. For example, when two polished glass plates are placed one on top of the other and are pressed together, they exhibit little tendency to adhere for reasons previously described. However, if a film of water is introduced between them, considerable difficulty is encountered in separating the two plates. The surface energy of the glass is sufficiently great to attract the molecules of water.

To produce adhesion in this manner, the liquid must flow easily over the entire surface and adhere to the solid. This characteristic is known as **wetting**. If the liquid does not wet the surface of the adherend, adhesion between the liquid and the adherend will be negligible or nonexistent. If there is a true wetting of the surface, adhesion failures should not occur. Failure in such instances actually occurs cohesively in the solid or in the adhesive itself, not along the interface where the solid and adhesive are in contact.

The ability of an adhesive to wet the surface of the adherend is influenced by a number of factors. The cleanliness of the surface is of particular importance. A film of water only one molecule thick on the surface of the solid may lower the surface energy of the adherend and prevent any wetting by the adhesive. Likewise, an oily film on a metallic surface may also inhibit the contact of an adhesive.

The surface energy of some substances is so low that few, if any, liquids wet their surfaces. Some organic substances, such as dental waxes, are of this type. Close packing of the structural organic groups and the presence of halogens may prevent wetting. Teflon (polytetrafluoroethylene), a commercial synthetic resin, is often used when it is desirable to prevent the adhesion of films to a surface. Metals, on the other hand, interact strongly with liquid adhesives because of their high surface energy.

In general, the comparatively low surface energies of organic and most inorganic liquids permit them to spread freely on solids of high surface energy. Formation of a strong adhesive joint requires good wetting.

CRITICAL QUESTION

You observe a lack of soft or hard tissue details in a gypsum model you have made from a hydrophobic impression material. What step(s) can be taken to eliminate this problem when using this impression material in the future?

Contact Angle of Wetting

The extent to which an adhesive wets the surface of an adherend may be determined by measuring the **contact angle** between the adhesive and the adherend. The contact angle is the angle formed at the interface of the adhesive and the adherend. If the molecules of the adhesive are attracted to the molecules of the adherend as much as, or more than, they are attracted to themselves, the liquid adhesive will spread completely over the surface of the solid, and no contact angle (θ = 0 degrees) will be formed (Fig. 2-16, *A*). Thus the forces of adhesion are stronger than the cohesive forces holding the molecules of the adhesive together. A dental material such as an elastomeric impression may not be ideal for replicating hard or soft oral tissues if an aqueous medium with a contact angle of greater than 90° is poured into this rubber-type mold. Under this condition the impression material is considered to be hydrophobic. To improve the wetting of the impression by an aqueous solution of a gypsum-forming model material, the manufacturer could change the formulation to render the material more hydrophilic or a **wetting agent** could be added to the aqueous gypsum-forming mixture.

However, if the energy of the adherend surface is reduced slightly by contamination or other means, the surface tension of the solid (γ_{SV}) decreases and a slight increase in the contact angle (θ) can be measured (Fig. 2-16, *B*). This increase in θ retains the force balance shown in Figure 2-16, *D*. Note that as θ increases from 0 to 90 degrees, the value of cos θ decreases from 1 to 0. If a monolayer film of a

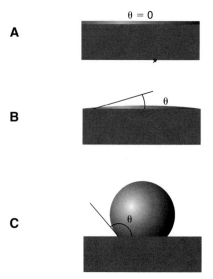

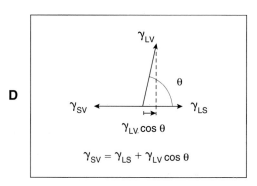

Fig. 2-16   Adhesion depends on wetting the surface. **A**, When the contact angle (θ) is 0 degrees, the liquid contacts the surface completely and spreads freely. **B**, Small contact angle on slightly contaminated surface. **C**, Large angle formed by poor wetting. **D**, The relationships among the surface tension of the solid (γ_{SV}), the liquid (γ_{LV}), and the contact angle (θ) can be used to determine the surface tension between the liquid and the solid (γ_{LS}) according to the equation, $\gamma_{SV} = \gamma_{LS} + \gamma_{LV} \cos\theta$. (Courtesy of K-J. Söderholm.)

contaminant is present over the entire surface, a medium angle might be obtained, whereas a very high angle would result on a solid of low surface energy (γ_{SV}), such as polytetrafluoroethylene (Fig. 2-16, *C*). Because the tendency for the liquid to spread increases as the contact angle decreases, the contact angle is a useful indicator of spreadability or **wettability** (Fig. 2-16, *D*). Complete wetting occurs at a contact angle of 0°, and no wetting occurs at an angle of 180°.

Thus the smaller the contact angle between an adhesive and an adherend, the better the ability of the adhesive to flow into and fill in irregularities within the surface of the adherend. The fluidity of the adhesive influences the extent to which these voids or irregularities are filled.

Solid "flat" surfaces are not actually planar. Surface imperfections represent a potential impediment to the achievement of an adhesive bond. Air pockets may be created during the spreading of the adhesive that prevent complete wetting of the entire surface (Fig. 2-17). When the adhesive interfacial region is subjected to thermal changes and mechanical stresses, **stress concentrations** develop around these voids. The stress may become so great that it initiates a separation in the adhesive bond adjacent to the void. This crack may propagate from one void to the next, and the joint may separate under stress.

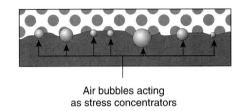

Fig. 2-17 Air voids created in surface irregularities. Such regions contribute to propagation of adhesive failure by concentration of stress at these sites. (Courtesy of K-J. Söderholm.)

Air bubbles acting
as stress concentrators

CRITICAL QUESTION

Micromechanical bonding of resin sealant to tooth enamel is usually quite effective in preventing pit and fissure areas from tooth decay. However, many factors can reduce the bonding effectiveness, resulting in partial or total loss of the sealant. Which of these factors are possible causes of debonding?

ADHESION TO TOOTH STRUCTURE

The fundamental principles of adhesion can be readily related to dental situations. For example, when contact angle measurements are used to study the wettability of enamel and dentin, it is found that the wettability of these surfaces is markedly reduced after the topical application of an aqueous fluoride solution. Transferring this information to the clinical setting, we find that the fluoride-treated enamel surface retains less plaque over a given period, presumably because of a decrease in surface energy. Thus, in addition to the recognized mechanism of reduced enamel solubility in an acidic environment, it is conceivable that fluoride products may be effective in reducing dental caries by providing a tooth surface that stays cleaner over a longer period.

Similarly, because of the higher surface energy of many restorative materials compared with that of the tooth surface, there is a greater tendency for the surface and margins of the restoration to accumulate debris. This may in part account for the relatively high incidence of secondary (recurrent) carious lesions seen in enamel at the margins of certain types of dental fillings.

The following chapters include discussions of the leakage that occurs between tooth structure and dental restorations. Under certain instances, secondary caries, pulpal sensitivity after placement of the filling or restoration, and deterioration at the margins of the restoration can be associated with a lack of adhesion between the restorative material and the tooth. Extensive research is in progress to develop adhesives that adhere to tooth structure. In subsequent chapters, we shall consider how traditional dental restorative procedures are affected by such adhesive systems.

By applying the principles that influence adhesion to dental structures, we can see that the problems associated with dental adhesives are indeed complex. The composition of tooth structures is not homogeneous. The amounts of both organic and inorganic components present in dentin differ from the amounts of these components present in enamel. A material that can adhere to the organic components may not adhere to the inorganic components, and an adhesive that bonds to enamel may not adhere to dentin to the same extent.

After the dentist has completed a tooth preparation for a filling, tenacious microscopic debris covers the enamel and dentin surfaces. This surface contamination, called the **smear layer**, reduces wetting. In addition, the instruments used to cut the cavity leave a rough surface that may increase air entrapment at the interface.

The greatest problems associated with bonding to tooth surfaces are the inadequate removal of etching debris and the contamination by water or saliva. The inorganic components of tooth structure have a strong affinity for water. The complete removal of water would require the heating of enamel and dentin to an unacceptable temperature. This means that a tooth cannot be safely dried at mouth temperature with the devices and agents currently available to the dentist. The presence of at least a monolayer of water on the surface of the prepared cavity must be accepted. This water layer reduces the surface energy, and it may reduce the wetting of the etched tooth surface by the adhesive restorative material.

In addition, fluid is exchanged through certain components of the tooth. The dental adhesive must displace the water, react with it, or wet the surface more effectively than the water already present on the surface and within the tooth structure. Furthermore, the adhesive must sustain long-term adhesion to tooth structure in an aqueous environment.

Although the obstacles are formidable, the progress of research in the field of adhesive materials is promising. To enhance adhesive bonding, manufacturers and dentists are developing and using more hydrophilic resins that are not as sensitive to the presence of moisture as materials previously in use. Certainly, these goals are worthy of the challenges presented. A truly adhesive filling material could replace many of those used in restorative dentistry. Likewise, the technique for placement of the material would be simplified, and the mechanical retention of the material in the cavity preparation would be unnecessary.

Even more intriguing is the possibility of developing a material capable of forming a thin, durable film on the tooth surface that could be topically applied to the intact enamel surface. Such a film with low surface energy could serve as a barrier to the formation of plaque, the development of caries, and even the deposition of calculus.

SELECTED READINGS

Buonocore MG: The Use of Adhesives in Dentistry. Springfield, IL, Charles C Thomas, 1975.

The problems associated with dental adhesives are well illustrated. Many of the procedures using bonding technology discussed in this text have since become commonplace.

Glantz P: On wettability and adhesiveness. Odont Rev 20:1(Suppl 17):1, 1969.

The first in a series of publications by this author suggesting that the use of topical fluorides provides an additional mechanism involved in reduction of dental caries, that is, lowering of the surface energy of tooth structure and thereby reducing plaque accumulation over a given interval.

Gordon JE: The New Science of Strong Materials, or Why You Don't Fall Through the Floor? 2nd ed. Princeton, NJ, Princeton University Press, 1984.

A general discussion of the strength of materials from a fundamental base. Structural materials such as timber, cellulose, teeth, and bone are particularly interesting.

Phillips RW, and Ryge G (eds): Proceedings on Adhesive Restorative Dental Materials. Spencer, IN, Owen Litho Service, 1961.

These historical transactions resulted from the first workshop on the problems of, and potential solutions to, the development of adhesive dental materials. The recommendations for critically important areas of research have provided an impetus for investigations in this area.

Van Vlack LH: Elements of Materials Science and Engineering, 5th ed. Reading, MA, Addison-Wesley, 1985.

An excellent text on materials science. Recommended for a more in-depth coverage of materials structure and properties.

Zisman WA: Influence of constitution on adhesion. Ind Eng Chem 55:19, 1963.

One of the pioneers in surface phenomena discusses parameters that influence wetting. Zisman was a leader in the use of contact angle measurements to screen the potential wetting of adhesives to selected adherends.

3

Physical Properties of Dental Materials

Kenneth J. Anusavice and William A. Brantley

OUTLINE

What Are Physical Properties?

Abrasion and Abrasion Resistance

Viscosity

Structural and Stress Relaxation

Creep and Flow

Color and Color Perception

Thermophysical Properties

Introduction to Tarnish and Corrosion

Causes of Tarnish and Corrosion

Classification of Corrosion

Electrochemical Corrosion

Protection Against Corrosion

Corrosion of Dental Restorations

Evaluation of Tarnish and Corrosion Resistance

Clinical Significance of Galvanic Currents

KEY TERMS

Chroma—Degree of saturation of a particular hue.

Coefficient of thermal expansion (linear coefficient of expansion)—Change in length per unit of original length of a material when its temperature is raised 1° K.

Color—Sensation induced from light of varying wavelengths reaching the eye.

Concentration cell—An electrochemical corrosion cell in which the potential difference is associated with the difference in concentration of a dissolved species, such as oxygen, in solution along different areas of a metal surface.

Corrosion—Chemical or electrochemical process in which a solid, usually a metal, is attacked by an environmental agent, resulting in partial or complete dissolution. Although glasses and other nonmetals are susceptible to environmental degradation, metals are generally more susceptible to such attack because of electrochemical reactions.

Creep—Time-dependent plastic strain of a material under a static load or constant stress.

Crevice corrosion—Accelerated corrosion in narrow spaces caused by localized electrochemical processes and chemistry changes, such as acidification and depletion in oxygen content. Crevice corrosion commonly occurs when microleakage takes place between a restoration and the tooth, under a pellicle layer, or under other surface deposits.

KEY TERMS—cont'd

Galvanic corrosion (electrogalvanism)—Accelerated attack occurring on a less noble metal when electrochemically dissimilar metals are in electrical contact within a liquid corrosive environment.

Galvanic shock—Pain sensation caused by the electric current generated when two dissimilar metals are brought into contact in the oral environment.

Hardness—Resistance of a material to being indented, cut, or scratched.

Hue—Dominant color of an object, for example, red, green, or blue.

Metamerism—Phenomenon in which the color of an object under one type of light appears to change when illuminated by a different light source.

Pitting corrosion—Highly localized corrosion occurring on base metals, such as iron, nickel, and chromium, which are protected by a naturally forming, thin film of an oxide. In the presence of chlorides in the environment, the film locally breaks down and rapid dissolution of the underlying metal occurs in the form of pits.

Rheology—Study of the deformation and flow characteristics of matter.

Sag—Irreversible (plastic) deformation of metal frameworks of fixed partial dentures in the firing temperature range of ceramic veneers.

Stress corrosion—Degradation caused by the combined effects of mechanical stress and a corrosive environment, usually exhibited as cracking.

Tarnish—Process by which a metal surface is dulled or discolored when a reaction with a sulfide, oxide, chloride, or other chemical causes a thin film to form.

Thermal conductivity (coefficient of thermal conductivity)—Property that describes the thermal energy transport in watts per second through a specimen 1 cm thick with a cross-sectional area of 1 cm^2 when the temperature differential between the surfaces of the specimen perpendicular to the heat flow is 1° K.

Thixotropic—Property of certain gels or other materials to become liquefied (less viscous) when shaken, stirred, patted, or vibrated.

Value—Relative lightness or darkness of a color.

Viscosity—Resistance of a fluid to flow.

Wear, abrasion, and erosion—Loss of material from a surface caused by a mechanical action or through a combination of chemical and mechanical actions.

WHAT ARE PHYSICAL PROPERTIES?

Physical properties are based on the laws of mechanics, acoustics, optics, thermodynamics, electricity, magnetism, radiation, atomic structure, or nuclear phenomena. **Hue, value**, and **chroma** are physical properties that are based on the laws of optics, which is the science that deals with phenomena of light, vision, and sight. **Thermal conductivity** and **coefficient of thermal expansion** are physical properties that are based on the laws of thermodynamics. The influence of the atomic or molecular nature of solids on these properties is discussed in Chapter 2. The following sections offer brief descriptions of physical properties, although some of these topics are presented in more detail in the chapters on specific materials. For example, **color** and thermal expansion coefficient are also discussed in the chapter on dental ceramics, flow is discussed in the chapter on impression materials, and **creep** is discussed in the amalgam chapter.

This chapter addresses properties that are defined in several other scientific fields. For example, **viscosity**, which is the resistance of a fluid to flow, is related to the fields of materials science and mechanics. Color, which is the sensation induced from light of varying wavelengths reaching the eye, is based on the laws of optics. Mechanical properties are a subset of physical properties, which are based on the laws of mechanics and are discussed in Chapter 4.

CRITICAL QUESTIONS

Hardness, which is the property of being difficult to indent, cut, or scratch, is sometimes used to predict the wear resistance of a material in a fixed or removable denture and its ability to abrade opposing dental structures. What factors other than hardness may be responsible for excessive wear of natural tooth enamel or prosthetic surfaces by a harder material such as a ceramic? How can a dentist prevent this problem?

ABRASION AND ABRASION RESISTANCE

Hardness has often been used as an index of the ability of a material to resist **abrasion** or **wear**. However, abrasion is a complex mechanism in the oral environment that involves an interaction among numerous factors. For this reason, the consideration of hardness as a predictor of abrasion resistance is of limited value. Hardness may be useful for comparing materials within a given classification, such as one brand of cast metal with another brand of the same type of casting alloy. However, hardness alone may be inappropriate for evaluating either the wear resistance or abrasiveness of different classes of materials, such as a metallic material compared with a synthetic resin.

A reliable in vitro test for abrasion resistance is one that is designed to simulate as closely as possible the particular type of abrasion to which the material will eventually be subjected in vivo. However, a simple in vitro wear test does not usually predict in vivo wear performance accurately because of the greater complexity of the clinical environment. The wear of enamel by ceramic and by certain base metal alloys is well known. However, the hardness of a material is only one of many factors that affect the wear of the contacting enamel surfaces. Other major factors include biting force, frequency of chewing, abrasiveness of the diet, composition of intraoral liquids, temperature changes, surface roughness, physical properties of the materials, and surface irregularities such as hard impurity particles, fine anatomic grooves, pits, or ridges. The excessive wear of tooth enamel by an opposing ceramic crown is more likely to occur in the presence of high biting forces and a rough ceramic surface. Although dentists cannot control the bite force of a patient, they can adjust the occlusion to create broader contact areas in order to reduce localized stresses, and they can polish the abrading ceramic surface to reduce the rate of destructive enamel wear.

VISCOSITY

Viscosity is the resistance of a liquid to flow. Up to this point, discussion of the physical properties of dental materials has been devoted to the room temperature or oral temperature behavior of solid materials that are subjected to various types of stress. However, dentists and dental office staff must also manipulate materials in a fluid state to achieve successful clinical outcomes when preventing caries or restoring teeth. Moreover, the success or failure of a given material may be as dependent on its properties in the liquid state as it is on its properties as a solid. For example, materials like cements and impression materials undergo a liquid-to-solid transformation in the mouth. Gypsum products used in the fabrication of models and dies are transformed from slurries into solid structures. Amorphous materials such as waxes and resins appear solid but actually are supercooled liquids that can flow plastically (irreversibly) under sustained loading or deform elastically (reversibly) under small stresses. The ways in which these materials flow or deform when subjected to stress are important to their use in dentistry. The study of flow characteristics of materials is the basis for the science of **rheology**.

Although a liquid at rest cannot support a shear stress (shearing force per unit shearing area), most liquids, when placed in motion, resist imposed forces that cause them to move. This resistance to fluid flow (*viscosity*) is controlled by internal frictional forces within the liquid. Thus viscosity is a measure of the consistency of a fluid and its inability to flow. A highly viscous fluid flows slowly. Dental materials have different viscosities depending on the preparation for their intended clinical application. Dental assistants, dentists, and dental students who have observed the more viscous nature of zinc polycarboxylate and resin cements compared with zinc phosphate cement when these materials have been properly mixed as luting cements are familiar with this viscosity difference.

Figure 3-1 helps to quantify this concept. A liquid occupies the space between two metal plates; the lower plate is fixed, and the upper plate is being moved to the right at a velocity (V). A force (F) is required to overcome the frictional resistance (viscosity) to fluid flow. As will be discussed in Chapter 4, *stress* is the force per unit area that develops within a structure when an external force is applied. This stress causes a deformation or strain to develop. Strain is calculated as a change in length divided by the initial reference length. If the plates have an area (A) in contact with the liquid, a shear stress (τ) can be defined as $\tau = F/A$. The shear strain rate, or rate of change of deformation, is $\varepsilon = V/d$, where d is the shear distance of the top plate relative to the fixed lower plate and V is the velocity of the top plate. As the shear force F increases, V increases, and a curve can be obtained for force versus velocity, analogous to the load versus displacement curves that are derived from static measurements on solids.

To explain the viscous nature of some materials, a shear stress versus shear strain rate curve can be plotted. The rheologic behaviors of four types of fluids are shown in Figure 3-2. An "ideal" fluid demonstrates a shear stress that is proportional to the strain rate. The plot is a straight line, indicating *Newtonian* behavior. Because the viscosity (η) is defined as the shear stress divided by the strain rate, τ/ε, a Newtonian fluid has a constant viscosity and exhibits a constant slope of shear stress plotted

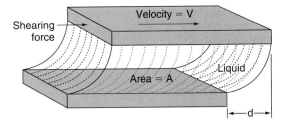

Fig. 3-1 Shear strain, d, of a viscous liquid between two plates caused by translation of the top plate at a velocity, V, relative to the rigid lower plate.

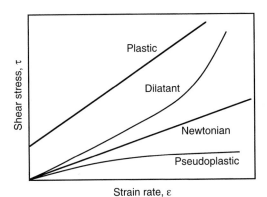

Fig. 3-2 Shear stress versus shear strain rate for fluids exhibiting different types of rheologic behavior.

against strain rate (see Fig. 3-2). The plot is a straight line and resembles the elastic portion of a stress-strain curve (see Chapter 4), with viscosity the analog of the elastic modulus (elastic stress divided by elastic strain). Viscosity is measured in units of MPa per second, or centipoise (cP). Pure water at 20° C has a viscosity of 1.0 cP, whereas the viscosity of molasses is approximately 300,000 cP. This value is similar to that of tempered agar hydrocolloid impression material (281,000 cP at 45° C). Of the elastomeric impression materials, light-body polysulfide has a viscosity of 109,000 cP compared with a value of 1,360,000 cP for heavy-body polysulfide at 36° C. Many dental materials exhibit *pseudoplastic* behavior, as illustrated by the change in slope of the plot in Figure 3-2. Their viscosity decreases with increasing strain rate until it reaches a nearly constant value. Liquids that show the opposite tendency are described as *dilatant*. These liquids become more rigid as the rate of deformation (shear strain rate) increases.

Finally, some classes of materials behave like a rigid body until some minimum value of shear stress is reached. This is represented by the offset along the shear stress axis. These fluids, which exhibit rigid behavior initially and then attain constant viscosity, are referred to as *plastic*. Ketchup is a familiar example—a sharp blow to the bottle is usually required to produce an initial flow.

The viscosity of most liquids decreases rapidly with increasing temperature. Viscosity may also depend on previous deformation of the liquid. A liquid of this type that becomes less viscous and more fluid under repeated applications of pressure is referred to as **thixotropic**. Dental prophylaxis pastes, plaster of Paris, resin cements, and some impression materials are thixotropic. The thixotropic nature of impression materials is beneficial because the material does not flow out of a mandibular impression tray until placed over dental tissues, and a prophylaxis paste does not flow out of a rubber cup until it is rotated against the teeth to be cleaned. If these materials are stirred rapidly and the viscosity is measured, a value is obtained that is lower than the value for a sample that has been left undisturbed.

The viscosity of a dental material may determine its suitability for a given application. Likewise, the nature of the shear stress versus shear strain rate curve can be important in determining the best way to manipulate a material. As explained in more detail later, the viscosity as a function of time can also be used to measure the working time of a material that undergoes a liquid-to-solid transformation.

STRUCTURAL AND STRESS RELAXATION

After a substance has been permanently deformed (plastic deformation), there are trapped internal stresses. For example, in a crystalline substance such as a metal, the atoms in the crystal structure are displaced, and the system is not in equilibrium. Similarly, in amorphous structures, some molecules are too close together and others too far apart when the substance is permanently deformed.

It is understandable that such situations are unstable. The displaced atoms are not in equilibrium positions. Through a solid-state diffusion process driven by thermal energy, the atoms can move back slowly to their equilibrium positions. The result is a change in the shape or contour of the solid as the atoms or molecules change positions. The material *warps* or *distorts*. This *stress relaxation* leads to distortion of elastomeric impressions.

The rate of relaxation increases with an increase in temperature. For example, if a wire is bent, it may tend to straighten out if it is heated to a high temperature. At room temperature, any such relaxation caused by rearrangement of metal atoms may be negligible. On the other hand, there are many noncrystalline dental materials (such as waxes, resins, and gels) that, when manipulated and cooled, can then undergo relaxation (distortion) at an elevated temperature. Considerable attention is given to this phenomenon in succeeding chapters, because such dimensional changes by relaxation may result in an inaccurate fit of dental appliances.

CREEP AND FLOW

If a metal is held at a temperature near its melting point and is subjected to a constant applied stress, the resulting strain will increase over time. **Creep** is defined as the time-dependent plastic strain of a material under a static load or constant stress. The related phenomenon of **sag** occurs in the permanent deformation of long-span metal bridge structures at porcelain-firing temperatures under the influence of the mass of the prosthesis. For a given thickness, a greater bridge mass is related to greater flexural stress and, thus, greater *flexural creep*. Metal creep usually occurs as the temperature increases to within a few hundred degrees of the melting range. Metals used in dentistry for cast restorations or substrates for porcelain veneers have melting points that are much higher than mouth temperatures, and they are not susceptible to creep deformation intraorally. However, some alloys used for metal-ceramic prostheses can creep at porcelain veneering temperatures. This phenomenon will be discussed further in Chapter 21.

Dental amalgams contain from 42 to 52 wt% Hg and begin melting at temperatures only slightly above room temperature. (The melting range of an alloy is discussed in Chapter 6.) Because of its low melting range, dental amalgam can slowly creep from a restored tooth site under periodic sustained stress, such as would be imposed by patients who clench their teeth. Because creep produces continuing plastic deformation, the process can be destructive to a dental prosthesis. The relationship of this property to the behavior of the amalgam restoration is discussed in Chapter 17. A creep test is required in American National Standards Institute/American Dental Association Specification No. 1 and Addendum 1a for dental amalgam products.

The term *flow*, rather than creep, has generally been used in dentistry to describe the rheology of amorphous materials such as waxes. The flow of wax is a measure of its potential to deform under a small static load, even that associated with its own mass. Although creep or flow may be measured under any type of stress, compression is usually employed in the testing of dental materials. A cylinder of prescribed dimensions is subjected to a given compressive stress for a specified time and temperature. The creep or flow is measured as the percentage decrease in length that occurs under these testing conditions. Creep may cause unacceptable deformation of dental restorations (such as low-copper dental amalgam) made from a material that is used clinically at a temperature near its melting point for an extended period. Creep may also lead to an unacceptable fit of fixed partial denture frameworks when a cast alloy with poor creep (sag) resistance is veneered with porcelain at relatively high temperatures (~1000° C).

COLOR AND COLOR PERCEPTION

The preceding sections have focused on those properties that are necessary to permit a material to restore the function of damaged or missing natural tissues. Another important goal of dentistry is to restore the *color* and appearance of natural dentition. Aesthetic considerations in restorative and prosthetic dentistry have received greater emphasis over the past several decades. The search for an ideal, general purpose, technique-insensitive, direct-filling, tooth-colored restorative material is one of the continuing challenges of current dental materials research.

Since aesthetic dentistry imposes severe demands on the artistic abilities of the dentist and technician, knowledge of the underlying scientific principles of color is essential. This is especially true for the increasingly popular restorations that involve ceramic materials (see Chapter 21). A more comprehensive treatment of this subject can be found in other texts (see the Selected Readings list at the end of this chapter).

Light is electromagnetic radiation that can be detected by the human eye. The eye is sensitive to wavelengths from approximately 400 nm (violet) to 700 nm (dark red), as shown in the color version of Figure 3-3 (see also color plates). The reflected light intensity and the combined intensities of the wavelengths present in incident and reflected light determine the appearance properties (hue, value, and chroma). For an object to be visible, it must reflect or transmit light incident on it from an external source. The incident light is usually polychromatic, that is, a mixture of the various wavelengths. Incident light is selectively absorbed or scattered (or both) at certain wavelengths. The spectral distribution of the transmitted or reflected light resembles that of the incident light, although certain wavelengths are reduced in magnitude.

The phenomenon of vision, and certain related terminology, can be illustrated by considering the response of the human eye to light reflected from an object. Light from an object that is incident on the eye is focused in the retina and is converted into nerve impulses that are transmitted to the brain. Cone-shaped cells in the retina are responsible for color vision. These cells have a threshold intensity required for color vision and also exhibit a response curve related to the wavelength of the incident light. Figure 3-4 illustrates such curves for individuals with normal color vision and for individuals with color-deficient vision. The normal observer curve shown in Figure 3-4 indicates the human visual responsiveness to light reflected or emitted from a particular source or object. This figure indicates that the eye is most sensitive

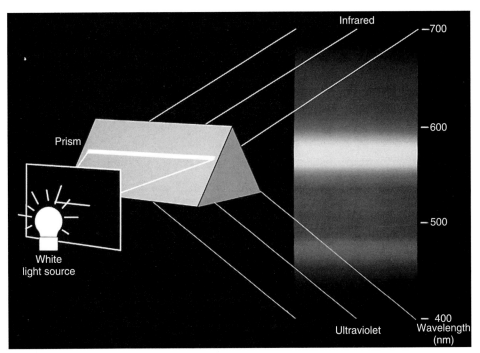

Fig. 3-3 Spectrum of visible light ranging in wavelength from 400 nm (violet) to 700 nm (red). The most visually perceptible region of the equal energy spectrum under daylight conditions is between wavelengths of 540 and 570 nm, with a maximum value of visual perceptibility at 555 nm (see Fig. 3-4). See also color plate.

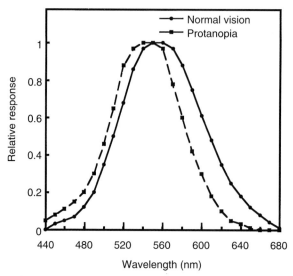

Fig. 3-4 Relative visual response of humans to wavelength of light for a normal observer and one with protanopia (red-green) color blindness. Protanopia is experienced by 1% of the male population and 0.02% of the female population.

to light in the green-yellow region (wavelength of 550 nm) and least sensitive at the red or blue regions of the color spectrum.

Because a neural response is involved in color vision, constant stimulation by a single color may result in color fatigue and a decrease in the eye's response. The signals from the retina are processed by the brain to produce the psychophysiological perception of color. Defects in certain portions of the color-sensing receptors result in the different types of color blindness, and thus, human observers vary greatly in their ability to distinguish colors. In a scientific sense, one might liken the normal human eye to an exceptionally sensitive differential colorimeter, a scientific instrument that measures the intensity and wavelength of light. Although the colorimeter is more precise than the human eye in measuring slight differences in colored objects, it can be extremely inaccurate when used on rough or curved surfaces. The eye is able to differentiate between two colors seen side by side on smooth or irregular surfaces, whether curved or flat.

CRITICAL QUESTION

Why do some tooth-colored restorations appear to be missing when viewed under "disco" lighting?

Three Dimensions of Color

Verbal descriptions of color are not precise enough to describe the appearance of teeth. For example, to describe a brownish-purple color called *puce*, Webster's Third New International Dictionary defines the word as "a dark red that is yellower and less strong than cranberry, paler and slightly yellower than average garnet, bluer, less strong, and slightly lighter than pomegranate, and bluer and paler than average wine." This definition is far too complex and imprecise to describe a desired color of a dental crown to a laboratory technician. Such a written description does not clearly and unambiguously allow one to perceive the color. Three variables must be measured to accurately describe our perception of light reflected from a tooth or restoration surface: hue, value, and chroma. **Hue** describes the dominant color of an object, for example, red, green, or blue. This refers to the dominant wavelengths present in the spectral distribution. The continuum of these hues creates the color solid shown in Figure 3-5 (see also color plates). **Value** increases toward the top (whiter) and decreases toward the bottom (darker or more black). Teeth and other objects can be separated into lighter shades (higher value) and darker shades (lower value). For example, the yellow of a lemon is lighter than is the red of a cherry. For a light-diffusing and light-reflecting object such as a tooth or dental crown, *value* identifies the lightness or darkness of a color, which can be measured independently of the hue. Figure 3-6 (see also color plates) represents a horizontal plane though the color solid in Figure 3-5. This color chart is based on the CIE L*a*b* color space in which L* represents the value of an object, a* is the measurement along the red-green axis, and b* is the measurement along the yellow-blue axis. The color of a red apple is shown by the letter A in the upper and lower charts. Its color appearance can be

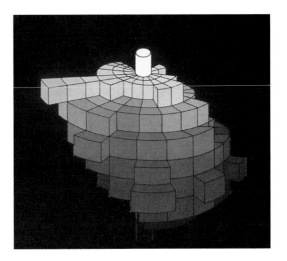

Fig. 3-5 Color solid that is used to describe the three dimensions of color. Value increases from black at the bottom center to white at the top center. Chroma increases from the center outward, and hue changes occur in a circumferential direction. See also color plate. (Courtesy of Minolta Corporation, Instrument Systems Division, Ramsey, NJ.)

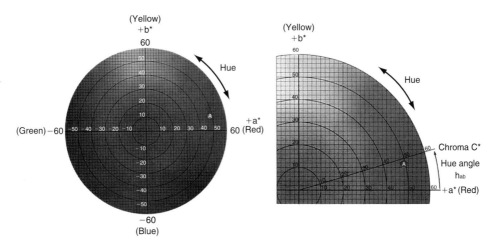
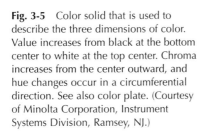

Fig. 3-6 L*a*b* color chart showing the color of a red apple at point A (top and bottom). For this chart, the appearance is expressed by L* (value) = 42.83; a* (red-green axis) = 45.04; and b* (yellow-blue axis) = 9.52. In contrast, the color of shade A2 porcelain can be described by L* = 72.99; a* = 1.00; and b* = 14.41. See also color plate. (Courtesy of Minolta Corporation, Instrument Systems Division, Ramsey, NJ.)

expressed by L* = 42.83, a* = 45.04, and b* = 9.52. In comparison, a dental body (gingival) porcelain of shade A2 can be described by a higher (lighter) L* of 72.99, a lower a* of 1.00, and a higher b* of 14.41.

The yellow color of a lemon is more "vivid" than that of a banana, which is a "dull" yellow. This is a difference in the color intensity. **Chroma** represents this degree of saturation of a particular hue. Just as value varies vertically, chroma varies radially (see Fig. 3-6, *bottom*). Colors in the center are dull (gray). In other words, the higher the chroma, the more intense the color. Chroma is not considered separately in dentistry. It is always associated with hue and value of dental tissues, restorations, and prostheses. In a similar manner, the adjustments on a color television set make use of these hue, value, and chroma principles.

In the dental operatory or laboratory, color matching is usually performed by the use of a *shade guide* such as the ceramic shade guide shown in Figure 3-7 (see also color plates) to select the color of ceramic veneers, inlays, or crowns to be made by a laboratory technician. The neck region of these shade tabs has been removed because its shade is darker and its presence would complicate the matching of the correct shade. Unfortunately, although a reasonable match can be achieved between a tooth (or restoration) and one of the shade guide tabs, it is difficult to describe this information to a laboratory technician who may not have a chance to see the patient. Furthermore, the thickness of the shade tab may be quite different from that of the prosthesis to be made, and the shade of one porcelain crown may look different from that of another crown made from the same batch of porcelain powder. Also, the porcelain of a given shade made by the same manufacturer may vary from batch to batch. Thus the challenges are formidable for the dentist and technician who work as a team to restore the proper appearance of teeth that are damaged, decayed, or defective.

The shade guide shown in Figure 3-7 was specially prepared by grinding away the necks of the porcelain tabs, because the correct shade is determined from the gingival half of the tab and not from the neck. These tabs are used in much the same way as paint chips are used to match the color of house paint. Using these shade tabs, one can specify the color characteristics (hue, value, chroma) and translucency to the technician who will produce the proper appearance in the laboratory. The tooth-shaped tabs in Figure 3-7 have been arranged in decreasing order of value (lightest

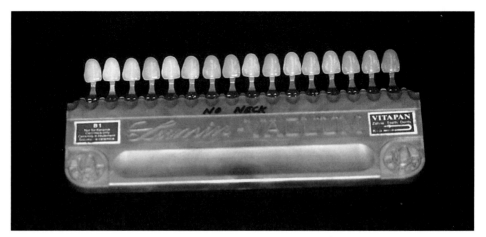

Fig. 3-7   Dental shade guide tabs of the Vita Lumin type arranged in decreasing order of value (lighter to darker). The necks of the tooth-shaped tabs have been ground away to facilitate the selection of tooth shades. See also color plate.

to darkest) from left to right rather than the standard grouping by hue (A1 to D4). This technique is based on the perception that the matching of tooth shades is simplified by the arrangement of tabs by value.

Obviously, if the technician can see the actual teeth, the probability of achieving an acceptable color match is even greater. However, patients often desire restorations of higher value than that of the natural teeth. As shown on the left side of Figure 3-8, *A,* the shade of the two central incisor metal-ceramic crowns with porcelain butt-joint margins is higher in value than that of the lateral incisor teeth. However, the patient was pleased with this result. A close-up view of the two metal-ceramic crowns is shown in Figure 3-8, *B* (see also color plates).

As stated previously, signals of color are sent to the human brain from three sets of receptors in the retina called *cones.* The cones are especially sensitive to red, blue, and green. Factors that interfere with the true perception of color generally include low or high light levels, fatigue of the color receptors, sex, age, memory, and cultural background. However, according to a recent study (Anusavice and Barrett, 1995), there appears to be no effect related to observer age, sex, or clinical experience relative to the accuracy of dental shade matching.

At low light levels, the rods of the human eye are more dominant than the cones, and color perception is lost. As the brightness becomes more intense, color appears to change (Bezold-Brucke effect). Also, if an observer looks at a red object for a reasonably long time, receptor fatigue causes a green hue to be seen when the observer then looks at a white background. For this reason, if a patient is observed against an intense-colored background, the dentist or clinician may select a tooth shade with a hue that is shifted somewhat toward the complementary color of the background color. For example, a blue background shifts color selection toward yellow, and an orange background shifts the color selection toward blue-green. Unfortunately, 8% of men and 0.5% of women exhibit color blindness. Most commonly, these people cannot distinguish red from green because of the lack of either green-sensitive or red-sensitive cones. However, this deficiency may not affect the shade selection of natural teeth.

Although the ranges of hue, chroma, and value ordinarily found in human teeth represent only a small portion of the standard color space (such as that shown in Fig. 3-5), the selectivity of the human eye is sufficient to make accurate color matching difficult when using a shade guide that contains only a small number of shades (Fig. 3-7). Spectrophotometric analysis of commercial shade guides has also demonstrated the absence of large regions of hue, value, and chroma when compared with the color space values determined for human teeth.

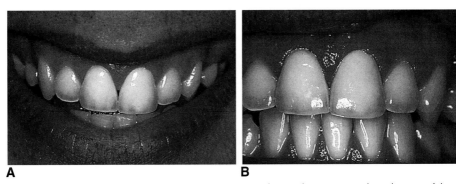

A **B**

Fig. 3-8 **A,** Two central incisor metal-ceramic crowns with porcelain margins. The value (L*) of these crowns is higher than that of the adjacent lateral incisor teeth. **B,** Close-up view of the metal-ceramic crowns on the left. See also color plate.

Because the spectral distribution of the light reflected from or transmitted through an object is dependent on the spectral content of the incident light, the appearance of an object is dependent on the nature of the light in which the object is viewed. Daylight, incandescent, and fluorescent lamps are common sources of light in the dental operatory or laboratory, and each of these has a different spectral distribution. Objects that appear to be color matched under one type of light may appear different under another light source. This phenomenon is called **metamerism**. Thus, if possible, color matching should be done under two or more different light sources, one of which should be daylight, and the laboratory shade-matching procedures should be performed under the same lighting conditions.

In addition to the processes already discussed, natural tooth structure absorbs light at wavelengths too short to be visible to the human eye. These wavelengths between 300 and 400 nm are referred to as *near-ultraviolet radiation*. Natural sunlight, photoflash lamps, certain types of vapor lamps, and ultraviolet lights used in decorative lighting are sources containing substantial amounts of near-ultraviolet radiation. The energy that the tooth absorbs is converted into light with longer wavelengths, in which case the tooth actually becomes a light source. This phenomenon is called *fluorescence*. The emitted light, a blue-white color, is primarily in the 400- to 450-nm range. Fluorescence makes a definite contribution to the brightness and vital appearance of a human tooth. As an example, a person with ceramic crowns or composite restorations that lack a fluorescing agent appears to be missing teeth when viewed under a black light in a nightclub.

The researcher developing a tooth-colored restorative material and the dentist and technician who fabricate them must be concerned with color matching under light sources that contain a sufficient near-ultraviolet component. Incandescent lighting contains little ultraviolet radiation. The dentist and laboratory technician must be aware of the importance of color matching under more than one source of light. Additional information on color and color perception is presented in Chapter 21 and in several reference books on color applications in dentistry.

THERMOPHYSICAL PROPERTIES
Thermal Conductivity

Heat transfer through solid substances most commonly occurs by means of conduction. The conduction of heat through metals occurs through the interactions of crystal lattice vibrations and by the motion of electrons and their interaction with atoms. **Thermal conductivity** (κ) is a thermophysical measure of how well heat is transferred through a material by conductive flow. The measurement of thermal conductivity is performed under *steady state conditions*. Under these conditions, temperatures in the system (i.e., the temperature gradient) do not change over time. The rate of heat flow through a structure is proportional both to the area (perpendicular to the heat flow direction) through which the heat is conducted and to the temperature gradient across the structure. Thus if significant porosity exists in the structure, the area available for conduction is reduced and the rate of heat flow is reduced. The thermal conductivity, or *coefficient of thermal conductivity*, is the quantity of heat in calories per second that passes through a specimen 1 cm thick having a cross-sectional area of 1 cm^2 when the temperature difference between the surfaces perpendicular to the heat flow of the specimen is 1° K. According to the second law of thermodynamics, heat flows from points of higher temperature to points of lower temperature.

Materials that have a high thermal conductivity are called *conductors*, whereas materials of low thermal conductivity are called *insulators*. The International System

(SI) unit or measure for thermal conductivity is watt per meter per second per degree Kelvin (W × m^{-1} × s^{-1} × K^{-1}). The higher the thermal conductivity, the greater is the ability of the substance to transmit thermal energy, and vice versa. Compared with a resin-based composite that has a low thermal conductivity, heat is transferred more rapidly away from the tooth when cold water contacts a metallic restoration because of its higher thermal conductivity. This increased conductivity of the metal compared with that of the resin composite induces greater pulpal sensitivity, which is experienced as a negligible, mild, moderate, or extreme discomfort, depending on previous tooth trauma and the pain response of the patient.

Thermal Diffusivity

The value of *thermal diffusivity* of a material controls the time rate of temperature change as heat passes through a material. It is a measure of the rate at which a body with a nonuniform temperature reaches a state of thermal equilibrium. Although the thermal conductivity of zinc oxide–eugenol is slightly less than that of dentin, its thermal diffusivity is more than twice that of dentin. The square root of thermal diffusivity is indirectly proportional to the thermal insulation ability, whereas the thickness of the cement base is directly related to its benefit as an insulator. Thus the thickness of the liner is a more important thermal insulation factor than the thermal diffusivity of the ceramic. The relevance of thermal diffusivity is explained in the following discussion.

In the oral environment, temperatures are not constant during the ingestion of foods and liquids. For these *unsteady state* conditions, heat transfer through the material decreases the thermal gradient. Under such conditions, thermal diffusivity is important. The mathematical formula that relates thermal diffusivity (h) to thermal conductivity (κ) is

$$h = \frac{\kappa}{c_p \rho} \qquad (1)$$

where κ is the thermal conductivity, c_p is the temperature-dependent specific heat at constant pressure (heat capacity), and ρ is the temperature-dependent density. Heat capacity is numerically equal to the more commonly used term *specific heat*. The SI unit of thermal diffusivity is typical of diffusion processes, that is, square meter per second. However, the unit of square centimeter per second is often used. As shown in Table 3-1, typical values of thermal diffusivity in units of 10^{-4} cm^2/sec are as follows: pure gold, 11,800; amalgam, 960; composite, 19–73, zinc phosphate cement, 30; glass ionomer, 22; dentin, 18–26; and enamel, 47. Thus for a patient drinking ice water, the low specific heat of amalgam and its high thermal conductivity suggest that the higher thermal diffusivity favors a thermal shock situation more than is likely to occur when only natural tooth structure is exposed to the cold liquid.

For a given volume of material, the heat required to raise the temperature a given amount depends on its *heat capacity* or specific heat (calorie per gram per degree Kelvin) and the density (gram per cubic centimeter). When the product of heat capacity and density ($c_p \rho$) is high, the thermal diffusivity may be low, even though the thermal conductivity is relatively high. Therefore, both thermal conductivity and thermal diffusivity are important parameters in predicting the transfer of thermal energy through a material. Because an unsteady state of heat transfer exists during the ingestion of hot or cold foods and liquids, the thermal diffusivity of a dental

| Table 3-1 | Density and Thermal Properties of Water, Enamel, Dentin and Dental Materials | | | |

Material	Density (g cm^{-3})	Specific heat (cal g^{-1} K^{-1})	Thermal conductivity (W m^{-1} K^{-1})	Thermal diffusivity (cm^2 s^{-1})
Water	1.00	1.00	0.44	0.0014
Dentin	2.14	0.30	0.57	0.0018–0.0026
Glass ionomer	2.13	0.27	0.51–0.72	0.0022
Zinc phosphate	2.59	0.12	1.05	0.0030
Composite	1.6–2.4	0.20	1.09–1.37	0.0019–0.0073
Enamel	2.97	0.18	0.93	0.0047
Amalgam	11.6	0.005	22.6	0.96
Pure gold	19.3	0.03	297	1.18

restorative material may be more important than its thermal conductivity. As noted in Table 3-1, enamel and dentin are effective thermal insulators. Their thermal conductivity and thermal diffusivity compare favorably with silica brick and water, in contrast with the markedly higher values for metals.

However, as for any thermal insulator, tooth structure must be present in sufficient thickness for insulating dental cements to be effective. When the layer of dentin between the bottom of the cavity floor and the pulp is too thin, the dentist should place an additional layer of an insulating base, as discussed in the chapter on dental cements. The effectiveness of a material in preventing heat transfer is directly proportional to the thickness of the liner and inversely proportional to the square root of the thermal diffusivity. Thus the thicknesses of the remaining dentin and the base are as important as, if not more important than, the thermal properties of the materials.

The low thermal conductivity of enamel and dentin aids in reducing thermal shock and pulpal pain when hot or cold foods are taken into the mouth. However, the presence of oral restorations of any type tends to change the environment. As discussed later, many restorative materials are metallic. Because of the free electrons present in solid metals (see Chapter 2), these materials are such good thermal conductors that the tooth pulp may be adversely affected by thermal changes. In many instances it is necessary to insert a thermal insulator between the restoration and the tooth structure. In this respect, a restorative material that exhibits a low thermal conductivity is more desirable.

On the other hand, artificial teeth are held in a denture base that ordinarily is constructed of a synthetic resin, which is a poor thermal conductor. In the upper denture, this base usually covers most of the roof of the mouth (hard palate). Its low thermal conductivity tends to prevent heat exchange between the supporting soft tissues and the oral cavity itself. Thus, the patient partially loses the sensation of hot and cold while eating and drinking. The use of a metal denture base may be more comfortable and pleasant from this standpoint.

Coefficient of Thermal Expansion

A thermal property that is important to the dentist is the **coefficient of thermal expansion**, which is defined as the change in length per unit of the original length

Table 3-2	Coefficients of Thermal Expansion (α) of Dental Materials Relative to That of Tooth Enamel and Dentin	
Material	α (ppm K^{-1})	$\alpha_{material}/\alpha_{tooth\ enamel}$
Aluminous porcelain	6.6	0.58
Dentin	8.3	0.75
Commercially pure titanium	8.5	0.77
Type II glass ionomer	11.0	0.96
Tooth enamel	11.4	1.00
Gold-palladium alloy	13.5	1.18
Gold (pure)	14.0	1.23
Palladium-silver alloy	14.8	1.30
Amalgam	25.0	2.19
Composite	14–50	1.2–4.4
Denture resin	81.0	7.11
Pit and fissure sealant	85.0	7.46
Inlay wax	400.0	35.1

of a material when its temperature is raised 1° K (see Thermal Energy in Chapter 2). Values of coefficients of thermal expansion of some materials of interest in dentistry are presented in Table 3-2. The units of α are typically expressed in units of μm/m°K or ppm/°K.

A tooth restoration may expand or contract more than the tooth during a change in temperature; thus there may be marginal microleakage adjacent to the restoration, or the restoration may debond from the tooth. According to the values in Table 3-2, restorative materials may change in dimension up to 4.4 times more than the tooth enamel for every degree of temperature change. However, although the dimensions of a wax pattern may change markedly when the temperature changes by 20C°, the relative contraction of an amalgam restoration that is 10 mm wide is only 5 μm when the oral temperature decreases by 20C° since the tooth enamel contracts by about 2.2 μm. Thus the net difference is only 2.7 μm, which is much smaller than the dimensional change of 220 μm between cusps that are subjected to mechanical stresses during the polymerization of resin-based composites.

The high thermal expansion coefficient of inlay wax is also important because it is highly susceptible to temperature changes. For example, an accurate wax pattern that fits a prepared tooth contracts significantly when it is removed from the tooth or a die in a warmer area and then stored in a cooler area. This dimensional change is transferred to a cast restoration that is made from the lost-wax process. Similarly, denture teeth that have been set in denture base wax in a relatively warm laboratory may shift appreciably in their simulated intraoral positions after the denture base is moved to a cooler room before the processing of a denture.

Thermal stresses produced from a thermal expansion or contraction difference are also important in the production of metal-ceramic restorations. Consider a porcelain veneer that is fired to a metal substrate (coping). It may contract to a greater extent than the metal during cooling and induce tangential tensile stresses or tensile hoop (circumferential) tensile stresses in the porcelain that may cause immediate or delayed crack formation. Although these thermal stresses cannot be eliminated completely, they can be reduced appreciably by selection of materials whose expansion or contraction coefficients are matched fairly closely (within 4%).

CRITICAL QUESTION

What factors in the oral environment promote the corrosion of metallic dental restorations and prostheses?

INTRODUCTION TO TARNISH AND CORROSION

In most cases **corrosion** is undesirable. However, in dental practice, a limited amount of corrosion around the margins of dental amalgam restorations may be beneficial, since the corrosion products tend to seal the marginal gap and inhibit the ingress of oral fluids and bacteria. Some metals and alloys are resistant to corrosion because of inherent nobility or the formation of a protective surface layer.

A common example of corrosion is rusting of iron, a complex chemical reaction in which iron combines with oxygen in air and water to form the hydrated oxide $Fe_2O_3 \bullet H_2O$. This oxide layer is porous, bulkier, weaker, and more brittle than the metal from which it formed. Loss of the nonadherent oxide exposes a fresh underlying metal surface, which enhances continuation of the corrosion process. One method to prevent this corrosion is to alloy iron with chromium, forming stainless steel (which also contains other alloying elements). As discussed in Chapter 20, the austenitic and martensitic stainless steel alloys have a variety of uses in dentistry.

High-noble alloys used in dentistry are so stable chemically that they do not undergo significant corrosion in the oral environment; the major components of these alloys are gold, palladium, and platinum. (Iridium, osmium, rhodium, and ruthenium are also classified as noble metals.) Silver is not considered noble by dental standards, since it will react with air, water, and sulfur to form silver sulfide, a dark discoloration product.

Metals undergo chemical or electrochemical reactions with the environment, resulting in dissolution or formation of chemical compounds. Commonly known as corrosion products, the chemical compounds may accelerate, retard, or have no influence on the subsequent deterioration of the metal surface. It is unfortunate that many of the most commonly used metals derive little or no protection from the corrosion products that form under normal circumstances. The familiar rusting of iron is an example of the effects that may be produced by such a process.

A primary requisite of any metal used in the mouth is that it must not produce corrosion products that will be harmful to the body. Some metals that are completely safe in the elemental state can form hazardous or even toxic ions or compounds. If the corrosion process is not too severe, these products may not be recognized easily.

Several aspects of the oral environment are highly conducive to corrosion. The mouth is warm and moist, and is continually subjected to fluctuations in temperature. Ingested foods and liquids have a wide range of pH. Acids are liberated during breakdown of foods, and the resulting debris often adheres tenaciously to the metallic restoration, providing a localized condition that promotes accelerated reaction between the corrosion products and the metal or alloy. Because it has the least tendency to become ionized, gold resists chemical attack very well. Thus it was natural that this most noble metal was employed early in modern dental history for the construction of dental appliances.

CAUSES OF TARNISH AND CORROSION

Tarnish is observable as a surface discoloration on a metal, or as a slight loss or alteration of the surface finish or luster. In the oral environment, tarnish often occurs from the formation of hard and soft deposits on the surface of the restoration. Calculus is the principal hard deposit, and its color varies from light yellow to brown. The soft deposits are plaques and films composed mainly of microorganisms and mucin. Stain or discoloration arises from pigment-producing bacteria, drugs containing such chemicals as iron or mercury, and adsorbed food debris. Although such deposits are the main cause of tarnish in the oral environment, surface discoloration may also arise on a metal from the formation of thin films, such as oxides, sulfides, or chlorides. This latter phenomenon may be only a simple surface deposit, and such a film may even be protective, as will be discussed subsequently. However, it can be an early indication of corrosion.

Corrosion is not merely a surface deposit. It is a process in which deterioration of a metal is caused by reaction with its environment. Frequently, the rate of corrosion attack may actually increase over time, especially with surfaces subjected to stress, with intergranular impurities in the metal, or with corrosion products that do not completely cover the metal surface. In due course, corrosion causes severe and catastrophic disintegration of the metal body. In addition, corrosion attack that is extremely localized may cause rapid mechanical failure of a structure, even though the actual volume loss of material is quite small.

This disintegration of a metal by the action of corrosion may occur through the action of moisture, atmosphere, acid or alkaline solutions, and certain chemicals. As noted previously, tarnish is often the forerunner of corrosion. The film that produces tarnish may in time accumulate elements or compounds that chemically attack the metallic surface. For example, eggs and certain other foods contain significant amounts of sulfur. Various sulfides, such as hydrogen or ammonium sulfide, corrode silver, copper, mercury, and similar metals present in dental alloys and amalgam. Also, water, oxygen, and chlorine ions are present in saliva and contribute to corrosion attack. Various acidic solutions such as phosphoric, acetic, and lactic acids are present at times and, at the proper concentration and pH, these can promote corrosion.

As will be seen in the later chapters, specific ions may play a major role in the corrosion of certain alloys. For example, oxygen and chlorine are implicated in the corrosion of amalgam at the tooth interface and within the body of the alloy. Sulfur is probably the most significant factor causing surface tarnish on casting alloys that contain silver, although chloride has also been identified as a contributor.

CLASSIFICATION OF CORROSION

Corrosion phenomena are often complex and incompletely understood. The more complex the environment and the more inhomogeneous the metal, the more complicated is the corrosion process. The microstructural phases and surface condition of the metal, as well as the chemical composition of the surrounding medium, determine the corrosion reactions. Other important variables affecting corrosion processes are the temperature, movement or circulation of the medium in contact with the metal surface, and the nature and solubility of the corrosion products. Despite these complexities, if the general corrosion mechanism is understood in a given situation, it is usually possible to recognize the controlling variables.

There are two general types of corrosion reactions. In *chemical corrosion* there is a direct combination of metallic and nonmetallic elements to yield a chemical compound through processes such as oxidation, halogenation, or sulfurization reactions. A good example is the discoloration of silver by sulfur, where silver sulfide forms by chemical corrosion. It can also be a corrosion product of dental gold alloys that contain silver. This mode of corrosion is also referred to as *dry corrosion*, since it occurs in the absence of water or another fluid *electrolyte* (i.e., an ionized solution that conducts electricity). Another example is the oxidation of silver-copper alloy particles that are mixed with mercury to prepare certain dental amalgam products. These alloy particles contain a silver-copper eutectic phase, and oxidation limits their reactivity with mercury, thereby affecting the setting reaction of the dental amalgam product. This is why it is prudent to store the alloy in a cool, dry location to ensure an adequate shelf life.

Chemical corrosion is seldom isolated and is almost invariably accompanied by *electrochemical* corrosion, which is also referred to as *wet corrosion*, since it requires the presence of water or some other fluid electrolyte. It also requires a pathway for the transport of electrons (i.e., an electrical current) if the process is to continue. This general mode of corrosion is much more important for dental restorations and will be the focus of the remainder of the chapter.

CRITICAL QUESTION

Which modes of electrochemical corrosion are possible for metallic dental restorations and prostheses?

ELECTROCHEMICAL CORROSION

The starting point for discussion of electrochemical corrosion is the electrochemical cell illustrated in Figure 3-9. Such a cell is composed of three essential components: an *anode*, a *cathode*, and an *electrolyte*. An apparatus is employed to measure the voltage and current between the two electrodes. In this example, the anode can be a dental amalgam restoration, a gold alloy restoration can represent the cathode, and saliva may serve as the electrolyte.

The anode is the surface or sites on a surface where positive ions are formed (i.e., the metal surface that is undergoing an *oxidation reaction* and corroding) with the production of free electrons. The reaction may be described as:

$$M^o \rightarrow M^+ + e^- \qquad (2)$$

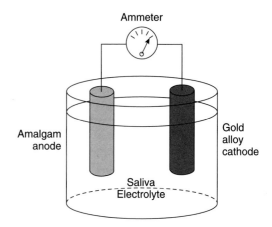

Fig. 3-9 Diagram of an electrochemical cell consisting of a simulated amalgam anode, a gold alloy cathode, and saliva as the electrolyte.

At the cathode or cathodic sites, a *reduction reaction* must occur that will consume the free electrons produced at the anode. Numerous possibilities exist that are dependent on the environment. For example, metal ions may be removed from the solution to form metal atoms, hydrogen ions may be converted to hydrogen gas, or hydroxyl ions may be formed:

$$M^+ + e^- \rightarrow M^o \tag{3}$$

$$2H^+ + 2e^- \rightarrow H_2\uparrow \tag{4}$$

$$2H_2O + O_2 + 4e^- \rightarrow 4(OH)^- \tag{5}$$

The electrolyte supplies the ions needed at the cathode and carries away the corrosion products at the anode. The external circuit serves as a conduction path to carry electrons (the electric current) from the anode to the cathode. If a voltmeter is placed into this circuit, an electrical potential difference, i.e., a voltage (V), can be measured. This voltage has considerable theoretical importance, as will be discussed next. It should also be pointed out that this simple electrochemical cell is, in principle, a battery since the flow of electrons in the external circuit is capable of lighting a light bulb in a flashlight or producing a physiological sensation such as pain.

In order for electrochemical corrosion to be an ongoing process, the production of electrons by the oxidation reactions at the anode must be exactly balanced by the consumption of electrons in the reduction reactions at the cathode. Often the cathodic reactions can be considered to be the primary driving force for electrochemical corrosion. This is a very important consideration in determining the rate of a corrosion process, and it can be used to advantage in order to reduce or eliminate corrosion.

The basis for any discussion of electrochemical corrosion of dental alloys is the *electromotive series* of the metals, which classifies the metals by their equilibrium values of *electrode potential*, thereby arranging them in the order of their dissolution tendencies in water. The electromotive series of elements that is useful for dental alloys is presented in Table 3-3. The potential value (V) for each element is calculated for a standard state, consisting of one atomic weight (g) of ions in 1000 mL of water at 25° C. Each of these standard half-cell potentials may be considered as the voltage of an electrochemical cell in which one electrode is the hydrogen electrode (equation 4), designated arbitrarily as zero potential, and the other electrode is the element of interest. (The hydrogen electrode is created by directing H_2 gas onto a platinum electrode.) The sign of the electrode potential in Table 3-3 indicates the polarity in such a cell, and metals with more positive potential have a lower tendency to dissolve in aqueous environments.

If two pure metals are immersed in an electrolyte and connected by an electrical conductor to form a galvanic cell, the metal with the lower electrode potential in Table 3-3 becomes the anode and undergoes oxidation, that is, its ions go into solution. As an example, for a galvanic cell composed of copper and zinc electrodes in an aqueous acidic solution, the zinc electrode becomes the anode and undergoes surface dissolution. In general, for galvanic cells having two different pure metal electrodes, the magnitude and direction of the current thus depend primarily on the electrode potentials of the individual metals.

It should be emphasized that the relative position of any element in the electromotive series is dependent not only on its inherent solution tendencies, but also on

Table 3-3	Electromotive Series of the Metals	
Metal	**Ion**	**Electrode potential (V)**
Gold	Au^+	+1.50
Gold	Au^{3+}	+1.36
Platinum	Pt^{2+}	+0.86
Palladium	Pd^{2+}	+0.82
Mercury	Hg^{2+}	+0.80
Silver	Ag^+	+0.80
Copper	Cu^+	+0.47
Bismuth	Bi^{3+}	+0.23
Antimony	Sb^{3+}	+0.10
Hydrogen	H^+	−0.00
Lead	Pb^{2+}	−0.12
Tin	Sn^{2+}	−0.14
Nickel	Ni^{2+}	−0.23
Cadmium	Cd^{2+}	−0.40
Iron	Fe^{2+}	−0.44
Chromium	Cr^{2+}	−0.56
Zinc	Zn^{2+}	−0.76
Aluminum	Al^{3+}	−1.70
Sodium	Na^+	−2.71
Calcium	Ca^{2+}	−2.87
Potassium	K^+	−2.92

the effective concentration of ions of that element that is present in the environment. As the ionic concentration of an element increases in the environment, the tendency for that element to dissolve decreases. It also should be emphasized that the electromotive series provides information only about whether a given corrosion reaction cannot occur. In an actual situation, it will predict neither the occurrence nor the rate of corrosion.

The increase in metal ion content in the environment may eventually prevent further corrosion. Sometimes a metal ceases corroding because its ions have saturated the immediate environment. This situation does not usually occur in dental restorations because dissolving ions are removed by food, fluids, and the toothbrush. Thus corrosion of the restorations will continue.

Many types of electrochemical corrosion are possible in the oral environment because saliva, with the salts it contains, is a weak electrolyte. The electrochemical properties of saliva depend on the concentrations of its components, pH, surface tension, and buffering capacity. Each of these factors may influence the strength of any electrolyte. Thus, the magnitude of the resulting corrosion process will be controlled by these variables.

In an environment in which a metal is corroding, both anodic and cathodic reactions take place simultaneously on the surface of the metal. Metal ions go into solution or form corrosion products because of the anodic reactions, and other ions are reduced in the cathodic reactions. These two reactions may occur at randomly distributed sites on the metal surface or, more frequently, there are anodic areas at which mostly the metal dissolves and cathodic areas at which mostly other ions are discharged. Several forms of electrochemical corrosion are based on the mechanisms that produce these inhomogeneous areas.

Dissimilar Metals

An important type of electrochemical corrosion occurs when combinations of *dissimilar metals* are in direct physical contact. Here the dental reference is to two adjacent restorations where the metal surfaces have different compositions. The alloy combinations that may produce **galvanic corrosion** or **electrogalvanism** through the flow of galvanic currents may or may not be in intermittent contact.

The effect of **galvanic shock** is well known in dentistry. For example, assume that a dental amalgam restoration is placed on the occlusal surface of a lower tooth directly opposing a gold inlay in an upper tooth. Because both restorations are wet with saliva, an electrical circuit exists, with a difference in potential between the dissimilar restorations (Fig. 3-10). When the two restorations are brought into contact, there is a sudden short-circuit through the two alloys, which may result in the patient experiencing a sharp pain. A similar effect may be observed by touching the tine of a silver fork to a gold foil or inlay restoration, and at the same time allowing some other portion of the fork to come in contact with the tongue. An undetected piece of aluminum foil in a baked potato can produce the same effect.

When the teeth are not in contact, there is still an electrical circuit associated with the difference in potential or electromotive force between the two restorations. The saliva forms the electrolyte, and the hard and soft tissues can constitute the external circuit, although the electrical resistance of the external circuit is considerable in comparison with that which exists when the two restorations are brought into contact. The current generated is inversely related to the electrical resistance of the metal

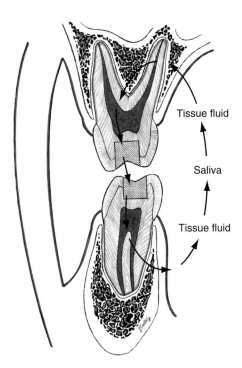

Tissue fluid

Saliva

Tissue fluid

Fig. 3-10 Possible path of a galvanic current in the mouth.

of interest. The electric currents measured under these conditions between a gold crown and an amalgam restoration in the same mouth, but not in contact, appear to be approximately 0.5 to 1 microampere (μA) with a corresponding potential difference of approximately 500 millivolts (mV). These oral galvanic currents are somewhat greater when dissimilar alloys are present, but they also occur between restorations of similar alloys, which never have exactly the same surface composition or structure.

A current is present even in a single isolated metallic restoration, although it is less intense. In this situation the electrochemical cell is generated as a result of the electrical potential differences created by the two electrolytes: saliva and tissue fluids. The term "tissue fluids" is used to denote the dentinal fluid, soft tissue fluid, and blood that provide the means for completing the external circuit. Because the chloride ion concentration is seven times higher than that of saliva, it is assumed that the interior surfaces of a dental restoration exposed to dentinal fluid will have a more active electrochemical potential. Possible current pathways are diagrammed in Figure 3-11.

Although the magnitude of these currents usually diminishes somewhat as the restoration ages, it remains indefinitely at the approximate value cited. The clinical significance of these currents, other than their influence on corrosion, will be discussed later in this chapter. Coating with a varnish tends to eliminate galvanic shock.

Heterogeneous Surface Composition

Another type of galvanic corrosion is associated with the *heterogeneous composition* of the surfaces of dental alloys, whose microstructures have been described in the preceding two chapters. Examples include the eutectic alloys and peritectic alloys (see Chapter 6). Commercial dental alloys generally contain more than three elements, and they can have complex microstructures that result in even more heterogeneous surface compositions.

The reason for the previous statement that the corrosion resistance of multiphase alloys is generally less than that of a single-phase solid solution should now be

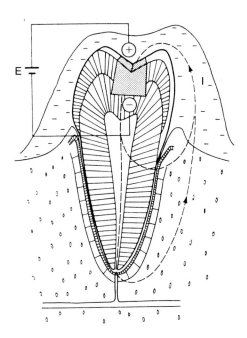

Fig. 3-11 Schematic illustration of a single metallic restoration showing two possible current pathways between an external surface exposed to saliva and an interior surface exposed to dentinal fluid. Because the dentinal fluid contains a higher Cl⁻ concentration than saliva, it is assumed that the electrode potential of the interior surface exposed to dentinal fluid is more active and is therefore given a negative sign (–). The potential difference between the two surfaces is represented by E. (From Metals Handbook, 9th ed, Vol. 13. Metals Park, OH, American Society for Metals, 1978, p 1342.)

evident. For example, when an alloy containing a two-phase eutectic microstructural constituent is immersed in an electrolyte, the lamellae of the phase with the lower electrode potential are attacked, and corrosion results.

In an alloy that is a single-phase solid solution, any cored structure is less resistant to corrosion than is the homogenized solid solution, because of differences in electrode potential caused by microsegregation and variations in composition between individual dendrites for those alloys with a dendritic microstructure (see Chapter 5). Even a homogenized solid solution is susceptible to corrosion at the grain boundaries, which are anodic to the cathodic grain interiors, because atomic arrangements at the grain boundaries are less regular and have higher energies (see Chapter 5). Solder joints between dental alloys also corrode because of differences in compositions of the alloy and solder.

Impurities in alloys enhance corrosion, and these impurities are typically segregated at the grain boundaries, as described in Chapter 5. Mercury impurities that can inadvertently contaminate gold alloys during handling by dental personnel have electrode potentials different from those of the bulk grains of the gold alloys. Finally, it follows from the preceding discussions that nominally pure metals, which do not contain significant quantities of impurities or secondary microstructural phases acting as miniature electrodes with different potentials, corrode at much slower rates than alloys.

Stress Corrosion

Since the imposition of stress increases the internal energy of an alloy, either through the elastic displacements of atoms or the creation of microstrain fields associated with dislocations (when permanent deformation occurs as described in Chapter 20), the tendency to undergo corrosion will be increased. It is plausible that, for most metallic dental appliances, the deleterious effects of stress and corrosion, called **stress corrosion**, are most likely to occur during fatigue or cyclic loading in the oral environment. Small surface irregularities, such as notches or pits, act as sites of stress concentration so that ordinary fatigue failure (in the absence of corrosion) occurs at nominal stresses below the normal elastic limit of the alloy. Stress corrosion has been proposed as a mechanism for the clinical failure of rubber dam clamps, and it may contribute to the clinical fracture of removable partial denture frameworks. Furthermore, any cold working of an alloy by bending, burnishing, or malleting causes localized permanent deformation in some parts of the appliance. Electrochemical cells consisting of the more deformed metal regions (anodic), saliva, and undeformed or less deformed metal regions (cathodic) are created, and the deformed regions will experience corrosion attack. This is one reason why excessive burnishing of the margins of metallic restorations is contraindicated.

CRITICAL QUESTION

How can a small pit in the surface of a metallic restoration become deeper and sustain aggressive, localized chemical attack?

Concentration Cell Corrosion

An important type of electrochemical corrosion is called **concentration cell** corrosion, which occurs whenever there are variations in the electrolytes or in the composition of the given electrolyte within the system. For example, there are often accumulations of food debris in the interproximal areas between the teeth, particularly if oral hygiene is poor. This debris then produces an electrolyte in that area, which is different from the electrolyte that is produced by normal saliva at the occlusal surface. Electrochemical corrosion of the alloy surface underneath the layer of food debris will take place in this situation.

A similar type of attack may occur from differences in the oxygen concentration between parts of the same restoration, with the greatest attack at the areas containing the least oxygen. Irregularities, such as pits, on restorations provide important examples of this phenomenon. The region at the bottom of such a concavity has a much lower oxygen concentration than that at the surface of the restoration, because the pit will typically be covered with food debris and mucin. The alloy at the bottom of the pit becomes the anode, and the alloy surface around the rim of the pit becomes the cathode, as diagrammed in Figure 3-12. Consequently, metal atoms at the base of the pit ionize and go into solution, causing the pit to deepen. The rate of such corrosion may be very rapid, since the area of the anodic region is much smaller than that of the cathodic region and there must be a balance of charge transport in both regions. Consequently, failure may occur much more rapidly than what would be anticipated from uniform surface attack. For this reason, all metallic dental restorative materials should be polished. An important category of concentration cell corrosion is **crevice corrosion**, in which preferential attack occurs at crevices in dental prostheses or at margins between tooth structure and restorations from the same causes that were previously discussed, namely changes in electrolyte and oxygen concentration caused by the presence of food debris and other deposits.

Seldom is any one of the preceding types of electrochemical corrosion found alone. Generally, two or more types act simultaneously, thereby compounding the problem. This phenomenon can be illustrated by considering the dissimilar metal corrosion between a cast gold inlay and an amalgam restoration. Because surface deposits can form during this type of electrochemical corrosion, differences in oxygen concentration will arise. Moreover, if the corrosion product layer is incomplete or porous, as is usually the case with metallic dental restorations, the resulting inhomogeneous surface produces new electrochemical cells for continued corrosion. It is evident that good oral hygiene, which prevents the formation of significant surface deposits, is essential for minimizing these corrosion processes.

In the very early stages of tarnish, concentration cells, and thus localized galvanic processes, may operate. Careful microscopic examination of the progress of tarnish on dental gold alloys reveals that the deposited film is initially discrete or discontinuous. The apparent continuity of the tarnish layer arises from an overlapping of these discrete regions, and this situation exists even when conditions remain constant. It is unfortunate that pH fluctuations in the oral environment, oral hygiene habits, characteristics of the saliva, and cyclic stresses can accelerate the multiple corrosion processes that act upon metallic restorations.

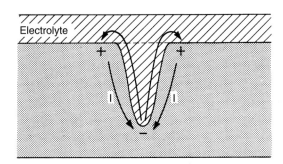

Fig. 3-12 A pit on a dental alloy as a corrosion cell. The region of the pit is an anode, and the surface around the rim of the pit is the cathode. The ionic current flows through the electrolyte and the electronic current flows through the metal. (With permission from Richman, MH: An Introduction to the Science of Metals. Waltham, MA, Blaisdell Publishing Co, 1967.)

PROTECTION AGAINST CORROSION

The strategy of gold coating is employed to enhance the appearance of many commercial nondental products. However, the noble metal is soft and, when its surface becomes scratched or pitted to such a depth that the base metal is exposed to the environment, the base metal will be corroded at a very rapid rate because concentration cells have been created and two dissimilar metals are in direct contact. Attempts to use metallic and nonmetallic coatings to provide corrosion protection for dental gold alloys have generally been ineffectual because such coatings: (1) were too thin, (2) were incomplete, (3) did not adhere to the underlying metal, (4) were readily scratched, or (5) were attacked by oral fluids.

However, in the case of two dissimilar metals in contact, paint or another nonconductive film can be used to advantage if it is applied to the more noble metal. The corrosion rate of the more active metal will be reduced because the surface area available for the reduction reaction has been decreased. A scratch in this type of coating will not lead to rapid attack of the active metal.

Certain metals develop a thin, adherent, highly protective film by reaction with the environment; such a metal is said to be passive. A thin surface oxide forms on chromium, which is a good example of a passivating metal, and stainless steels contain sufficient amounts of chromium added to iron (and other elements) to passivate the alloy, as will be described in Chapter 20. Iron, steel, and certain other metals that are subject to corrosion may also be electroplated with nickel followed by chromium for corrosion protection and esthetic reasons. However, it should be pointed out that tensile stress and certain ions, such as chloride ions, can disrupt the protective oxide film, leading to rapid corrosion. Chromium-passivated metals can be susceptible to stress corrosion and **pitting corrosion**, and patients should be warned against using household bleaches for cleaning partial denture frameworks or removable orthodontic appliances that are alloyed with chromium. Titanium also forms a passivating titanium oxide film, which is of interest since both commercially pure (CP) titanium and alloys in which titanium is a major component element are being used for a variety of dental applications, such as cast restorations, implants, orthodontic wires and endodontic instruments, to be described in Chapters 19, 20, and 23.

Noble metals resist corrosion because their electromotive force is positive with regard to any of the common reduction reactions found in the oral environment. In order to corrode a noble metal under such conditions, an external current (overpotential) is required.

CORROSION OF DENTAL RESTORATIONS

It is apparent that the oral environment and dental structures present complex conditions that can promote tarnish and corrosion. Variations in diet, bacterial activity, drugs, smoking, and oral hygiene habits unquestionably account for most of the differences in corrosion often noted for patients in whom the same dental alloy, handled in the same manner, was employed.

Corrosion resistance is a highly important consideration in the composition of dental alloys, since the release of significant amounts of corrosion products may adversely affect the biocompatibility of an alloy. Unfortunately, there is no laboratory test that duplicates oral conditions in a way that can accurately predict the susceptibility of the material to corrosion. Various accelerated tests using sulfide, chloride, and other solutions have been advocated to evaluate tarnish and corrosion resistance. For example, the noble metal content, particularly gold, influences the resistance to sulfide tarnishing.

A guideline that has been employed by manufacturers for many dental alloys is that at least half the atoms should be noble metals (gold, platinum, and palladium) to ensure against corrosion. Palladium has been found to be effective in reducing the susceptibility to sulfide tarnishing for alloys containing silver. If noble metals are used to avoid corrosion, it is important that the more active constituents of the alloy be uniformly dispersed in a random solid solution, since the formation of a second phase that is enriched in an active metal will produce a galvanic corrosion cell.

Base metals, such as stainless steels, nickel-chromium alloys, cobalt-chromium alloys, and titanium are virtually immune to sulfide tarnishing. However, these alloys are susceptible to localized attack in the presence of chlorides, and it is important that the corrosion testing of these alloys evaluate their resistance to pitting and crevice corrosion. Generally, titanium and its alloys are superior in their resistance to chloride attack, compared with the other dental base metal alloys.

CRITICAL QUESTION

How can potentiodynamic polarization tests provide information about the relative in vitro corrosion behavior of different dental alloys in the same electrolyte?

EVALUATION OF TARNISH AND CORROSION RESISTANCE

High-gold casting alloys tarnish very slowly, and a sodium sulfide immersion test to accelerate this process was developed three decades ago. Many investigations of the in vitro tarnishing behavior of a wide variety of dental alloys have been published since that time. The most reliable method to evaluate tarnish and corrosion resistance is by clinical studies, which may require several years. Articles listed in the references should be consulted for the research methodology.

Potentiodynamic polarization tests have been frequently employed to evaluate the in vitro corrosion behavior of dental alloys. Three electrodes are required: an experimental electrode prepared from the dental alloy, a counter electrode (typically platinum) to complete the electrochemical cell, and a reference electrode (usually a saturated calomel electrode or a saturated Ag|AgCl electrode). Several electrolytes have been used by investigators: saline solution at an appropriate chloride ion concentration, Fusayama solution, Ringers solution, or other chemical media designed to simulate the oral environment or body fluid. A potentiostat (high-precision power supply with a voltmeter and an ammeter) slowly varies the potential between the experimental electrode and the reference electrode from a relatively high negative value to a relatively high positive value (typically from –1000 mV to +1000 mV). For a typical scanning rate (voltage change) in the range of 1 mV/s, the entire range back to the starting negative potential (cyclic polarization) will be completed in less than 1 hr. However, a much longer testing time is required, since the open-circuit potential (OCP) of the alloy relative to the reference electrode in the absence of an external voltage is first allowed to stabilize before scanning is commenced, and time periods for stabilization of up to 24 hr have been used by investigators.

A highly schematic potentiodynamic polarization diagram for the in vitro corrosion testing of a dental alloy that shows active-passive behavior is presented in Figure 3-13. The potential for the alloy relative to the reference electrode is shown on the vertical axis (typically in units of mV or V) using a linear scale, and the horizontal axis shows the current density (typically in units of $\mu A/cm^2$ or mA/cm^2) plotted on a logarithmic scale. The lower and upper portions of the diagram are, respectively, the curves for cathodic and anodic polarization of the alloy, where potentials other than the OCP have been applied. These curves represent the summation of all electrochemical processes, whether they are Faradaic processes involving charge transfer, such as metal ionization and formation of passive films, or non-Faradaic processes that do not involve charge transfer, such as adsorption of species, reorientation of surface molecules, and diffusion effects. The intersection of the tangent lines to these curves at very low current density defines the corrosion potential (E_{corr}) and corrosion current density (i_{corr}). (It is not possible to indicate a zero value of current density on this diagram because of the logarithmic scale for the horizontal axis.) With increasing potential beyond E_{corr} (active region), where the polarization curve has an S-shape, the anodic current in the specimen first increases and then begins to decrease at the primary passive potential (E_{pp}) to a lower value, as a passive film forms on the alloy surface. After formation of the surface film, there is minimal change or a small increase in current density with increasing voltage (upper portion of the passive region in Fig. 3-13), until the breakdown potential (E_b) for the film is reached. Thereafter, in the transpassive region, the current density rapidly increases with further increases in potential.

These diagrams can be used to compare the in vitro corrosion resistance of two dental alloys when the same electrolyte and scanning conditions are used. The more electrochemically active alloy will have a lower potential value for E_{corr}, and the current density will be higher at a given value of potential in the active anodic region. For dental alloys that have naturally occurring passive surface films, such as the stainless steel and titanium alloys, a high breakdown potential is observed. If the initial scanning is performed over a narrow potential range, such as from −20 mV to +20 mV relative to the OCP, the cathodic and anodic polarization curves are approximately linear, and the polarization resistance (R_p) can be determined from the slope of these curves as a measure of the corrosion resistance of

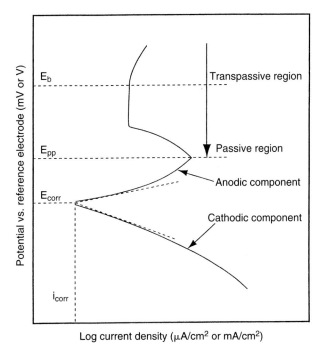

Fig. 3-13 Schematic potentiodynamic polarization diagram for the in vitro corrosion testing of a dental alloy that exhibits active-passive behavior.

the alloy. Figure 3-14 shows the cyclic polarization diagram for a high-palladium alloy in Fusayama solution, where the very low values of current density are indicative of excellent in vitro corrosion resistance. The reverse scan in this diagram, beginning with +1000 mV and ending at −1000 mV relative to the reference electrode, does not retrace the forward scan from −1000 mV to +1000 mV, because the forward scan caused alterations in the specimen surface.

Recently, electrochemical impedance spectroscopy has been employed to gain insight into the corrosion mechanisms for dental casting alloys. A small sinusoidal potential variation, such as ± 10 mV, is imposed on the test specimen in the region of the OCP or a selected active potential of interest, over a wide frequency range from 0.01 Hz to 10 kHz, and the current is collected and analyzed for phase relationships with the voltage. Using equivalent electrical circuit modeling for the electrochemical system, specific information can be obtained about the Faradaic and non-Faradaic corrosion mechanisms that is not possible to obtain from potentiodynamic polarization methods. The reader should consult corrosion textbooks for additional information about this technique.

A recently developed experimental apparatus for observing the corrosion behavior of dental alloys is the scanning electrochemical microscope (SECM), in which the current and position are recorded as a microelectrode is scanned over a metallurgically polished alloy surface. The SECM can image microelectrochemical processes on alloy surfaces where charge transfer reactions are occurring. Figure 3-15 represents an SECM image that illustrates the formation of a pit in a low-copper dental amalgam. (See also color plates.)

In closing this section, it is important to note that the International Organization for Standardization (ISO) has approved Standard 10271, which requires alloy specimens to be immersed in an aqueous corrosion testing solution of lactic acid and NaCl and the concentrations of the released elements to be measured. Future studies are needed to compare the results from this immersion test with those from potentiodynamic polarization evaluations of corrosion properties.

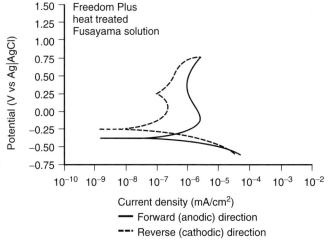

Fig. 3-14 Cyclic potentiodynamic polarization diagram for a Pd-Cu-Ga alloy in Fusayama solution. The alloy has been subjected to heat treatment simulating the porcelain firing cycles. (From Sun D, Monaghan P, Brantley WA, and Johnston WM: Potentiodynamic polarization study of the in vitro corrosion behavior of 3 high-palladium alloys and a gold-palladium alloy in 5 media. J Prosthet Dent 87:86-93, 2002.)

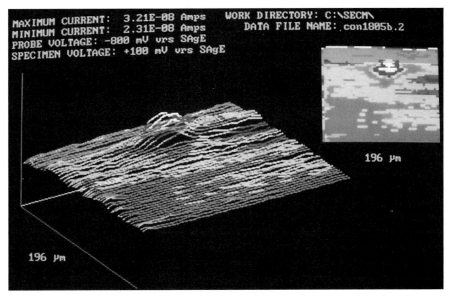

MAXIMUM CURRENT: 3.21E-08 Amps   WORK DIRECTORY: C:\SECM\
MINIMUM CURRENT: 2.31E-08 Amps   DATA FILE NAME: con1805b.2
PROBE VOLTAGE: -800 mV vrs SAgE
SPECIMEN VOLTAGE: +100 mV vrs SAgE

196 µm

196 µm

Fig. 3-15 Scanning electrochemical microscope image of a pit in a low-copper dental amalgam. (Courtesy of P. Monaghan. From Ph.D. Thesis, Northwestern University, Chicago, 1996.)

CRITICAL QUESTION

Why are in vitro methods of measuring electrochemical corrosion behavior unable to predict in vivo evaluation of corrosion resistance for dental alloys?

CLINICAL SIGNIFICANCE OF GALVANIC CURRENTS

It has been proven that small galvanic currents associated with electrogalvanism are continually present in the oral cavity. Their influence on corrosion was discussed earlier. As long as metallic dental restorative materials are employed, there seems to be little possibility that these galvanic currents can be eliminated. The cement base, although a good thermal insulator, has little effect in minimizing the current that is carried into the tooth and through the pulp. Although many of these base materials are effective electrical insulators when they are dry, they lose this property when they become wet through marginal microleakage or from moisture in the dentin. Until materials or techniques are developed that will provide perfect adaptation to the cavity walls, the possibility of blocking such currents is highly improbable. For all practical purposes, the metallic restoration cannot be isolated electrically from the tooth.

Although postoperative pain caused by galvanic shock is not a common occurrence in the dental office, it can be a source of discomfort to an occasional patient. However, such postoperative pain usually occurs immediately after insertion of a new restoration, and generally it gradually subsides and disappears in a few days. It is likely that the physiological condition of the tooth is the primary factor responsible for the pain resulting from this current flow. Once the tooth has responded from the injury of preparing the cavity and has returned to a more normal physiological condition, the current flow then produces no response. Practically, the best method for reducing or eliminating galvanic shock seems to be to paint a coating varnish on the surface of the metallic restoration. As long as the varnish remains, the restoration is insulated from saliva and no electrochemical cell is established. By the time the varnish has worn away, the pulp has usually healed sufficiently so that no pain persists.

Although it has been suggested that these oral galvanic currents, or the metallic ions that are liberated from restorations because of the galvanic currents, could account for many types of dyscrasias, such as lichenoid lesions, ulcers, leukoplakia, cancer, and kidney disorder, research has failed to find any correlation between dissimilar metals and tissue irritation. While it is the opinion of the majority of research workers in pathology and dental materials that these galvanic currents are probably deleterious only from the standpoint of patient discomfort on rare occasions, dentists should avoid clinical procedures that exacerbate the condition, such as insertion of an amalgam restoration directly in contact with a gold crown. Mercury released from the corroding amalgam (the anode) may interact with the gold alloy (the cathode) and weaken it. A discoloration of both restorations may also occur, and whether it is harmful or not, a metallic taste is present subsequent to the dental operation and may persist indefinitely. For further reading on this topic, consult the articles by Marek and Mueller listed under Additional Readings on Corrosion.

SELECTED READINGS

American Dental Association: Esthetic dentistry: A new direction. J Am Dent Assoc, Dec (Special issue), 1987.

A series of papers covering the many facets of selecting materials and clinical procedures used in aesthetic dentistry. Depicted are the improved services available through bonding technology, with particular emphasis on the organization of color in the design and fabrication of restorative materials.

Antonson SA, and Anusavice KJ: Contrast ratio of veneering and core ceramics as a function of thickness. Int J Prosthodont 14:316-320, 2001.

Barna GJ, Taylor JW, King GE, and Pelleu GB Jr: The influence of selected light intensities on color perception within the color range of natural teeth. J Prosthet Dent 46:450, 1981.

Based on a study of the influence of light intensity on the ability to discriminate color differences within the color range of natural teeth. A significant number of the dentists in the study were found to be color-deficient. In such instances, the dentist should obtain assistance when matching tooth shades.

Goldstein RE: Change Your Smile, 2nd ed. Chicago, Quintessence, 1988.

Although this book is written for the patient, it is a useful reference for dentists to illustrate aesthetic and reconstructive changes that are possible. The color illustrations before and after restorative treatment are evidence of the satisfactory end result when based on an appreciation of parameters involved in color phenomena.

Jacobs SH, Goodacre CJ, Moore BK, and Dykema RW: Effect of porcelain thickness and type of metal-ceramic alloy on color. J Prosthet Dent 57:138-145, 1987.

Johnston WM, and Kao EC: Assessment of appearance by visual observation and clinical colorimetry. J Dent Res 68:819-22, 1989.

Judd DB and Wyszecki G: Color in Business, Science, and Industry. New York, John Wiley & Sons, 1975.

This book, developed for a variety of businesses, reviews the principles of color vision, color matching, color deficiencies, colorimetry, and the physics of colorant layers.

McLean JW: The Science and Art of Dental Ceramics. Vol. 1: The Nature of Dental Ceramics and Their Clinical Use. Amador City, CA, Quintessence, 1979.

Essential reading for those interested in an in-depth discussion of principles of color as related to dental ceramics. Basic fundamentals are clearly interwoven with clinical procedures.

Miller LL: A Scientific approach to shade matching. In: Proceedings of the Fourth International Symposium on Ceramics. Chicago, Quintessence, 1988, p 193.

It is unfortunate that commercial shade guides do not cover all the areas of value, hue, and chroma present in tooth structure. A definitive analysis of the problem is presented.

Miller LL: Shade matching. J Esthet Dent 5:143-153, 1993.

Mörmann WH, Link C, and Lutz F: Color changes in veneer ceramics caused by bonding composite resins. Acta Med Dent Helv 1:97-102, 1996.

O'Brien WJ: Biomaterials Properties Database, University of Michigan: http://www.lib.umich.edu/dentlib/Dental tables/. University of Michigan, Ann Arbor, Michigan.

This superb database provides an electronic reference to the following properties of dental materials: strength between restorative materials and tooth structures, Brinell hardness number, coefficient of friction, coefficient of thermal expansion (linear), color range of natural teeth, colors of dental shade guides, contact angle, creep of amalgam, critical surface tension, density, dynamic modulus, elastic modulus, flow, heat of fusion, heat of reaction, Izod impact strength, index of refraction, Knoop hardness number, melting temperatures and ranges, Mohs' hardness, penetration coefficient, percent elongation, permanent deformation, Poisson's ratio, proportional limit, shear strength, Shore A hardness, solubility and disintegration in water, specific heat, strain in compression, surface free energy, surface tension, tear energy, tear strength, thermal conductivity, thermal diffusivity, transverse strength, ultimate compressive strength, ultimate tensile strength, vapor pressure, Vickers hardness, water sorption, yield strength, and zeta potential.

O'Brien WJ, Nelson D, and Lorey RE: The assessment of chroma sensitivity to porcelain pigments. J Prosthet Dent 49:63-66, 1983.

Ruyter JE, Nilner K, and Moller B: Color stability of dental composite resin materials for crown and bridge veneers. Dent Mater 3:246-251, 1987.

ADDITIONAL READINGS ON CORROSION

Berzins DW, Kawashima I, Graves R, and Sarkar NK: Electrochemical characteristics of high-Pd alloys in relation to Pd-allergy. Dent Mater 16:266-273, 2000.

In vitro electrochemical evaluations of a variety of palladium-containing alloys provide insight into the mechanism of palladium allergy for some patients.

Burse AB, Swartz ML, Phillips RW, and Dykema RW: Comparison of the in vitro and in vivo tarnish of three gold alloys. J Biomed Mater Res 6:267-277, 1972.

This classic article describes an experimental protocol for in vivo tarnish evaluation and shows the importance of the proper elemental ratio in gold alloy compositions.

Fontana MG: Corrosion Engineering, 3rd ed. New York, McGraw-Hill, 1986.

The primary corrosion textbook used by engineers. Basic and advanced theory is presented in readable format, and specific metal-environment interactions are included.

Gilbert JL, Smith SM, and Lautenschlager EP: Scanning electrochemical microscopy of metallic biomaterials: Reaction rate and ion release imaging modes. J Biomed Mater Res 27:1357-1366, 1993.

The underlying principles for the scanning electrochemical microscope are presented, and several materials and specimen geometries are examined.

Marek M: The corrosion of dental materials. In: Scully JC (ed): Treatise on Materials Science and Technology. New York, Academic Press, 1983, pp 331-394.

A detailed treatment of corrosion phenomena associated with dental amalgam.

Meyer J-M, and Reclaru L: Electrochemical determination of the corrosion resistance of noble casting alloys. J Mater Sci: Mater Med 6:534-540, 1995.

The in vitro corrosion resistance is compared for a large number of noble casting alloys.

Mills RB: Study of incidence of irritation in mouths having teeth filled with dissimilar metals. Northwest Univ Bull 39:18, 1939.

Analysis of a large group of patients did not show a relationship between the presence of dissimilar metals and tissue irritation, casting doubt on the validity of this hypothesis.

Mueller HJ: Tarnish and corrosion of dental alloys. In: Metals Handbook, 9th ed, Vol. 13. Metals Park, Ohio, American Society for Metals, 1987, pp 1336-1366.

An excellent overview of corrosion behavior of many dental alloy systems based on data from both in vitro and in vivo studies.

Phillips RW, Schnell RJ, and Shafer WG: Failure of galvanic current to produce leukoplakia in rats. J Dent Res 47:666, 1968.

A high galvanic current generated in the mouths of rats did not induce tissue changes, again suggesting that oral dyscrasia is more likely associated with other causes.

Reed GJ, and Willmann W: Galvanism in the oral cavity. J Am Dent Assoc 27:1471, 1940.

One of the first studies demonstrating the presence of galvanic currents in the oral cavity, and approximate values for the magnitude were established.

Sarkar NK: The Electrochemical Behavior of Dental Amalgams and Their Component Phases. Ph.D. Thesis, Northwestern University, Chicago, 1973. (Available through University Microfilms International.)

An excellent description of laboratory testing of the corrosion behavior of dental amalgam. Its technical nature requires a fundamental understanding of corrosion theory.

Sarkar NK, Fuys RA Jr, and Stanford JW: The chloride corrosion of low-gold casting alloys. J Dent Res 58:568-575, 1979.

A classic article that first presented the application of cyclic polarization experiments to the corrosion of low-gold dental casting alloys.

Sturdevant JR, Sturdevant CM, Taylor DF, and Bayne SC. The 8-year clinical performance of 15 low-gold casting alloys. Dent Mater 3:347-352, 1987.

An important article that reports the tarnish and corrosion behavior of numerous gold casting alloys of known compositions over a prolonged period of time.

Sun D, Monaghan P, Brantley WA, and Johnston WM. Electrochemical impedance spectroscopy study of high-palladium dental alloys. Part I: Behavior at open-circuit potential. Part II: Behavior at active and passive potentials. J Mater Sci: Mater Med 13:435-442 and 443-448, 2002.

The experimental procedure and interpretation of results at potentials of clinical interest are described for the technique of electrochemical impedance spectroscopy.

Tait WS: An Introduction to Electrochemical Corrosion Testing for Practicing Engineers and Scientists. Racine, WI, 1994, Pair O Docs Publications.

A readable and concise account of electrochemical corrosion testing procedures and the underlying theory.

Tufekci E, Mitchell JC, Olesik JW, Brantley WA, Papazoglou E, and Monaghan P: Inductively coupled plasma-mass spectroscopy measurements of elemental release from 2 high-palladium dental casting alloys into a corrosion testing medium. J Prosthet Dent 87:80-85, 2002.

A highly sensitive analytical technique shows that the release of individual elements over a one-month period appears to be correlated with microstructural phases in the alloys.

Tuccillo JJ, and Nielsen JP: Observations of onset of sulfide tarnish on gold-base alloys. J Prosthet Dent 25:629-637, 1971.

This classic article presents the sodium sulfate immersion test for evaluation of tarnish resistance, which has been used in many subsequently published studies.

Seghi RR, Johnston WM, and O'Brien WJ: Spectrophotometric analysis of color differences between porcelain systems. J Prosthet Dent 56:35-40, 1986.

4

Mechanical Properties of Dental Materials

Kenneth J. Anusavice

OUTLINE

What Are Mechanical Properties?

Stresses and Strains

Mechanical Properties Based on Elastic Deformation

Strength Properties

Mechanical Properties of Tooth Structure

Mastication Forces and Stresses

Other Mechanical Properties

Stress Concentration Factors

Criteria for Selection of Restorative Materials

KEY TERMS

Brittleness—Relative inability of a material to deform plastically.

Compressive stress—Ratio of compressive force to cross-sectional area perpendicular to the axis of applied force.

Compressive strength—Compressive stress within a compression test specimen at the point of fracture.

Ductility—Relative ability of a material to deform plastically under a tensile stress before it fractures.

Elastic strain—Deformation that is recovered upon removal of an externally applied force or pressure.

Elastic modulus (Modulus of elasticity or Young's modulus)—Relative stiffness of a material; ratio of elastic stress to elastic strain.

Flexural strength (Bending strength or Modulus of rupture)—Force per unit area at the point of fracture of a test specimen subjected to flexural loading.

Flexural stress (Bending stress)—Force per unit area of a material subjected to flexural loading.

Fracture toughness—The critical stress intensity factor at the beginning of rapid crack propagation in a solid containing a crack of known shape and size.

Hardness—Resistance of a material to plastic deformation typically measured under an indentation load.

Percent elongation—Maximum amount of plastic strain a tensile test specimen can sustain before it fractures (See **Ductility**).

Plastic strain—Deformation that is not recoverable when the externally applied force is removed.

Pressure—Force per unit area acting on the external surface of a material.

Proportional limit—Maximum stress at which stress is proportional to strain and above which plastic deformation occurs.

KEY TERMS—cont'd

Resilience—The relative amount of elastic energy per unit volume released on unloading of a test specimen.

Shear stress—Ratio of force to the original cross-sectional area parallel to the direction of the force applied to a test specimen.

Shear strength—Maximum shear stress at the point of fracture of a test specimen.

True stress—Ratio of applied force to the actual cross-sectional area; however, for convenience stress is often calculated as the ratio of applied force to the initial cross-sectional area.

Stress—Force per unit area within a structure subjected to an external force or pressure (See **Pressure**).

Stress concentration—Area or point of significantly higher stress associated with a structural discontinuity such as a crack or pore or a marked change in dimension of a structure.

Strain—Change in length per unit initial length.

Stress intensity factor—A measure of the relative amount of increased stress at the tip of a crack of a given shape and size when the crack surfaces are displaced in the opening mode (See also **Fracture toughness**).

Strain hardening (Work hardening)—Increase in strength and hardness and corresponding decrease in ductility of a metal that is caused by plastic deformation.

Strain rate—Change in strain per unit time during loading of a structure.

Strength—Maximum stress that a structure can withstand without sustaining a specific amount of plastic strain (yield strength) or stress at the point of fracture (ultimate strength).

Tensile stress—Ratio of tensile force to the original cross-sectional area perpendicular to direction of applied force.

Tensile strength (Ultimate tensile strength)—Tensile stress (in a tensile test specimen) at the point of fracture.

Toughness—Ability of a material to absorb elastic energy and to deform plastically before fracturing; measured as the total area under a plot of tensile stress vs. tensile strain.

Yield strength—The stress at which a test specimen exhibits a specific amount of plastic strain.

WHAT ARE MECHANICAL PROPERTIES?

This chapter focuses on the mechanical properties of materials. Mechanical properties are defined by the laws of mechanics, that is, the physical science that deals with energy and forces and their effects on bodies. The discussion centers primarily on static bodies—those at rest—rather than on dynamic bodies that are in motion. Thus all mechanical properties are measures of the resistance of a material to deformation or fracture under an applied force.

An important factor in the design of a dental prosthesis is **strength**, a mechanical property of a material that ensures that the prosthesis serves its intended functions effectively, safely, and for a reasonable time period. In a general sense, strength is the ability of the prosthesis to resist induced **stress** without fracture or permanent deformation (plastic strain). Plastic deformation occurs when the elastic stress limit (proportional limit) within the prosthesis is exceeded.

By the end of the section on **stress concentration** factors, you should have developed a conceptual foundation of the causes of fracture of restorative materials and an understanding of design features that will increase or decrease fracture resistance in the oral environment. This knowledge will allow you to differentiate the potential causes of clinical failures that may be attributed to material deficiencies, dentist errors, technician errors, or patient factors.

The failure potential of a prosthesis under applied forces is related to the mechanical properties of the prosthetic material. Mechanical properties are the measured responses, both elastic (reversible on force removal) and plastic (irreversible or nonelastic), of materials under an applied force, distribution of forces, or pressure. Mechanical properties are expressed most often in units of **stress** and/or **strain**. They can represent measurements of: (1) elastic or reversible deformation (i.e., **proportional limit**, **resilience**, and **modulus of elasticity**); (2) plastic or irreversible deformation (e.g., **percent elongation** and **hardness**); or (3) a combination of elastic and plastic deformation, such as **toughness** and **yield strength**. To discuss these properties, one must first understand the concepts of stress and strain.

CRITICAL QUESTION

What are the main factors that affect the strength of a material?

STRESSES AND STRAINS

Stress is the force per unit area acting on millions of atoms or molecules in a given plane of a material. Except for certain flexural situations, such as four-point bending specimens, and certain nonuniform object shapes, stress typically decreases as a function of distance from the area of the applied force or applied **pressure**. For dental applications, there are several types of stress that develop according to the nature of the applied forces and the object shape. These include **tensile stress**, **shear stress**, and **compressive stress**. The strength of a material is defined as the average level of stress at which a material exhibits a certain amount of initial plastic deformation or at which fracture occurs in test specimens of the same shape and size. The strength is dependent on several factors including the (1) **strain rate**, (2) the shape of the test specimen, (3) the surface finish (that controls the relative size and number of surface flaws), and (4) the environment in which a material is tested. However, the clinical strength of brittle materials (such as ceramics, amalgams, composites, and cements) may appear to be low when large flaws are present or if stress concentration areas exist because of improper design of a prosthetic component (such as a notch along a section of a clasp arm on a partial denture). Under these conditions a clinical prosthesis may fracture at a much lower applied force because the localized stress exceeds the strength of the material at the critical location of the flaw (stress concentration).

When a patient chews with a gold crown in place, the atomic structure of the crown is slightly deformed elastically by the forces of mastication. If only elastic deformation occurs, the surface of the crown will recover completely when the forces are removed. Elastic stresses in materials do not cause permanent (irreversible) deformation. On the other hand, stresses above the proportional limit cause permanent deformation and, if high enough, they may cause fracture of a material. For brittle materials that exhibit only elastic deformation and can sustain no plastic deformation, stresses at or slightly above the maximum elastic stress (proportional limit) result in fracture. These mechanical properties of dental materials are important for the dentist to understand when designing a restoration or making adjustments to a prosthesis. The differences between mechanical properties are easier to visualize through the use of a stress-strain diagram, as described later.

When an external force acts on a solid, a reaction occurs to oppose this force that is equal in magnitude but opposite in direction to the external force. The stress produced within a material is equal to the applied force divided by the area over which it acts. A tensile force produces **tensile stress**; a compressive force produces **compressive stress**; and a shear or bending force produces **shear stress**. A bending force can produce all three types of stress in a structure, but in most cases fracture occurs because of the tensile stress component. In this situation, the tensile and compressive stresses are principal axial stresses, whereas the shear stress represents a combination of tensile and compressive components.

Whenever a stress is present, deformation or strain is induced. As an illustration, assume that a stretching or tensile force of 200 N is applied to a wire 0.000002 m^2 in cross-sectional area. The *tensile stress* (σ), by definition, is the tensile force per unit area perpendicular to the force direction,

$$\sigma = \frac{200 \text{ N}}{0.000002 \text{ m}^2} = 100 \times 10^6 \frac{\text{N}}{\text{m}^2} = 100 \frac{\text{MN}}{\text{m}^2} = 100 \text{ MPa} \tag{1}$$

Because the wire has fractured at this stress level, the **tensile strength** of this wire is 100 MPa. In the English system of measurement, the stress is expressed in pounds per square inch. However, the megapascal unit is preferred because it is consistent with the SI system of units. (SI stands for Systéme Internationale d' Unités [International System of Units] for length, time, electric current, thermodynamic temperature, luminous intensity, mass, and amount of substance.)

To illustrate the magnitude of 1 MPa, consider a McDonald's quarter-pound hamburger suspended from a 1.12-mm-diameter monofilament fishing line. The stress per unit area within the line is approximately 1 MPa. If the wire above is 0.1 m long, and if it stretches 0.001 m under the load, the strain (ε), by definition, is the change in length, Δl, per unit original length, l_o, or,

$$\varepsilon = \frac{\Delta l}{l_o} = \frac{0.001 \text{ m}}{0.1 \text{ m}} = \frac{0.0001 \text{ m}}{\text{m}} = 0.01\% \tag{2}$$

We can conclude that the wire fractures at a tensile stress of 100 MPa and at a *tensile strain* of 0.01%. Note that although strain is a dimensionless quantity, units such as meter per meter or centimeter per centimeter are often used to remind one of the system of units employed in the actual measurement. The accepted equivalent in the English system is inch per inch, foot per foot, and so forth.

CRITICAL QUESTION

Why is the maximum elastic strain of a cast alloy used for an inlay or crown an important factor when burnishing a margin? Use a sketch of a gap (e.g., Fig. 4-4) between a crown and the tooth margin or a stress-strain diagram (e.g., Fig. 4-3) to explain your answer.

Strain, or the change in length per unit length, is the relative deformation of an object subjected to a stress. Strain may be either elastic or plastic or elastic and plastic. **Elastic strain** is reversible. The object fully recovers its original shape when the force is removed. **Plastic strain** represents a permanent deformation of the material that does not decrease when the force is removed. When a prosthetic component such as a clasp arm on a partial denture is deformed past the elastic limit into the plastic deformation region, only the elastic strain is recovered when the force is released. Thus, when an adjustment is made by bending an orthodontic wire, a margin of a metal crown, or a denture clasp, the plastic strain is permanent, but the wire, margin, or clasp springs back a certain amount as elastic strain recovery occurs.

As previously described, a stress is described by its magnitude and the type of deformation it produces. Three types of "simple" stresses can be classified: *tensile*, *compressive*, and *shear*. Complex stresses, such as those produced by applied forces that cause flexural or torsional deformation, are discussed in the section on **flexural stress.**

Tensile Stress

A *tensile stress* is caused by a load that tends to stretch or elongate a body. A tensile stress is always accompanied by *tensile strain*. There are few pure tensile stress situations in dentistry. However, a tensile stress can be generated when structures are flexed. The deformation of a bridge and the diametral compression of a cylinder that are described later represent examples of these complex stress situations. In fixed prosthodontics clinics, a sticky candy can be used to remove crowns by means of a tensile force when patients try to open their mouths. However, tensile, compressive, and shear stresses can also be produced by a bending force as shown in Figure 4-1 as discussed in the following sections. Because most dental materials are quite brittle, they are highly susceptible to crack initiation in the presence of surface flaws when subjected to tensile stress, such as when they are subjected to flexural loading. Although some brittle materials can be strong, they fracture with little warning because little or no plastic deformation occurs to indicate high levels of stress.

Compressive Stress

If a body is placed under a load that tends to compress or shorten it, the internal resistance to such a load is called a *compressive stress*. A compressive stress is associated with a *compressive strain*. To calculate either tensile stress or compressive stress, the applied force is divided by the cross-sectional area perpendicular to the force direction.

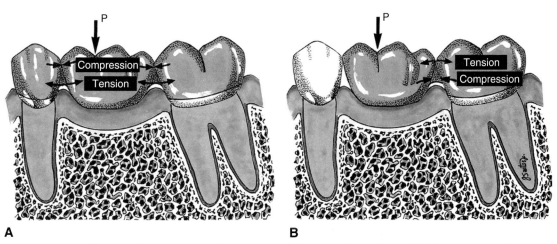

A   **B**

Fig. 4-1 A, Stresses induced in a three-unit bridge by a flexural force (P). **B,** Stresses induced in a two-unit cantilever bridge. Note that the tensile stress develops on the gingival side of the three-unit bridge and on the occlusal side of the cantilever bridge. See also color plates.

CRITICAL QUESTION

Although the shear bond strength of dental adhesive systems is often reported in manufacturers' advertisements, most dental prostheses and restorations are not likely to fail because of pure shear stresses. Which two factors tend to prevent the occurrence of pure shear failure?

Shear Stress

A *shear stress* tends to resist the sliding or twisting of one portion of a body over another. Shear stress can also be produced by a twisting or torsional action on a material. For example, if a force is applied along the surface of tooth enamel by a sharp-edged instrument parallel to the interface between the enamel and an orthodontic bracket, the bracket may debond by shear stress failure of the resin luting agent. Shear stress is calculated by dividing the force by the area parallel to the force direction.

In the oral environment shear failure is unlikely to occur for at least four reasons: (1) many of the brittle materials in restored tooth surfaces generally have rough, curved surfaces. (2) The presence of chamfers, bevels, or changes in curvature of a bonded tooth surface would also make shear failure of a bonded material highly unlikely. (3) To produce shear failure the applied force must be located immediately adjacent to the interface, as shown in Figure 4-2, *B*. This is quite difficult to accomplish, even under experimental conditions under which polished, flat interfaces are used. The farther away from the interface the load is applied, the more likely that tensile failure rather than shear failure will occur because the potential for bending stresses would increase. (4) Because the tensile strength of brittle materials is usually well below their **shear strength** values, tensile failure is more likely to occur.

Flexural (Bending) Stress

Examples of flexural stresses that are produced in a three-unit bridge or fixed partial denture (FPD) and a two-unit cantilever FPD are illustrated in Figures 4-1, *A* and 4-1, *B*, respectively. These stresses are produced by bending forces in dental appliances in one of two ways: (1) by subjecting a structure such as an FPD to three-point loading, whereby the endpoints are fixed and a force is applied between these endpoints, as in Figure 4-1, *A*; and (2) by subjecting a cantilevered structure that is supported at only one end to a load along any part of the unsupported section Figure 4-1, *B*. Also, when a patient bites into an object, the anterior teeth receive forces that are at an angle to their long axes, thereby creating flexural stresses within the teeth.

As shown in Figure 4-1, *A*, tensile stress develops on the tissue side of the FPD, and compressive stress develops on the occlusal side. Between these two areas is the neutral axis that represents a state with no tensile stress and no compressive stress. For a cantilevered FPD such as shown in Figure 4-1, *B*, the maximum tensile stress develops with the occlusal surface or the surface that is becoming more convex (indicating a stretching action). If you can visualize this unit bending downward toward the tissue, the upper surface becomes more convex or stretched (tensile region), and the opposite surface becomes compressed. As explained in the section

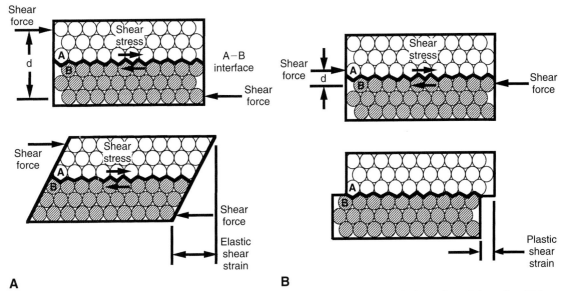

Fig. 4-2 Atomic model illustrating elastic shear deformation (**A**) and plastic shear deformation (**B**) for a unit length of a material structure.

on stress concentration, these areas of tension represent potential fracture initiation sites in most materials, especially in brittle materials that have little or no plastic deformation potential.

Shown in Figure 4-2 is a bonded two-material system with the white atoms of material A shown above the interface and the shaded atoms of material B shown below the interface. The atoms are represented over six atom planes, although dental structures have millions of atom planes. However, the principles of stress and strain apply in both cases. In the upper section of Figure 4-2, *A* a shear force is applied at a distance d/2 from interface A-B. As this force increases in magnitude, it first produces an elastic shear strain (lower section of Figure 4-2) that will return to zero when the shear force is removed. As shown in Figure 4-2, *B*, if the shear force on the external surface is increased sufficiently, a permanent or plastic deformation will be produced.

For the case in Figure 4-2, *B*, the force is applied along interface A-B and not at a distance away, as shown in Figure 4-2, *A*. Because of this application of force along the interface, pure shear stress and shear strain develop only within the interfacial region, and localized plastic deformation has also occurred. In the lower section of Figure 4-2, *B*, the force has been released, and a permanent strain of one atom space has occurred. For Figure 4-2, *A*, the stress induced is not pure shear since the force is applied at a distance from the interface. This is the reason why most shear bond tests do not actually measure shear strength, but a tensile component of bending stress.

MECHANICAL PROPERTIES BASED ON ELASTIC DEFORMATION

There are several important mechanical properties and parameters that are measures of the elastic strain or **plastic strain** behavior of dental materials. These are **elastic modulus** (also called **Young's modulus** or **modulus of elasticity**), *dynamic Young's modulus* (determined by measurement of ultrasonic wave velocity), *shear modulus, flexibility, resilience,* and *Poisson's ratio.* Other properties that are determined from stresses at the end of the elastic region of the stress-strain or within the initial plastic deformation region *(proportional limit, elastic limit,* and *yield strength)* are described in the following section on strength properties.

Elastic Modulus (Young's Modulus or Modulus of Elasticity)

Elastic modulus describes the relative stiffness or rigidity of a material, which is measured by the slope of the elastic region of the stress-strain graph. Shown in Figure 4-3 is a stress-strain graph for a stainless steel orthodontic wire that has been subjected to a tensile force. The ultimate tensile strength, yield strength (0.2% off-set), proportional limit, and elastic modulus are shown in the figure. This figure represents a plot of **true stress** versus strain because the force has been divided by the changing cross-sectional area as the wire was being stretched. The straight-line region represents reversible elastic deformation, because the stress remains below the proportional limit of 1020 MPa, and the curved region represents irreversible plastic deformation that is not recovered when the wire fractures at a stress of 1625 MPa. However, the elastic strain (approximately 0.52%) is fully recovered when the force is released or after the wire fractures. We can see this easily by bending a wire in our hands a slight amount and then reducing the force. It straightens back to its original shape as the force is decreased to zero, assuming that the induced stress has not exceeded the proportional limit.

This principle of elastic recovery is illustrated in Figure 4-4 for a burnishing procedure of an open metal margin (top, left) where a dental abrasive stone is shown rotating against the metal margin (top, right) to close the marginal gap as a result of elastic plus plastic strain. However, after the force is removed, the margin springs back an amount equal to the total elastic strain. Only by removing the crown from a tooth or die can total closure be accomplished. Because we must provide at least

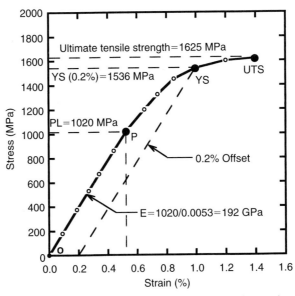

Fig. 4-3 Stress-strain plot for a stainless steel orthodontic wire that has been subjected to tension. The proportional limit (PL) is 1020 MPa. Although not shown, the elastic limit is approximately equal to this value. The yield strength (YS) at a 0.2% strain offset from the origin (O) is 1536 MPa and the ultimate tensile strength (UTS) is 1625 MPa. An elastic modulus value (E) of 192,000 MPa (192 GPa) was calculated from the slope of the elastic region.

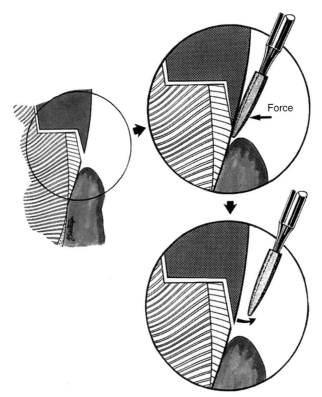

Fig. 4-4 Schematic illustration of a procedure to close an open margin of a metal crown **(top, left)** by burnishing with a rotary instrument **(top, right)**. Note that after the rotating stone is removed **(bottom)**, the elastic strain has been recovered and a slight marginal discrepancy remains. See also color plate.

25 µm of clearance for the cement, total burnishing on the tooth or die is usually adequate since the amount of elastic strain recovery is relatively small.

A stress-strain graph is shown in Figure 4-5 for enamel and dentin that have been subjected to compressive stress. These curves were constructed from typical values of elastic moduli, proportional limit, and ultimate **compressive strength** reported in the scientific literature. If the tensile stress below the proportional limit in Figure 4-3 or the compressive stress (below the proportional limit) in Figure 4-5 is divided by its corresponding strain value, that is, tensile stress/tensile strain or compressive stress/compressive strain, a constant of proportionality will be obtained that is known as the *elastic modulus, modulus of elasticity*, or *Young's modulus*. These terms are designated by the letter *E*. The slope of the straight-line region (elastic range) of the stress-strain graph is a measure of the relative *rigidity* or *stiffness* of a material. Although the stiffness of a dental prosthesis can increase by increasing its thickness, the elastic modulus does not change. The elastic modulus has a constant value that describes a material's relative stiffness as determined from a stress-strain graph.

Differing values of proportional limit, elastic modulus, and ultimate compressive strength have been reported for enamel and dentin, depending on the area of the tooth from which the test specimens were obtained. Note that the proportional limit, ultimate compressive strength, and elastic modulus of enamel are greater than the corresponding values for dentin (see Fig. 4-5). In fact, the elastic modulus of enamel is about three times greater than that of dentin and, depending on the study cited, it can be as much as seven times higher. Dentin is capable of sustaining significant plastic deformation under compressive loading before it fractures.

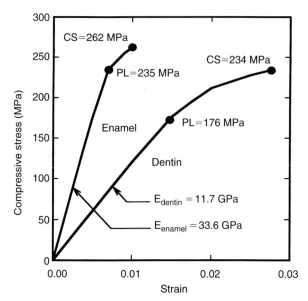

Fig. 4-5   Stress-strain plot for enamel and dentin that have been subjected to compression. The ultimate compressive strength (CS), proportional limit (PL), and elastic modulus (E) values are shown. (Data from Stanford JW, Weigel KV, Paffenbarger GD, and Sweeney WT: Compressive properties of hard tooth tissue. J Am Dent Assoc 60:746, 1960.)

Thus, enamel is a stiffer and more brittle material than dentin. Conversely, dentin is more flexible and tougher.

Since the elastic modulus of a material is a constant, it is unaffected by the amount of elastic or plastic stress that is induced in the material. It is independent of the **ductility** of a material since it is measured in the linear region of the stress-strain plot, and it is not a measure of its plasticity or strength. Materials with a high elastic modulus can have either high or low strength values. Although a compressive test was selected to measure the properties of tooth structures in Figure 4-5, the elastic modulus can also be measured by means of a tensile test.

Because the elastic modulus represents the ratio of the elastic stress to the elastic strain, it follows that the lower the strain for a given stress, the greater the value of the modulus. For example, if one wire is much more difficult to bend than another of the same shape and size, considerably higher stress must be induced before a desired strain or deformation can be produced in the stiffer wire. Such a material would possess a comparatively high modulus of elasticity. A polyether impression material has a greater stiffness (elastic modulus) than all other elastomeric impression materials. Thus a greater force is needed to remove an impression tray from undercut areas in the mouth. Modulus of elasticity is given in units of force per unit area, typically giganewtons per square meter (GN/m^2), or gigapascals (GPa). This property is indirectly related to other mechanical properties. For example, two materials may have the same proportional limit but may have elastic moduli that differ considerably.

The elastic modulus of a tensile test specimen can be calculated as follows:
Where
    E is the elastic modulus
    P is the applied force or load
    A is the cross-sectional area of the material under stress
    Δl is the increase in length
    l_o is the original length

By definition:

$$\text{Stress} = P / A = \sigma \tag{3}$$

$$\text{Strain} = \Delta l / l_o = \varepsilon \tag{4}$$

Thus,

$$E = \frac{\text{Stress}}{\text{Strain}} = \frac{\sigma}{\varepsilon} = \frac{(P / A)}{\Delta l / l_o} \tag{5}$$

Dynamic Young's Modulus

Elastic modulus can be measured by a dynamic method as well as the static techniques that were described in the previous section. Since the velocity at which sound travels through a solid can be readily measured by ultrasonic longitudinal and transverse wave transducers and appropriate receivers, the velocity of the sound wave and the density of the material can be used to calculate the *elastic modulus* and *Poisson's ratio* values. This method of determining dynamic elastic moduli is less complicated than conventional tensile or compressive tests, but the values are often found to be higher than the values obtained by static measurements. For most purposes, these values are acceptable.

If, instead of uniaxial tensile or compressive stress, a shear stress was induced, the resulting shear strain could be used to define a shear modulus for the material. The shear modulus (G) can be calculated from the elastic modulus (E) and Poisson's ratio (ν) using equation 6:

$$G = \frac{E}{2(1 + \nu)} = \frac{E}{2(1 + 0.3)} = 0.38E \tag{6}$$

A value of 0.3 for Poisson's ratio is typical. Thus, the shear modulus is usually about 38% of the elastic modulus.

Flexibility

In the case of dental appliances and restorations, a high value for the elastic limit (the stress above which a material will not recover to its original state when the force is released) is a necessary requirement for the materials from which they are fabricated, because the structure is expected to return to its original shape after it has been stressed and the force is removed (elastic recovery). Usually a moderately high modulus of elasticity is also desirable, because only a small deformation will develop under a considerable stress, such as in the case of an inlay or an impression material.

There are instances, however, in which a larger strain or deformation may be needed with a moderate or slight stress. For example, in an orthodontic appliance, a spring is often bent a considerable distance under the influence of a small stress. In such a case, the structure is said to be *flexible* and it possesses the property of *flexibility*. The *maximum flexibility* is defined as the flexural strain that occurs when the material is stressed to its proportional limit.

Resilience

As the interatomic spacing increases, the internal energy increases. As long as the stress is not greater than the proportional limit, this energy is known as *resilience*. Popularly, the term *resilience* is associated with "springiness," but it connotes something more than this. On the basis of the previous discussion, resilience can be defined as the amount of energy absorbed within a unit volume of a structure when it is stressed to its proportional limit. The resilience of two or more materials can be compared by observing the areas under the elastic region of their stress-strain plots, assuming that they are plotted on the same scale. The material with the larger elastic area has the higher resilience.

Shown in Figure 4-6 is a stress-strain diagram that illustrates the concepts of resilience and toughness. The area bounded by the elastic region is a measure of resilience, and the total area under the stress-strain curve is a measure of toughness. This figure is explained further in the following section.

Work is the product of the force times the distance through which the force acts. When work is performed on a body, energy is imparted to it. Consequently, when a dental restoration is deformed, it absorbs energy. If the induced stress is not greater than the proportional limit (the oral structure is not permanently deformed) only elastic energy is stored in the structure.

When a dental restoration is deformed during mastication, the chewing force acts on the tooth structure, the restoration, or both, and the magnitude of the structure's strain (deformation) is determined by the induced stress. In most dental restorations, large strains are precluded because of the proprioceptive response of neural receptors in the periodontal ligament. The pain stimulus causes the force to be

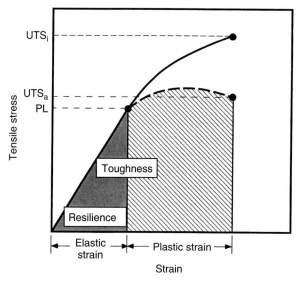

Fig. 4-6   Conventional tensile stress-strain curve **(bold dashed line)** in the plastic deformation region calculated on the basis of the initial cross-sectional area of a rod. The *solid line* (above the **dashed line**) represents the calculated stress values based on the actual reduced area of the rod as deformation increases. The resilience can be calculated by measuring the area within the elastic region. The toughness is related to the total area within the elastic and plastic regions. In this case, the proportional limit (PL) remains constant, but the toughness and ultimate strength (UTS$_i$) are different.

decreased and the induced stress to be reduced, thereby preventing damage to the teeth or restorations. For example, a proximal inlay might cause excessive movement of the adjacent tooth if large proximal strains developed during compressive loading on the occlusal surface. Hence, the restorative material should exhibit a moderately high elastic modulus and relatively low resilience, thereby limiting the elastic strain that is produced.

Poisson's Ratio

When a tensile force is applied to a cylinder or rod, the object becomes longer and thinner. Conversely, a compressive force acts to make the cylinder or rod shorter and thicker. If an axial tensile stress, σ_z, in the z (long axis) direction of a mutually perpendicular xyz coordinate system produces an elastic tensile strain, and accompanying elastic contractions in the x and y directions (ε_x and ε_y, respectively), the ratio of $\varepsilon_x / \varepsilon_z$ or $\varepsilon_y / \varepsilon_z$ is an engineering property of the material called *Poisson's ratio* (ν).

$$\nu = -\frac{\varepsilon_x}{\varepsilon_z} = -\frac{\varepsilon_y}{\varepsilon_z} \tag{7}$$

Poisson's ratio can be similarly determined in an experiment involving an axial compressive stress. Poisson's ratio is related to the nature and symmetry of the interatomic bonding forces described in Chapter 2. For an ideal isotropic material of constant volume, the ratio is 0.5. Most engineering materials have values of approximately 0.3.

CRITICAL QUESTION

Is it possible for a stiff material with a high modulus of elasticity to fail with no plastic deformation and at a lower strength than a more flexible material? Explain your answer.

STRENGTH PROPERTIES

Strength is the stress necessary to cause either fracture (*ultimate strength*) or a specified amount of plastic deformation (*yield strength*). When we describe the strength of an object or a material, we are most often referring to the maximum stress that is required to cause fracture. Both types of deformational behavior can be described by strength properties, but we should use proper strength terms to differentiate between the stress to cause permanent deformation and that required to produce fracture.

For specific dental materials, particularly metals, we are equally interested in the maximum stress that a structure can sustain before it becomes permanently or plastically deformed. This stress can be described either by the *proportional limit* or *elastic limit*. At stresses above these limits, plastic deformation occurs.

The strength of a material can be described by one or more of the following properties: (1) *proportional limit*, the stress above which stress is no longer proportional to strain; (2) *elastic limit*, the maximum stress a material can withstand before it becomes plastically deformed; (3) *yield strength* or *proof stress*, the stress required to produce a given amount of plastic strain; and (4) **ultimate tensile strength, shear strength, compressive strength,** and *flexural strength*, each of which is a measure of stress required to fracture a material. Strength is not a measure of individual atom-to-atom attraction or repulsion, but rather it is a measure of the interatomic forces collectively over the entire wire, cylinder, implant, crown, pin, or whatever structure is stressed. Furthermore, the ultimate strength may not necessarily be equal to the actual instantaneous average stress at fracture since the original cross-sectional area has changed in size.

CRITICAL QUESTION

Why is the ultimate tensile strength sometimes less than the maximum stress?

Shown in Figure 4-6 is a stress-strain plot of a metal rod that has been subjected to a tensile test. The stress is calculated by dividing the applied force at any instant by the original cross-sectional area and is represented by the bold dashed line above the lightly shaded area. However, the diameter actually decreases as the metal is stretched. The true stress is calculated as the force divided by the actual cross-sectional area at each measured strain value and is represented in Figure 4-6 by the bold line in the plastic deformation region above the dashed curve.

It is evident that the cross section of the wire decreases as it lengthens under tensile stress. Because of the reduction in area, the force required to increase deformation actually decreases. Thus the stress calculated for testing purposes (force per unit initial area) decreases, and the ultimate tensile strength based on the initial area (lower UTS value) as indicated in Figure 4-6 is less than the maximum tensile stress that occurs at the peak of the curve.

Although the true stress-strain curve represents the situation more accurately, the stress-strain curve as indicated by the dashed line in Figure 4-6 is commonly used. When we calculate the tensile strength of a certain wire, we wish to know the maximum stress it supports in tension without regard to the small changes that may occur in the cross-sectional area. Therefore the ultimate tensile strength is defined as the tensile stress within a structure at the point of rupture.

Brittle materials have a tensile strength that is markedly lower than the corresponding compressive strength, because of their inability to plastically deform and reduce the tensile stress at flaw tips. This is true of all brittle dental materials, such as amalgams, composites, cements, and ceramics. The failure of these materials in clinical usage is most often associated with their low tensile strengths and the presence of flaws within the tensile stress region.

Proportional Limit

As a wire is stretched steadily in tension, the wire eventually fractures. However, in dentistry we are also interested in the stress at which plastic deformation begins to develop. One method to determine this point is to plot a stress-strain diagram similar to that in Figures 4-3, 4-5, or 4-6. If the material obeys Hooke's law, the elastic stress will be proportional to elastic strain. For such a material, the stress-strain diagram shown in Figure 4-3 starts from the origin (O) as a straight line. Along this line the material behaves elastically, and it springs back to its initial shape and size at the instant the force is removed. When a certain stress value corresponding to point P is exceeded, the line becomes nonlinear, and stress is no longer proportional to strain. If a straight edge is laid along the straight-line portion of the curve from O to P, the stress value at P, the point above which the curve digresses from a straight line, is known as the *proportional limit*.

For a material to satisfy Hooke's law, the elastic stress must be directly proportional to the elastic strain. The initial region of the stress-strain plot must be a straight line. Because direct proportionality between two quantities is graphically represented by a straight line, the linear portion of the graph in Figures 4-3, 4-5, and 4-6 satisfies this law. Because the proportional limit (stress corresponding to point P) is the greatest elastic stress possible in accordance with this law, it represents the maximum stress above which stress is no longer proportional to strain. For the stress-strain curve of dentin that is shown in Figure 4-5, the strain corresponding to the proportional limit is important because it represents the percent deformation that can be sustained in dentin before it becomes deformed permanently.

Elastic Limit

If a small tensile stress is induced in a wire, the wire will return to its original length when the load is removed. If the load is increased progressively in small increments and then released after each increase in stress, a stress value will be reached at which the wire does not return to its original length after it is unloaded. At this point the wire has been stressed beyond its *elastic limit*. The elastic limit of a material is defined as the greatest stress to which a material can be subjected such that it returns to its original dimensions when the force is released. Although tensile stress was used in the example, similar elastic limit measurements can be made for any type of stress, although different values of elastic limit are obtained in tension, compression, and shear.

CRITICAL QUESTION

Yield strength is a commonly reported property for metals and alloys but not for ceramics. Why is it not possible to measure the yield strength of ceramics or other purely brittle materials? Use a stress-strain plot to explain your answer.

Yield Strength (Proof Stress)

The conditions assumed for the definitions of elastic limit and proportional limit are not always realized under practical conditions. If the measuring instruments are sufficiently sensitive, irregularities on the straight-line region of the stress versus strain plot represent minor deviations from Hooke's law and cause some uncertainty in determining the precise point at which the selected line deviates from linearity (proportional limit). Thus, a different property, *yield strength*, is used in such cases when the proportional limit cannot be determined with sufficient accuracy.

Yield strength often is a property that represents the stress value at which a small amount (0.1% or 0.2%) of plastic strain has occurred. A value of either 0.1% or 0.2% of the plastic strain is often selected and is referred to as the *percent offset*. The yield strength is the stress required to produce the particular offset strain (0.1% or 0.2%) that has been chosen. As seen in Figure 4-3, the yield strength for 0.2% offset is greater than that associated with an offset of 0.1%. If yield strength values for two materials tested under the same conditions are to be compared, identical offset values should be used. To determine the yield strength for a material at 0.2% offset, a line is drawn parallel to the straight-line region (see Fig. 4-3), starting at a value of 0.002, or 0.2% of the plastic strain, along the strain axis, and is extended until it intersects the stress-strain curve. The stress corresponding to this point is the yield strength. Although the term *strength* implies that the material has fractured, it actually is intact, but it has sustained a specific amount of plastic strain (deformation).

For brittle materials such as dental ceramics, the stress-strain plot is a straight line with no plastic region. Thus, a determination of yield strength is not practical at either a 0.1% or 0.2% strain offset because there can be no intercept of straight line offset parallel to the elastic deformation line.

Elastic limit, proportional limit, and *yield strength* are defined differently, but their values (of stress) are fairly close to each other in many cases. Elastic and proportional limits are usually assumed to be identical, although their experimental values may differ slightly. As shown in Figure 4-3, the yield strength (proof stress) is greater than the proportional limit. These values are important in the evaluation of dental materials, because they represent the stress at which permanent deformation of the structure begins. If they are exceeded by mastication stresses, the restoration or appliance may no longer function as originally designed.

Permanent (Plastic) Deformation

As shown in Figure 4-3, the stress-strain graph is no longer a straight line above the proportional limit (PL), but rather it curves until the structure fractures. The stress-strain graph shown in Figure 4-3 is more typical of actual stress-strain curves for ductile materials. Unlike the linear portion of the graph at stresses below the proportional limit, the shape of the curve above P is not possible to extrapolate because stress is no longer proportional to strain.

If the material is deformed by a stress at a point above the proportional limit before fracture, the removal of the applied force will reduce the stress to zero, but the strain does not decrease to zero because plastic deformation has occurred. Thus, the object does not return to its original dimension when the force is removed. It remains bent, stretched, compressed, or otherwise plastically deformed.

Cold Working (Strain Hardening or Work Hardening)

When a metal had been stressed beyond its proportional limit, the hardness and strength of the metal increase at the area of deformation, but the ductility of the metal decreases. As dislocations move and pile up along grain boundaries, further plastic deformation in these areas becomes more difficult. As a result, repeated plastic deformation of the metal, such as occurs during bending of orthodontic wire or adjustment of a clasp arm on a removable partial denture, can lead to brittleness of the wire and it will fracture when further permanent adjustment is attempted. Since the elastic modulus remains constant, the stress-strain curve of the deformed area would extend above the level of ultimate strength of the metal, but the plastic deformation part of the curve would be decreased progressively with each bend of a wire or clasp arm. The key to minimize the risk of reduced plasticity (embrittlement) is to deform the metal in small increments so as not to plastically deform the metal excessively.

Diametral Tensile Strength

Tensile strength is generally determined by subjecting a rod, wire, or dumbbell-shaped specimen to tensile loading (a uniaxial tension test). Since such a test is quite difficult to perform for brittle materials because of alignment and gripping problems, another test has become popular for determining this property for brittle dental materials. It is referred to as the *diametral compression test,* which is represented schematically in Figure 4-7. This test should be used only for materials that exhibit predominantly elastic deformation and little or no plastic deformation.

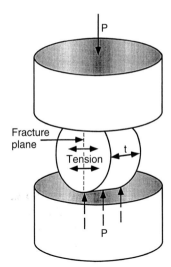

Fig. 4-7 Diametral compression test. Although a compressive force is applied along the side of the disk, a tensile fracture is produced. The tensile strength is calculated from the fracture load P, the disk diameter D, and the thickness t.

In this method, the compressive load is placed by a flat plate against the side of a short cylindrical specimen (disk), as illustrated in Figure 4-7. The vertical compressive force along the side of the disk produces a tensile stress that is perpendicular to the vertical plane that passes through the center of the disk. Fracture occurs along this vertical plane (the dashed vertical line on the disk). In such a situation, the tensile stress is directly proportional to the compressive load applied. It is computed by the following formula:

$$\text{Tensile stress} = \frac{2P}{\pi Dt} \qquad (8)$$

where P is the applied load, D is the diameter, and t is the thickness.

This test is simple to conduct and provides excellent reproducibility of results. However, use of this test on materials that exhibit appreciable plastic deformation before fracture results in erroneously high tensile strength determinations. The fracture of the specimen into several pieces rather than the ideal fragmentation into two segments suggests an unreliable test result.

Flexure Strength

Flexure strength, transverse strength, or *modulus of rupture,* as this property is variously called, is essentially a strength test of a bar supported at each end, or a thin disk supported along a lower support circle, under a static load. For the disk specimen, the failure stress value is referred to as the *biaxial flexure strength* and the theory involved is beyond the scope of this textbook. For a bar subjected to three-point flexure (upper central loading), the mathematical formula for computing the flexure strength is as follows:

$$\sigma = \frac{3Pl}{2bd^2} \qquad (9)$$

where σ is the flexural strength, l is the distance between the supports, b is the width of the specimen, d is the depth or thickness of the specimen, and P is the maximum load at the point of fracture.

The units of stress are force per unit area, most often given in SI units of megapascals (MPa). This test is, in a sense, a collective measurement of tensile, compressive, and shear stresses simultaneously; however, for sufficiently thin specimens, it is usually dominated by the tensile stress that develops along the lower surface. When the load is applied, the specimen bends. For a flat strip specimen, the resulting strain is represented by a decrease in length of the top surface (compressive strain) of the specimen and an increase in the length of the lower surface (tensile strain). Consequently, the principal stresses on the upper surface are compressive, whereas those on the lower surface are tensile. Obviously, the stresses change direction within the specimen between the top and the bottom surfaces, with both stress and strain being zero at the region of change. This neutral surface does not change in dimension and is known as the *neutral axis*. Shear stress is also produced near the supported ends of the specimen, but it does not play a significant role in the fracture process. For brittle materials such as ceramics, flexure tests are preferred to the diametral compressive test because they more closely simulate the stress distributions in dental prostheses such as cantilevered bridges and multiple-unit fixed partial dentures (FPDs or bridges), and clasp arms of removable partial dentures (RPDs).

Fatigue Strength

Strength values obtained from a measurement of the failure load described earlier may be quite misleading if they are used to design a structure that is subjected to repeated or cyclic loading. Few clinical fractures occur during a single-load application. If such fractures were common, these products would be withdrawn from the market soon after their introduction. This is a good reason why one should not be the first to buy a new restorative material, but rather allow sufficient time for clinical data to be reported. Most prosthetic and restoration fractures develop progressively over many stress cycles after initiation of a crack from a critical flaw and subsequently by propagation of the crack until a sudden, unexpected fracture occurs. Stress values well below the ultimate tensile strength can produce premature fracture of a dental prosthesis because microscopic flaws grow slowly over many cycles of stress. This phenomenon is called *fatigue failure*. Normal mastication induces several thousands of stress cycles per day within a dental restoration. For glasses and certain glass-containing ceramics, the induced tensile stress and the presence of an aqueous environment further reduce the number of cycles to cause dynamic fatigue failure.

Fatigue behavior is determined by subjecting a material to a cyclic stress of a maximum known value and determining the number of cycles that are required to produce failure. As shown in Figure 4-8, a plot of the failure stress versus the number of cycles to failure enables calculation of a *maximum service stress* or an *endurance limit*—the maximum stress that can be maintained without failure over an infinite number of cycles. For brittle materials with rough surfaces, the endurance limit is lower than it would be if the surfaces were more highly polished (see Fig. 4-8). For a given applied stress, the rougher material would fail in fewer cycles of stress.

Some materials or prosthetic appliances exhibit *static fatigue*, a phenomenon attributed to the interaction of a constant tensile stress with structural flaws over time. The influence of flaw size on the stress to cause failure is shown in Figure 4-9. Note that for a given flaw size, less stress is required to produce failure if the stress is dynamically cycled between high and low values. Furthermore, aqueous solutions are known to corrosively degrade dental ceramics by converting surface flaws to one or more cracks over time in the presence of tensile stress. This environmental factor

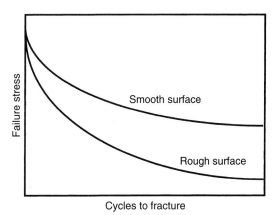

Fig. 4-8 Dynamic fatigue failure stress for a brittle material as a function of surface roughness and number of stress cycles.

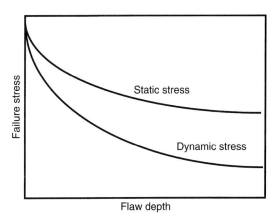

Fig. 4-9 Dynamic and static fatigue failure stress for a brittle material as a function of flaw depth.

further reduces the magnitude of tensile stress that can be sustained by ceramics over time.

Ceramic orthodontic brackets and activated wires within the brackets represent a clinical system that can exhibit *static fatigue failure*. The delayed fracture of molar ceramic crowns that are subjected to periodic cyclic forces may be caused by *dynamic fatigue failure*. Thus, dental restorative materials can exhibit either static or dynamic fatigue failure, depending on the nature of the loading or residual stress situation. In either case, the failure begins as a flaw that propagates until catastrophic fracture occurs.

Impact Strength

Impact strength may be defined as the energy required to fracture a material under an impact force. The term *impact* is used to describe the reaction of a stationary object to a collision with a moving object. A Charpy-type impact tester is usually used to measure impact strength. A pendulum is released that swings down to fracture the center of a bar specimen that is supported at both ends. The energy lost by the pendulum during the fracture of the specimen can be determined by a comparison of the length of its swing after the impact with that of its free swing when no impact occurs. The energy units are joules, foot-pounds, inch-pounds, and so forth. Unlike most mechanical tests, the dimensions, shape, and design of the specimen to be tested should be identical for uniform results.

For another impact device, called the *Izod impact tester,* the specimen is clamped vertically at one end. The blow is delivered at a certain distance above the clamped end instead of at the center of the specimen supported at both ends as described for the Charpy impact test.

With appropriate values for the velocities and masses involved, a blow by a fist to the lower jaw can be considered an impact situation. In the impact process, the external forces and resulting stresses change rapidly, and a static property such as the proportional limit is not useful in predicting the resulting deformations. However, a moving object possesses a known amount of kinetic energy. If the struck object is not permanently deformed, it stores the energy of the collision in an elastic manner. This ability is reflected by the *resilience* of a material, which is measured by the area under the elastic region of the stress-strain diagram. Thus, a material with a low elastic modulus and a high tensile strength is more resistant to impact forces. A low elastic modulus and a low tensile strength suggest low-impact resistance. For dental materials of low-impact resistance, the elastic moduli and tensile strengths, respectively, are as follows:

Dental porcelain:	40 GPa and 50-100 MPa
Amalgam:	21 GPa and 27-55 MPa
Resin-based composite:	17 GPa and 30-90 MPa
Poly(methylmethacrylate):	3.5 GPa and 60 MPa
Alumina ceramic:	350-418 GPa and 120 MPa

Thus, if one simply calculates the area under the stress versus strain graph, the greatest resilience is associated with the composite, followed in decreasing order by the porcelain, PMMA, amalgam, and alumina.

MECHANICAL PROPERTIES OF TOOTH STRUCTURE

Many of the mechanical properties of human tooth structure have been measured, but the reported values vary markedly from one study to another. Undoubtedly, the differences are attributed to the technical problems associated with preparing and testing such small specimens, which in some instances are less than 1 mm in length. The results reported in one study are shown in Table 4-1. This study analyzed the effect of enamel rod orientation by propagating cracks in the occlusal surface and in axial sections, in directions parallel and perpendicular to the occlusal surface. The cracks in the axial enamel section were longer in the direction perpendicular rather than parallel to the occlusal surface. The cracks that propagated toward the dentinoenamel junction (DEJ) were arrested and did not penetrate the DEJ into dentin. The **fracture toughness** of dentin varied by a factor of 3 as a function of enamel rod orientation. The elastic modulus of enamel also varied between the occlusal surface and the axial section. The results of this study suggest that, since the mechanical properties of tooth structure are a function of structural orientation, values of elastic modulus and fracture toughness should be selected based on the structural features in the areas of interest. The indentation energy is a recently introduced property that is used to predict the machinability and wear behavior of ceramics. Research data suggest that during indentation or cutting, brittle enamel may be removed by microfracture, whereas dentin may be removed by formation of ductile chips.

Although the data in Table 4-1 indicate a variation in the properties of enamel and dentin from one type of tooth to another, the difference probably is more the result of variations within individual teeth than between teeth. The properties of enamel vary somewhat with its position on the tooth, that is, cuspal enamel is stronger than enamel on other surfaces of the tooth. Also, the properties vary

Table 4-1	Properties of Tooth Structure (Human Third Molars)		
Microhardness indentation method	Enamel occlusal section	Enamel axial section	Dentin
Hardness (GPa)	3.23	3.03	0.58
Toughness (MPa·m$^{\frac{1}{2}}$)	0.77	0.52 ($\perp$) 1.30 ($\parallel$)	—
Modified microhardness indentation method	Enamel occlusal section	Enamel axial section	Dentin
Hardness (GPa)	3.62	3.37	0.57
Elastic modulus (GPa)	94	80	20
Indentation energy (μJ)	2.6	2.7	7.5

From Xu HHK, Smith DT, Jahanmir S, Romberg E, Kelly JR, Thompson VP, and Rekow ED: Indentation damage and mechanical properties of human enamel and dentin. J Dent Res 77(3):472-80, 1998.
$\perp$: Enamel axial section perpendicular to occlusal surface; $\parallel$: enamel axial section parallel to occlusal surface

according to the histological (microscopic) structure. For example, enamel is stronger under longitudinal compression than when subjected to lateral compression. On the other hand, the properties of dentin appear to be independent of structure, regardless of the direction of compressive stress.

The tensile properties of tooth structure have also been measured. Dentin is considerably stronger in tension (50 MPa) than is enamel (10 MPa). Although the compressive strengths of enamel and dentin are comparable, the proportional limit and modulus of elasticity of enamel are higher than the corresponding values for dentin. The higher modulus of elasticity results in less resilience of enamel in comparison with dentin.

MASTICATION FORCES AND STRESSES

Because of their dynamic nature, the biting stresses during mastication are difficult to measure. A number of studies have been made to determine the biting force. The *Guinness Book of Records* (1994) lists the highest biting force as 4337 N (975 pounds) sustained for 2 sec. The average maximum sustainable biting force is approximately 756 N (170 pounds). However, the range of biting forces varies markedly from one area of the mouth to another and from one individual to another. For the molar region, bite forces range from 400 to 890 N (90 to 200 pounds); in the premolar area, they range from 222 to 445 N (50 to 100 pounds); in the cuspid region, they vary from 133 to 334 N (30 to 75 pounds); and in the incisor region, they vary from 89 to 111 N (20 to 55 pounds). Although there is considerable overlap, biting force generally is higher for males than for females and is greater in young adults than in children.

If one assumes that if a force of 756 N (170 pounds) is applied to a cusp tip over an area equivalent to 0.039 cm^2 (0.006 square inch), the compressive stress would be 193 MPa (28,000 psi). If the area is smaller, then the stress within the cusp would be proportionately greater.

Normally, the energy of the bite is absorbed by the food bolus during mastication, as well as by the teeth, periodontal ligament, and bone. Nevertheless, the design of the tooth is an engineering marvel in that the tooth is generally able to absorb significant static as well as dynamic (impact) energies. As can be seen in

Figure 4-5, the modulus of resilience of dentin is greater than that of enamel and, thus, it is better able to absorb impact energy. Enamel is a brittle substance with a comparatively high modulus of elasticity, a low proportional limit in tension, and a low modulus of resilience. However, although it is supported by dentin with significant ability to deform elastically, teeth seldom fracture under normal occlusion.

OTHER MECHANICAL PROPERTIES
Toughness

Toughness is defined as the amount of elastic and plastic deformation energy required to fracture a material. It is a measure of the energy required to propagate critical flaws in the structure. As previously noted, the *modulus of resilience* is the energy required to stress a structure to its proportional limit. It can be measured as the area under the elastic, straight-line portion of the stress-strain curve. Toughness is indicated as the total area under the stress-strain graph (such as shown in Fig. 4-6) from zero stress to the fracture stress. Toughness increases with increases in strength and ductility. The greater the strength and the higher the ductility (total plastic strain), the greater the toughness. Thus, it can be concluded that a tough material is generally strong, although a strong material is not necessarily tough.

Fracture Toughness

The strength of ductile materials such as gold alloys and some composites is useful for determining the maximum stress that restorations of these materials can withstand before a certain amount of plastic deformation or fracture occurs. For brittle materials such as dental ceramic, strength values are of only limited value in the design of ceramic prostheses. Small defects (porosity and microcracks) are randomly distributed in location and in size throughout a ceramic, causing large strength variations in otherwise identical ceramic specimens. Furthermore, surface flaws caused by grinding, such as from coarse-grit, medium-grit, or fine-grit diamond particles, can greatly weaken an otherwise strong ceramic, especially in the presence of tensile stress in the area of these flaws. The strength is inversely proportional to the square root of the flaw depth into the surface. Fracture toughness, or the critical stress intensity, is a mechanical property that describes the resistance of brittle materials to the catastrophic propagation of flaws under an applied stress. Fracture toughness is given in units of stress times the square root of crack length, that is, MPa·m$^{\frac{1}{2}}$ or the equivalent form, MN·m$^{-\frac{3}{2}}$.

CRITICAL QUESTION

Is a stiff material (high elastic modulus) stronger than a more flexible material? Explain your answer by sketching a stress-strain plot.

Brittleness

Shown in Figure 4-10 are three stress-strain curves of materials with variable strength, elastic modulus, and percent elongation. Material A is stronger, stiffer, and more ductile than materials B or C. Material B has less ductility than material A and is thus more brittle. Material C has no ductility and is perfectly brittle; it is also the weakest of the three materials. Brittleness is the relative inability of a material to sustain plastic deformation before fracture of a material occurs. For example,

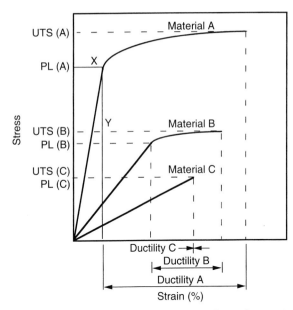

Fig. 4-10 Stress-strain plots of materials that exhibit different mechanical properties. UTS, ultimate tensile stress; PL, proportional limit.

amalgams, ceramics, and composites are brittle at oral temperatures (5 to 55° C). They sustain little or no plastic strain before they fracture. In other words, a brittle material fractures at or near its proportional limit. This behavior is shown by material C in Figure 4-10.

However, a brittle material is not necessarily weak. For example, a cobalt-chromium partial denture alloy may have a percent elongation of less than 1.5% elongation, but an ultimate tensile strength of 870 MPa. The tensile strength of a glass-infiltrated alumina core ceramic (In-Ceram Alumina) is moderately high (450 MPa), but it has 0% elongation.

If a glass is drawn into a fiber with very smooth surfaces and insignificant internal flaws, its tensile strength may be as high as 2800 MPa (400,000 psi), but it will have no ductility (0% elongation). Thus, dental materials with low or zero percent elongation, including amalgams, composites, ceramics, and nonresin luting agents, will have little or no burnishability, because they have no plastic deformation potential.

CRITICAL QUESTION

What is the difference in appearance between a stress-strain graph for a material that has high strength, high stiffness, and high ductility and one for a material that is weak, flexible, and more brittle?

Ductility and Malleability

When a structure is stressed beyond its proportional limit, it becomes permanently deformed. If a material sustains tensile stress and considerable permanent deformation without rupture, it is ductile. *Ductility* represents the ability of a material to sustain a large permanent deformation under a tensile load before it fractures. For example, a metal that can be drawn readily into a long, thin wire is considered to be *ductile*.

Examples of three materials with different amounts of ductility (percent elongation) are shown in Figure 4-10. Material A is the most ductile as shown by the longest plastic strain range (curved region). Material C is typical of brittle materials because no plastic deformation is possible and fracture occurs at the proportional limit.

The ability of a material to sustain considerable permanent deformation without rupture under compression, as in hammering or rolling into a sheet, is termed *malleability*. Gold is the most ductile and malleable pure metal, and silver is second. Of the metals of interest to the dentist, platinum ranks third in ductility, and copper ranks third in malleability.

Ductility is the maximum plastic deformation a material can withstand when it is stretched at room temperature. It is quite important from a dental standpoint. Its magnitude can be assessed by the amount of permanent deformation indicated by the stress-strain curve. For example, the plastic strain indicated in Figure 4-10 is an estimation of the ductility of the substance. After fracture, the mechanical stress is reduced to zero, and the residual strain represents the amount of permanent deformation that has been produced in the object.

Measurement of Ductility

There are three common methods for measurement of ductility: (1) the percent elongation after fracture; (2) the reduction in area of tensile test specimens; and (3) the maximum number of bends performed in a cold bend test. Probably the simplest and most commonly used method is to compare the increase in length of a wire or rod after fracture in tension to its length before fracture. Two marks are placed on the wire or rod a specified distance apart and this distance is designated as the *gauge length*. For dental materials, the standard gauge length is usually 51 mm. The wire or rod is then pulled apart under a tensile load. The fractured ends are fitted together, and the gauge length is again measured. The ratio of the increase in length after fracture to the original gauge length, expressed in percent, is called the *percent elongation* and represents the quantitative value of ductility.

Another manifestation of ductility is the necking or cone-shaped constriction that occurs at the fractured end of a ductile wire after rupture under a tensile load. The percentage of decrease in cross-sectional area of the fractured end in comparison to the original area of the wire or rod is referred to as the *reduction in area*.

A third method for the measurement of ductility is known as the *cold bend test*. The material is clamped in a vise and bent around a mandrel of a specified radius. The number of bends to fracture is counted, and the greater the number, the greater the ductility. The first bend is made from the vertical to the horizontal, but all subsequent bends are made through angles of 180 degrees.

CRITICAL QUESTION

Hardness is a property that is used to predict the wear resistance of a material and its ability to abrade opposing dental structures. What other factors may be responsible for excessive wear of natural tooth enamel or prosthetic surfaces by a hard material?

Hardness

The term *hardness* is difficult to define. In mineralogy the relative hardness of a substance is based on its ability to resist scratching. In metallurgy, and in most other disciplines, the concept of hardness that is most generally accepted is the "resistance to indentation." It is on this precept that most modern *hardness* tests are designed.

The indentation produced on the surface of a material from an applied force of a sharp point or an abrasive particle results from the interaction of numerous properties. Among the properties that are related to the hardness of a material are compressive strength, proportional limit, and ductility.

Knowledge of the hardness of materials is useful to the engineer and furnishes valuable information to the dentist. Hardness tests are included in numerous American Dental Association (ADA) specifications for dental materials. There are several types of surface hardness tests. Most are based on the ability of the surface of a material to resist penetration by a diamond point or a steel ball under a specified load. The tests most frequently used in determining the hardness of dental materials are known by the names *Barcol, Brinell, Rockwell, Shore, Vickers,* and *Knoop.* The selection of the test should be determined by the material being measured.

The Brinell hardness test is one of the oldest tests employed for determining the hardness of metals. In the Brinell test, a hardened steel ball is pressed under a specified load into the polished surface of a material, as diagrammed in Figure 4-11. The load is divided by the area of the projected surface of the indentation, and the quotient is referred to as the *Brinell hardness number,* usually abbreviated as BHN. Thus, for a given load, the smaller the indentation, the larger is the number, and the harder is the material.

The Brinell hardness test has been used extensively for determining the hardness of metals and metallic materials used in dentistry. In addition, the BHN is related to the proportional limit and the ultimate tensile strength of dental gold alloys. Because the test is a relatively simple one, it may often be conveniently used as an index of properties that involve more complicated test methods.

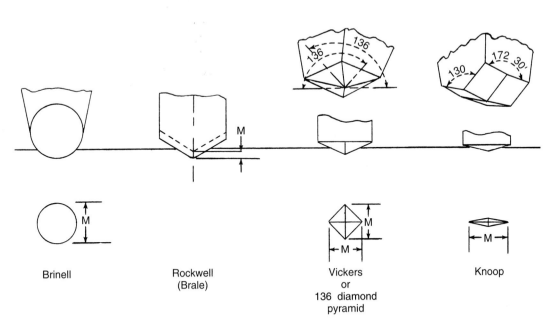

Fig. 4-11 Shapes of hardness indenter points **(upper row)** and the indentation depressions left in material surfaces **(lower row)**. The measured dimension M that is shown for each test is used to calculate hardness. The following tests are shown: *Brinell test*—a steel ball is used, and the diameter of the indentation is measured after removal of the indenter. *Rockwell test*—a conical indenter is impressed into the surface under a minor load **(dashed line)** and a major load **(solid line),** and M is the difference between the two penetration depths. *Vickers* or *136-degree diamond pyramid test*—a pyramidal point is used, and the diagonal length of the indentation is measured. *Knoop test*—a rhombohedral pyramid diamond tip is used, and the long axis of the indentation is measured.

The Rockwell hardness test is somewhat similar to the Brinell test in that a steel ball or a conical diamond point is used, as diagrammed in Figure 4-11. Instead of measuring the diameter of the impression, the depth of penetration is measured directly by a dial gauge on the instrument. A number of indenting points with different sizes are available for testing a variety of different materials. The *Rockwell hardness number* (abbreviated as RHN) is designated according to the particular indenter and load employed.

The convenience of the Rockwell test, with direct reading of the depth of the indentation, has led to its wide usage in industry. Neither the Brinell test nor the Rockwell test is suitable for brittle materials.

The Vickers hardness test employs the same principle of hardness testing that is used in the Brinell test. However, instead of a steel ball, a square-based pyramid is used (see Fig. 4-11). Although the impression is square instead of round, the method for computation of the *Vickers hardness number* (usually abbreviated as HV) is the same as that for the BHN in that the load is divided by the projected area of indentation. The lengths of the diagonals of the indentation are measured and averaged. The Vickers test is employed in the ADA specification for dental casting gold alloys. The test is suitable for determining the hardness of brittle materials; therefore, it has also been used for measuring the hardness of tooth structure.

The Knoop hardness test employs a diamond-tipped tool that is cut in the geometric configuration shown in Figure 4-11. The impression is rhombic in outline, and the length of the largest diagonal is measured. The projected area is divided into the load to give the *Knoop hardness number* (usually abbreviated as KHN). When the indentation is made, and the indenter is subsequently removed, the shape of the Knoop indenter causes elastic recovery of the projected impression to occur primarily along the shorter diagonal. The stresses are distributed in such a manner that only the dimensions of the minor axis are subject to change by relaxation. Thus, the hardness value is virtually independent of the ductility of the tested material. The hardness of tooth enamel can be compared with that of gold, porcelain, resin, and other restorative materials. Also, the load may be varied over a wide range, from 0.1 kg to more than 1 kg, so that values for both exceedingly hard and soft materials can be obtained by this test.

The Knoop and Vickers tests are classified as microhardness tests in comparison with the Brinell and Rockwell macrohardness tests. Both Knoop and Vickers tests employ loads less than 9.8 N. The resulting indentations are small and are limited to a depth of less than 19 μm. Hence, they are capable of measuring the hardness in small regions of thin objects. The Rockwell and Brinell tests give average hardness values over much larger areas. Other less sophisticated measurement methods, such as the Shore and the Barcol tests, are sometimes employed for measuring the hardness of rubber and plastic types of dental materials. These tests use compact portable indenters of the type generally used in industry for quality control. The principle of these tests is also based on resistance to indentation. The equipment generally consists of a spring-loaded metal indenter point and a gauge from which the hardness is read directly. The hardness number is based on the depth of penetration of the indenter point into the material.

CRITICAL QUESTION

Why do prostheses sometimes fail under a very small force, even though the strength of the prosthetic material is relatively high?

STRESS CONCENTRATION FACTORS

Although dental prostheses are designed to resist plastic deformation and fracture, unexpected fractures occur occasionally even when high-quality materials have been used. As stated previously, these failures result from locally high stresses in specific areas even though the average stress in the structure is low. The cause of this strength reduction is the presence of small microscopic flaws or microstructural defects on the surface or within the internal structure. These flaws are especially critical in brittle materials in areas of tensile stress because the stress at the tips of these flaws is greatly increased and may lead to crack initiation and broken bonds. Shown in Figure 4-12 is a theoretical tensile stress distribution in a brittle and a ductile material. Although the tensile stress has increased at the flaw tip in each case, it has increased by a smaller amount in the ductile material (center illustration of Fig. 4-12) in which plastic deformation has occurred with subsequent widening of the flaw tip, thereby reducing the magnitude of localized tensile stress. As shown on the left side of Figure 4-12, the tensile stress in a brittle material cannot be relieved by plastic deformation at the flaw tip and a crack develops as the stress increases to a critical level. Note the increased level of tensile stress at the tip of the flaw. However, the stress at areas far away from these flaws will be much lower if flaws are absent in these areas. The flaw does not play a significant role when the material is subjected to an external compressive force, as shown in the center of Figure 4-12. In this case the **compressive stress** that develops in the material tends to close the crack, and this stress distribution is more uniform.

There are two important aspects of these flaws: (1) the stress intensity increases with the length of the flaw, especially when it is oriented perpendicular to the direction of tensile stress, and (2) flaws on the surface are associated with higher stresses than are flaws of the same size in interior regions. Thus surface finishing of brittle materials such as ceramics, amalgams, and composites is extremely important in areas subjected to tensile stress.

Localized areas of stress enhancement can also result from factors other than the inherent microscopic flaws on the surface or interior of a material. Areas of high stress concentration are caused by one or more of the following factors:
1. surface flaws, such as porosity, grinding roughness, and machining damage
2. interior flaws such as voids or inclusions

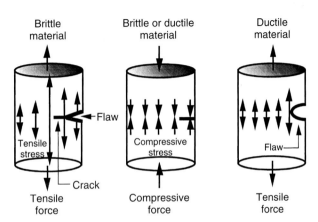

Fig. 4-12 Influence of tensile and compressive stresses on flaws in brittle and ductile materials.

3. marked changes in contour, such as the point of attachment of a clasp arm to a partial denture framework or a sharp internal angle at the pulpal-axial line angle of a tooth preparation for an amalgam or composite restoration

4. a large difference in elastic moduli or thermal expansion coefficient across a bonded interface

5. a Hertzian load (or point contact)

There are several ways to minimize stress concentrations and thus reduce the risk of clinical fracture. Relative to factor 1, the surface can be polished to reduce the depth of the flaws. Little can be done for interior flaws other than to improve the quality of the structure or increase the size of the object. For factor 3, the design of any prosthesis should vary gradually rather than abruptly. Notches should be avoided. Internal line angles of tooth preparations should be well rounded to minimize the risk of cusp fracture. For factor 4, the most brittle material should have the lower elastic modulus so that more stress is transferred to the material with the higher elastic modulus. If this is not possible, the elastic moduli of the two materials should be more closely matched. For factor 4, the materials must be closely matched in their coefficients of expansion or contraction. If a thermal mismatch cannot be avoided, the weaker, more brittle material should have a slightly lower expansion or contraction coefficient so that a protective compressive stress is sustained in its structure next to the interface. Relative to factor 5, the cusp tip of an opposing crown or tooth should be well rounded such that occlusal contact areas in the brittle material are large.

CRITICAL QUESTIONS

Fracture toughness is a more precise measure of the fracture resistance of a brittle material than its tensile strength. Why is tensile strength of brittle materials such as dental amalgam, composite, ceramic, and inorganic cements so variable? Which one of a series of reported tensile strength values should be used when considering the selection of a new product of one of these materials?

CRITERIA FOR SELECTION OF RESTORATIVE MATERIALS

We have discussed the variability of tensile strength in earlier sections. Because brittle materials are so susceptible to surface flaws and internal defects when tensile stresses are present and because they cannot plastically deform to reduce stress concentrations, their tensile strengths are far lower than their compressive strengths. For convenience, compressive strengths are reported even though most brittle materials rarely fail under compressive stresses. However, when tensile strength values are not available, flexural strength values should be used since they reflect a tensile mode of fracture. When tensile strength, flexure strength, or fracture toughness data are not available, compressive strength values may be useful when comparisons are to be made of the fracture resistance of a similar family of brittle materials, such as groups of amalgams, composites, or cements. Significantly lower values indicate a potentially higher risk of clinical failure although this hypothesis should be validated with clinical data.

Because the physical properties described earlier have been obtained using specimen shapes and sizes quite different than those of tooth restorations, we must select materials intuitively on the basis of these property comparisons. Engineers employ similar criteria for the selection of materials to be used for the construction of a bridge. Engineers have an advantage over dentists in this respect, because they know beforehand the maximum "average" stresses that structures are expected to sustain before fracture occurs. Furthermore, these expected stress values are multiplied by a "safety factor" to ensure that the structure may be able to withstand a certain amount of excess stress. However, the tensile strength values reported for restorative materials represent the average stress values below which 50% of the test specimens have fractured and above which only 50% have survived. Because this is an unacceptable failure rate for restorative dentistry, the range of measured values should be known. From an ultraconservative viewpoint, the lowest strength values, not mean values, should be used to compare materials and also to design a prosthesis to resist fracture at a high level of confidence.

It is unfortunate that the magnitudes of mastication forces are not known for any given patient to the extent that the dentist can predict the stresses that will be induced in restorative appliances. However, knowledge of the relationships between the properties of restorative materials that are known to exhibit excellent long-term survival performance is reinforced by clinical experience. As is true for the field of engineering, the dental profession is also aware that the best test of a successful restorative material is the test of time under actual clinical conditions.

When clinical survival data over a 3-year period or longer are not known for a restorative material, we should first investigate whether reliable short-term (less than 3-year) clinical data are available. In the absence of such clinical data, a new material should be evaluated on the basis of whether it meets minimal property requirements identified in dental materials specifications and standards such as those that have been developed by the ADA and the International Organization for Standardization. If a new material meets these requirements, dentists can be reasonably confident that the material will perform satisfactorily if it is used properly.

SELECTED READINGS

Frechette VD: Failure Analysis of Brittle Materials, 1990, Westerville, OH, The American Ceramic Society.

This classic textbook on fracture surface analysis provides an excellent pictorial overview on basic fractographic techniques. Since many dental materials are brittle in nature, the identification of fracture patterns and the crack origin may be useful to identify the principal sites of crack initiation.

Guinness Book of Records, 1994 edition, New York, Facts on File, p 168.

This book cites the highest bite force recorded in a human.

Metals Handbook, Desk Edition, Sixth Printing, 1991, Metals Park, OH, American Society for Metals.

Starting with a glossary of over 3,000 engineering terms, this handbook provides a comprehensive overview of metals and metal technology including properties and selection criteria, processing information, and testing and inspection guidelines on failure analysis, mechanical testing, nondestructive testing, metallography, fractography, and quality control.

O'Brien WJ: Dental Materials: Properties and Selection. Chicago, IL, Quintessence, 1989.

The appendix contains a complete listing of tabulated values of the physical and mechanical properties of dental materials and tooth structures.

O'Brien WJ: University of Michigan: Biomaterials Properties Database, *http://www.lib.umich.edu/dentlib/Dental_tables/*, University of Michigan, Ann Arbor, MI

This database provides an electronic reference to the following properties of dental materials: bond strength between restorative materials and tooth structures, Brinell hardness number, coefficient of friction, coefficient of thermal expansion, color range of natural teeth, colors of dental shade guides, contact angle, creep of amalgam, critical surface tension, density, dynamic modulus, elastic modulus, flow, heat of fusion, heat of reaction, Izod impact strength, index of refraction, Knoop hardness number, melting temperatures and ranges, Mohs' hardness, penetration coefficient, percent elongation, permanent deformation, Poisson's ratio, proportional limit, shear strength, Shore A hardness, solubility and disintegration in water, specific heat, strain in compression, surface free energy, surface tension, tear energy, tear strength, thermal conductivity, thermal diffusivity, transverse strength, ultimate compressive strength, ultimate tensile strength, vapor pressure, Vickers hardness, water sorption, yield strength, and zeta potential.

Stanford JW, Weigel KV, Paffenbarger GD, and Sweeney WT: Compressive properties of hard tooth tissue. J Am Dent Assoc 60:746, 1960.

Although this study data was published in 1960, it remains one of the most authoritative references on the mechanical properties of tooth structure.

Van Vlack LH: Elements of Materials Science and Engineering, 5th ed. Reading, MA, Addison-Wesley, 1985.

This text was also cited in Chapter 2 as one of the best reference books on the structure of matter, the properties of materials, and engineering.

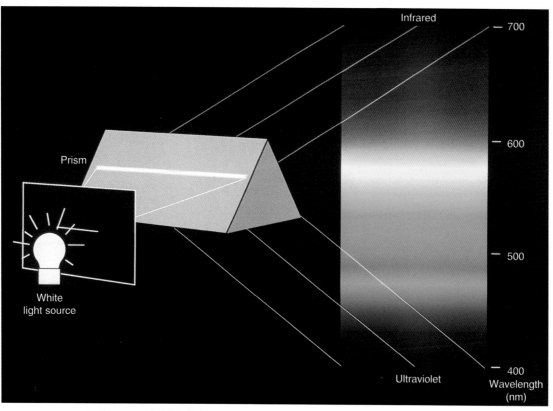

1 Spectrum of visible light ranging in wavelength from 400 nm (violet) to 700 nm (red). The most visually perceptible region of the equal energy spectrum under daylight conditions is between wavelengths of 540 and 570 nm, with a maximum value of visual perceptibility at 555 nm.

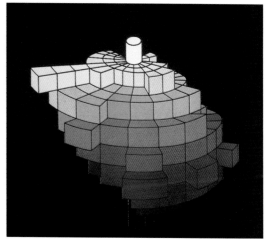

2 Color solid that is used to describe the three dimensions of color. Value increases from black at the bottom center to white at the top center. Chroma increases from the center outward, and hue changes occur in a circumferential direction. (Courtesy of Minolta Corporation, Instrument Systems Division, Ramsey, NJ.)

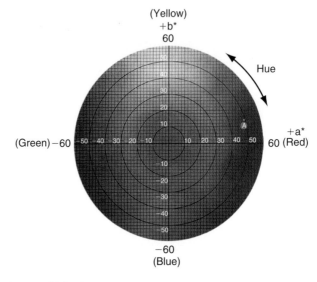

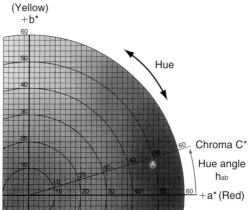

3 L*a*b* color chart showing the color of a red apple at point A (top and bottom). For this chart, the appearance is expressed by L* (value) = 42.83; a* (red-green axis) = 45.04; and b* (yellow-blue axis) = 9.52. In contrast, the color of shade A2 porcelain can be described by L* = 72.99; a* = 1.00; and b* = 14.41. (Courtesy of Minolta Corporation, Instrument Systems Division, Ramsey, NJ.)

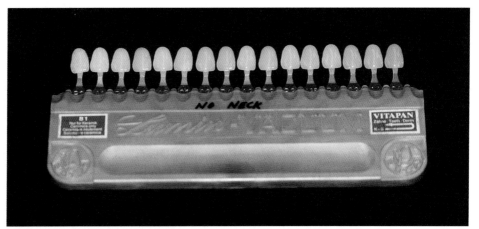

4 Dental shade guide tabs of the Vita Lumin type arranged in decreasing order of value (lighter to darker). The necks of the tooth-shaped tabs have been ground away to facilitate the selection of tooth shades.

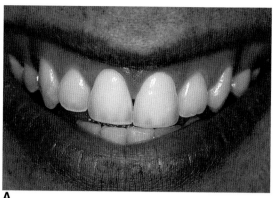 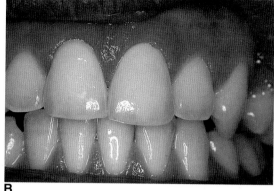

A **B**

5 **A,** Two central incisor metal-ceramic crowns with porcelain margins. The value (L*) of these crowns is higher than that of the adjacent lateral incisor teeth. **B,** Close-up view of the metal-ceramic crowns on the left.

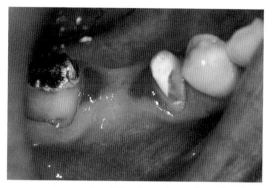

6 Example of an inflammatory response (mesial to the molar and distal to the premolar) to either the metal in a bridge or the temporary restoration in a 30-year-old female. The cause of the inflammation is not known; it could be either an allergic response or a nonspecific inflammatory response. Causes of reactions such as this are often difficult to determine with certainty. In any case, the response is caused by release of agents from the materials into the adjacent tissues. It is often suspected that reactions such as this contribute to periodontal inflammation caused by plaque, but this is difficult to prove. (Photograph courtesy of Dr. Kevin Frazier, Medical College of Georgia School of Dentistry).

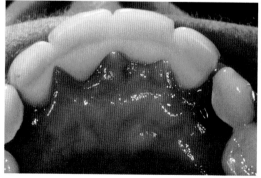

7 Example of nickel allergy around metal-ceramic crowns in a female patient. Significant inflammation is present in the lingual gingiva, especially around teeth numbers 6 (13), 7 (12), 10 (22), and 11 (23). The allergic reaction, which occurs even though the majority of the nickel alloy is covered with porcelain, is caused by release of nickel ions from the crowns into the adjacent tissues. Allergic reactions such as this are often very difficult to differentiate from gingivitis, periodontal disease, or general irritation from toxicity. (Photograph courtesy of Dr. Michael Myers, Medical College of Georgia School of Dentistry.)

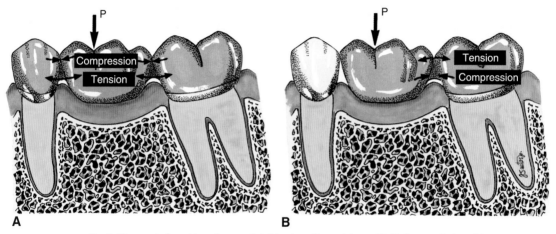

8 **A,** Stresses induced in a three-unit bridge by a flexural force (P). **B,** Stresses induced in a two-unit cantilever bridge. Note that the tensile stress develops on the gingival side of the three-unit bridge and on the occlusal side of the cantilever bridge.

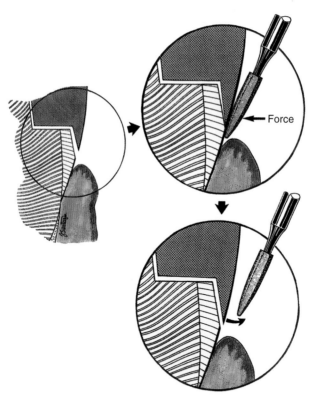

9 Schematic illustration of a procedure to close an open margin of a metal crown **(top, left)** by burnishing with a rotary instrument **(top, right).** Note that after the rotating stone is removed **(bottom),** the elastic strain has been recovered and a slight marginal discrepancy remains.

5

Solidification and Microstructure of Metals

William A. Brantley

OUTLINE
Metals
Metallic Bonds
Alloys
Solidification of Metals

KEY TERMS

Alloy—A crystalline substance with metallic properties that is composed of two or more chemical elements, at least one of which is a metal.

Dendritic microstructure—A cast alloy microstructure consisting of highly elongated crystals with a branched morphology rather than equiaxed grains.

Equiaxed grain microstructure—A cast alloy microstructure in which all of the grains have similar dimensions.

Grain—A microscopic single crystal in the microstructure of a metallic material.

Heterogeneous nucleation—Formation of solid nuclei on the mold walls or on particles within the molten metal.

Homogeneous nucleation—Formation of solid nuclei that takes place at random locations within a supercooled molten metal in a clean, inert container.

Metal—An element or alloy whose atomic structure readily loses electrons to form positively charged ions, and which exhibits metallic bonding (through a spatial extension of valence electrons), opacity, good light reflectance from a polished surface, and high electrical and thermal conductivity.

Microstructure—Structural appearance of a metal revealed by microscopic imaging of the chemically or electrolytically etched surface of a flat, polished specimen.

Nucleus—Stable cluster of atoms of a new phase that forms within a parent phase, such as during the solidification of a metal.

Phase—A homogeneous, physically distinct, and mechanically separable region of a metal microstructure.

Chapters 5, 6, 12, and 19 provide an introduction to cast **metals** and **alloys** and physical metallurgy. Although the use of cast metals has decreased in recent years because of increased consumer demand for aesthetics over durability, a knowledge of the structure and properties of cast metals and alloys is essential to ensure proper handling of these materials in clinical practice and to diagnose clinical failures of cast restorations should they occur. Furthermore, cast metals are used as copings or substructures for metal-ceramic restorations, the most common crown and bridge prostheses and the most durable of all aesthetic restorations, especially when used to restore posterior teeth. In this chapter, the principles of equilibrium **phase** formation during the solidification of cast metals are presented. Take careful note of the key terms for this chapter. These terms will facilitate the understanding of phase transformations in dental casting alloys.

CRITICAL QUESTIONS

Why are metals with similar properties found in the same region of the periodic table? What transition metals are important components in dental alloys?

METALS

In dentistry, metals represent one of the four major classes of materials used for the reconstruction of damaged or missing oral tissues. Although metals are readily distinguished from ceramics, polymers, and composites, it is not easy to define the word *metal* because of the wide variation in properties of metallic materials. *The Metals Handbook* (1992) defines a metal as "an opaque lustrous chemical substance that is a good conductor of heat and electricity and, when polished, is a good reflector of light." An alloy is a substance with metallic properties that consists of two or more chemical elements, at least one of which is a metal. Gallium and mercury, elements commonly used in dental alloys, are liquid at body temperature. However, all metals and alloys used as restorative materials in dentistry are crystalline solids. Metals can also be described in terms of qualitative and quantitative properties such as their luster, malleability, ductility, electrical conductivity, thermal conductivity, specific gravity, and ability to make a ringing sound when struck.

With the exception of pure gold foil, commercially pure (CP) titanium, and endodontic silver points, metals used for dental restorations, partial denture frameworks, orthodontic wires, and endodontic instruments are alloys. The wide variety of complex dental alloy compositions are described in Chapters 6, 17, 19, and 20 and consist of the following: (1) dental amalgams containing the major elements mercury, silver, tin, and copper; (2) noble metal alloys in which the major elements are some combination of gold, palladium, silver, and important secondary elements including copper, platinum, tin, indium, and gallium; and (3) base metal alloys with a major element of nickel, cobalt, iron, or titanium and many secondary elements that are found in the alloy compositions. Moreover, CP titanium, which is classified in four different grades, may also technically be considered as an alloy, because small percentages of other elements are allowed as impurities as specified by a standard set by the American Society for Testing and Materials (ASTM) for each grade.

A clean metallic surface exhibits a luster that is difficult to duplicate in other types of solid materials. Most metals emit a metallic sound ("ring") when they are struck, although certain silica compounds can be made to produce a similar sound. A unique characteristic of metals is that they are good thermal and electrical conductors. Compared with ceramics, polymers, and composites, metals have a high fracture toughness (K_{Ic}), that is, the ability to absorb energy and inhibit crack propagation under increasing tensile stress. This property is a measure of the resistance of a material to crack propagation. For example, K_{Ic} for most metals varies between 25 and 60 MPa·m$^{1/2}$, compared with a range of 0.75 to 5.0 MPa·m$^{1/2}$ for dental ceramics. Generally, solid metals are stronger and denser than other nonmetallic elements. Most metals also are more ductile and malleable than nonmetals, which are generally brittle. A few metals (iron, nickel, and cobalt), which are component elements of dental alloys, can be magnetized, but they can also be produced in a nonmagnetic state.

Although many metals are resistant to chemical attack in air at room temperature, some metals require alloying elements to resist tarnish and corrosion in the oral environment. For example, chromium is required as an alloying element in alloys based on iron, nickel, or cobalt to provide passivation of the alloy through the formation of a thin surface layer of chromium oxide. Noble metals (gold, iridium, osmium, palladium, platinum, rhodium, and ruthenium) are highly resistant to corrosion and oxidation and do not require alloying elements for this purpose. However, pure noble metals must be alloyed to provide sufficient resistance to deformation and fracture when they are used for cast restorations. Small additions of oxidizable elements, such as iron, tin, and indium, are added to noble alloys used for metal-ceramic prostheses to promote bonding between the ceramic veneer and the metal oxide on the metal surface.

Of the 115 elements currently listed in most recent versions of the periodic tables of the elements, about 81 can be classified as metals. (Additional elements that have been created with nuclear reactors have short half-lives.) It is of scientific interest that the metallic elements can be grouped according to density, ductility, melting point, and nobility. This indicates that the properties of metals are closely related to their valence electron configuration. The groupings of pure metal elements can be seen in Figure 5-1, the periodic chart of the elements. Several metals of importance for dental alloys are *transition elements*, in which the outermost electron subshells are occupied before the interior subshells are completely filled. The student should refer to a standard chemistry textbook to review the several series of transition elements.

To the chemist and physicist, all metallic elements have one common characteristic: the outermost electrons around the neutral atom are loosely bound. For example, the chemist knows that sodium, zinc, and aluminum atoms tend to lose their valence electrons and become positive ions in solution. Also, if two different metals form the electrodes of a galvanic cell, the more easily oxidized metal becomes the anode and supplies electrons to an external circuit.

Most metals have a "white" appearance (e.g., aluminum, silver, nickel, palladium, tin, and zinc.) However, there are slight differences in hue and chroma among the white metals. Two nonwhite metals in the periodic table are gold and copper, both of which are important components of cast dental alloys.

The properties of the pure elements do not change abruptly from metallic to nonmetallic as one moves to the right side of the periodic chart (see Figure 5-1). Rather, the boundary between metals and nonmetals is somewhat arbitrary, and the elements near the boundary exhibit characteristics of both metals and nonmetals. The elements carbon, boron, and silicon are often combined with metals to form commercially important engineering materials. Silicon and germanium are termed *semiconductors* because their electrical conductivity is intermediate between that of a metal and that of an insulator. These two elements form the basis for many electronic devices. However, in dentistry the most common casting alloys used for dental appliances and prostheses are based on a majority of one of the following elements: cobalt, gold, iron, nickel, palladium, silver, and titanium.

CRITICAL QUESTION

Why are the general physical and mechanical properties of metallic dental materials different from those of ceramic and polymeric dental materials?

Periodic chart of elements

Light metals: I A, II A · Heavy metals: III B – II B (High melting; Brittle; Ductile; Noble; Low melting) · Nonmetals: III A – VII A · Inert gases: VIII A

I A	II A	III B	IV B	V B	VI B	VII B	VIII B	VIII B	VIII B	I B	II B	III A	IV A	V A	VI A	VII A	VIII A
1 H 1.00794 $1s^1$																1 H 1.00794 $1s^1$	2 He 4.002602 $1s^2$
3 Li 6.941 (He) $2s^1$	4 Be 9.012182 (He) $2s^2$											5 B 10.811 (He) $2s^2 2p^1$	6 C 12.011 (He) $2s^2 2p^2$	7 N 14.00674 (He) $2s^2 2p^3$	8 O 15.9994 (He) $2s^2 2p^4$	9 F 18.9984032 (He) $2s^2 2p^5$	10 Ne 20.1797 (He) $2s^2 2p^6$
11 Na 22.989768 (Ne) $3s^1$	12 Mg 24.3050 (Ne) $3s^2$											13 Al 26.981539 (Ne) $3s^2 3p^1$	14 Si 28.0855 (Ne) $3s^2 3p^2$	15 P 30.973762 (Ne) $3s^2 3p^3$	16 S 32.066 (Ne) $3s^2 3p^4$	17 Cl 35.4527 (Ne) $3s^2 3p^5$	18 Ar 39.948 (Ne) $3s^2 3p^6$
19 K 39.0983 (Ar) $4s^1$	20 Ca 40.078 (Ar) $4s^2$	21 Sc 44.955910 (Ar) $3d^1 4s^2$	22 Ti 47.88 (Ar) $3d^2 4s^2$	23 V 50.9415 (Ar) $3d^3 4s^2$	24 Cr 51.9961 (Ar) $3d^5 4s^1$	25 Mn 54.93805 (Ar) $3d^5 4s^2$	26 Fe 55.847 (Ar) $3d^6 4s^2$	27 Co 58.93320 (Ar) $3d^7 4s^2$	28 Ni 58.6934 (Ar) $3d^8 4s^2$	29 Cu 63.546 (Ar) $3d^{10} 4s^1$	30 Zn 65.39 (Ar) $3d^{10} 4s^2$	31 Ga 69.723 (Ar) $3d^{10} 4s^2 4p^1$	32 Ge 72.61 (Ar) $3d^{10} 4s^2 4p^2$	33 As 74.92159 (Ar) $3d^{10} 4s^2 4p^3$	34 Se 78.96 (Ar) $3d^{10} 4s^2 4p^4$	35 Br 79.904 (Ar) $3d^{10} 4s^2 4p^5$	36 Kr 83.80 (Ar) $3d^{10} 4s^2 4p^6$
37 Rb 85.4678 (Kr) $5s^1$	38 Sr 87.62 (Kr) $5s^2$	39 Y 88.90585 (Kr) $4d^1 5s^2$	40 Zr 91.224 (Kr) $4d^2 5s^2$	41 Nb 92.90638 (Kr) $4d^4 5s^1$	42 Mo 95.94 (Kr) $4d^5 5s^1$	43 Tc (98.9063)[a] (Kr) $4d^5 5s^2$	44 Ru 101.07 (Kr) $4d^7 5s^1$	45 Rh 102.90550 (Kr) $4d^8 5s^1$	46 Pd 106.42 (Kr) $4d^{10}$	47 Ag 107.8682 (Kr) $4d^{10} 5s^1$	48 Cd 112.411 (Kr) $4d^{10} 5s^2$	49 In 114.818 (Kr) $4d^{10} 5s^2 5p^1$	50 Sn 118.710 (Kr) $4d^{10} 5s^2 5p^2$	51 Sb 121.757 (Kr) $4d^{10} 5s^2 5p^3$	52 Te 127.60 (Kr) $4d^{10} 5s^2 5p^4$	53 I 126.90447 (Kr) $4d^{10} 5s^2 5p^5$	54 Xe 131.29 (Kr) $4d^{10} 5s^2 5p^6$
55 Cs 132.90543 (Xe) $6s^1$	56 Ba 137.327 (Xe) $6s^2$	57 La* 138.9055 (Xe) $5d^1 6s^2$	72 Hf 178.49 (Xe) $4f^{14} 5d^2 6s^2$	73 Ta 180.9479 (Xe) $4f^{14} 5d^3 6s^2$	74 W 183.84 (Xe) $4f^{14} 5d^4 6s^2$	75 Re 186.207 (Xe) $4f^{14} 5d^5 6s^2$	76 Os 190.23 (Xe) $4f^{14} 5d^6 6s^2$	77 Ir 192.22 (Xe) $4f^{14} 5d^7 6s^2$	78 Pt 195.08 (Xe) $4f^{14} 5d^9 6s^1$	79 Au 196.96654 (Xe) $4f^{14} 5d^{10} 6s^1$	80 Hg 200.59 (Xe) $4f^{14} 5d^{10} 6s^2$	81 Tl 204.3833 (Xe) $4f^{14} 5d^{10} 6s^2 6p^1$	82 Pb 207.2 (Xe) $4f^{14} 5d^{10} 6s^2 6p^2$	83 Bi 208.98037 (Xe) $4f^{14} 5d^{10} 6s^2 6p^3$	84 Po (209.9828)[a] (Xe) $4f^{14} 5d^{10} 6s^2 6p^4$	85 At (209.9871)[a] (Xe) $4f^{14} 5d^{10} 6s^2 6p^5$	86 Rn (222.0176)[a] (Xe) $4f^{14} 5d^{10} 6s^2 6p^6$
87 Fr (223.0197)[a] (Rn) $7s^1$	88 Ra (226.0254)[a] (Rn) $7s^2$	89 Ac † (227.0278)[a] (Rn) $6d^1 7s^2$	104 ?[b] (261)[a] (Rn) $5f^{14} 6d^2 7s^2$	105 Ha[b] (262.114)[a] (Rn) $5f^{14} 6d^3 7s^2$													

a Value in parentheses denotes mass number of most stable known isotope.
b Name and symbols are not officially accepted. Kurchatovium, Ku, has been proposed by Russian investigators and rutherfordium, Rf, by American investigators for element 104.

Atomic weights have been updated according to Vocke RD: Atomic weights of the elements 1997. Pure Appl Chem 1999; 71:1594-1607.

Rare earth elements
*** Lanthanoid Series**

58 Ce 140.115 (Xe) $4f^2 6s^2$	59 Pr 140.90765 (Xe) $4f^3 6s^2$	60 Nd 144.24 (Xe) $4f^4 6s^2$	61 Pm (144.9127)[a] (Xe) $4f^5 6s^2$	62 Sm 105.36 (Xe) $4f^6 6s^2$	63 Eu 151.965 (Xe) $4f^7 6s^2$	64 Gd 157.25 (Xe) $4f^7 5d^1 6s^2$	65 Tb 158.92534 (Xe) $4f^9 6s^2$	66 Dy 162.50 (Xe) $4f^{10} 6s^2$	67 Ho 164.93032 (Xe) $4f^{11} 6s^2$	68 Er 167.26 (Xe) $4f^{12} 6s^2$	69 Tm 168.93421 (Xe) $4f^{13} 6s^2$	70 Yb 173.04 (Xe) $4f^{14} 6s^2$	71 Lu 174.967 (Xe) $4f^{14} 5d^1 6s^2$

Radioactive elements
† Actinoid Series

90 Th 232.0381 (Rn) $6d^2 7s^2$	91 Pa (231.03588)[a] (Rn) $5f^2 6d^1 7s^2$	92 U 238.0508 (Rn) $5f^3 6d^1 7s^2$	93 Np (237.0482)[a] (Rn) $5f^4 6d^1 7s^2$	94 Pu (244.0642) (Rn) $5f^6 7s^2$	95 Am (243.0614)[a] (Rn) $5f^7 7s^2$	96 Cm (247.0703)[a] (Rn) $5f^7 6d^1 7s^2$	97 Bk (247.0703)[a] (Rn) $5f^8 6d^1 7s^2$	98 Cf (251.0796)[a] (Rn) $5f^{10} 7s^2$	99 Es (252.083)[a] (Rn) $5f^{11} 7s^2$	100 Fm (257.0951)[a] (Rn) $5f^{12} 7s^2$	101 Md (256.094)[a] (Rn) $5f^{13} 7s^2$	102 No (259.1009)[a] (Rn) $5f^{14} 7s^2$	103 Lr (260.11)[a] (Rn) $5f^{14} 6d^1 7s^2$

Fig. 5-1. Periodic Chart of the Elements. (From Burtis, CA, and Ashwood, ER: Tietz Fundamentals of Clinical Chemistry, 5 ed. Philadelphia, WB Saunders, 2001.)

METALLIC BONDS

In addition to covalent and ionic bonds, atoms in a solid can be held together by a primary interaction known as the *metallic bond*. One of the chief characteristics of a metal is the ability to conduct heat and electricity, which is associated with the mobility of the *free electrons* present in these materials.

Since the outer-shell valence electrons can be removed easily from atoms in metals, the nuclei containing the balance of the bound electrons form positively charged ionic cores. The unbound or free valence electrons form a "cloud" or "gas," resulting in electrostatic attraction between the free electron cloud and the positively charged ionic cores. Closed-shell repulsion from the outer electrons of the ionic cores balances this attractive force at the equilibrium interatomic spacing for the metal. Metallic bonding can be contrasted with the ionic and covalent modes of bonding, in which valence electrons are localized near the parent atoms.

The free electrons act as conductors of both thermal energy and electricity. They transfer energy by moving readily from areas of higher energy to those of lower energy, under the influence of either a thermal gradient or an electrical field (potential gradient). Metallic bonding is also responsible for the luster, or mirror-reflecting property, of polished metals and their typical capability of undergoing significant permanent deformation (associated with the properties of ductility and malleability) at sufficiently high mechanical stresses. These characteristics are not found in ceramic and polymeric materials in which the atomic bonding occurs through a combination of the covalent and ionic modes. The formation of positive ions (cations) from metals in solution is a consequence of the ionic cores that are associated with metallic bonding.

ALLOYS

The use of pure metals is quite limited in dentistry. Pure metals also have limited use in engineering applications, because they are apt to be soft and, like iron, many tend to corrode rapidly. The metals most useful to civilization, along with some of their physical constants, are listed in Table 5-1. It is fortunate that metallic elements maintain their metallic behavior even when they are not pure and that they can often tolerate a considerable addition of other elements when they solidify from the liquid to the solid state.

To optimize properties, most metals commonly used in engineering and dental applications are mixtures of two or more metallic elements or, in some cases, one or more metals and/or nonmetals. Although such mixtures can be produced in a number of ways, they are generally prepared by fusion of the elements above their melting points. A solid material formed by combining a metal with one or more other metals or nonmetals is called an alloy. For example, a small amount of carbon is added to iron to form steel. A certain amount of chromium is added to iron, carbon, and other elements to form stainless steel, an alloy that is highly resistant to corrosion. As previously noted, chromium is also used to impart corrosion resistance to nickel or cobalt alloys, which comprise two of the major groups of base metal alloys used in dentistry. Chromium provides this corrosion resistance by forming a very thin, adherent surface oxide that prevents the diffusion of oxygen or other corroding species to the underlying bulk metal. Although pure gold is also highly resistant to corrosion, copper is added to gold for many dental alloys to increase their strength and resistance to permanent deformation. Early dental and engineering alloys evolved by trial and error, but currently developed special-purpose alloys are the result of technological advances.

In this chapter, the term *metal* is used all-inclusively to include alloys as well as pure metals. If the concept being discussed does not apply to both alloys and pure

| Table 5-1 | Physical Constants of the Alloy-forming Elements | | | | |

Element	Symbol	Atomic weight	Melting point (°C)	Boiling point (°C)	Density (g/cm³)	Linear coefficient of thermal expansion (10⁻⁴/°C)
Aluminum	Al	26.98	660.2	2450	2.70	0.236
Antimony	Sb	121.75	630.5	1380	6.62	0.108
Bismuth	Bi	208.98	271.3	1560	9.80	0.133
Cadmium	Cd	112.40	320.9	765	8.37	0.298
Carbon	C	12.01	3700.0	4830	2.22	0.06
Chromium	Cr	52.00	1875.0	2665	7.19	0.062
Cobalt	Co	58.93	1495.0	2900	8.85	0.138
Copper	Cu	63.54	1083.0	2595	8.96	0.165
Gold	Au	196.97	1063.0	2970	19.32	0.142
Indium	In	114.82	156.2	2000	7.31	0.33
Iridium	Ir	192.2	2454.0	5300	22.5	0.068
Iron	Fe	55.85	1527.0	3000	7.87	0.123
Lead	Pb	207.19	327.4	1725	11.34	0.293
Magnesium	Mg	24.31	650.0	1107	1.74	0.252
Mercury	Hg	200.59	−38.87	357	13.55	0.40
Molybdenum	Mo	95.94	2610.0	5560	10.22	0.049
Nickel	Ni	58.71	1453.0	2730	8.90	0.133
Palladium	Pd	106.4	1552.0	3980	12.02	0.118
Platinum	Pt	195.09	1769.0	4530	21.45	0.089
Rhodium	Rh	102.91	1966.0	4500	12.44	0.083
Silicon	Si	28.09	1410.0	2480	2.33	0.073
Silver	Ag	107.87	960.8	2216	10.49	0.197
Tantalum	Ta	180.95	2996.0	5425	16.6	0.065
Tin	Sn	118.69	231.9	2270	7.298	0.23
Titanium	Ti	47.90	1668.0	3260	4.51	0.085
Tungsten	W	183.85	3410.0	5930	19.3	0.046
Zinc	Zn	65.37	420.0	906	7.133	0.397

Data from Lyman T (ed): Metals Handbook, 8th ed., Vol. 1. Cleveland, American Society for Metals, 1964.

metals, that distinction will be clearly stated. In Chapters 19 and 20, the physical and chemical properties of alloys are discussed in some detail. However, before proceeding to alloys, a discussion of the fundamentals of how a solid is formed from the molten (liquid) state is warranted.

SOLIDIFICATION OF METALS

Pure metals, in common with other chemical elements, can be identified by their specific melting points and boiling points and by their basic physical and chemical properties. Some of these properties for metals of dental interest are tabulated in Table 5-1.

For instructional purposes, we will first consider the solidification phenomena that occur during the freezing of a pure metal in a clean container. Some aspects of the freezing of alloys are briefly considered in this chapter, but details of the solidification process for alloys are discussed in Chapter 6. If a pure metal is melted and allowed to cool to room temperature in a clean (and inert) container, and if its temperature during cooling is plotted as a function of time, a graph similar to that in Figure 5-2 results. Note that the temperature decreases steadily from point A to point B'. An increase in temperature then occurs from point B' to point B, at which time the temperature remains constant until the time indicated at point C is reached. Subsequently, the temperature of the metal decreases steadily to room temperature.

The temperature T_f, as indicated by the straight or "plateau" portion of the curve at BC, is the freezing point, or solidification temperature of the pure metal. This is also the melting point, or *fusion temperature*. During melting, the temperature remains constant. During freezing or solidification, heat is released as the metal changes from the higher-energy liquid state to the lower-energy solid state. This energy difference is the *latent heat of solidification* and is equal to the heat of fusion studied in physics courses. It is defined as the number of calories of heat liberated from 1 gram of a substance when it transforms from the liquid state to the solid state.

To interpret the curve in Figure 5-2, one must recognize that all temperatures above T_f, as indicated by the plateau BC, are associated with the molten metal. After point C, all temperatures below T_f are associated with the solid metal. The initial cooling of the liquid metal from T_f to point B' is termed *supercooling*. During the supercooling process, crystallization begins for the pure metal. Once the crystals begin to form, release of the latent heat of fusion causes the temperature to rise to T_f, where it remains until crystallization is completed at point C. It is important to emphasize that supercooling of pure metals only occurs in clean and inert containers, that is, under circumstances in which heterogeneous nucleation (to be discussed later) is not possible.

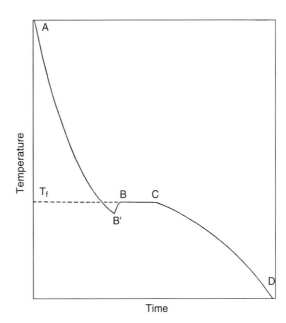

Fig. 5-2. A time-temperature cooling curve for a pure metal that illustrates supercooling.

The fusion temperatures of metals and alloys, as well as their solidification behavior, are of considerable interest to the dentist and the dental laboratory, since many metallic dental structures are prepared by casting. As will be described in Chapter 12, a wax or plastic *pattern* is prepared that is an exact replica of the dental restoration or prosthesis to be cast. Using a highly accurate dental investment, a mold is prepared from the pattern, into which the molten alloy is cast or poured under pressure. When the alloy solidifies, the original pattern is precisely reproduced as a metal *casting*. The casting procedures and materials involved are discussed in Chapters 12 and 19.

CRITICAL QUESTION

Why are dental alloys expected to begin freezing by heterogeneous nucleation, rather than by homogeneous nucleation?

Nucleus Formation

Although the surface tension of liquid metals is approximately 10 times greater than that of water, the structures of liquid metals are not much different from those of other liquids. Similar to what occurs with other liquids, metal atoms can migrate in the liquid state at a rapid rate determined by the diffusion coefficient of approximately 10^{-5} cm^2/sec. Liquid metals do not differ in structure from one another as much as do solid metals, and they exhibit a tendency towards an atomic arrangement characterized by short-range order.

As the molten metal approaches its freezing temperature (plateau BC in Fig. 5-2), its energy relationships change. Figure 5-3 provides a description of this solidification process from the viewpoint of thermodynamics. Solidification begins with the

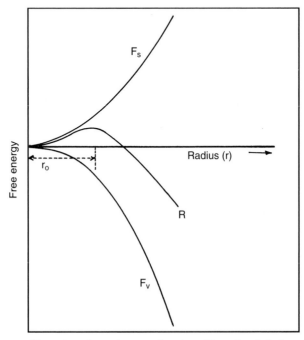

Fig. 5-3. Free energy of formation of a nucleus as a function of its radius. F_v is the volume free energy of the embryo, F_s is the free surface energy, and R is the resultant free energy.

formation of embryos in the molten metal, in which an *embryo* is a small cluster of atoms that has the same arrangement as the long-range atomic order found in the solidified metal. At temperatures above T_f (the fusion temperature), such embryos will also form spontaneously in the molten metal, but they are unstable since the liquid state has a lower free energy than the solid state.

It is important to consider the contributions of the *surface free energy* and the *volume free energy* to the overall free energy of these embryos as a function of the embryo size. The surface free energy (F_S) of an embryo is greater than its internal or bulk energy because the unequal attraction of the surface atoms tends to draw these atoms closer together, causing an increase in surface tension. Thus work is required to create the surface of an embryo, which is the basis of the surface energy contribution. For the usual assumption of spherical embryos, this surface free energy increases as the square of the embryo radius. The volume free energy contribution (F_V) is the difference in the free energies of the solid and liquid states, and the solid state has lower free energy when the temperature is below the equilibrium freezing temperature (T_f). Thus, F_V becomes increasingly negative (more energetically favorable) as the temperature of the supercooled liquid is decreased below T_f. For a given temperature below T_f, F_V varies as the third power of the spherical embryo radius.

At a specific temperature of the supercooled liquid metal, the overall or resultant (R) free energy of an embryo as a function of its radius is the sum of the surface free energy (positive) and the volume free energy change (negative) contributions. The curve for R in Figure 5-3 shows that, at small values of embryo radius, F_S is dominant and the overall free energy for the formation of the embryo is positive (energetically unfavorable). At larger values of the embryo radius, F_V becomes dominant and the overall free energy of the embryo is negative (energetically favorable). There is a critical *nucleus* size, designated as r_0 in Figure 5-3, that corresponds to the maximum point in the total free energy of the embryos as a function of radius. For an embryo of radius (r_0), the overall free energy (R) decreases with the addition of another atom and continues to decrease as the embryo grows. Hence, embryos with radii smaller than r_0 are unstable and spontaneously form and disappear in the liquid metal, whereas embryos with radii larger than r_0 are stable nuclei and continue to grow during the solidification process.

It follows that the greater the amount of supercooling, or equivalently, the greater the rate of temperature reduction below T_f, the smaller is the critical radius r_0, because the value of F_V for a given embryo size becomes increasingly negative. (The value of F_S per unit area is not greatly affected by the amount of supercooling.) This effect is shown in Figure 5-4, which illustrates the small values of r_0 that occur for the freezing of metals. Hence, an increasing number of embryos become stable as the supercooling is increased, and these embryos have reduced surface energy because of their decreased radii. If the molten metal is cooled so rapidly that solidification must occur at a much lower temperature than T_f, there is a tendency for many, very small, stable nuclei or solidification centers to form. If a single crystal is desired, little supercooling is needed, and the molten metal must be cooled very slowly. This method of nucleus formation in the bulk liquid metal is called *homogeneous nucleation*, since it occurs in the absence of some surface that would promote heterogeneous nucleation, as discussed in the next section. Homogeneous nucleation is a random process, having equal probability of occurring at any point in the molten metal.

Another method for reducing the surface energy of the embryo is for the atoms to contact the surface of some particle in the molten metal or area on the mold surface that they can wet. Because the surface area of the embryo in contact with the molten metal is thereby reduced, the surface energy is decreased, facilitating the

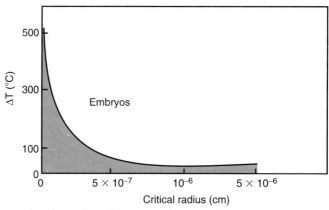

Fig. 5-4. The critical nucleus radius of copper as a function of the degree of supercooling. ΔT denotes the number of degrees of supercooling below T_f (584° C). The shaded area represents nuclei; the unshaded area represents the embryos. (From Eisenstad, M: Introduction to Mechanical Properties of Materials, 1971. Pearson Education, Inc., Upper Saddle River, New Jersey.)

formation of stable embryos. Such a process is known as *heterogeneous nucleation* because a foreign body "seeded" the nucleus. For example, if the solidifying metal is gold, very fine particles of gold sifted into the molten metal can cause nucleation. As stated previously, the mold walls or particles of dust and other impurities in the molten metal may produce heterogeneous nucleation. It is important to note that supercooling is not required for heterogeneous nucleation, which generally occurs with cast dental alloys.

CRITICAL QUESTION

Why is the grain size or the microstructural scale of a cast dental alloy significantly decreased by a substantial increase in the rate of solidification?

Solidification Modes and Effects on Properties

The crystallization of solid metals from the liquid state is controlled by atomic diffusion from the molten metal to the nuclei. The crystals do not form regularly along one plane at a time, but rather by atomic diffusion to irregular positions in the crystal structure, with structural discontinuities and imperfections constantly being formed in a random manner.

Characteristically, a pure metal crystallizes from nuclei in a pattern that often resembles the branches of a tree, yielding elongated crystals that are called *dendrites*. In three dimensions, their general appearance is similar to that of the two-dimensional frost crystals that form on a windowpane in the winter. After their nucleation, typically at mold walls for castings, dendrites grow during the solidification of pure metals by the mechanism of *thermal supercooling*. Extensions or elevated areas (termed *protuberances*) form spontaneously on the advancing front of the solidifying metal and grow into regions of *negative temperature gradient*. (Macroscopically, a positive temperature gradient exists for the solidifying metal, in which the temperature increases from a minimum value at the mold walls to a maximum value in the molten metal at the center of the mold.) In these regions of negative temperature gradient, the temperature is higher in the liquid adjacent to the frozen metal because of the latent heat of fusion released during freezing. The protuberances rapidly grow in the adjacent supercooled regions that lie farther away in the molten metal; growth is along specific crystallographic directions. The latent heat released by the solidifying metal also lowers the amount of supercooling at the liquid-solid interface, hindering growth in regions adjacent to the protuberances and resulting in separated, highly elongated crystals. A similar growth mechanism subsequently occurs at lateral sites along the protuberances and later at lateral sites along the secondary branches, resulting in the three-dimensional dendritic structure.

Dendrites in cast alloys form by a different mechanism of *constitutional supercooling*, which will be discussed in the next chapter. Nonetheless, at this point it is worthwhile to consider the **microstructures** and implications of dendrites in cast dental alloys. Figure 5-5 shows the dendritic structure of an as-cast palladium-based alloy that has been polished and etched. The light areas are the dendrites, and the dark areas are interdendritic regions. *Dendritic microstructures* are not generally desirable for cast dental alloys, since the interdendritic regions can serve as sites for facile crack propagation. Figure 5-6 shows the room-temperature fracture surface of a cast tensile test specimen prepared from a base metal alloy for removable partial denture frameworks, where such crack propagation is evident in the distinctive dendritic microstructure. Another example occurs with the cooling of some high–palladium-content alloys that have a dendritic as-cast microstructure. *Hot tears* (microcracks) can form at elevated temperatures in thin areas of castings prepared from these alloys, where there is insufficient bulk metal to resist the stresses imposed by the stronger casting investment, and these cracks will degrade the mechanical properties of the restorations. To avoid hot tears,

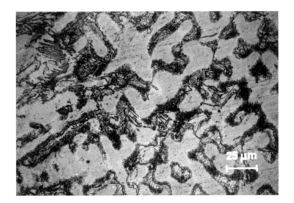

Fig. 5-5. Optical microscopic image of a polished and etched palladium-based alloy with a dendritic as-cast microstructure. (From Carr AB, and Brantley WA. New high-palladium casting alloys: Part 1. Overview and initial studies. Int J Prosthodont 4:265, 1991. Reproduced with permission from Quintessence Publishing Company, Inc.)

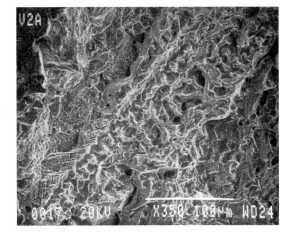

Fig. 5-6. SEM image of the fracture surface of a cast base metal alloy for removable partial denture frameworks, showing the pattern of crack propagation in the pronounced dendritic microstructure. (From Bridgeport DA, Brantley WA, and Herman PF. Cobalt-chromium and nickel-chromium alloys for removable prosthodontics, Part 1. Mechanical properties of as-cast alloys. J Prosthodont 2:144, 1993. Reproduced with permission.)

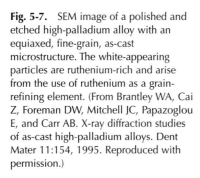

Fig. 5-7. SEM image of a polished and etched high-palladium alloy with an equiaxed, fine-grain, as-cast microstructure. The white-appearing particles are ruthenium-rich and arise from the use of ruthenium as a grain-refining element. (From Brantley WA, Cai Z, Foreman DW, Mitchell JC, Papazoglou E, and Carr AB. X-ray diffraction studies of as-cast high-palladium alloys. Dent Mater 11:154, 1995. Reproduced with permission.)

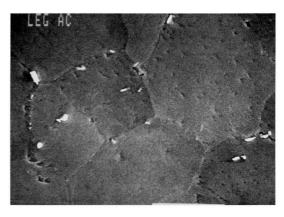

castings need to have adequate thickness, and an alloy should be selected that has an **equiaxed grain structure** in the as-cast condition, rather than a dendritic structure. A lower burnout temperature (Chapter 12) may also be advantageous, because the alloy will have greater elevated-temperature strength at the lower mold temperature.

Although dental base metal casting alloys typically solidify with a dendritic microstructure, most noble metal casting alloys solidify with an *equiaxed polycrystalline microstructure*, such as that shown in Figure 5-7. The microstructural features in this figure are called *grains*, and the term *equiaxed* means that the three dimensions of each grain are similar, in contrast to the elongated morphology of the dendrites in Figures 5-5 and 5-6. The grains in Figure 5-7 have dimensions ranging from approximately 10 to 20 μm (microns), where 1 μm = 10^{-6} m or 10^{-3} mm.

A highly schematic representation of the development of an equiaxed grain structure in two dimensions is shown in Figure 5-8. Solidification starts from isolated nuclei in the molten metal, and these crystals gradually become larger by the aggregation of atoms. Progressively, the crystals grow toward one another. When the adjacent crystals eventually impinge, their growth is stopped, as diagrammed in Figure 5-8, *E*. Figure 5-8, *F*, is a schematic illustration of the resulting microstructure, after the surface of the solidified metal has been polished and etched. It can be seen that each grain is a microscopic single crystal that has a different orientation from adjacent grains. It is important to appreciate the highly schematic nature of Figure 5-8, *E*. For example, with a grain size of 20 μm and a separation of 2 Å (0.2 nm) between atomic planes, the width of a grain would span 100,000 atomic planes.

Two other important aspects of grain boundaries must also be emphasized. First, from Figure 5-8, *E*, it is evident that a given atomic plane is discontinuous at a grain boundary. As discussed in Chapter 20, this has enormous significance for the movement of dislocations on their slip planes during the permanent deformation of ductile dental alloys. The dislocations cannot cross from one grain into an adjacent grain, and they will subsequently pile up at the grain boundaries. When this occurs, further deformation in these regions will require greater stress. Second, from Figure 5-8, *E*, it is also evident that the grain boundary regions are the final sites to undergo freezing for a molten metal that forms an equiaxed grain structure. Consequently, low-melting phases, precipitates, and porosity are typically found at the grain boundaries of cast dental alloys. The same principle is also applicable in the interdendritic regions of dental alloys with as-cast dendritic microstructures. These regions are the final microstructural areas to undergo freezing, and a complex interdendritic structure can be seen for a palladium-based alloy in Figure 5-5.

As previously noted for Figures 5-5 and 5-7, the microstructure of a metal can be revealed by polishing the surface and etching with an appropriate chemical solution

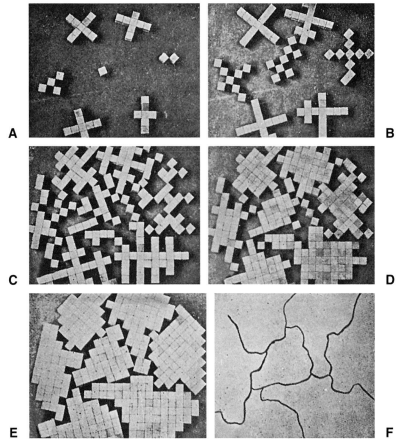

Fig. 5-8. Stages in the formation of metallic grains during the solidification of a molten metal. (From Rosenhain W: Introduction to Physical Metallurgy, 3rd ed. London, Constable and Co, Ltd, 1935. Reproduced with permission.)

and technique. A series of successively finer abrasives (typically aluminum oxide or silicon carbide) are employed. For the initial grinding stages, abrasives embedded in polishing papers are used; the later polishing stages are performed with slurries of water and abrasive powders. Generally, for the final polishing stage, an abrasive with a particle size of 0.05 μm is used, since the width of the resulting scratches will be about an order of magnitude smaller than the wavelength of visible light, and thus they will not be visible by eye or in the optical microscope. The chemical or electrolytic etching medium preferentially removes atoms and creates grooves at the grain boundaries, because these atoms are in a less regular arrangement and have higher energy compared with atoms in the interiors of grains. As a consequence, the grain boundaries have a darker appearance than the bulk grains in the optical microscope because of light scattering by these grooves. In an analogous manner, differences in electron scattering by the grain boundaries and bulk grains in etched metals result in a topographic contrast when viewed in a scanning electron microscope.

CRITICAL QUESTION

How does the grain size affect the properties of cast dental alloys?

Grain Refinement and Grain Size

Modern dental noble metal casting alloys generally have *equiaxed fine-grain microstructures* because of the incorporation of small amounts of iridium, ruthenium, or rhenium as grain-refining elements (generally less than about 1 wt% for palladium alloys and much smaller quantities for gold alloys). Although the precise mechanism for grain refinement is uncertain, these three elements have much higher melting temperatures than palladium and gold, and elemental analyses based on transmission electron microscopy have shown that the microstructures of high–palladium-content alloys contain pure ruthenium particles. The grain size is expected to be important for noble metal casting alloys, since the yield strength of engineering alloys has been found to vary inversely with the square root of grain size (Hall-Petch equation). It should be noted that the formation of fine grain sizes in noble metal alloys may be aided by the rapid solidification conditions that occur during dental casting, as discussed in Chapters 6 and 12, because the time during which solidification occurs would be insufficient for the growth of large crystals. The compositional uniformity and corrosion resistance of a cast dental alloy will be superior for a fine grain size, because there is less opportunity for microsegregation, as discussed in the next chapter.

The linear intercept method can be used to estimate the grain size of an alloy. Random lines of known length, such as 10 cm, are placed on a series of photomicrographs obtained at a standardized magnification for the polished and etched alloy. The total number of grain boundary intersection points, divided by the total length of the lines used, multiplied by the magnification, yields the number of grain boundaries intercepted per centimeter. The reciprocal of this number is used as a measure of the grain size, which is usually expressed in microns.

For dental base metal casting alloys, in which nickel, cobalt, iron and titanium are the principal elements, the use of grain-refining elements has not been reported, and these alloys typically have dendritic as-cast microstructures. It is important to distinguish between mechanisms of dendrite formation in cast pure metals and alloys that do not contain grain-refining elements. Dendrites form during the freezing of pure metals by *thermal supercooling*. During this process, crystals are nucleated at the investment walls and dendrites grow perpendicular to the walls toward the mold center along the directions of heat flow. In contrast, dendrites in alloys form by the mechanism of *constitutional supercooling*. Additional details on this process are presented in Chapter 6.

SELECTED READINGS

Brantley WA, Cai Z, Vermilyea SG, Papazoglou E et al: Effects of solidification conditions and heat treatment on the microstructure and Vickers hardness of Pd-Cu-Ga dental alloys. Cells Mater 6:127, 1996.

This article shows that the incidence of hot tears in a high–palladium alloy with a dendritic as-cast microstructure is much greater when the alloy is quenched rather than bench-cooled. The path of crack propagation is between adjacent inter-dendritic regions.

Carr AB, Cai Z, Brantley WA, and Mitchell JC: New high-palladium casting alloys: Part 2. Effects of heat treatment and burnout temperature. Int J Prosthodont 6:233, 1993.

This article discusses the formation of hot tears in a high-palladium alloy with a dendritic as-cast microstructure and the potential role of burnout temperature on their formation.

Metals Handbook, Desk Edition. Metals Park, OH, American Society of Metals, 1992.

A comprehensive reference book on the structure, properties, and processing of metals. This book also describes testing methods for metals and provides and an excellent review of fractographic analysis procedures for the study of fractured metals.

Nielsen JP, and Tuccillo JJ: Grain size in cast gold alloys. J Dent Res 45:964, 1966.

Although there may be uncertainty about the suggested homogeneous nucleation mechanism, this is the classic reference on grain refinement in dental gold alloys.

Reed-Hill RE, and Abbaschian R: Physical Metallurgy Principles, 3rd ed. Boston, PWS Publishing, 1994. (Order through Thomson Learning, Florence, KY. ISBN/ISSN 0-534-92173-6.)

An excellent textbook on physical metallurgy that discusses the solidification of metals and alloys and the formation of equiaxed polycrystalline and dendritic microstructures.

Periodic Table of the Elements web sites:
http://www.shef.ac.uk/~chem/web-elements/
http://chemserv.bc.edu/web-elements/web-elements-home.html
http://www.chemicalelements.com

6

Equilibrium Phases in Cast Alloys

William A. Brantley

OUTLINE

Classification of alloys

Solid Solutions

Constitution or Equilibrium Phase Diagrams

Eutectic Alloys

Physical Properties

Peritectic Alloys

Solid State Reactions

Other Binary Systems

Ternary and Higher-Order Alloy Systems

KEY TERMS

Alloy system—All possible alloyed combinations of two or more elements, at least one of which is a metal. For example, the gold-silver system includes all possible alloys of gold and silver, varying from 100% gold to 100% silver.

Binary alloy—An alloy that contains two chemical elements.

Coring—A microstructural condition in which a composition gradient exists between the center and the surface of a structural component such as a dendrite, grain, or particle.

Phase diagram (constitution diagram)—A graph of the phase field limits as a function of temperature and composition. Phase diagrams usually represent equilibrium conditions or approximations of equilibrium conditions, although metastable conditions and phases may also be shown.

Quaternary alloy—An alloy that contains four chemical elements.

Solid solution (metallic)—A solid crystalline phase containing two or more elements, at least one of which is a metal, that are intimately combined at the atomic level.

Ternary alloy—An alloy that contains three chemical elements.

The production of dental prostheses made with a core or framework of metal usually involves the casting of a molten pure metal or an **alloy** into a refractory mold. The mold is formed around a wax or plastic pattern of the prosthesis that will be produced from the cast metal. The wax or plastic is subsequently eliminated at an elevated burnout temperature, and the molten metal is cast into the mold under centrifugal force. Additional details on casting methodology and the solidification process are described in Chapters 12 and 5, respectively.

CRITICAL QUESTION

Why should a dentist or lab technician consider both the weight percent and the atomic percent of potentially toxic elements when selecting an alloy for dental prostheses?

Most alloys solidify over a range of temperatures in which solid and liquid **phases** coexist, rather than at a single temperature as does a pure metal. The presence of atoms of more than one metal may also cause certain reactions in the solid state that cannot occur with a pure metal; these reactions directly affect the properties of the alloy. When observed with the optical microscope, the grains of such alloys may resemble those of pure metals.

To specify a particular alloy, it is necessary to list the elements contained in the alloy and the amount of each element that is present. The concentration of each element can be expressed as a weight percentage (wt%) or as an atomic percentage (at%). As an example, the $AuCu_3$ phase, which can form during slow cooling of molten Au-Cu alloys in a specific composition range, contains 51 wt% gold and 49 wt% Cu, but on an atomic basis, it contains 25 at% gold and 75 at% Cu. Unless stated otherwise, compositions of dental alloys are usually specified in weight percent.

Another important example of the difference between atomic and weight percentages occurs with predominantly nickel-based alloys that contain an apparently small amount (1.8 wt%) of beryllium, a relatively toxic element. However, these nickel-chromium-molybdenum-beryllium alloys contain a much larger atomic proportion of beryllium (approximately 11 at%). For alloys with elements that differ considerably in atomic weight, the weight percentage composition and atomic percentage composition will differ substantially. Usually, the properties of an alloy relate more directly to the atomic percentage rather than the weight percentage of each element.

From a metallurgical standpoint, an alloy *phase* is any homogeneous, physically distinct, and mechanically separable portion of the **microstructure**. The existence of matter in three different physical states or phases—solid, liquid, or gas—is a familiar concept. However, in metallurgy, more than one phase is frequently present in the solid state. For example, grains (crystals) of two or more different compositions, which are mechanically separable, may be present in an alloy. As described in Chapter 5, the region between any two grains is called a grain boundary.

Polycrystalline metals and alloys generally never attain true time-invariant, minimal energy *equilibrium* conditions in the solid state because of very slow solid-state atomic diffusion rates and other factors. For example, if an alloy has been cooled very rapidly from a high temperature at which the rate of atomic diffusion is considerable (the situation for dental casting conditions, as described in Chapter 12), an unstable structure may appear to be stable at room temperature. Nevertheless, in this chapter, equilibrium conditions will be assumed unless stated otherwise. Equilibrium conditions are approached in the research laboratory when there is very slow cooling with prolonged times at temperatures sufficiently high to allow ample opportunity for solid-state diffusion to occur.

CLASSIFICATION OF ALLOYS

Cast dental alloys can be classified according to the following five categories: (1) use (all-metal inlays, crowns and bridges, metal-ceramic prostheses, posts and cores, removable partial dentures, and implants), (2) major elements (gold-based, palladium-based, silver-based, nickel-based, cobalt-based, and titanium-based), (3) nobility (high noble, noble, and predominantly base metal), (4) principal three elements (such as Au-Pd-Ag, Pd-Ag-Sn, Ni-Cr-Be, Co-Cr-Mo, Ti-Al-V, and Fe-Ni-Cr), and (5) dominant phase system (single phase [isomorphous], eutectic, peritectic, and intermetallic).

If two metals are present, a **binary alloy** is formed; if three or four metals are present, **ternary** and **quaternary alloys**, respectively, are produced, and so on. As the number of metals increases beyond two, the alloy structure becomes increasingly complex. Consequently, only binary alloys will be studied in detail in this chapter.

The simplest alloy is a **solid solution**, in which atoms of two metals are located in the same crystal structure, such as face-centered cubic (fcc), body-centered cubic (bcc), and hexagonal close-packed (hcp). When observed with the optical microscope, the grains of such alloys may resemble those of pure metals. The structure may appear to be entirely homogeneous since only one phase is formed during solidification. For example, most gold alloys used in clinical dentistry are predominantly solid solutions, although they contain more than two metals.

When two metals are not completely soluble in each other, more complex **alloy systems** result, and the solid state is a mixture of two or more phases. Important examples are the *eutectic alloys* and *peritectic alloys*, which will be discussed later. *Intermediate phases* can exist, which have a range of compositions different from the solid solutions formed by the nearly pure metals. In some alloy systems *intermetallic compounds* that have a fixed composition can also be formed.

SOLID SOLUTIONS

By far the greatest number of alloys that are useful for dental restorations are based on solid solutions. A liquid solution of sugar and water is a homogeneous system in which molecules of sugar diffuse and intermingle at random with those of water. The same is true of a molten solution of silver in palladium. If this solution is frozen, the silver atoms will be distributed randomly in the face-centered cubic structure of solid palladium, thereby forming a solid solution. Because the silver atoms enter into the crystal structure of palladium, the system is not mechanically separable, and only one solid phase is formed. However, the atoms of silver may not be randomly located in the palladium crystal structure because of the rapid temperature decrease during the dental casting procedure. To produce a homogeneous structure, heat treatment at appropriately high temperatures and for suitably long periods of time promotes sufficient solid-state diffusion so that the distribution of palladium and silver atoms becomes uniform.

Solutes and Solvents

When sugar is dissolved in water, the water is referred to as the solvent and the sugar as the solute. When two metals are mutually soluble in the solid state, the solvent is that metal whose crystal structure persists. In palladium-silver alloys, the two metals are completely soluble in all proportions and the same type of crystal structure occurs throughout the alloy system. In such a case, the solvent is defined as the metal whose atoms occupy the majority of the total number of positions in the crystal structure.

The atomic arrangement within binary solid solutions may be of several types. In the *substitutional solid solution*, the atoms of the solute metal occupy the positions in the crystal structure that are normally occupied by the solvent atoms in the pure metal. For a palladium-silver alloy in which palladium is the solvent metal, the silver atoms replace the palladium atoms randomly in the crystal structure. These concepts can be extended to solid solutions in which atoms of several solute metals are randomly located in the crystal structure of the solvent metal.

Another type of solid solution of considerable importance is the *interstitial solid solution*. In this case, the solute atoms are present in random positions (interstices) between the atoms in the crystal structure of the solvent metal. This type of solid solution ordinarily requires that the solute atoms be much smaller in diameter than the solvent atoms, and these solid solutions usually are limited to relatively small concentrations of solute. The interstitial solid solution of carbon in iron is important, since it forms the basis for the family of engineering alloys called carbon steels. The commercially pure (CP) titanium alloys, which are important for implant and restorative dentistry, consist of high-purity (99 wt% or higher) titanium, with oxygen, carbon, nitrogen and hydrogen atoms dissolved interstitially.

In gold-copper substitutional solid solutions, the solvent and solute atoms have some affinity for each other at low temperatures, such that a random arrangement of gold and copper atoms represents a higher energy state than if the atoms were situated (ordered) to have like nearest neighbors. For such an alloy, if sufficient time is available, small movements of the gold and copper atoms may cause an ordering of the solid solution that exists at elevated temperatures, where these atom species are randomly located. Thus at high temperatures, gold-copper alloys are *disordered solid solutions* with a face-centered cubic crystal structure (Fig. 6-1, *A*). If an alloy containing 50.2 wt% gold and 49.8 wt% copper is allowed to cool slowly below 400° C (752° F), the $AuCu_3$ structure forms, in which the gold atoms are located at the corners of the face-centered cubic (fcc) unit cells and the copper atoms are located at the centers of the faces (Fig. 6-1, *B*). This unit cell is equivalent to $AuCu_3$, since two adjacent unit cells share each of the six copper atoms at the centers of each of the six faces of the cube and eight unit cells share each of the eight gold corner atoms. This *ordered structure* is termed a *superlattice*. The structure of $AuCu_3$ is simple cubic, rather than fcc, because of the loss of symmetry in the gold crystal structure caused by the presence of the copper atoms.

Conditions for Solid Solubility

In any substitutional solid solution, the average distance between the solvent atoms changes according to the size of the solute atom species, and the entire crystal structure may be expanded or contracted, sometimes nonuniformly. Generally, however,

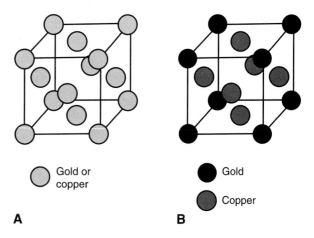

Fig. 6-1. Structure of $AuCu_3$. In a unit cell of the face-centered cubic crystal structure for a disordered gold-copper substitutional solid solution, **A,** the positions of the gold atoms cannot be distinguished from the positions of the copper atoms. In the superlattice or ordered arrangement, **B,** the gold atoms are situated at the corners, and the copper atoms are on the faces of the cube.

Gold or copper

Gold

Copper

A

B

such changes in atomic distances are not great because one of the primary requisites for two or more metals to form solid solutions is that their atomic diameters be similar.

At least four factors determine the extent of solid solubility of metals: atom size, valence, chemical affinity, and chemical structure.

Atom Size. If the sizes of two metallic atoms differ by less than approximately 15% (first noted by Hume-Rothery), they possess a favorable size factor for solid solubility. If the size factor is greater than 15%, multiple phases appear during solidification. No metal is completely lacking in solid solubility with another metal, and even if this solid solubility is only a fraction of one percent, such limited solubility can be of importance in certain instances.

Valence. Metals of the same valence and size are more likely to form extensive solid solutions than are metals of different valences. The valence difference between the solvent and solute atoms determines the electron-to-atom (e/a) ratio for the alloy, and a given alloy structure typically can tolerate only a small change in the value of e/a before transforming to a different, lower energy structure. As an example, for alloys of copper with metals of higher valence, the maximum solid solubility decreases as the valence of the solute metal increases.

Chemical Affinity. When two metals exhibit a high degree of chemical affinity, they tend to form an intermetallic compound upon solidification rather than a solid solution. As has been noted for gold and copper, metals with some affinity can form ordered structures at lower temperatures.

Crystal Structure. Only metals with the same type of crystal structure can form a complete series of solid solutions. For example, the important gold-copper and palladium-silver alloy systems for noble metal prostheses form a continuous series of solid solutions, in which all alloys have the fcc structure.

Although the diameter of the copper atom differs as much as 12% from that of the gold, silver, palladium, and platinum atoms in dental gold casting alloys for all-metal prostheses (Table 6-1), copper is an important component and provides significant strengthening for these alloys. As will be discussed later, copper forms a limited series of solid solutions with silver. There is complete solid solubility of copper in gold and palladium at high temperatures. Upon cooling to an appropriate

Table 6-1	Atomic Diameters of Metals of Dental Interest	
Metal	**Atomic diameter (angstroms)**	**Crystal structure**
Gold	2.882	Face-centered cubic
Platinum	2.775	Face-centered cubic
Palladium	2.750	Face-centered cubic
Silver	2.888	Face-centered cubic
Copper	2.556	Face-centered cubic
Tin	3.016	Body-centered tetragonal
Zinc	2.665	Close-packed hexagonal
Silicon	2.351	Diamond cubic

From Lyman T (ed): Metals Handbook, 8th ed., Vol. I. Cleveland, American Society for Metals, 1964.

lower temperature range, ordering takes place for some gold-copper compositions, as already discussed for the formation of the $AuCu_3$ superlattice.

According to Table 6-1, the difference between the atomic diameters of silver and tin is only approximately 4%. However, these two metals differ in valence and have different crystal structures, and it will be shown in Chapter 17 that there is limited solid solubility for tin in silver. As the tin content increases, an intermetallic compound (Ag_3Sn) forms, which is an important constituent of dental amalgams.

Physical Properties of Solid Solutions

Whenever a solute atom substitutes for a solvent atom in the crystal structure of a metal, the different size of the solute atom results in a localized distortion, and the movement of dislocations becomes more difficult, as discussed in Chapter 20. The strength, proportional limit, and hardness are increased, and the ductility is usually decreased. Thus, solid solution alloying can be a highly efficient means of strengthening a metal. The general effects of this *solid solution strengthening* are the same as those achieved with the mechanical deformation by cold working (strain hardening) that will be discussed in Chapter 20.

For example, pure gold is not an acceptable material for low–stress-bearing restorations unless it is strain-hardened, as in the compaction of direct-filling gold. Although pure gold in the cast condition is also too weak for restorations, if as little as 5 wt% copper is alloyed with gold, the latter loses practically none of its ability to resist tarnish and corrosion, yet adequate strength and hardness are imparted so that the gold-copper alloy can be used for the casting of small inlays. It will be seen in Chapter 19 that dental gold casting alloys have more complex compositions, particularly those used for larger inlays, onlays, crowns, and endodontic posts, for which much greater strength is necessary.

The solid solution strengthening of an alloy is increased with greater concentrations of the solute atoms and with increasingly dissimilar sizes of the solvent and solute atoms, provided that the solid solubility limit is not exceeded. Generally, for two metals that form a continuous series of solid solutions, the maximal hardness is reached at approximately 50 at% of each metal. As would be expected from a solid solution that impedes dislocation movement (see Chapter 20), the ductility of the alloy usually decreases progressively as the strength and hardness increase.

CRITICAL QUESTION

Why is the study of binary phase diagrams important, even though dental alloys contain more than three elements and conditions during solidification and cooling after casting are far removed from equilibrium?

CONSTITUTION OR EQUILIBRIUM PHASE DIAGRAMS

Constitution or equilibrium **phase diagrams** are of central importance to the metallurgy of alloys, since they show the phases that are present in an alloy system for different compositions and temperatures. For engineering materials, these plots are simply referred to as phase diagrams. With the restriction of a two-dimensional format, only binary phase diagrams for alloy systems prepared from two component metals can be completely presented. For ternary alloy systems, a three-dimensional phase diagram would be required to completely portray variations in temperature and the compositions of two component metals, and phase diagrams for alloy systems with more than three component metals can be exceedingly complex.

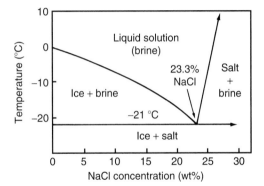

Fig. 6-2. Solubility of NaCl in brine **(right upward-sloping line)** and solubility of ice in brine **(left curve)**. (Redrawn from Van Vlack, L H: Elements of Materials Science and Engineering, 4th ed. Reading, MA, Addison-Wesley Publishing Co, 1980, p 332. Used with permission of the publisher.)

As discussed in more detail later, there are useful strategies for displaying the relevant phase information for these multicomponent alloy systems. A more fundamental problem exists when one extrapolates predictions of compositions and phases from a phase diagram, which portrays equilibrium relationships, to a cast dental alloy in which solidification and cooling to room temperature occur under conditions far removed from equilibrium. Nonetheless, binary phase diagrams are useful for understanding the structure of dental alloys and can provide microstructural predictions when some cast dental alloys are subjected to heat treatment.

We introduce the concept of a constitution or equilibrium phase diagram by using the table salt-water system (Fig. 6-2). The dissolution of NaCl in water to form liquid brine is the starting point for the discussion. It is observed that at a particular temperature, a solubility or miscibility limit exists on how much salt can be dissolved in brine before salt crystals begin to settle out. Note that a pure single-phase liquid (brine) becomes a two-phase solid-liquid mixture (salt and brine) as the solubility limit of salt in water is exceeded. If the temperature of the system is increased, the amount of salt that can be dissolved in water increases. If the temperature is decreased sufficiently, another solid phase (ice) eventually appears. Although pure water solidifies to form ice at 0° C, it is well known that the addition of salt to water will depress its freezing point. This information for the salt-water system can be assembled as a "map," showing what phases are present at a particular temperature and composition (amount of salt).

It should be emphasized that this diagram assumes equilibrium conditions have been established, a reasonable assumption for diffusion in this particular system. Figure 6-2 can be subdivided into four regions: one single-phase liquid region (brine); two liquid-solid, two-phase regions (ice plus brine and salt plus brine); and one solid-solid, two-phase region (ice plus salt). As the temperature of a salt solution is lowered for salt concentrations less than 23.3%, almost pure water freezes in the solution to form the ice-brine mixture. Note that a liquid solution containing 23.3% salt freezes directly at −21° C to yield the ice-salt mixture, without passing through an intervening two-phase region.

Now consider a solid solution alloy system of pure metal A and pure metal B. As previously noted, such a system is composed of all possible combinations of A and B, ranging from 100 wt% A to 100 wt% B. For this solid solution system, A and B are completely soluble at all compositions in both the solid and liquid states.

Cooling curve experiments such as the ones discussed in the previous chapter will now be performed on a series of alloys from the A-B system as follows: (1) 100% A; (2) 80% A–20% B; (3) 60% A–40% B; (4) 40% A–60% B; (5) 20% A–80% B; and (6) 100% B. The resulting cooling curves are shown in Figure 6-3, *A*. Curves 1 and 6 for pure metals A and B are familiar from the previous chapter, showing the usual

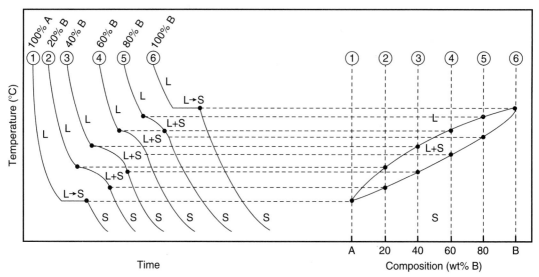

Fig. 6-3. Determination of a phase diagram by thermal analysis. **A,** Cooling curves of six alloys of various compositions are determined experimentally. Temperature is shown on the vertical axis as a function of time on the horizontal axis. **B,** The fusion temperature and the liquidus and solidus temperatures are then plotted as a function of composition to form the phase diagram. (With permission from Richman, M: An Introduction to the Science of Metals. Waltham, MA, Blaisdell Publishing Co, 1967, p 213.)

situation of isothermal freezing with essentially no supercooling. Curves 2 through 5 illustrate that solid solution alloys do not have a single freezing temperature, but instead solidify over a temperature range. The region labeled (L + S) on each cooling curve is a two-phase region composed of a liquid and a solid, where the alloy is undergoing solidification.

These cooling curves can now be used to determine the equilibrium phase diagram for the A-B alloy system. The temperature at which the first solid forms (called the *liquidus temperature*) for each composition is determined from the cooling curves in Figure 6-3, *A* and is then plotted on a temperature-composition diagram. Similarly, the temperature at which the last liquid solidifies (called the *solidus temperature*) is determined and plotted on the same diagram. When these points are connected with smooth curves, the *equilibrium phase diagram* (Fig. 6-3, *B*) results.

The upper curve in Figure 6-3, *B*, is called the *liquidus*, since the alloys in this system are entirely liquid for temperatures and compositions above this curve. The lower curve is called the *solidus*, since the alloys are entirely solid for temperatures and compositions below this curve. The region between the two curves is the two-phase liquid plus solid region, defined by the range of temperatures in which alloy compositions are undergoing freezing.

Consider now an alloy system that has considerable dental interest and resembles the theoretical system just described. Figure 6-4 presents the palladium-silver phase diagram. These metals exhibit complete solubility in both liquid and solid states. Note the liquid, liquid-solid, and solid regions, separated by the liquidus and solidus curves.

Interpretation of the Phase Diagram

As an illustration of how this phase diagram can be used, consider the cooling of an alloy composition of 65% palladium and 35% silver, as indicated by the dashed line

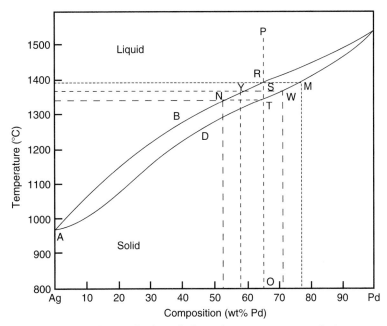

Fig. 6-4. Equilibrium phase diagram for the palladium-silver system (wt%). Only the percentage composition for palladium is given; the percentage composition for silver is determined by subtracting the palladium composition from 100.

PO, which is perpendicular to the base line or horizontal composition axis (see Fig. 6-4). If the point on the line PO that corresponds to the temperature of 1500° C (2732° F) is considered, the alloy is clearly in the liquid state.

When the temperature decreases to approximately 1400° C (2552° F), the vertical line PO touches the liquidus curve at point R, and the first solid forms. However, the composition of these first crystals is different from the 65% palladium and 35% silver parent alloy. To determine the composition of the first solid that forms, follow *tie line* RM from point R on the liquidus curve, parallel to the base line, until it intersects the solidus curve at point M. Now project this point of intersection to the base line to determine that the composition of the first solid is 77 wt% palladium, compared with the composition of 65% wt% palladium for the liquid phase at point R.

When the temperature decreases to approximately 1370° C (2498° F), denoted by point S, the alloy is about midway through its freezing range. The compositions of the solid and liquid may be determined by drawing tie line YW and locating its points of intersection with the solidus and liquidus curves. The approximate composition of the liquid is now 57% palladium, given by the projection of point Y on the base line, and that of the solid is 71% palladium, determined by projecting point W to the base line. At the temperature corresponding to point T (approximately 1340° C or 2444° F), the last portion of liquid that solidifies has the composition of 52% palladium (point N). The solid phase is 65% palladium (point T). In the absence of grain-refining elements, the alloy will freeze in a dendritic structure, as described in the Chapter 5.

When the temperature decreases below point T, the 65% palladium alloy is entirely solid. The chemical composition of any phase in the palladium-silver system at any temperature can be obtained in a similar manner. When an alloy composition is undergoing equilibrium solidification, the percentages of the liquid and solid phases present at a given temperature can be calculated by the *lever rule*. As an illustrative example, at 1370° C (2498° F) the amount of liquid phase is given by the quotient of segment length SW and the length of the entire tie line YW, expressed as a percentage, or approximately 44%. The percentage of the solid phase at this temperature under equilibrium conditions is therefore approximately 56%. Alternatively, the percentage of solid phase could have been determined first as the quotient of segment length YS and the length of the entire tie line YW.

In general, to find the percentages of two phases in equilibrium at a given temperature, the point of intersection of the vertical line for the alloy composition with the tie line across the two-phase field becomes the fulcrum. Then the ratio of the length of the tie line segment *opposite* a given boundary curve to the total length of the tie line connecting the two boundary curves is the percentage of the phase whose composition limit is defined by the given boundary curve. Remember that Figure 6-4 is an equilibrium phase diagram and that for the diagram to be valid, the alloy system would have to be held at each of these temperatures for a time sufficient for diffusion to produce equilibrium conditions. This means that, *at each temperature,* the composition would be the same throughout each of the solid phase crystals and the composition of the liquid phase (when present) would not vary at any position in the alloy. After equilibrium has been achieved, the compositions and amounts of the liquid and solid phases present are stable.

CRITICAL QUESTION

Why is the development of microsegregation in cast alloys more pronounced when there is a greater difference between the liquidus and solidus temperatures?

Coring

From Figure 6-4 and the summary in Table 6-2, it is evident that the composition of a rapidly cooled dendrite will not be uniform. For example, the first stable nucleus that forms at the temperature R (or slightly below) in Figure 6-4 is rich in palladium. As the temperature decreases, the palladium content decreases in each succeeding "layer" that solidifies on this nucleus, with an increase in the silver content. The palladium content of the liquid phase also decreases, and its silver content increases, as the solidification temperature is approached.

At the solidus temperature T in Figure 6-4, the composition of the outermost "layer" of the dendrite is 65% palladium and 35% silver. In the **coring** process the

Table 6-2	Chemical Compositions and Phase Amounts of a 65% Palladium (Pd) and 35% Silver (Ag) Alloy			
Temperature			**Chemical composition**	
°C	**°F**		**Liquid (% Pd)**	**Solid (% Pd)**
1500	2732		65	*
1400	2552		65	77
1370	2498		57	71
1340	2444		52	65
900	1652		*	65

*Phase not present at this temperature.

last liquid to solidify is richer in silver (point N) and solidifies between the dendrites, as described in the preceding chapter. Thus under rapid freezing conditions, the alloy has a *cored structure*. The *core* consists of the dendrites composed of compositions with higher solidus temperatures, and the *matrix* is the portion of the microstructure between the dendrites that contains compositions with lower solidus temperatures.

An excellent example of a cored structure can be observed in the photomicrograph in Figure 6-5, *A*, for an as-cast copper-silver alloy. The light, relatively broad microstructural features are the dendrites (core) with the higher melting compositions. The dark, narrow features are the *interdendritic regions* (matrix), which have lower melting temperatures. (Compare Fig. 6-5, *A*, with Fig. 5-5 in Chapter 5.) A *homogenization heat treatment*, which allows atomic diffusion to occur, can eliminate as-cast compositional nonuniformity. Figure 6-5, *B*, shows that the microstructure now consists of equiaxed grains with small dark regions, which are casting defects (porosity), as discussed in Chapter 12, as well as perhaps precipitate particles that formed during the heat treatment. Figure 6-5, *A*, represents the situation found for dental base metal alloys, which generally have dendritic as-cast microstructures. Some noble alloys for metal-ceramic applications, which have equiaxed polycrystalline as-cast microstructures, show substantial *microsegregation*, in which the solidified grains have nonuniform compositions and the grain boundaries have an indistinct appearance in the etched microstructure. For these alloys, the microsegregation is greatly reduced, with the appearance of distinct grain boundaries, after homogenization heat treatment.

Homogenization

For homogenization heat treatment, the cast alloy is held at a temperature near its solidus to achieve the maximum amount of diffusion without melting. (This process required 6 hr for the alloy shown in Fig. 6-5, *B*.) Little or no grain growth occurs when a casting receives this type of heat treatment, because the grain boundaries are largely immobilized by secondary or impurity elements and phases. Higher temperatures are employed than would be used with isothermal heat treatment (*annealing*) of a wrought alloy, as discussed in Chapter 20.

It has already been noted in Chapter 3 that an inhomogeneous dental gold alloy is more subject to tarnish and corrosion than the same alloy after homogenization. This is also important for silver-palladium alloys, since silver-rich phases tend to

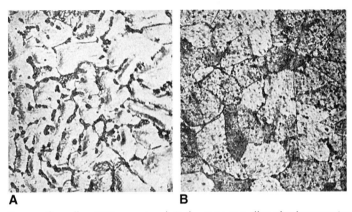

A　　　　　　　　**B**

Fig. 6-5. **A,** Copper-silver alloy (1%) as-cast and, **B,** the same cast alloy after homogenization heat treatment. (×100.)

tarnish readily in the oral environment. In Chapter 20 it will be shown that alloys with heterogeneous microstructures have greater resistance to permanent deformation than similar alloys with homogeneous microstructures. Consequently, the ductility of an alloy usually increases after homogenization heat treatment.

Dendrite Formation in Alloys

Now that the preceding background has been established, we can briefly describe the constitutional supercooling mechanism for the formation of dendrites during the solidification of a solid solution alloy. As the alloy composition freezes (see Fig. 6-4), there is a difference in the solute atom concentration in the liquid adjacent to the solid surface compared with that in the bulk liquid, and there is insufficient time with normal rates of solidification for the solute atoms to become uniformly distributed in the liquid. When the temperature gradient in the liquid is considered, there is generally a region adjacent to the solid surface at which the temperature is lower than the equilibrium freezing temperature for the given solute concentration. Protuberances (i.e., extensions) that form on the freezing alloy surface, which always arise because of random fluctuations, will lie in this supercooled liquid region and grow rapidly. The same mechanism will result in rapid growth of secondary protuberances that form at lateral sites on the original protuberances, followed by rapid growth of tertiary protuberances that form at lateral sites on the secondary protuberances. Thus this process yields three-dimensional branched dendrites. The growth of these branches takes place along specific crystallographic directions for different crystal structures.

CRITICAL QUESTIONS

What are the advantages and disadvantages of alloys that have eutectic microstructural constituents? How do properties vary for the different groups of alloy compositions in binary eutectic systems?

EUTECTIC ALLOYS

Many binary alloy systems do not exhibit complete solubility in both the liquid and the solid states. The eutectic system is an example of an alloy for which the component metals have limited solid solubility. Two metals, A and B, which are completely insoluble in each other in the solid state, provide the simplest illustration of a eutectic alloy. In this case, some grains are composed solely of metal A, and the remaining grains are composed of metal B. The situation is analogous to a frozen brine solution. Although the salt and water molecules intermingle randomly in solution, the result upon freezing is a mixture of salt crystals and ice crystals that form independently of each other.

However, all metals are soluble in one another in the solid state to at least some extent (which can be very small in certain cases). Therefore, a binary eutectic system, in which the two metals are partially soluble in each other, will be used for purposes of illustration. Such a system of interest to dentistry is the silver-copper system.

Silver-Copper System

The phase diagram for this system is presented in Figure 6-6, where 3 phases are found: (1) a liquid phase (L), (2) a silver-rich substitutional solid solution phase (α) containing a small amount of copper atoms, and (3) a copper-rich substitutional solid

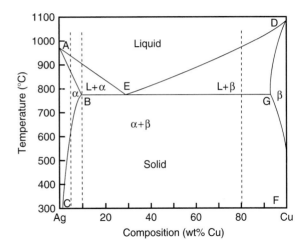

Fig. 6-6. Equilibrium phase diagram for the silver-copper system (wt%).

solution phase (β) containing a small amount of silver atoms. The α and β phases are sometimes referred to as *terminal solid solutions* because of their locations at the left and right sides of the phase diagram. The solidus can be identified as the boundary line ABEGD, since the liquid phase is not found below this line. The liquidus can be identified as AED, since there are no solid phases above this line. The major portion of the diagram below 780° C is composed of a two-phase (α + β) region, which represents a mixture of the silver-rich and copper-rich phases in the alloy microstructures.

The first difference to be noted when comparing Figure 6-6 with the solid solution system of Figure 6-4 is that the liquidus and solidus meet at E. This composition (72% silver and 28% copper) is known as the *eutectic composition* or simply the *eutectic*. The following characteristics of this special composition should be noted:

- The temperature at which the eutectic composition melts (779° C or 1435° F) is lower than the fusion temperature of silver or copper (*eutectic* literally means "lowest melting") and is the lowest temperature at which any alloy of silver and copper is entirely liquid.
- There is no solidification range for composition E. The eutectic liquid composition freezes at a constant temperature, similar to a pure metal, but the solid consists of two phases (α and β). Eutectic alloys are often used when a lower fusion temperature is desired, such as for dental solders (see Chapter 19). However, eutectic alloys are inferior in other important properties compared with solid solution alloys. This will be discussed in more detail later.

When a binary eutectic solidifies, atoms segregate to form regions of the two nearly pure parent metals. A layered or *lamellar structure* is typically formed, as seen in Figure 6-7, *A*, because the least amount of diffusion is required to produce atom segregation; however, rod-shaped eutectic morphologies are observed for some alloys. This structure is also referred to as the *eutectic constituent*, in which the term *constituent* means a distinctive microstructural feature.

The eutectic reaction is sometimes written schematically as follows:

$$\text{Liquid} \rightarrow \alpha \text{ solid solution} + \beta \text{ solid solution} \qquad (1)$$

This reaction is referred to as an *invariant transformation*, because it occurs at a single temperature and composition.

Another important aspect of the phase diagram in Figure 6-6 is the manner in which two portions (AB and DG) of the solidus slope toward the third portion, the

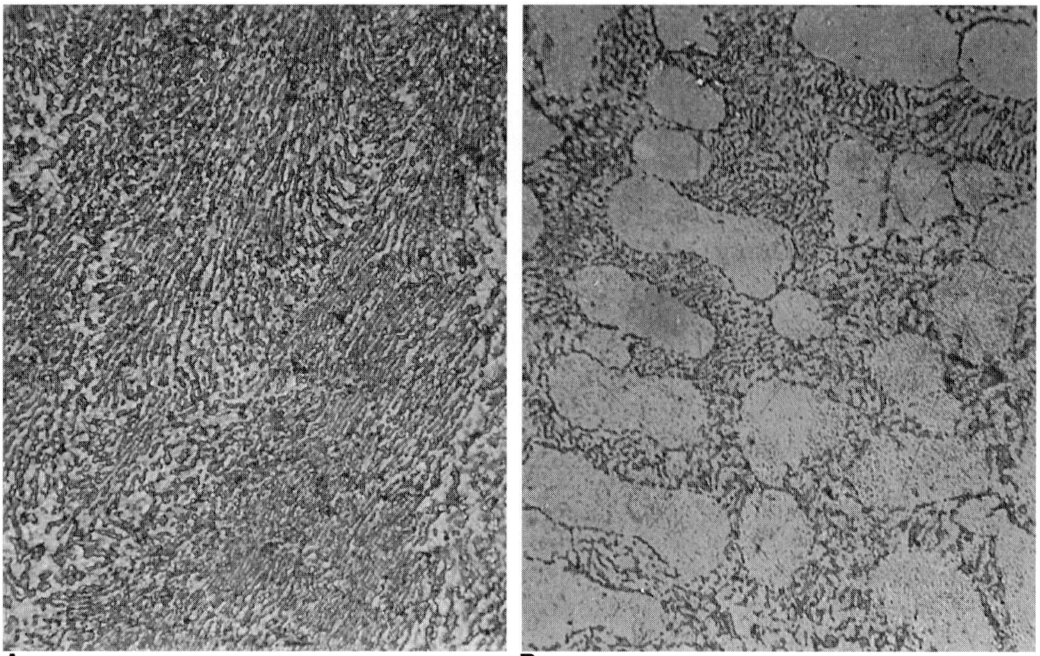

Fig. 6-7. Microstructure of two lead-tin alloys. **A,** The alloy has the eutectic composition 62% Sn–38% Pb. The structure is composed of alternating layers (lamellae) of solid solution **(dark)** that is Pb-rich and β solid solution **(light)** that is Sn-rich. (×1280.) **B,** The alloy has a high tin content (75% Sn–25% Pb). The light islands are primary β phase that solidified first. They are surrounded by the eutectic structure that solidified when the eutectic temperature was reached. (×560.) (Courtesy of P.G. Winchell.)

horizontal line BEG. At the left side of the diagram from A to B, the copper content of the silver-rich α phase varies from 0% to nearly 9%. At the right side of the diagram from D to G, the silver content of the copper-rich β phase varies from 0% to approximately 8%.

The phase diagram in Figure 6-6 contains *solvus lines* CB and FG that are not present in phase diagrams for solid solution systems. Solvus line CB shows that under equilibrium conditions the solid solubility of copper in the α phase increases from about 1% at 300° C to nearly 9% at B. Solvus line FG shows that the equilibrium solid solubility of silver in the β phase increases from an extremely small value at 300° C to a maximum of approximately 8% at point G. (This value is measured in the left direction, starting with the value of 0% Ag at the right end of the horizontal composition axis.)

The compositions of the phases that form during equilibrium cooling for the various alloys of silver and copper can be determined in the same manner as for solid solutions of silver and palladium. For example, if an alloy containing 10% copper is melted at a temperature above the liquidus and allowed to cool under equilibrium conditions (second dashed vertical line from the left in Figure 6-6), crystals of the first solid form in the liquid phase at approximately 900° C (1652° F). If a horizontal tie line is drawn from the liquidus (AE) to the solidus (AB), it is found that this first solid is the α solid solution, with an approximate composition of 4% copper and 96% silver.

If the temperature of this alloy is allowed to decrease further to 850° C (1562° F), another tie line drawn at this temperature between the solidus and liquidus indicates that under equilibrium conditions all α solid solution crystals have the approximate composition of 5% copper and the remaining liquid has a uniform composition of approximately 15% copper. When the temperature of the alloy reaches the eutectic temperature of 779° C, the tie line becomes BE. The last liquid to solidify has the eutectic composition of 72% silver and 28% copper, and it forms alternating layers of the α and β phases, similar to those shown in Figure 6-7, A.

If the starting molten alloy composition contains a greater percentage of copper than that for the eutectic, the changes in composition during cooling are similar, except that now the first solid to form (as crystals) in the liquid phase is the β solid solution. The changes in composition of the liquid and β phases during the equilibrium cooling of an alloy containing 80% copper and 20% silver, represented by the right dashed vertical line in Figure 6-6, can be determined by constructing tie lines (including EG) at several temperatures across the (L + β) phase field.

In summary, the first crystals to form during the equilibrium freezing of silver-copper alloys whose compositions lie between points B and G are either the solid solution α or the solid solution β (referred to as *primary* α or β). The final portion of the molten alloy to freeze will form regions of the eutectic structure. The grains (called *primary grains*) that form by the growth of these starting primary α or β crystals are large, compared with the dimensions of the alternating layers of α and β phases comprising the eutectic. As described previously for the silver-palladium solid solution system, application of the lever rule will give the percentages of the two phases at any temperature in the (L + α) or (L + β) phase fields during the equilibrium cooling process.

The cooling of solidified alloy compositions below the eutectic temperature can be illustrated by the equilibrium cooling of the molten alloy composition containing 5% copper, as indicated by the first vertical dashed line at the left in Figure 6-6. This alloy freezes completely as the α solid solution at approximately 860° C (1580° F), where the vertical dashed line intersects AB. As the temperature continues to decrease below the eutectic temperature of 779° C, the composition of this solid solution phase remains unchanged until a temperature of approximately 630° C (1166° F) is reached (intersection of the vertical dashed line with CB). Then the copper-rich β solid solution begins to precipitate from the α solid solution, because the solid solubility limit of copper in the latter solid solution has been exceeded. It must be emphasized that this occurs only if very slow cooling has permitted equilibrium to be achieved. In this case, application of the lever rule will give the percentages of the α and β phases at any temperature in this two-phase field. However, rapid cooling of the 5% copper alloy will not allow sufficient time for atomic diffusion and it will result in an alloy consisting of almost entirely α phase at room temperature.

If the starting molten alloy contains between approximately 9% and 92% copper (compositions lying between vertical lines passing through B and G), the lamellar eutectic structure will form during equilibrium solidification. Alloy compositions lying to the left of B or to the right of G will form either primary α phase crystals or primary β phase crystals, respectively, during freezing, which is completed when the temperature decreases below AB or DG, respectively. Then, as the solidified alloy cools under equilibrium conditions to room temperature, precipitates of the other solid solution phase will form (typically at the grain boundaries) when the temperature decreases below the solvus line (CB or FG, respectively). The molten eutectic alloy composition (point E) freezes at the single temperature of 779° C (1435° F) to directly yield the two-phase α + β structure, similar to that shown in Figure 6-7, A.

PHYSICAL PROPERTIES

Unlike the palladium-silver system, in which the mechanical properties of the solid solution alloys are found to vary nearly linearly with small to moderate changes in composition, more complex relationships occur for alloy compositions in eutectic systems. Alloys in these systems with a composition less than that of the eutectic are called *hypoeutectic alloys*, and those with a composition greater than the eutectic are known as *hypereutectic alloys*. Therefore, the primary crystals of the hypoeutectic alloys in the silver-copper system of Figure 6-6 consist of the α solid solution, whereas those of the hypereutectic alloys consist of the β solid solution. Hypoeutectic or hypereutectic alloys that contain the eutectic constituent in their microstructures (compositions between B and G) are relatively brittle, whereas alloys with microstructures lacking this constituent (compositions to the left of B or to the right of G) are ductile. This is because the alternating lamellae of the α and β phases inhibit the movement of dislocations, which is responsible for the permanent deformation of these alloys, as discussed in Chapter 20. However, the strength, and sometimes the hardness, of alloys containing the eutectic constituent may surpass those of the pure component metals because of the composite structure of the alloy.

There has been some use of α solid solution casting alloys of silver and copper in pediatric dentistry. The tarnish resistance of these alloys is superior to that of the alloys containing the eutectic constituent, as discussed in Chapter 3. The silver-copper eutectic is found as the admixed component in some types of high-copper amalgam alloys (Chapter 17). Another example of the potential importance of eutectic compositions occurs near the gold end of the Au-Ir system, in which the eutectic composition at approximately 0.005% Ir has been considered relevant for the grain refinement of dental gold casting alloys by iridium. However, as noted in Chapter 5, there may be some uncertainty about the mechanism for this grain refinement.

PERITECTIC ALLOYS

In addition to the eutectic system, limited solid solubility of two metals can result in a *peritectic transformation*. The silver-tin system, which is the basis for the original dental amalgam alloys, is a peritectic system. Silver and platinum, which are found in many gold casting alloys, exhibit a peritectic transformation. Also, palladium and ruthenium have a peritectic reaction at 16.5 wt% Ru. Ruthenium is an important grain-refining element for palladium casting alloys.

Like the eutectic transformation, the peritectic reaction is an invariant reaction, occurring at a particular composition and temperature. The reaction can be written as:

$$\text{Liquid} + \beta \text{ solid solution} \rightarrow \alpha \text{ solid solution} \tag{2}$$

Figure 6-8 is the phase diagram for the silver-platinum alloy system. The α phase is silver-rich, the β phase is platinum-rich, and the two-phase (α + β) region results from the limited solid solubility (less than approximately 12% at 700° C) of silver in platinum. (See Fig. 6-8, which shows that the equilibrium solid solubility of platinum in silver is approximately 56% at 700° C.) The peritectic transformation occurs at point P, where the liquid (composition at β) and the platinum-rich β phase (composition at point D) transform into the silver-rich α phase (composition at point P). For a hypoperitectic composition, such as exists for alloy I, cooling through the peritectic temperature results in the following transformation:

$$\text{Liquid} + \beta \rightarrow \text{Liquid} + \alpha \tag{3}$$

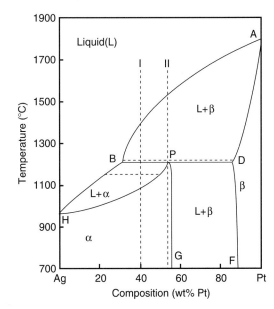

Fig. 6-8. Equilibrium phase diagram of the platinum-silver system (wt%).

It can be seen from Fig. 6-8 that the two liquid phases involved in transformation (3) have different compositions. For both transformations (2) and (3), the α phase forms at the interface between the liquid and β phase, and because substantial diffusion in these phases is required for transformation, peritectic alloys are especially prone to coring during rapid cooling. From the discussions in Chapters 3 and 20, it follows that this cored structure has inferior corrosion resistance and is more brittle than the homogeneous α solid solution phase.

SOLID STATE REACTIONS

Solid state reactions provide an important mechanism that can be used to strengthen some dental alloys. The most well-known example is the ordering in gold-copper alloys, which is relevant for Types III and IV gold casting alloys for all-metal restorations (see Chapter 19). As previously described, although the gold and copper atoms are completely soluble in the liquid state and at high temperatures in the solid state, at lower temperatures the attraction of these two atom species can convert regions of the random solid solution into an ordered solid phase for some compositions.

CRITICAL QUESTION

How does copper provide strengthening and hardening of gold casting alloys by two different mechanisms?

Gold-Copper System

Figure 6-9 illustrates the phase diagram for the gold-copper system. The melting range is very narrow for all compositions, and the liquidus and solidus curves touch at 80.1 wt% gold. At the right side of this diagram, note that the addition of 10 wt% copper to gold lowers the liquidus temperature substantially. These facts are advantageous in the use of gold alloy compositions based on this system for dental casting procedures.

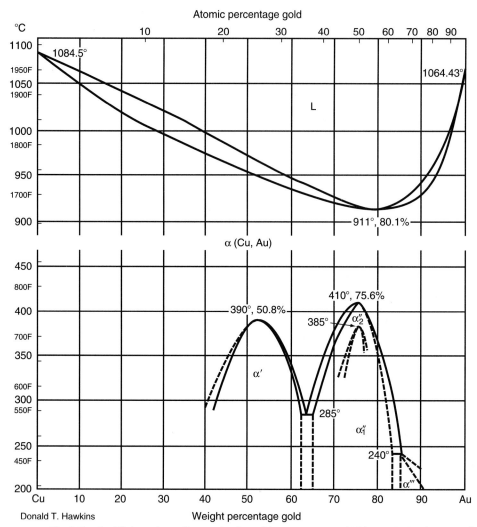

Fig. 6-9.   Equilibrium phase diagram for the gold-copper system. (With permission from Metals Handbook, Vol 8, 8th ed. Metals Park, OH, American Society for Metals, 1973, p 267.)

At temperatures below the solidus temperature, but above 410° C, gold and copper have complete mutual solid solubility and all alloys initially solidify as the α disordered solid solution, in which the atoms of each species are randomly located in the fcc crystal structure. However, when alloys of appropriate compositions are subsequently cooled under conditions approaching equilibrium, solid-state ordering transformations occur.

As shown in Figure 6-9, when alloys containing between approximately 40 wt% and 65 wt% gold are cooled below 390° C under equilibrium conditions, the ordered phase α' forms. This is the $AuCu_3$ structure that was shown in Figure 6-1. As previously noted, because of the greatly differing atomic weights of gold and copper, the $AuCu_3$ structure is approximately 50 wt% gold.

On the other hand, when alloys containing between approximately 65 wt% and 85 wt% gold are cooled below 410° C under equilibrium conditions, Figure 6-9 shows that a different ordered structure forms (α₂″, which is referred to as AuCu II). With further equilibrium cooling below 385° C, the α₂″ structure transforms to the α₁″ ordered structure, which is referred to as AuCu I. Under normal slow cooling

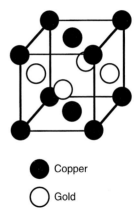

● Copper

○ Gold

Fig. 6-10. Unit cell of the face-centered tetragonal superlattice of AuCu.

conditions for gold-copper alloys in this composition range, the α_1'' structure is found. It should be noted that the equiatomic AuCu structure contains approximately 75 wt% gold.

The gold and copper atoms, which were randomly located in the fcc structure of the α phase at higher temperatures, occupy alternating planes in the α_1'' superlattice (Fig. 6-10). This ordered structure has a face-centered tetragonal unit cell because the lattice parameter in one of the three axial directions (vertical direction, as shown in Fig. 6-10) is different from that in the other two directions, because of the unequal atomic radii of gold and copper. The α_2'' superlattice has an unusual orthorhombic unit cell. Referring to Figure 6-10, the unit cell for AuCu II may be visualized as consisting of five tetragonal AuCu I unit cells similar to the one illustrated and joined to five more tetragonal AuCu I unit cells, in which the copper atoms are now located at the midplane rather than the top and bottom faces.

Regions of ordered structure provide substantial strengthening of dental gold casting alloys, in addition to that arising from several solute atom species in the disordered fcc gold solid solution matrix. Because the crystal structure of the ordered phase differs from that of the gold solid solution, each region of ordered phase is surrounded by a localized elastic strain field, which is necessary to maintain continuity of atomic bonds across the interface with the matrix. Consequently, the movement of dislocations (described in Chapter 20) through gold casting alloys containing regions of ordered structure is substantially impeded. A full description of the complex strengthening mechanism associated with ordering is beyond the scope of this book, and interested readers should refer to articles listed in the Selected Readings at the end of this chapter.

The *quenching* procedure (rapid cooling in a room-temperature water bath or an ice-water bath), which is performed under normal dental laboratory conditions (see Chapter 12), does not allow sufficient time for atomic movement to form the ordered structure. The disordered solid solution is retained at room temperature, and the gold alloy is relatively soft and ductile, which facilitates adjustments of the casting at the dental laboratory or chairside with the patient. Bench-cooling the Type III or IV gold alloy casting through the ordering temperature range allows enough atomic movement for partial transformation. Although the alloy will be stronger and harder compared with the quenched condition, more time is required for removal of adherent investment from the bench-cooled casting, and this slow-cooling procedure is not commonly performed. Alternatively, after adjustments have been completed on a Type III or IV gold alloy casting in the quenched condition, the casting may be given an *age-hardening heat treatment*. The alloy is heated to a temperature within the ordering range for a period of time as recommended by the manufacturer and then it is quenched. This procedure is also not commonly performed, because of the additional time involved. For commercial Type III and IV dental gold casting alloys, the Vickers hardness increases by 50 to 100 after age hardening. (The amount of copper in the Type I and II dental gold casting alloys is insufficient for age hardening.)

If desired, another furnace heat treatment may be used to restore hardened Type III or IV gold alloy castings to their softened condition. This procedure, termed *solution heat treatment*, involves heating the casting to a temperature below the solidus temperature, (e.g., 700° C or 1292° F), holding for a short period of time (typically 10 min) so that the alloy returns to a random substitutional solid solution, and then quenching to retain this atomic arrangement at room temperature. The softened casting can later be given the previously described age-hardening heat treatment and quenched, returning to a stronger, but less ductile alloy.

Under normal clinical conditions, cast gold restorations are cemented on prepared teeth using the alloy in the softened condition. It has been found that significant aging of a commercial Type IV gold alloy takes place slowly over a 2-week period at intraoral temperature. The accompanying dimensional changes in the gold alloy castings do not have clinical significance. Such behavior might be expected for Type III and other Type IV gold alloys at 37° C, since the ordered structure is present under equilibrium conditions. It would be of interest to investigate the hardness and dimensional changes in a variety of Types III and IV gold alloys aged at 37° C for longer periods of time.

Transmission electron microscopic observations at high magnifications have been performed on traditional commercial high-gold Types III and IV casting alloys, in which the maximum hardness was achieved in 1 to 4 hr after isothermal annealing at elevated temperatures (230° to 350° C) recommended by the manufacturers. The ordered platelets in the gold solid solution matrix after annealing for 25 hr were less than 10 nm in size. An optical microscope photomicrograph at a much lower magnification of the microstructure of a dental gold alloy that was subjected to a prolonged period of aging is shown in Figure 6-11. In many studies of the mechanisms for age hardening of dental gold casting alloys, prolonged heat treatments

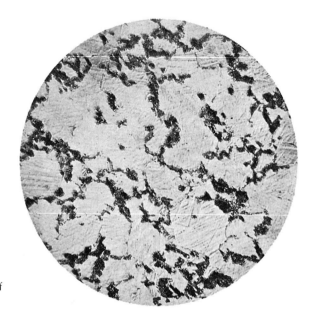

Fig. 6-11. A photomicrograph of a dental gold alloy that was age hardened at 450° C for a prolonged period of 100 hr. (× 250.) (Courtesy of E.M. Wise.)

have been used to increase the precipitate size for more convenient transmission electron microscopic observations.

Silver-Copper System

A 92.5% silver–7.5% copper alloy, sometimes used for inlay purposes in deciduous teeth, is known as sterling silver. This alloy is used extensively in fine silverware and was the basis for silver coinage. Using the phase diagram in Figure 6-6, note that 7.5% copper alloy solidifies as the α solid solution on slow cooling from the melt, and the copper-rich β phase precipitates on continued cooling. If a specimen of this alloy were solution heat-treated at 775° C (1427° F) for 30 min, quenched to room temperature, and reheated at 325° C (617° F) for 2 hr, age-hardening would yield finely dispersed precipitates in the microstructure and the alloy would be significantly strengthened. Silversmiths use this procedure, because the solution heat-treated alloy is soft and has high ductility, permitting it to be readily shaped by cold working. The finished utensil can then be subjected to age hardening, adding significantly to its durability.

OTHER BINARY SYSTEMS
Gold Alloys

As previously noted, dental gold casting alloys may contain as many as four important solute metals (copper, silver, palladium, and platinum) that provide solid solution strengthening. Other elements in amounts less than 1 wt %, such as zinc and iridium, are present as well. Because many of these metals in binary combinations can form precipitates leading to age hardening, assuming that the precipitate sizes are optimum (see Chapters 19 and 20), it is useful to briefly consider the platinum-gold, palladium-copper and platinum-copper binary systems. Comparisons of these diagrams provides information about phases that might be present in the multicomponent commercial gold alloys.

In the platinum-gold system at temperatures below the solidus, a large two-phase region develops in a manner similar to a eutectic structure. The palladium-copper system contains two superlattice transformations, leading to the formation of PdCu and $PdCu_3$. The platinum-copper system contains at least two intermediate phases: PtCu and $PtCu_3$. These phase diagrams and their potential relevance to alloy properties can be analyzed by the same approaches that have been previously discussed. Note that phases might exist in cast dental alloys that would not occur under equilibrium conditions with the alloy compositions, because of elemental microsegregation during rapid solidification and cooling. Furthermore, the compositions of phases in multicomponent alloys will generally be more complex than those for binary compositions.

A particularly effective age-hardening constituent in gold alloys is an iron-platinum intermetallic compound ($FePt_3$). $FePt_3$ is useful in strengthening high-gold alloys for metal-ceramic prostheses, in which platinum is employed to increase the melting range and lower the coefficient of thermal expansion of the alloy. Such alloys are discussed in Chapter 19.

CRITICAL QUESTION

Why are there substantial differences between the microstructures and strengthening mechanisms for the high-palladium alloys and the palladium-silver alloys?

Palladium Alloys

High-palladium alloys have been popular for metal-ceramic prostheses since their inception in the early 1980s because of their excellent mechanical properties and good adherence to dental porcelain. Although the unit metal cost of these alloys was formerly less than half that of alternative gold alloys, their clinical selection has diminished in recent years because of the price volatility of palladium. These alloys are based on the Pd-Ga system, in which there is a eutectic composition at the high-palladium side of the phase diagram and complex precipitation reactions at lower temperatures in the current version of the diagram. For the originally introduced Pd-Cu-Ga alloys, both the rapid cooling rate during solidification and the addition of copper shift the eutectic composition to higher percentages of palladium and result in formation of a Pd_2Ga eutectic constituent in the as-cast microstructure. Both the Pd-Cu-Ga alloys and the subsequently developed Pd-Ga alloys have a fine submicron tweed structure observed by transmission electron microscopy. This structure appears to form by a martensitic phase transformation (see Chapter 19) in the fcc palladium solid solution matrix and is stable during heat treatment that simulates the firing cycles for dental porcelain. Strengthening of these alloys occurs by the solid solution mechanism and by the formation of Pd_5Ga_2 precipitates in some Pd-Cu-Ga alloy compositions.

With this recent price volatility of palladium, the popularity of the palladium-silver alloys (Chapter 19) has increased. Although the starting point for these alloys is the palladium-silver phase diagram in Figure 6-4, additional elements that provide adequate mechanical properties and metal oxides for porcelain bonding cause the formation of secondary phases in the microstructures. The appropriate binary diagrams may be useful for predicting the occurrence of these phases. Because the precipitate sizes are generally too small for accurate determination of their compositions using a scanning electron microscope or the electron microprobe, elemental analysis using a transmission electron microscope is required.

TERNARY AND HIGHER-ORDER ALLOY SYSTEMS

Most dental gold alloys are ternary alloys of gold, silver, and copper, containing minor additions of such metals as platinum, palladium, and zinc. A majority of these alloys, which form single-phase solid solutions when quenched after solidification, can be strengthened and hardened by heat treatment. A variety of age-hardening mechanisms have been found, depending on the alloy composition. Uzuka et al have portrayed the composition regions for the different phase transformations in the Au-Cu-Ag system, using a triangular phase diagram corresponding to an isothermal cross-section at 300° C through the three-dimensional diagram.

There are many other ternary combinations, quaternary combinations, and higher-order multicomponent alloy systems used for restorative dentistry. Such systems are complex, and the phase diagram information available is limited, with the exception of the Ag-Hg-Sn ternary system for dental amalgams that is discussed in Chapter 17.

Binary phase diagrams are often useful in predicting the influence of individual component elements in casting alloys, although such equilibrium diagrams must always be interpreted with caution, given the nonequilibrium conditions associated with the dental casting process. Pseudobinary phase diagrams, in which the concentration of one or more of the components is fixed, are frequently employed to study the phases present in higher-order alloy systems.

SELECTED READINGS

Brantley WA, Cai Z, Carr AB, and Mitchell JC: Metallurgical structures of as-cast and heat-treated high-palladium dental alloys. Cells Mater 3:103, 1993.

High-palladium alloys with equiaxed polycrystalline and dendritic microstructures are described. Careful study of the micrographs is useful for comparing the potential structural integrity and some properties of these alloys.

Cullity BD: Principles of X-Ray Diffraction, 2nd ed. Reading, MA, Addison-Wesley Publishing Co, 1978.

A description of x-ray diffraction techniques used to determine crystal structures of metallic materials. Chapter 13 in this book summarizes the ordered structures in gold-copper alloys.

Flinn R, and Trojan P: Engineering Materials and Their Applications, 3rd ed. Boston, MA, Houghton Mifflin Co, 1986, pp 116-169.

A discussion of equilibrium (phase diagram) and nonequilibrium conditions in systems as related to properties. Excellent photographs and examples.

Metals Handbook, Desk Edition. Metals Park, OH, American Society of Metals, 1991.

A comprehensive reference book on the casting, structure, and properties of metals, including a section on metallography procedures.

Nitta SV, Clark WAT, Brantley WA, Grylls RJ, and Cai Z: TEM analysis of tweed structure in high-palladium dental alloys. J Mater Sci Mater Med 10:513, 1999.

The characteristic submicron tweed structure and microtwins in these alloys are described.

Porter DA, and Easterling KE: Phase Transformations in Metals and Alloys, 2nd ed. London, Chapman & Hall, 1992.

This undergraduate engineering textbook describes phase transformations and the structure and properties of interfaces.

Uzuka T, Kanzawa Y, and Yasuda K: Determination of the AuCu superlative formation region in gold-copper-silver ternary system. J Dent Res 60:883, 1981.

A classic article that presents the solid-state transformations in this important ternary alloy system.

Van Vlack LH: Elements of Materials Science and Engineering, 6th ed. Reading, MA, Addison-Wesley, 1989.

An excellent first textbook on materials science. Chapter 5 describes phase diagrams, and Chapters 8 and 9 present deformation and strengthening mechanisms for alloys.

Vermilyea SG, Huget EF, and Vilca JM: Observations on gold-palladium-silver and gold-palladium alloys. J Prosthet Dent 44:292, 1980.

Excellent examples of microsegregation in as-cast noble dental alloys are shown.

Watanabe I, Atsuta M, Yasuda K, and Hisatsune K: Dimensional changes related to ordering in an AuCu-3 wt% Ga alloy at intraoral temperature. Dent Mater 10:369, 1994.

Intraoral ordering and the clinical significance of resulting dimensional changes are reported for an experimental gold casting alloy and a commercial Type IV gold alloy.

Wu Q, Brantley WA, Mitchell JC, Vermilyea SG, Xiao J, and Guo W: Heat-treatment behavior of high-palladium dental alloys. Cells Mater 7:161, 1997.

Evidence is presented for the contribution of a very hard phase to the strengthening of some high-palladium alloys, and the formation of discontinuous precipitates is described.

Yasuda K, and Ohta M: Difference in age-hardening mechanism in dental gold alloys. J Dent Res 61:473, 1982.

A comprehensive description of the ordered structures and other phases that provide age hardening of ternary gold-silver-copper alloys.

Yasuda K, Van Tendeloo G, Van Landuyt J, and Amelinckx S: High-resolution electron microscopic study of age-hardening in a commercial dental gold alloy. J Dent Res 65:1179, 1986.

This article shows the unique ability of high-resolution transmission electron microscopy to reveal the complex ordered structures in a commercial dental gold casting alloy.

7

Dental Polymers

H. Ralph Rawls

OUTLINE
Applications of Resins in Dentistry

Classification

Requisites for Dental Resins

Fundamental Nature of Polymers

Physical Properties of Polymers

Chemistry of Polymerization

Copolymerization

Acrylic Dental Resins

KEY TERMS
Backbone—The main chain of a polymer.

Block copolymer—A polymer made of two or more monomer species and identical monomer units occurring in relatively long sequences along the main polymer chain.

Chain transfer—A stage of polymerization in which the growing end of a chain is transferred to another molecule, initiating further chain growth.

Curing—Chemical reaction in which low–molecular-weight monomers or small polymers are converted into higher–molecular-weight materials to attain desired properties.

Elastic recovery—Reduction or elimination of elastic strain when an applied force is removed; elastic solids recover elastic strain immediately on removal of the applied force whereas viscoelastic materials recover elastic strain over time.

Final set—Stage at which the curing process is complete.

Free radical—A compound with an unpaired electron that is used to initiate polymerization.

Graft or branched copolymer—A polymer in which sequences of one type of mer unit are attached as a graft (branched) onto the backbone of a second type of mer unit.

Initial set (of a polymer)—The stage of polymerization during which the polymer retains its shape.

Induction—Activation of free radicals, which in turn initiate growing polymer chains.

Monomer—A chemical compound capable of reacting to form a polymer.

Plastic flow (of a polymer)—Irreversible deformation that occurs when polymer chains slide over one another and become relocated within the material.

Polymer—Chemical compound consisting of large organic molecules formed by the union of many repeating smaller monomer units.

Polymerization—Chemical reaction in which monomers of a low molecular weight are converted into chains of polymers with a high molecular weight:

$$\text{Monomer} + \text{Monomer} + \text{Monomer} + \text{Monomer} \xrightarrow{\text{Polymerization}} -\text{Mer} - \text{Mer} - \text{Mer} - \text{Mer} -$$

KEY TERMS—cont'd

Propagation—Stage of polymerization during which polymer chains continue to grow to high molecular weights.

Random copolymer—Polymer made of two or more monomer species but with no sequential order between the mer units along the polymer chain.

Setting (of a polymer)—The extent to which polymerization has progressed.

Thermoplastic polymer—Polymeric material made of linear and/or branched chains that softens when heated above the glass-transition temperature (T_g), at which molecular motion begins to force the chains apart.

Thermosetting polymer—Polymeric material that becomes permanently hard when heated above the temperature at which it begins to polymerize and that does not soften again on reheating to the same temperature.

Termination—Stage of polymerization during which polymer chains cease to grow.

Viscoelastic—Ability of a polymer to behave as an elastic solid (spring) and as a viscous liquid (dashpot).

APPLICATIONS OF RESINS IN DENTISTRY

Synthetic resins are used in a variety of dental applications. Typical uses include the following:

- Dentures (bases, liners, and artificial teeth)
- Cavity-filling materials ("composites")
- Sealants
- Impression materials
- Equipment (mixing bowls)
- Cements (resin-based)

Dental resins are used mainly to restore and replace tooth structure and missing teeth. These resins can be bonded with other resins directly to tooth structure or to other restorative materials. If all teeth are missing, a denture base (the part of the denture that rests on the soft tissues overlying the maxillary and mandibular jawbone in the mouth) with attached denture teeth can be made to restore chewing ability.

CLASSIFICATION

Dental resins solidify when they polymerize. **Polymerization** occurs through a series of chemical reactions by which the macromolecule, or the **polymer**, is formed from large numbers of molecules known as **monomers**. Synthetic resins are often called *plastics*. A plastic material is a substance that, although dimensionally stable in normal use, was plastically reshaped at some stage of manufacture. Resins are composed of very large molecules. The particular form and morphology of the molecule determine whether the resin is a fiber, a rigid material, or a rubberlike product. Polymers have had an enormous impact on dentistry, and they are now used as sealants (prophylactic material used to seal fissures against the ingress of cariogenic bacteria), bonding materials, restorative materials, veneering materials, denture bases, denture teeth, and impression materials.

The utility of plastics is derived from their ability to be formed into complex shapes, often by the application of heat and pressure. Based on their thermal behavior, they can be divided into **thermoplastic** and **thermosetting polymers**, depending on whether they soften when heated.

A third group of polymeric materials are the *elastomers*. The modern elastomer industry was founded on the naturally occurring latex isolated from the *Hevea brasiliensis* tree. Since the early 20th century, chemists have been attempting to synthesize materials whose properties duplicate or at least simulate those of natural rubber. This has led to the production of a wide variety of synthetic elastomers, some of which are used in dentistry as impression materials. Elastomers readily undergo deformation and exhibit extensive reversible elongation under small, applied stresses; that is, they exhibit elasticity.

In dentistry, most resins are based on methacrylates, particularly methyl methacrylate. However, because the field is dynamic and new types of resins are being developed on a regular basis, a dentist's knowledge must include basic concepts of resin chemistry so that new developments in the field can be critically evaluated. This chapter provides a brief review of the fundamentals of resin chemistry.

REQUISITES FOR DENTAL RESINS

Methacrylate polymers have earned great popularity in dentistry because (1) they can be processed easily using relatively simple techniques, (2) they are aesthetic, and (3) they are economical. Because of their biological, physical, aesthetic, and handling properties, methacrylate polymers are capable of providing an excellent balance of performance features and characteristics needed for use in the oral cavity. Ideally, these characteristics include (1) biological compatibility, (2) physical properties, (3) ease of manipulation, (4) aesthetic qualities, (5) relatively low cost, and (6) chemical stability in the mouth.

Biological Compatibility

The resin should be tasteless, odorless, nontoxic, nonirritating, and otherwise not harmful to the oral tissues. To fulfill these requirements, a resin should be completely insoluble in saliva or in any other fluids taken into the mouth and should be impermeable to oral fluids to the extent that the resin does not become unsanitary or disagreeable in taste or odor. If the resin is used as a filling or cementing material, it should set fairly rapidly and bond to tooth structure to prevent microbial ingrowth along the tooth-restoration interface. A more comprehensive overview of the biocompatibility of dental materials is presented in Chapter 8.

Physical Properties

The resin should possess adequate strength and resilience, as well as resistance to biting or chewing forces, impact forces, and excessive wear that can occur in the oral cavity. The material should also be dimensionally stable under all conditions of service, including thermal changes and variations in loading. When used as a denture base for maxillary dentures, the resin should have a low specific gravity.

Manipulation

The resin should not produce toxic fumes or dust during handling and manipulation. It should be easy to mix, insert, shape, and cure, and it must have a relatively short **setting** time and be insensitive to variations in these handling procedures. Clinical complications, such as oxygen inhibition, saliva contamination, and blood contamination, should have little or no effect on the outcome of any handling procedure. In addition, the final product should be easy to polish, and in case of unavoidable breakage, it should be possible to repair the resin easily and efficiently.

Aesthetic Properties

The material should exhibit sufficient translucency or transparency so that it can be made to match the appearance of the oral tissues it replaces. The resin should be capable of being tinted or pigmented, but there should be no change in color or appearance of the material subsequent to its fabrication.

Economic Considerations

The cost of the resin and its processing method should be relatively low, and processing should not require complex and expensive equipment.

Chemical Stability

Although methacrylate polymers fulfill the aforementioned requirements reasonably well, no resin has yet met all of these ideal criteria. The conditions in the mouth are highly demanding, and only the most chemically stable and inert materials can withstand such conditions without deterioration.

CRITICAL QUESTION

How do the mechanical properties of a polymer change as the molecular weight increases?

FUNDAMENTAL NATURE OF POLYMERS

The most significant features of polymers are that they consist of very large molecules and that their molecular structure is capable of virtually limitless configurations and conformations. Chain length, the extent of chain branching and cross-linking, and the organization of the chains are fundamental features of polymers that determine the properties of polymeric materials. Polymerization is a repetitive intermolecular reaction that is functionally capable of proceeding indefinitely. Because any chemical compound possessing a molecular weight in excess of 5000 is considered to be a macromolecule, most polymer molecules can be described as macromolecules. In some instances, the molecular weight of the polymer molecule can be as high as 50 million.

In addition to the traditional polymers, macromolecules can consist of inorganic polymers such as the silicon dioxide network found in several ceramics and resin composites used in dentistry. The discussion in this chapter is limited to organic polymers.

Chain Length and Molecular Weight

The longer the polymer chain, the greater is the number of entanglements (temporary connections) that can form among chains. Therefore, the longer the chain length, the more difficult it is to distort the polymeric material, and thus such properties as rigidity, strength and the melting temperature increase with increasing chain length (Fig. 7-1). Consider the analogy between the behavior of a group of polymer molecular chains and a plate of spaghetti. The longer the strands or chains, the more difficult it is to separate them. Cutting them up—that is, reducing the chain length—makes them easier to separate.

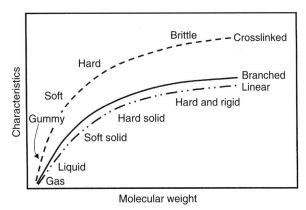

Fig. 7-1 Effect of polymer chain length, branching, and cross-linking on mechanical and physical properties. Rigidity, strength, and melting temperature increase as polymer chain length grows and molecular weight increases.

Synthetic resins polymerize randomly from local sites that have been activated. Thus, depending on the ability of the chains to grow from their local activation sites, the molecular chains that form within a polymeric material consist of chains that vary in length. Therefore, an average value is needed to express the molecular weight of polymers. Two types of average are commonly used, the number average, $\overline{M}_n$, based on the average number of mer repeating units in a chain, and the weight average, $\overline{M}_w$, based on the molecular weight of the average chain.

The number average molecular weight for various commercial dental denture polymers typically varies from 8,000 to 39,000, but molecular weights as high as 600,000 have been reported. Denture teeth with *cross-linked* resin (see below) may have even higher molecular weight.

Biologically, it is important to realize that polymerization seldom is entirely complete and that residual monomer molecules can be leached from polymeric materials. These low–molecular-weight compounds sometimes can cause adverse reactions, primarily allergic reactions. The residual monomer also has a pronounced effect on the molecular weight of the polymer. For example, 0.9% of residual monomer molecules in a polymer with a theoretical number average molecular weight of 22,400 if completely cured, will reduce the molecular weight of the polymer to 7,300.

The expression $\overline{M}_w$ implies that larger molecules are weighted more in the calculation. Therefore, $\overline{M}_w$ is always greater than $\overline{M}_n$, except when all molecules are of the same length; then $\overline{M}_w = \overline{M}_n$. Considering the concepts just discussed, the ratio $\overline{M}_w/\overline{M}_n$ (called the *polydispersity*) is a measure of the range and distribution of chain sizes. Polymers with equal value of $\overline{M}_w$ but different values of polydispersity will exhibit somewhat different properties. For example, higher polydispersity polymers will begin to melt at a lower temperature and have a larger temperature range of melting.

Chain Branching and Cross-Linking

In the ideal situation, polymerization should yield *linear* macromolecules. However, in practice, molecular chains that are exclusively linear are seldom realized. Structural units of the polymer are often connected together in a manner to form a nonlinear, *branched* or *cross-linked* polymer (Fig. 7-2). Branching is analogous to extra arms growing out of a polymer chain; the probability of entanglement, or

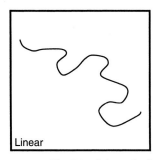
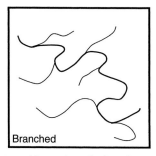
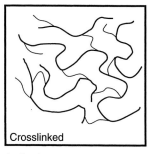

Fig. 7-2   Schematic diagrams of linear, branched, and cross-linked polymers.

temporary connections, increases. *Cross-links* are permanent connections between chains. A highly cross-linked polymeric material can consist of a single giant molecule or a few giant molecules.

In cross-linked polymers, some of the structural units must have at least two sites where reactions can occur. For example, during **curing** of polysulfide impression material, or during the formation of calcium alginate from sodium alginate, linear polymers are joined, or bridged, through certain reactive side chains to form cross-linked molecular networks (Fig. 7-3).

Cross-linking forms bridges between chains and dramatically increases molecular weight. Consequently, physical and mechanical properties vary with the composition and extent of cross-linking for a given polymer system. The three-dimensional network of cross-linked polymers increases rigidity and resistance to solvents. Cross-linking of a low–molecular-weight polymer increases the softening temperature, known as the *glass-transition temperature* (T_g), compared with that of a high–molecular-weight polymer (see Fig. 7-1). On the other hand, cross-linking has only modest influence on strength.

Copolymer Structures.   Polymers that have only one type of repeating unit (mer) are *homopolymers*; those with two or more types of mer units are known as *copolymers*. There are three different types of copolymers:

- **Random copolymer**—No sequential order exists among the two (or more) mer units along the polymer chain.

... ABBABABAAABAAAABABBBBABAAAABABABB ...

- **Block copolymer**—Identical monomer units occur in relatively long sequences along the main polymer.

... AAAAABBBBBBBAAAABBBBBBBAAAABBBAAAA ...

- **Graft or branched copolymer**—Sequences of one type of mer unit are attached as a graft (branched, Fig. 7-2) onto a **backbone** of a second type of mer unit.

... AAAAAAAAAAAAA ...
| |
B B
B B
B B

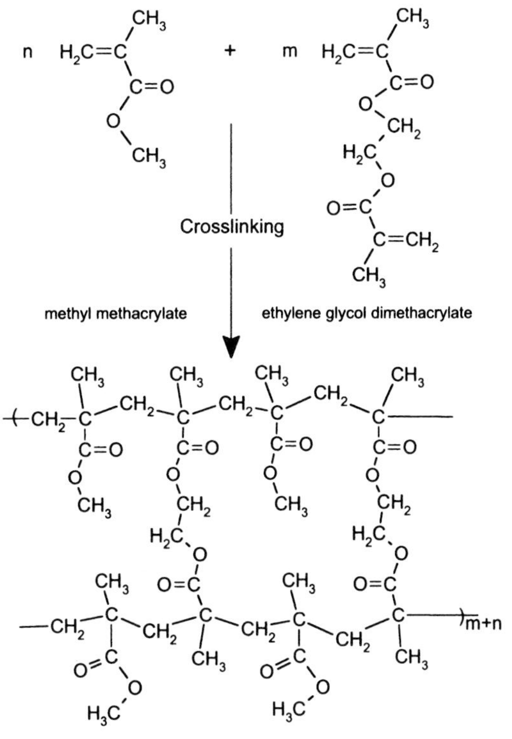

Fig. 7-3 A crosslinked structure is formed by copolymerization, with at least one of the comonomers being multifunctional. In this illustration methyl methacrylate is copolymerized with the difunctional monomer ethylene glycol dimethacrylate.

Molecular Organization

In some polymers the chains are randomly coiled and entangled in a very disordered pattern known as an amorphous structure (Fig. 7-4, left side). In others, the chains can align themselves to form a highly ordered, or crystalline, structure (Fig. 7-4, right side). Most polymeric materials combine these two forms of organization in greater or lesser proportions. Characteristically, the linear dental polymers are predominantly amorphous with little or no crystallinity. The polymer chains form a tangled mass, comparable with cooked spaghetti in which each string is a mile or so long. Such polymer segments have little chance to migrate and are immobile in the solid state. As in the case of glass, a short-range order results.

However, many polymers have regions of long-range ordering that produce a degree of crystallinity, depending on the secondary bonds that can be formed, the structure of the polymer chain, the degree of ordering, and the molecular weight (see Fig. 7-4). Although polymer crystallinity may increase tensile strength, it may also reduce ductility—that is, increase the brittleness—of the resin and increase its melting temperature.

Factors that reduce or prevent crystallinity include the following:

■ Copolymerization, which decreases the ability of polymer chains to align themselves.

■ Long branched polymers, which inhibit polymer chains from becoming aligned.

■ Random arrangement of substituent groups, particularly large side groups that keep polymer chains separated.

■ Plasticizers, which tend to separate the chains (see the following section).

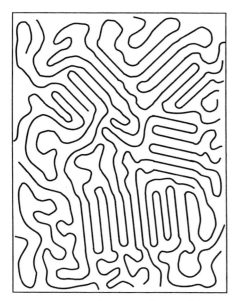 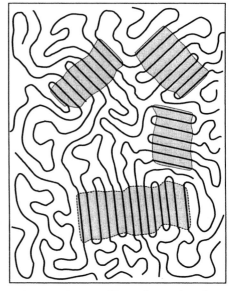

Fig. 7-4 Schematic diagram **(left)** of a polymer that contains crystalline and amorphous intermolecular and intramolecular organization and combinations of both amorphous and crystalline regions **(shaded areas on right).**

PHYSICAL PROPERTIES OF POLYMERS
Deformation and Recovery

Applied forces produce stresses within polymers that can cause elastic strain, plastic strain, or a combination of elastic plus plastic strain.

- *Plastic* deformation is irreversible and results in a new permanent shape.
- *Elastic* deformation is reversible and will be completely recovered when the stress is eliminated.
- *Viscoelastic* deformation results in a combination of elastic and plastic strain, but recovery of only elastic strain occurs as the stress is decreased. The recovery, however, is not instantaneous once the stress is eliminated; The process of recovery occurs over time. The amount of deformation that does not recover at the moment the stress is eliminated may be regarded as plastic deformation, as described in Chapter 4.

CRITICAL QUESTIONS

What is the difference between elastomers and plastics? What causes some polymers to respond elastically to stresses and others to act viscoelastically?

Rheometric Properties

The rheometry, or *flow* behavior, of solid polymers involves a combination of elastic and plastic deformation (*viscous* flow) and **elastic recovery** when stresses are eliminated. This combination of elastic and plastic changes is termed *viscoelasticity*. The chain length, number of cross-links, temperature, and rate of force application (fast impact versus extrusion) determine which type of behavior dominates.

- **Plastic flow:** Irreversible strain behavior that occurs when polymer chains slide over one another and become relocated within the material, resulting in *permanent* deformation.
- **Elastic recovery:** Reversible strain behavior that occurs in the amorphous regions of polymers when the randomly coiled chains straighten and then recoil, like springs that return to their original location without sliding past one another when an applied force is removed (Fig. 7-5).

Plastic and elastic properties are used to describe *ideal* materials. However, actual dental polymeric materials are deformed by a combination of elastic plus plastic strain processes. Thus elastomers do not always recover fully and retain a small degree of plastic deformation, whereas plastics exhibit a high level of plastic deformation, but they also have at least some small degree of elastic recovery. This phenomenon is called *viscoelastic recovery* (Fig. 7-6).

CRITICAL QUESTION

What effects are likely if a plasticizer is leached out of a polymer?

Solvation Properties

Polymers are usually slow to dissolve, are seldom clearly either soluble or insoluble in any given liquid, and their solvation characteristics are very sensitive to $\overline{M}_w$,

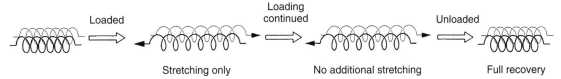

Fig. 7-5 Elastic recovery: springlike behavior (rapid and reversible). Chains uncoil, but they do not slip past one another because of crystalline regions, entanglements, or cross-links. Thus when unloaded, they recoil completely.

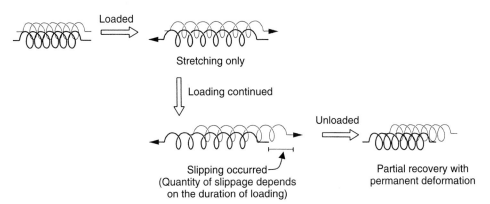

Fig. 7-6 Viscoelastic recovery: chains stretch and uncoil and also slip past one another, producing plastic, irreversible, permanent distortion and partial recovery when unloaded.

$\overline{M}_w/\overline{M}_n$ (*polydispersity*), cross-linking, crystallinity, and chain branching. The following characteristics describe the general nature of polymers:

- The longer the chains (the higher the molecular weight), the more slowly a polymer dissolves.
- Polymers tend to *absorb* a solvent, swell, and soften, rather than dissolve.
- Cross-linking prevents complete chain separation and retards dissolution.
- Highly cross-linked polymers cannot be dissolved.
- Elastomers swell more than plastics.
- A small amount of swelling of dental polymeric devices can have undesirable results on the fit of prostheses.
- Absorbed molecules (e.g., water) spread polymer chains apart and facilitate slip between chains. This lubricating effect is called *plasticization*.

Cross-linkage provides a sufficient number of bridges between linear macromolecules to form a three-dimensional network that decreases water sorption, decreases solubility, and increases the strength and rigidity of the resin. For example, cross-linkage has been used widely in the manufacture of acrylic teeth to increase their resistance to degradation by alcohol and other solvents, and the surface stresses produced by solvents. Crystalline regions act as physical cross-links, reducing solubility.

Plasticizers are often added to resins to reduce their softening or fusion temperatures. It is possible to plasticize a resin that is normally hard and stiff at room temperature to a condition in which it is flexible and soft by including a plasticizer in the resin. For example, PVC pipe is hard and rigid and contains very little plasticizer, whereas PVC tubing is soft and elastic and contains a very high level of plasticizer.

A plasticizer acts to partially neutralize secondary bonds or intermolecular forces that normally prevent the resin molecules from slipping past one another when the material is stressed. In some cases, the action is analogous to that of a solvent, with the plasticizing agent penetrating between the macromolecules and increasing the intermolecular spacing. This type of plasticizer is referred to as an *external plasticizer* because it is not a part of the polymer structure. Its molecular attraction to the polymer should be extremely high so that it does not volatilize or otherwise leach out during the fabrication or subsequent use of the resin. Such a condition is seldom realized in practice, so this type of plasticizer is used sparingly in dental resins.

Plasticizing of a resin can also be accomplished by copolymerization with a suitable comonomer. In this case, the plasticizing agent becomes part of the polymer and thus acts as an *internal plasticizer*. For example, when butyl methacrylate is added to methyl methacrylate before polymerization, the polymerized resin is plasticized internally by the butyl methacrylate segments (see Fig. 7-14). The function of the butyl methacrylate molecules is to increase intermolecular spacing via pendant groups. Plasticizers usually reduce the strength, hardness, and the softening point of the resin.

CRITICAL QUESTIONS

What is the difference between thermosetting and thermoplastic polymers? Which involves a reversible physical change and which involves an irreversible change?

Thermal Properties

The physical properties of a polymer are influenced by changes in temperature and environment and by the composition, structure, and molecular weight of the polymer. In general, the higher the temperature, the softer and weaker the polymer becomes. Polymers can be formed into many desired shapes, using processes that depend on whether the polymeric material is a "thermoset" or a "thermoplastic" type.

Thermoplastic polymers are made of linear and/or branched chains. They soften when heated above the glass transition temperature (T_g), at which molecular motion begins to force the chains apart. The resin can then be shaped and molded and, upon cooling, will harden in this form. However, on reheating, they soften again and can be reshaped if required before hardening as the temperature decreases. This cycle can be carried out repeatedly. Thermoplastic resins are fusible (i.e., they melt) and they are usually soluble in organic solvents.

Thermosetting polymers undergo a chemical change and become permanently hard when heated above the temperature at which they begin to polymerize, and do not soften again on reheating to the same temperature. They are usually cross-linked in this state, and thus, they are insoluble and infusible, decomposing instead. Thermosetting plastics generally have superior abrasion resistance and dimensional stability compared with thermoplastic polymers, which have better flexural and impact properties.

A temperature of particular interest in polymer science is the glass-transition temperature, T_g. An understanding of T_g and how it is affected by the polymer structure requires a discussion of the interatomic bonds that hold the different polymer chains together in a polymer. Along each single polymer chain, valence electrons continuously move back and forth. Because of these electron movements, varying electron densities exist along the chain at different times and locations. Adjacent chains adapt their electron densities along the chains to balance these differences in charge density. Because of these interactions, interatomic **induction** forces (known as *van der Waals* and *London forces*) are developed between the chains. These forces, as well as hydrogen bonding, form polar bonds between the polymer chains, bonds that are much weaker than the primary bonds along the polymer chains. When a polymer is heated to its T_g or to a higher temperature, the weak polar bonds are broken and the polymer molecular chains can move more freely relative to each other. The increased mobility has a strong impact on many physical properties, such as strength, modulus of elasticity, and thermal expansion. Strength and elastic modulus decrease as the temperature approaches T_g, whereas thermal expansion increases.

If two similar polymers consisting of straight polymer chains are compared, the one with the higher molecular weight will also have a higher T_g. If the straight-polymer chain length is increased, the number of polar bond sites increase along that chain. In addition, the longer chain length increases the chance for chain entanglements. Thus the increased number of polar bond sites along each chain and their increased chain entanglements explain why polymers with a higher molecular weight need more thermal energy to reach their T_g.

From a mechanical point of view, chain slippage also decreases as the chain length increases. At a certain chain length, though, the polar bonds and the entanglements are strong enough to resist dislodgment of the individual chain. For this critical chain length, the applied force first breaks the cohesive bond of the chain rather than dislodging chains. This balance between the strength of the polar bonds and the covalent bond of the chain explains why the physical and mechanical properties of the polymer increase with increased molecular weight to a certain point. Subsequently, increased molecular weight becomes less important.

The number average molecular weight is indicative of both T_g and the strength of the polymer. As mentioned previously, the value for the number average molecular weight is lowered markedly by the presence of a relatively few monomer molecules, which lowers T_g and weakens the resin considerably.

Although dependent on its type, a resin generally possesses mechanical strength only when its degree of polymerization is relatively high, that is, in the range of approximately 150 to 200 recurring units. Above this molecular weight, there is very little increase in strength with further polymerization, as explained previously. Likewise, the molecular-weight distribution of the polymer plays an important role in determining physical properties. In general, a narrow distribution of molecular weight yields the most useful polymers.

Long side chains protruding from the monomer molecule generally produce a weaker resin with a lower softening temperature in comparison with the properties of a polymer that possesses a straight-chain structure. This weakened effect is caused by the side chains separating the main chains, thus reducing the effectiveness of the polar bonds along the main chain. This is similar to the plasticizing effect discussed in the previous section. However, if the side chains can react with adjacent chains to form a cross-linked polymer, the strength of the polymer is increased.

Based on the preceding description of a polymer, heat should have a significant impact on the properties of a polymer. As the temperature increases, the rotation of polymer segments increases. These rotations, coupled with thermal expansion, increase chain separation, break polar bonds, and facilitate chain disentanglement. These factors in turn facilitate chain slippage and explain the thermoplastic behavior of a resin when it reaches T_g. If cross-linkages exist, slippage cannot occur, and the material becomes more difficult to soften.

CRITICAL QUESTION

What are the benefits and drawbacks of a heavily cross-linked polymer?

If a cross-linked resin is softened, it will not easily change shape permanently. The material becomes rubbery in consistency. Thus an elastomeric dental impression material can be described as a cross-linked polymeric structure with a T_g lower than room temperature. The low T_g implies that the chain segments are thermally agitated at room temperature. In this manner, the chains are rendered more flexible. In fact, almost any means can be used to impart elastomeric qualities through which the polymer molecules are rendered more mobile. Another requisite is that some degree of cross-linking must be present so that any deformation is readily reversible. Such cross-linking must occur only occasionally between the chains. If a high degree of cross-linking is present, a network configuration prevails, and the resin becomes rigid and useless as an impression material. The situation is analogous to that described in the formation of calcium alginate in alginate gels. Such cross-linked bonds cause the polymer to return to its original shape after the load is released, as in the case of the gels.

CHEMISTRY OF POLYMERIZATION

Monomers may be joined via one of two types of reaction: *addition* polymerization and *step-growth* or condensation polymerization. In addition, polymerization monomers are activated one at a time and add together in sequence to form a growing chain. In step-growth polymerization the components are difunctional and all are, or become, reactive simultaneously. Chains then grow by the stepwise linking of bifunctional monomers that often, but not always, produces a low molecular weight byproduct such as water or an alcohol.

Addition Polymerization

Most dental resins are polymerized by a mechanism in which monomers add sequentially to the end of a growing chain. Addition polymerization starts from an active center, adding one monomer at a time to rapidly form a chain. In theory, the chain can grow indefinitely until the entire monomer is exhausted. The process is simple, but it is not easy to control.

Compared with step-growth polymerization (discussed on page 161), addition polymerization can readily produce giant molecules of almost unlimited size. There is no change in composition during addition polymerization. The macromolecules are formed from smaller units, or monomers, without change in composition, because the monomer and the polymer have the same empirical formulas. In other words, the structure of the monomer is repeated many times in the polymer.

CRITICAL QUESTIONS

What are the rates of activation and free radical initiation and curing? Which three activation processes are used for dental polymers?

Stages in Addition Polymerization

Four distinct stages in the addition polymerization chain reaction process: **induction, propagation, chain transfer**, and **termination**.

Induction. Two processes control the induction stage: *activation* and *initiation*. For an addition polymerization process to begin, a source of **free radicals**, R•, is required. Free radicals can be generated by *activation* of radical-producing molecules using a second chemical, heat, visible light, ultraviolet light, or energy transfer from another compound that acts as a free radical (Fig. 7-7). Of these, chemical agents, heat, and visible light are most often used in dentistry.

$$R\text{—}R + \text{external energy} \rightarrow 2\ R\bullet \tag{1}$$

One of the requisites of an addition-polymerizable compound is the presence of an unsaturated group, that is, a *double bond*, as well as a source of free radicals. Theoretically, R• can be almost any free radical. A free radical is an atom or group of atoms possessing an unpaired electron (•). The unpaired electron confers electron-withdrawal ability to the free radical. When the free radical and its unpaired

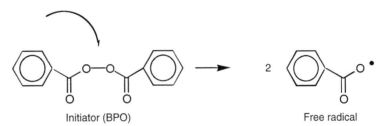

Initiator (BPO) Free radical

Fig. 7-7 Activation (heat or chemical) of benzoyl peroxide (BPO). During activation, the—O—O— bond is broken, and the electron pair is split between the two fragments. The dot adjacent to the oxygen of the free radical symbolizes the unpaired electron.

electron approach a monomer with its high-electron-density double bond, an electron is extracted, and it pairs with the R• electron to form a bond between the radical and the monomer molecule, leaving the other electron of the double bond unpaired. Thus the original free radical bonds to one side of the monomer molecule and forms a new free radical site at the other end. The reaction is now *initiated*.

Ethylene, $H_2C=CH_2$, the simplest monomer capable of addition polymerization, can be used for illustration:

$$R\bullet + H_2C=CH_2 \rightarrow RH_2C-CH_2\bullet \tag{2}$$

Initiation of the important dental resin, methyl methacrylate, is shown in Fig. 7-8.

The free radical–forming chemical used to start the polymerization is *not* a catalyst (although it is often incorrectly described by this term), because it enters into the chemical reaction and becomes part of the final chemical compound. It is more accurately called an *initiator* because it is used to start the reaction. A number of substances capable of generating free radicals are potent initiators for the polymerization of poly(methyl methacrylate) and other methacrylate-type resins used extensively in dentistry (see below and Chapters 15 and 22). The most commonly employed initiator is benzoyl peroxide, which is activated rapidly between 50° and 100° C to release two free radicals per benzoyl peroxide molecule (see reaction 1 and

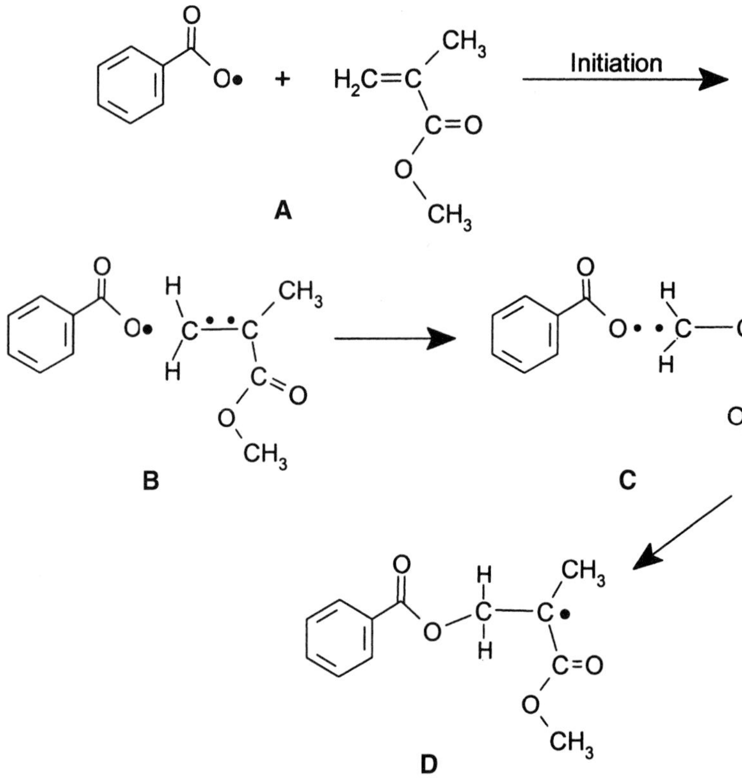

Fig. 7-8 Initiation of a methyl methacrylate molecule. As the unpaired electron of the free radical approaches the methyl methacrylate molecule (**A** and **B**), one of the electrons in the double bond is attracted to the free radical to form an electron pair and a covalent bond between the free radical and the monomer molecule (**C** and **D**). When this occurs, the remaining unpaired electron makes the new molecule a free radical (**D**).

Fig. 7-7). Induction is the period during which initiator molecules become energized and break down into free radicals, followed by these radicals reacting with monomer molecules to initiate chain growth (see reactions 2 and 3 and Fig. 7-8). This period is greatly influenced by the purity of the monomer. Any impurities present that are able to react with activated groups can increase the length of this period by consuming the activated initiator molecules. However, the higher the temperature, the more rapid the formation of free radicals and, consequently, the shorter the induction period.

The polymerization processes useful for dental resins are commonly activated by one of three energy sources: heat, chemicals, and light. Most denture base resins are polymerized by heat activation, as explained previously, producing two free radicals, which then initiate and propagate the polymerization of methyl methacrylate monomer, as shown in reactions 1, 2, 3, and 4.

A second type of induction system is chemically activated at ambient oral temperature. Such a system consists of at least two reactants that, when mixed together, undergo a chemical reaction that generates free radicals. During storage, these components must be separated from each other; hence chemically induced systems always consist of two or more parts. An example of such a system is the tertiary amine (the *activator*) and benzoyl peroxide (the *initiator*), which are mixed together to initiate the polymerization of so-called "self-cured" dental resins at room temperature. This process, in fact, is a special case of heat activation, because the presence of the amine reduces the thermal energy required to break the initiator into free radicals at ambient temperature (i.e., room temperature or mouth temperature). The amine forms a complex with benzoyl peroxide, which reduces the thermal energy (and thus the temperature) needed to split it into two free radicals.

A third type of induction system is light-activated. In this system, photons from a light source activate the initiator to generate free radicals that, in turn, can initiate the polymerization process. When this system was first introduced to dentistry, ultraviolet light was used. However, because of concerns about the effect of ultraviolet light on the retina and unpigmented oral tissues, its limited penetration depth, and the loss in intensity of the ultraviolet light source over time, initiator systems were subsequently developed that are activated by visible light. In the visible light–cured dental restoratives, camphorquinone and an organic amine (e.g., dimethyl-aminoethylmethacrylate) generate free radicals when irradiated by light in the blue-to-violet region. Light with a wavelength of about 470 nm is needed to trigger this reaction. Because no appreciable polymerization takes place at ambient temperature in the dark, such compositions can be one-part systems, provided that they are stored where they are not exposed to light. However, factors such as light intensity, angle of illumination, and distance of resin from the light source can significantly affect the number of free radicals that are formed, thereby making this system technique sensitive.

Propagation. The resulting free radical-monomer complex then acts as a new free radical center when it approaches another monomer to form a *dimer*, which also becomes a free radical. This reactive species, in turn, can add successively to a large number of ethylene molecules so that the polymerization process continues through the propagation of the reactive center.

$$RH_2C—CH_2• + H_2C=CH_2 \rightarrow RH_2C—CH_2—H_2C—CH_2• \qquad (3)$$

$$RH_2C—CH_2—H_2C—CH_2• + H_2C=CH_2 \rightarrow$$
$$RH_2C—(CH_2—H_2C)_2—CH_2•....etc. \qquad (4)$$

Propagation reactions are further illustrated in Figure 7-9. Because little energy is required once chain growth begins, the process continues with evolution of heat and leads to large polymer molecules within seconds. Theoretically, the chain reactions should continue until all of the monomer has been converted to a polymer between the **initial set** and the **final set**. The process continues to complete the formation of the desired polymer. However, the polymerization reaction is never quite completed.

The growth of the polymer chain ceases when the reactive center is destroyed by one of a number of possible termination reactions (as discussed later). The entire addition polymerization process can be pictured as a series of chain reactions. The process occurs rapidly, almost instantaneously. The reactions are *exothermic,* and considerable heat is evolved.

Chain Transfer. In this process, the active free radical of a growing chain is transferred to another molecule (e.g., a monomer or inactivated polymer chain) and a new free radical for further growth is created. For example, a monomer molecule may be activated by a growing macromolecule in such a manner that termination occurs in the latter (Fig. 7-10) Thus a new nucleus for growth results. In the same manner, an already terminated chain might be reactivated by chain transfer, and it will continue to grow (Fig. 7-11). These processes differ from the termination reactions described below.

Termination. Although chain termination can result from chain transfer, addition polymerization reactions are most often terminated either by direct coupling of two free radical chain ends or by the exchange of a hydrogen atom from one growing chain to another.

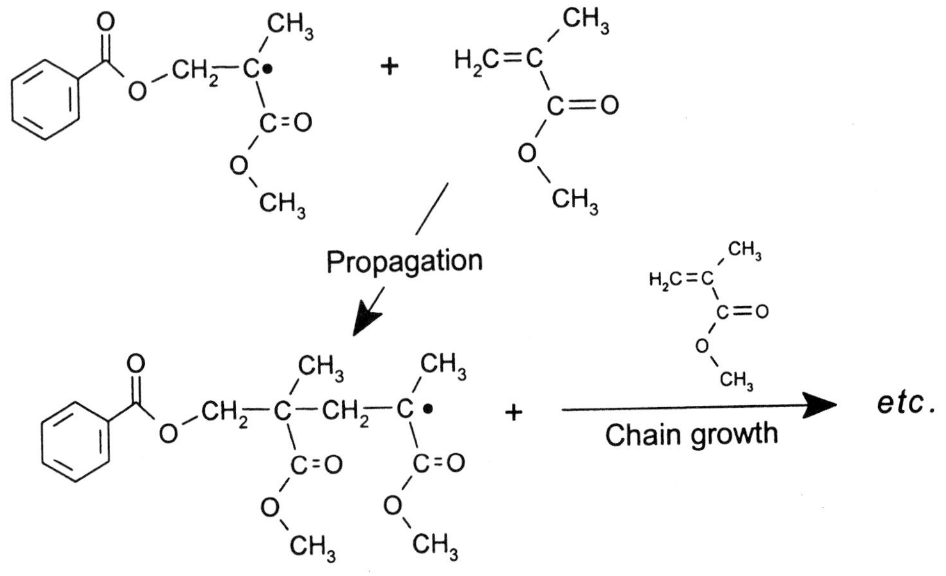

Fig. 7-9   Propagation and chain growth. As the initiated molecule approaches other methyl methacrylate molecules, the free electron interacts with the double bond of the methyl methacrylate molecule, and a new, longer free radical is formed.

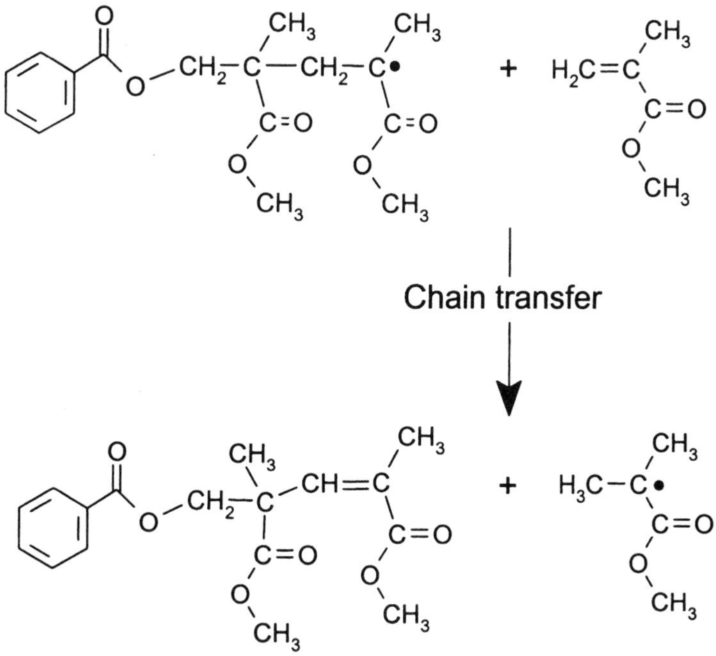

Fig. 7-10 Chain transfer occurs when a free radical approaches a methyl methacrylate molecule and donates a hydrogen atom to the methyl methacrylate molecule. This causes the free radical to rearrange to form a double bond and become unreactive, and the MMA monomer to form a free radical that can participate in a chain-propagation reaction.

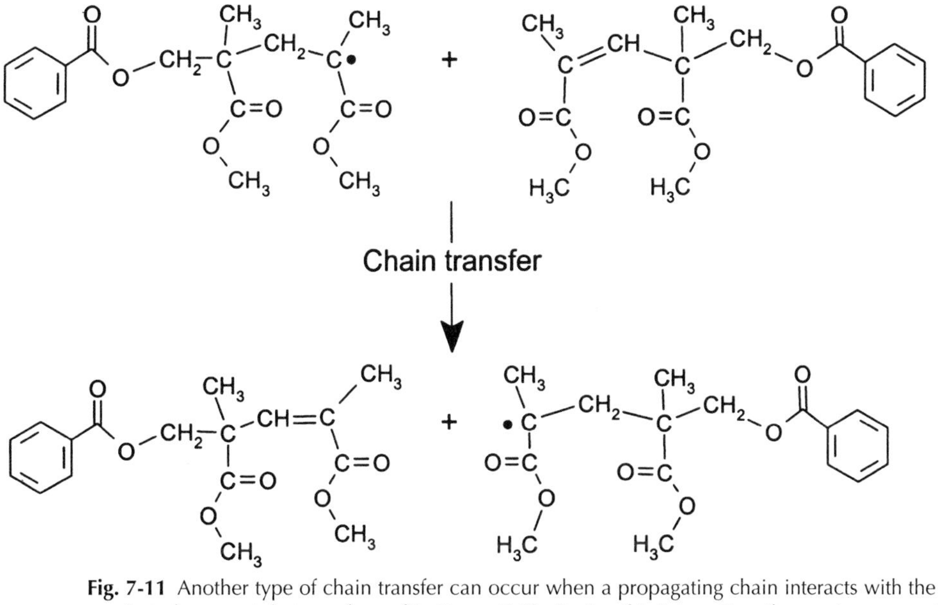

Fig. 7-11 Another type of chain transfer can occur when a propagating chain interacts with the passivated segment that was formed in Figure 7-10. During this interaction, the passive segment becomes active, while the active segment becomes passive.

Termination by direct coupling can be illustrated by the ethylene addition reaction. Continuing from the propagation reaction (see reaction 4), if a growing chain with *m* monomer units encounters another growing chain with *n* units, then:

$$RH_2C-(CH_2-H_2C)_m-CH_2\bullet + \bullet H_2C-(CH_2-H_2C)_n-CH_2 R \rightarrow$$
$$RH_2C-(CH_2-H_2C)_m-CH_2-H_2C-(CH_2-H_2C)_n-CH_2R \quad (5)$$

Both molecules combine and become deactivated by formation of a covalent bond (Fig. 7-12).

Another means by which such an energy exchange can occur is the transfer of a hydrogen atom from one growing chain to another (Fig. 7-13). In this case, a double bond is produced when the hydrogen atom is transferred.

CRITICAL QUESTIONS

What mechanisms are responsible for inhibition of polymerization? What are the benefits of inhibitors in dental resins? What role does O_2 play as an inhibitor?

Inhibition of Addition Polymerization

As noted in the previous section, the polymerization reactions are not likely to result in a complete exhaustion of the monomer, nor do they always form polymers of high molecular weight. Impurities in the monomer often inhibit such reactions.

Any impurity in the monomer that can react with free radicals inhibits or retards the polymerization reaction. An impurity can react with the activated initiator or with an activated growing chain to prevent further growth. The presence of such

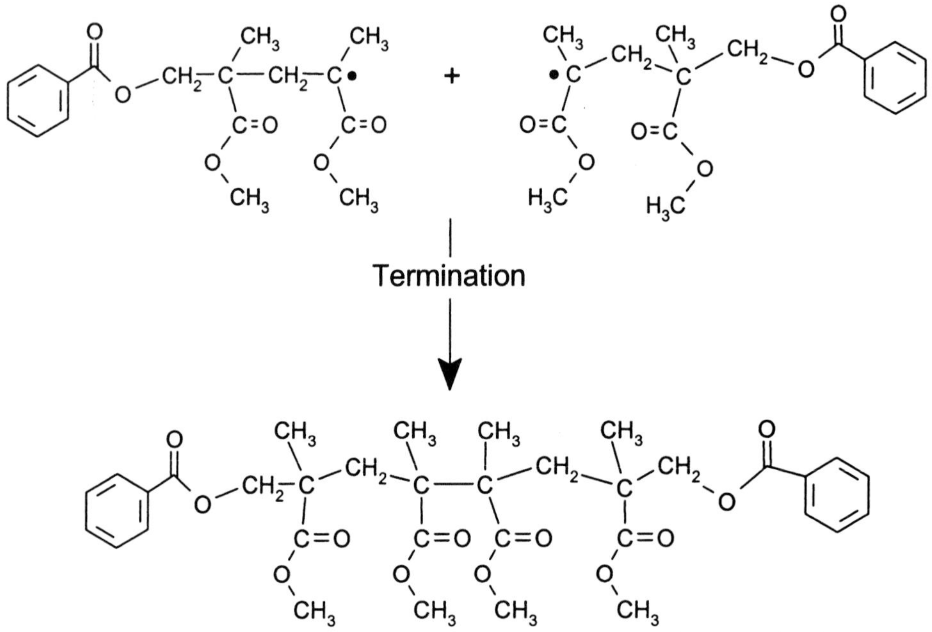

Fig. 7-12 Termination occurs when two free radicals interact and form a covalent bond.

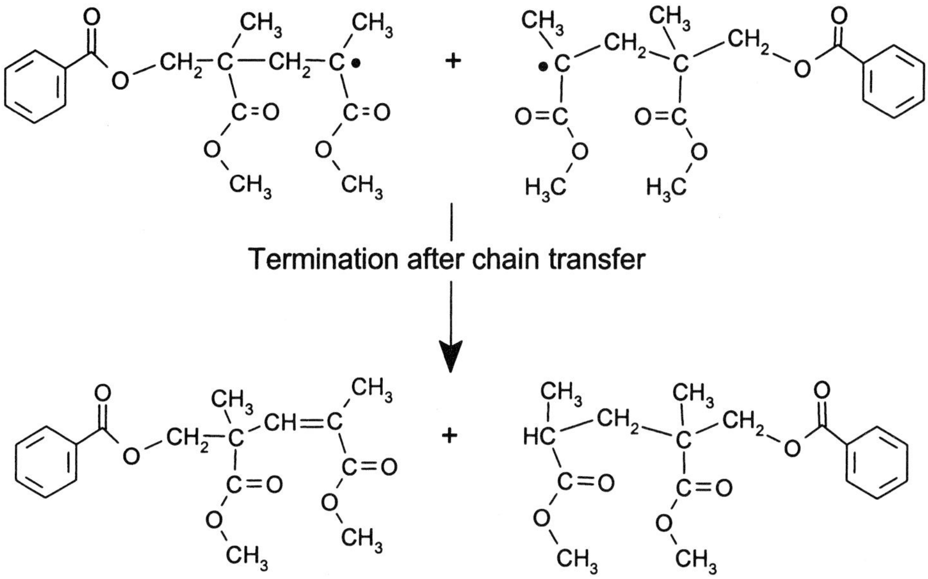

Fig. 7-13 When two free radicals approach each other, a new double bond may be formed on the molecule that donates a hydrogen atom to the other free radical.

inhibitors markedly influences the length of the induction period, as well as the degree of polymerization.

For example, the addition of a small amount of a common inhibitor, such as hydroquinone, to the monomer inhibits spontaneous polymerization if no initiator is present and retards the polymerization in the presence of an initiator. Thus inhibitors affect both the storage stability and the working time of a dental resin. For this reason, commercial dental resins commonly contain a small amount (approximately 0.006% or less) of an inhibitor such as the methyl ether of hydroquinone to aid in the prevention of polymerization during storage and, in the case of two-part (self-cure) systems, to provide adequate time for mixing and placement.

Oxygen reacts rapidly with free radicals, and its presence retards the polymerization reaction. It has been shown, for example, that the reaction velocity and the degree of polymerization are decreased if polymerization is conducted in open air in comparison with the higher values obtained when the reaction is carried out in an oxygen-deficient environment. The influence of oxygen on polymerization is governed by many factors, such as its concentration, the temperature, and light intensity. It is important to be aware of the inhibiting effect of oxygen on the polymerization process. Thus air thinning of bonding resins should be avoided to optimize curing in important regions of a restoration. A common clinical practice is to use a matrix material, which helps to shape the resin and acts as a barrier to prevent contact with oxygen during curing. Such a matrix strip prevents a sticky, air-inhibited layer from forming on the surface.

Step-Growth Polymerization

The reactions that produce step-growth polymerization can progress by any of the chemical reaction mechanisms that join two or more molecules in producing a simple, nonmacromolecular structure. The primary compounds react, often with the formation of by-products such as water, alcohols, halogen acids, and ammonia.

The formation of these by-products is the reason step-growth polymerization often is called *condensation polymerization*. The structure of the monomers is such that the process can repeat itself and build macromolecules. This mechanism is also the one used in biological tissues to produce proteins, carbohydrates, deoxyribonucleic acid, and ribonucleic acid, which are exclusively formed via step-growth polymerization reactions.

In step-growth polymerization, a linear chain of repeating mer units is obtained by the stepwise intermolecular condensation or addition of the reactive groups in which *bifunctional* or trifunctional monomers are all simultaneously activated, as opposed to the activation of one monomer at a time in chain-growth addition polymerization. For example:

$$HO—(Silicone)—OH + n \ HO—(Silicone)—OH \rightarrow$$
$$HO—(Silicone)—(O—Silicone)_n—OH + n \ H_2O\uparrow \qquad (6)$$

This type of reaction is also illustrated in Chapter 9. In one reaction, water is removed in the process of joining trimercaptans to form a polysulfide rubber (see Fig. 9-4), and in the other case, ethanol is removed in the process of joining siloxane molecules to form silicone rubber (see Fig. 9-5). At each step in the reaction a new bi- or trifunctional higher–molecular-weight compound is formed. As the reaction proceeds, progressively longer chains form until ultimately the reaction contains a mixture of polymer chains of large molar masses. In the case of the trifunctional reaction for a polysulfide impression material, a structure forms that is both branched and cross-linked (see Fig. 9-4).

As polymer science has progressed, the classification of condensation-polymerized resins has broadened. Because the goal is to minimize classification uncertainties, the term *step-growth polymerization* (rather than *condensation polymerization*) is preferred. Step-growth polymerized resins are those in which polymerization is accompanied by repeated elimination of small molecules. The formation of polymers by step growth is rather slow because the reaction proceeds in a stepwise fashion from monomer to dimer to trimer, and so forth, until large polymer molecules containing many monomer molecules are eventually formed. Such a polymerization process tends to stop before the chain has reached a truly great size, because as the chains grow, they become less mobile and less numerous.

CRITICAL QUESTION

What are the practical benefits of using copolymer resins for dental applications?

COPOLYMERIZATION

In many of the polymerization reactions described above, the macromolecule was formed by the polymerization of a single type of structural unit. However, two or more chemically different monomers, each with some desirable property, can be combined to yield specific physical properties of a polymer. As defined earlier, the polymer formed is a *copolymer*, and its process of formation is known as *copolymerization* (Fig. 7-14). In a copolymer, the relative number and position of the different type of repeating units may vary among the individual macromolecules.

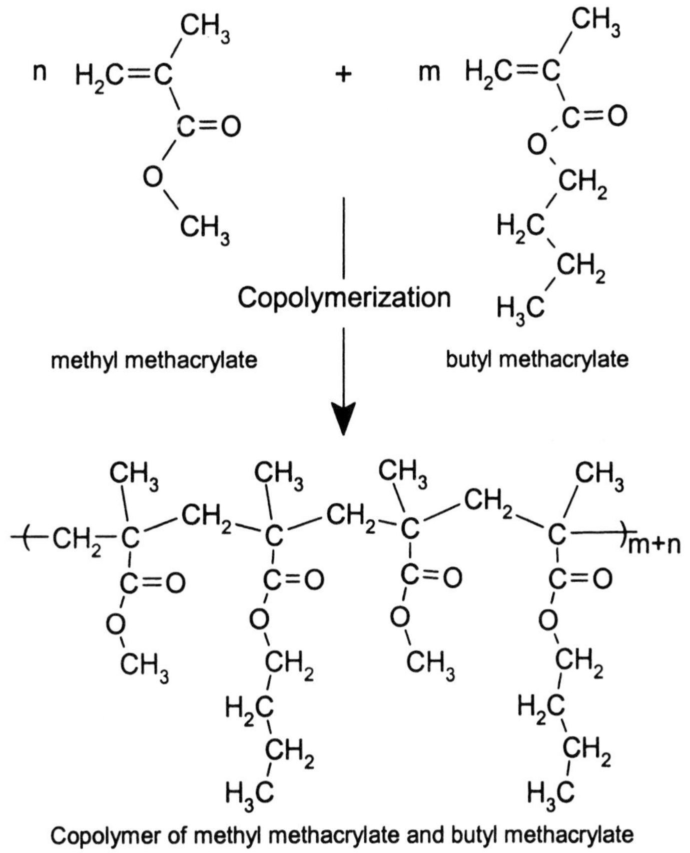

Fig. 7-14 Copolymerization between butyl methacrylate and methyl methacrylate. Because the butyl methacrylate molecules increase the backbone separation of the polymer molecules, the intermolecular interactions decrease, as does the glass transition temperature.

Copolymerization is most easily illustrated with two monomers, although it is possible to incorporate more than two monomers. For example, two monomers ($H_2C=CHR^1$ and $H_2C=CHR^2$) consisting of ethylene derivatives can be incorporated, with either R^1 or R^2 substituted for one of the H-atoms, as shown below:

$$n\, H_2C=CHR^1 + m\, H_2C=CHR^2 \rightarrow$$
$$(H_2C-CHR^1-H_2C-CHR^2)_{n+m} \qquad (7)$$

This copolymer structure is highly idealized because the occurrence of alternately placed radicals in the chain would seldom occur. It is more probable that the positions of the radicals are random—a matter of probability. The composition of the copolymer depends on the relative reactivities of the two (or more) different monomers, as well as the relative reactivity of like monomers among themselves. For example, if the tendency of $H_2C=CHR^1$ to homopolymerize (polymerization with itself) is so great that it polymerizes independently of $H_2C=CHR^2$, no copolymerization will occur, and the resulting resin will consist of a mixture of two polymers:

$$n\, H_2C=CHR^1 + m\, H_2C=CHR^2 \rightarrow$$
$$(H_2C-CHR^1)_n + (H_2C-CHR^2)_m \qquad (8)$$

Such an extreme condition seldom, if ever, occurs. In most instances, the cured polymer consists of a mixture of polymers and copolymers, with varying degrees of polymerization or copolymerization. Furthermore, as explained above, copolymers can vary in the molecular sequence and arrangement among the repeating random block and graft units. Copolymerization can have a very strong influence on the physical and mechanical properties of the resulting resin, changing them considerably from those of the respective homopolymers.

Many useful resins are manufactured by copolymerization. Methyl methacrylate, acrylic esters, and methacrylic esters all copolymerize readily, with little inhibition between monomer pairs. For example, small amounts of ethyl acrylate may be copolymerized with methyl methacrylate to alter the flexibility and fracture resistance of a denture.

Grafting of various polymer segments onto a linear chain provides an important mechanism for modifying or tailor-making macromolecules to obtain required properties for specific uses. For example, block and graft polymers (see Fig. 7-2) often show improved impact strength. In small quantities, these polymers can modify the adhesive properties of resins, as well as their surface characteristics.

ACRYLIC DENTAL RESINS

As previously mentioned, for a synthetic resin to be useful in dentistry, it must exhibit exceptional qualities regarding its chemical and dimensional stability and yet it must also possess properties that render it relatively easy to process. It must be strong and hard, but not brittle. A few acrylic resins used in dentistry are discussed in the following.

Acrylic Resins

The acrylic resins are derivatives of ethylene and contain a vinyl ($-C=C-$) group in their structural formula:

$$H_2C=CHR \tag{9}$$

There are at least two acrylic resin series that are of dental interest. One series is derived from acrylic acid, $CH_2=CHCOOH$, and the other from methacrylic acid, $CH_2=C(CH_3)COOH$. Both of these compounds polymerize by addition in the usual manner. Although the polyacids are hard and transparent, their polarity, related to the carboxyl group, causes them to imbibe water. The water tends to separate the chains and to cause a general softening and loss of strength. The esters of these polyacids, however, are of considerable dental interest. For example, if **R** represents any ester radical, the polymerization reaction for poly(methacrylate) will be:

$$CH_2=C(CH_3) \rightarrow -CH_2-C(CH_3)-CH_2-C(CH_3)- \tag{10}$$
$$\underset{COOR}{|} \qquad \underset{COOR}{|} \qquad \underset{COOR}{|}$$

Because R can be almost any organic or inorganic radical, it is evident that thousands of different acrylic resins are capable of formation. Such a consideration does not include the possibilities of copolymerization, which are even greater.

The effect of esterification on the softening point of a few of the poly(methacrylate) compounds is shown in Table 7-1.

For short chain lengths, increasing the length of the side chain lowers the softening point or glass transition temperature. For example, poly(methyl methacrylate) is

Table 7-1	Softening Temperatures of Polymethacrylate Esters
Poly(methacrylate)	**T_g (° C)**
Methyl	125
Ethyl	65
n-Propyl	38
Isopropyl	95
n-Butyl	33
Isobutyl	70
sec-Butyl	62
tert-Amyl	76
Phenyl	120

the hardest resin of the series with the highest softening temperature. Poly(ethyl methacrylate) possesses a lower softening point and surface hardness, and poly(*n*-propyl methacrylate) has an even lower softening point and hardness.

Methyl Methacrylate

Poly(methyl methacrylate) by itself is not used in dentistry to a great extent in molding procedures. Rather, the liquid monomer methyl methacrylate (Fig. 7-15) is mixed with the polymer, which is supplied in the powdered form. The monomer partially dissolves the polymer to form a plastic dough. This dough is packed into the mold, and the monomer is polymerized by one of the methods discussed previously. Consequently, the monomer methyl methacrylate is of considerable importance in dentistry.

Methyl methacrylate is a transparent liquid at room temperature with the following physical properties:

- Molecular weight = 100
- Melting point = −48° C
- Boiling point = 100.8° C (note how close this is to the boiling point of water)
- Density = 0.945 g/mL at 20° C
- Heat of polymerization = 12.9 kcal/mol

Methyl methacrylate exhibits a high vapor pressure and is an excellent organic solvent. Although the polymerization of methyl methacrylate can be initiated by visible light, ultraviolet light, or heat, it is commonly polymerized in dentistry by the use of a chemical initiator, as described previously.

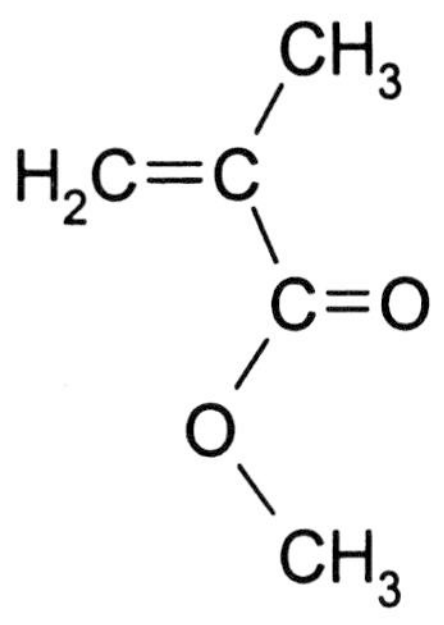

$$H_2C=C \begin{smallmatrix} CH_3 \\ \\ C=O \\ / \\ O \\ \\ CH_3 \end{smallmatrix}$$

Fig. 7-15 Methyl methacrylate molecule.

The conditions for the polymerization of methyl methacrylate are not critical, provided that the reaction is not carried out too rapidly. The degree of polymerization varies with the conditions of polymerization, such as the temperature, method of activation, type of initiator, initiator concentration, purity of chemicals, and similar factors. Because they polymerize readily under the conditions of use, the methacrylate monomers are particularly useful in dentistry. Many other resin systems do not polymerize at room temperature in the presence of air. A volume shrinkage of 21% occurs during the polymerization of the pure methyl methacrylate monomer.

Poly(methyl Methacrylate)

Poly(methyl methacrylate)[1] (see Fig. 7-15) is a transparent resin of remarkable clarity; it transmits light in the ultraviolet range to a wavelength of 250 nm. It is a hard resin with a Knoop hardness number of 18 to 20. It has a tensile strength approximately 60 MPa, a density of 1.19 g/cm^3, and a modulus of elasticity of approximately 2.4 GPa (2400 MPa).

This polymer is extremely stable. It does not discolor in ultraviolet light, and it exhibits remarkable aging properties. It is chemically stable to heat and softens at 125° C, and it can be molded as a thermoplastic material. Between 125° and 200° C, depolymerization takes place. At approximately 450° C, 90% of the polymer depolymerizes to form the monomer. Poly(methyl methacrylate) of high molecular weight degrades to a lower polymer at the same time that it converts to the monomer.

Like all acrylic resins, poly(methyl methacrylate) exhibits a tendency to absorb water by a process of imbibition. Its noncrystalline structure possesses a high internal energy. Thus molecular diffusion can occur in the resin, because less activation energy is required. Furthermore, the polar carboxyl group, even though esterified, can form a hydrogen bridge to a limited extent with water. Because poly(methyl methacrylate) is a linear polymer, it is soluble in a number of organic solvents that may be found in a dental laboratory or operatory, such as chloroform and acetone.

Multifunctional Methacrylate and Acrylate Resins

The backbone of the molecule formed in this system can have any shape, but methacrylate groups are found at the ends of the chain or at the end of branching chains. One of the first multifunctional methacrylates used in dentistry was Bowen's resin, or bis-GMA (Fig. 7-16). The bis-GMA resin can be described as an aromatic ester of a dimethacrylate, synthesized from an epoxy resin (ethylene glycol of *bis*-phenol A) and methyl methacrylate. Because bis-GMA has two —OH groups that form hydrogen bonds between the monomers, it is extremely viscous. A low-viscosity dimethacrylate, such as triethyleneglycol dimethacrylate (TEGDMA), is blended with it to reduce viscosity (Fig. 7-17).

The rigid central core of two aromatic groups reduces the ability of bis-GMA molecules to rotate during polymerization and thereby to participate efficiently in the polymerization process. Therefore, one of the methacrylate groups reacts often,

---

1. The nomenclature of *poly(methyl methacrylate)* has been retained throughout this chapter. Frequently, it is referred to as *polymethyl methacrylate* or *methyl methacrylate polymer*. However, the present rules of the International Union of Pure and Applied Chemistry state: "A polymer of unspecified chain length is named with the prefix 'poly' followed by, in parentheses or brackets, as appropriate, the name of the smallest repeating unit. The generic name for a single-stranded linear polymer is thus poly(bivalent radical)." (Macromolecules 1:19, 1968.)

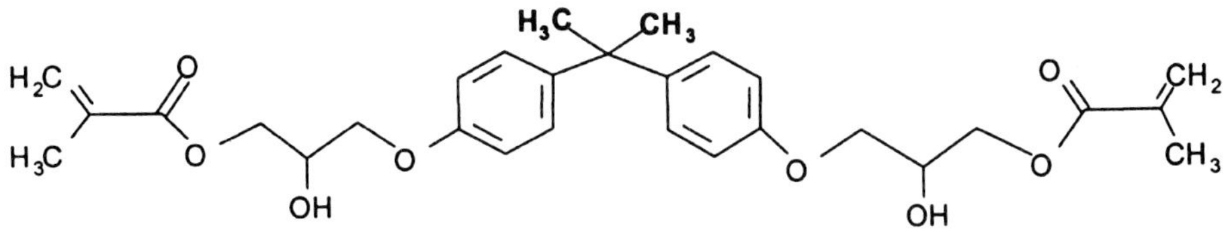

Fig. 7-16 Bis-GMA molecule. The central part of the molecule becomes stiff because of restricted rotational ability of the two rings.

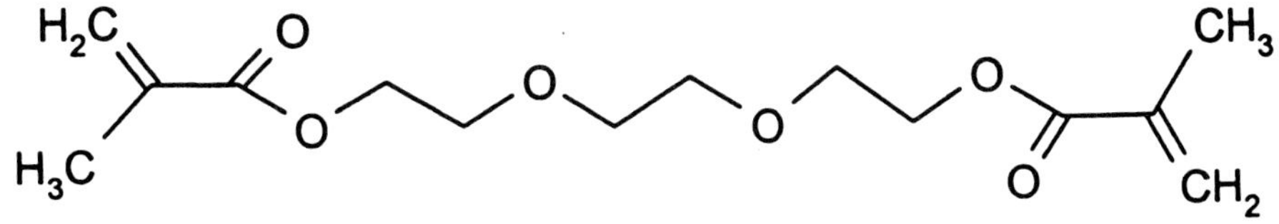

Fig. 7-17 TEGDMA molecule. The backbone structure is flexible, which facilitates molecular interaction during polymerization and increases the degree of conversion.

whereas the other does not. This process results in a bis-GMA molecule that forms a branch, or pendant group, along the polymer chain. Some of these branches cross-link with adjacent chains, and some do not. To quantify the efficiency of polymerization and cross-linking, the clinician determines the ratio, R, of unreacted methacrylate groups before and after polymerization. The *degree of conversion*, expressed in percentage of consumed methyl methacrylate groups, can be determined from the formula:

$$(1 - R) \times 100 = \text{degree of conversion} \tag{11}$$

Various dimethacrylate resin combinations have been explored through the years in attempts to reduce viscosity and to increase the degree of conversion. One resin group that has shown promise is *urethane dimethacrylate* (UDMA). This UDMA group can be described as any monomer chain containing one or more urethane groups and two methacrylate end groups (Fig. 7-18).

In addition to the dimethacrylates mentioned previously, other multifunctional resins have been introduced to dentistry during the last few years. For example, in some dentin bonding agents a monomer called dipentaerythiol penta-acrylate monophosphate (PENTA-P) is used (Fig. 7-19). As seen from the PENTA-P formula, this monomer contains as many as five acrylate groups per monomer molecule.

Another multifunctional resin that has been used extensively during the last few years is poly(acrylic acid), to which hydroxyethyl methacrylate (HEMA) has been grafted (Fig. 7-20). Such a modified poly(acrylic acid) (PAA) is used in light-curable glass ionomer cements (see Chapter 16). During light exposure, free radical polymerization is initiated, causing the methacrylate groups to react. The reaction that cross-links the PAA molecules constitutes the **initial setting** reaction. After this reaction, the carboxylate groups continue to react with the glass particles through an acid-base reaction. During this reaction, the PAA releases the hydrogen ions and the PAA chains become negatively charged (see Fig. 16-11 and Fig. 16-17).

These negative charges, however, are balanced by cations leached from the glass. These cations, such as Ca^{2+} and Al^{3+}, form ionic bonds between the chains that now also become ionically cross-linked. In addition, the negatively charged PAA chains also form bonds to tooth tissues containing cations such as Ca^{2+}.

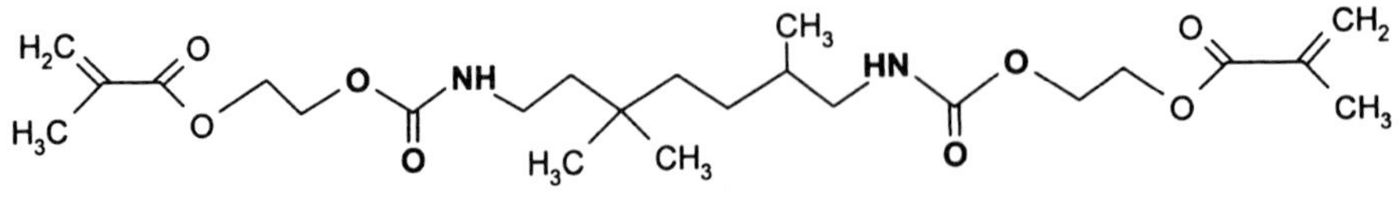

Fig. 7-18   UDMA molecule, which has two urethane groups. Otherwise, the backbone structure is flexible.

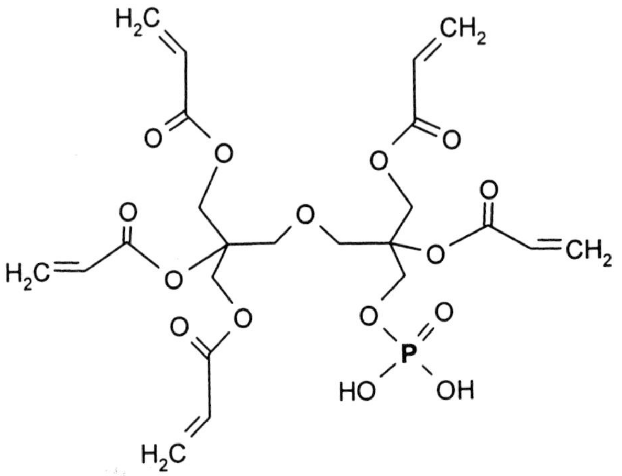

Fig. 7-19   PENTA-P molecule. This molecule has a phosphate group and five acrylate groups. The phosphate group can etch enamel and dentin surfaces, whereas the five acrylate groups increase reactivity and cross-linking ability.

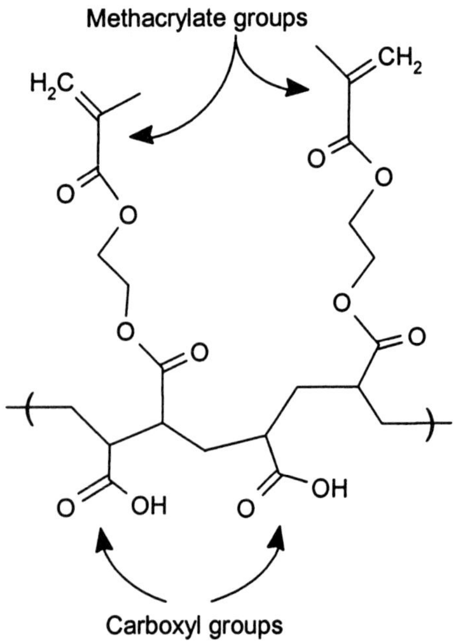

Fig. 7-20   Polyacrylic acid with grafted ethyl methacrylate groups. The carboxyl groups can etch dentin and enamel by giving up their hydrogen ions. When this occurs, the molecule becomes negatively charged and bonds to positive ions, such as calcium, present at the tooth surface. This ionic bond formation can also occur between polyacrylic acid chains, causing the material to set. Another setting mechanism that can be used is addition polymerization. This polymerization reaction can be initiated by light, which causes the methacrylate groups to react.

By observing this modified PAA molecule, you can see that as the number of methacrylate groups increase, the number of carboxylate groups decreases. This is important because fewer carboxylate groups reduce the extent of the acid-base reaction and weaken the enamel-dentin interaction. Thus a light-cured glass ionomer consists of a combination of both addition polymerization and acid-base reactivity, yielding a so-called hybrid material. Further development using acidic monomers instead of HEMA-modified PAA has led to a new material called a *compomer*, which shows physical properties similar to those of composite materials, as well as the ability to release fluoride in a manner similar to that of glass ionomer cements.

SELECTED READINGS

Cowie JMG: Polymers: Chemistry and Physics of Modern Materials. Aulesbury, Intertext, 1973.

An excellent introduction to polymer science, written so that knowledge is nicely blended with humor.

Morrison RT, and Boyd RN: Organic Chemistry, 5th ed. Boston, Allyn and Bacon, 1987.

A classic textbook in organic chemistry. The book gives the reader a fundamental understanding of the different mechanisms that affect the molecular structure of organic compounds used in different fields of science, including dentistry.

Sun SF: Physical Chemistry of Macromolecules: Basic Principles and Issues. New York, John Wiley, 1994.

This textbook unites biophysical chemistry and physical polymer chemistry. It offers a good overview of molecular structure, physical properties, and modern experimental techniques.

Ward IM: Mechanical Properties of Solid Polymers, 2nd ed. New York, Wiley-Interscience, 1983.

This textbook establishes the mechanics of the polymer behavior and also discusses molecular and structural phenomena.

Useful Web Sites for Dental Resins:

http://www.psrc.usm.edu/macrog/index.html
http://abalone.cwru.edu/tutorial/enhanced/files/textbook.htm

http://www.irc.leeds.ac.uk/iaps/mod1/mod1.html

8

Biocompatibility of Dental Materials

John C. Wataha

OUTLINE

Biocompatibility: Historical Background

Adverse Effects from Dental Materials

Biological Response in the Dental Environment

Measuring the Biocompatibility of Materials

Current Biocompatibility Issues in Dentistry

Clinical Guidelines for Selecting Biocompatible Materials

KEY TERMS

Allergy—Abnormal antigen-antibody reaction to a substance that is harmless to most individuals (see **Hypersensitivity**).

Biocompatibility—Ability of a material to elicit an appropriate biological response in a given application in the body.

Biointegration—Process in which bone or other living tissue becomes integrated with an implanted material with no intervening space.

Estrogenicity—Ability of a chemical to act in the body in a manner similar to that of estrogen, the female sex hormone.

Hypersensitivity—Abnormal clinical reaction or exaggerated immune response to a foreign substance that is manifested by one or more of the following signs and symptoms (among others): breathing difficulty, erythema, itching, sneezing, swelling, and vesicles. The most relevant dental situations are Type I hypersensitivity (immediate reaction) and Type IV hypersensitivity (delayed reaction) according to the Gell and Coombs classification of immune responses.

Osseointegration—Process in which living bony tissue forms to within 100 Å of the implant surface without any intervening fibrous connective tissue.

Sensitization—Process that produces an allergy antibody, which reacts specifically to the causative foreign substance.

Toxicity—Dose-related potential of a material to cause cell or tissue death.

Xenoestrogen—A chemical, not indigenous to the body, that acts in the body in a manner similar to that of estrogen.

The **biocompatibility** of dental materials is a complex topic that draws on knowledge from biology, patient risk factors, clinical experience, and engineering. Although ignored for many years, biocompatibility is now recognized as a fundamental requirement for any dental restorative material. This chapter discusses the definition of biocompatibility, the types of biological responses that materials may cause, and the anatomical aspects of the oral cavity that influence or modify biological responses to materials. Methods used to measure biocompatibility are described, along with the regulations that govern these methods and the difficulty in interpreting the results of biocompatibility tests. Finally, a short review of several dental biocompatibility issues is presented with recommendations for clinicians on making clinical judgments when assessing the biological safety of restorative materials.

CRITICAL QUESTION

How has the ethical view on testing of new materials for their biological properties changed in dentistry over the past century?

BIOCOMPATIBILITY: HISTORICAL BACKGROUND

Although the concept of the ethical treatment of patients extends back to the time of Hippocrates (460–377 B.C.), the idea that new dental materials must be tested for safety and efficacy before clinical use is much more recent. As late as the mid 1800s, dentists tried new materials for the first time by putting them into patients' mouths. Many exotic formulations were used. For example, Fox developed a "fusible metal" that consisted of bismuth, lead, and tin, which he melted and poured into the cavity preparation at a temperature of approximately 100° C. Even G.V. Black used patients to test many of his new ideas for restorative materials, such as early amalgams. The concept of protecting the patient as a research subject is only 30 to 40 years old, and many of the regulations and ethics in this area are still being challenged and defined today. In most cases, a committee of clinicians, basic scientists, and laypersons regulate and oversee the testing of new materials in humans. These committees are generally, but not always, university-based and are called IRBs (Institutional Review Boards). Regulations for IRBs are maintained by the Department of Health and Human Services, an agency of the U.S. federal government.

Using humans as research subjects today without some previous testing or knowledge of the biological properties of a material is unethical and illegal. Still, every new material must be inserted into a human for the first time at some point. Therefore, many alternative tests have been developed to try to minimize the risks to humans. The current philosophy about testing the biological properties of dental materials in a systematic way evolved in the 1960s as the need to protect patients became politically acute and as the number of new materials increased. Public outcry against the use of nonconsenting humans as research subjects—for example, the use of nonconsenting U.S. citizens for radiation experiments by the Department of Energy (1931–1994) and the use of institutionalized mentally retarded children for hepatitis research (1963-1966)—drove the development of regulations to protect humans in research. The oversight for this testing now rests largely with the Food and Drug Administration (FDA—www.fda.gov), but these activities also are regulated by organizations such as the American National Standards Institute (ANSI—www.ansi.org), the American Dental Association (ADA—www.ada.org) and the International Organization for Standardization (ISO—www.iso.ch). In spite of these oversights, there is still an experimental aspect to the use of all materials in dentistry (and medicine), and despite good clinical research, materials are still used before their biological properties can be fully ascertained.

Biological testing of materials has evolved significantly over the past 40 years. Initially, most biological reactions to materials were categorized empirically and relied on animal models. Many studies between the 1950s and the 1970s involved the use of premolar teeth that were scheduled for orthodontic extraction. As cell-culture techniques developed, research focused on the mechanisms that affected biological responses to materials. In the past decade, new molecular biological and imaging techniques have been applied to assist our understanding of the biological response to materials. Today, the field of biocompatibility testing has reached a point where some prediction of biological properties is possible and the future will likely provide the ability to design materials that elicit customized biological responses.

CRITICAL QUESTION

Because titanium has been successful biologically as a femoral hip implant, can we assume that it will also perform with good biocompatibility when used for a dental endosseous implant?

Implicit in the definition of biocompatibility is an interaction between the body and the material (Fig. 8-1). Placement of a material in the body creates an interface that is normally not present. This interface is not static; rather, it is the site of many dynamic interactions between the material and the body through which the body may alter the material or the material may alter the body. The dynamics of these interactions will determine both the biological response to the material (its biocompatibility) and the ability of the material to survive or resist degradation or corrosion in the body. Because every biological interface is active, it is not possible to have a material that is inert. The activity of this interface depends on the location of the material, its duration in the body, the properties of the material, and health of the host.

Also implicit in the definition of biocompatibility is the concept that it is not simply a property of a material. In this sense, biocompatibility is much like color. The color of an object relies on the properties of the material, the source of light,

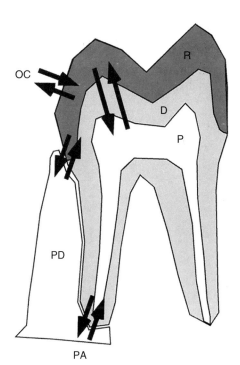

Fig. 8-1 The placement of a restoration **(R)** onto a tooth creates an interface between the material and the tissues adjacent to the material. In dentistry, these interfaces **(arrows)** may be between materials and the pulp **(P)** via the dentin **(D)**, the periodontium **(PD)**, the periapical bone **(PA)**, or the oral cavity **(OC)** in general. Wherever an interface exists, it is active and dynamic, involving two-way interactions that allow the tissue to influence the material or the material to influence the tissue.

and how the reflected light is perceived by the viewer. Thus color is an interactive property, and biocompatibility shares this attribute. Biocompatibility depends on the condition of the host, the properties of the material, and the context in which the material is used. Therefore, we cannot necessarily say that because a material is biocompatible as an implant it will also be so as a crown and bridge material. Furthermore, biocompatibility in a young person may differ from that in an older adult (or in a patient with diabetes versus one without diabetes). Ultimately, the biological response depends on the interactions that result from the biological interface created when the material is placed in the body.

ADVERSE EFFECTS FROM DENTAL MATERIALS
Toxicity, Inflammation, Allergy, and Mutagenicity

There are a number of possible biological reactions to materials, although not all of them have been documented for dental materials. Classically, these reactions have been separated into toxic, inflammatory, allergic, and mutagenic reactions. The division between these reactions is based on traditional histological and pathological analysis of tissues. In reality, the boundaries between these categories are gray—and the more we know about the molecular control of cells and tissues, the grayer these boundaries become.

Of the biological responses to materials, toxicity was the earliest response studied. Even today, the first screening test used for almost all materials is a toxicity test (Fig. 8-2). Materials may be capable of releasing substances into a patient's body, and the release of certain substances in adequate amounts can cause overt toxicity. For example, early dental materials containing lead posed a real risk to the patient because of the toxic properties of the lead that leached into the patient's body. Fortunately, most materials capable of causing overt toxicity are no longer used in dentistry.

Inflammation is a second fundamental type of biological response to a material. The inflammatory response is complex but involves the activation of the host's immune system to ward off some threat. Inflammation may result also from toxicity (Fig. 8-3) or from **allergy**, and often the inflammatory response precedes toxicity. Histologically, the inflammatory response is characterized by edema of the tissue with an infiltration of inflammatory cells such as neutrophils (in the short-term) or monocytes and other lymphocytic cells (in the long-term) (Fig. 8-4). Current biocompatibility research attempts to determine whether materials may cause or contribute to inflammation in the host even if no toxicity is evident (Fig. 8-5).

Fig. 8-2 Example of an in vitro toxicity test for dental alloys. A cell-culture tray has 24 wells, each containing cells and an alloy specimen. A different alloy has been used in each row, with six replicates. The alloy and cells are allowed to interact for 72 hr, after which the cells are treated with a chemical that turns dark blue if the cells have active mitochondria. The alloys in the bottom two rows have allowed the cells to survive, whereas the alloy in the second row has killed the cells. The alloy in the top row has allowed limited cellular activity. Toxicity tests such as this are used to screen dental materials for appropriate biocompatibility in the early stages of material development.

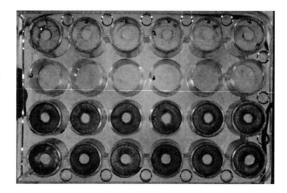

Fig. 8-3 Example of an animal test for material biocompatibility. Polyethylene **(PE)** or nickel wire **(Ni)** specimens about 1 cm long and 1 mm in diameter were inserted subcutaneously in mice for 7 days. The control site **(C)** had no material. After 7 days, the tissue was dissected from the mouse and photographed, with the external surface facing away. The control site shows no evidence of inflammation, and the polyethylene site shows mild inflammation with some enlargement of blood vessels. However, the nickel site shows severe inflammation that results from release of large amounts of nickel into the tissue. Animal tests such as this are often used in the biocompatibility assessment for dental materials.

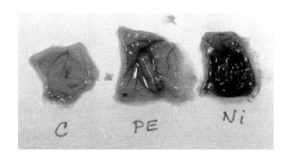

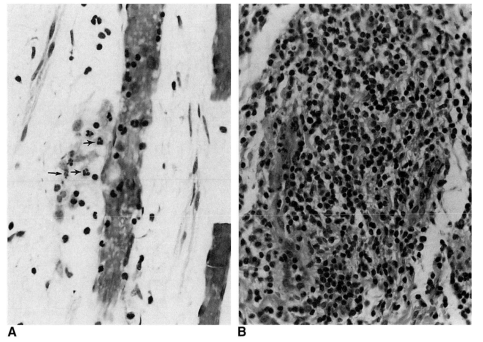

A　　　　　　　　　　　**B**

Fig. 8-4 Examples of acute **(A)** and chronic **(B)** inflammatory responses in the dental pulp. In **A,** neutrophils, characteristic of the acute response, have escaped **(arrows)** through an injured blood vessel wall and can be seen in the pulp connective tissue. Hematoxylin-eosin stain. (×450.) In **B,** a chronic inflammation of the pulp is characterized by a massive cellular infiltrate of lymphocytes, eosinophils, plasma cells, and macrophages. Hematoxylin-eosin stain. (×400.) (Adapted from Stanley HR: Dental Iatrogenesis. Int Dent J 44:3-18, 1994).

The contribution of dental materials to inflammatory reactions is especially important because pulpal and periodontal diseases are largely chronic inflammatory responses to long-term infections.

Although *allergic responses* to materials are perhaps the most familiar to the lay public, these responses are not simple to define in practice. Classically, an allergic reaction occurs when the body specifically recognizes a material as foreign and reacts disproportionately to the amount of the material present. The reaction

Fig. 8-5 Example of an inflammatory response (mesial to the molar and distal to the premolar) to either the metal in a bridge or the temporary restoration in a 30-year-old female. The cause of the inflammation is not known; it could be either an allergic response or a nonspecific inflammatory response. Etiologies of reactions such as this are often difficult to determine with certainty. In any case, the response is caused by release of agents from the materials into the adjacent tissues. It is often suspected that reactions such as this contribute to periodontal inflammation caused by plaque, but this is difficult to prove. See also color plate. (Photograph courtesy of Dr. Kevin Frazier, Medical College of Georgia School of Dentistry).

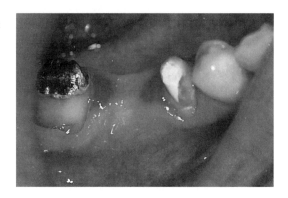

typically involves all dimensions of the immune system including T and B lymphocytes and monocytes or macrophages. An allergic reaction results histologically in an inflammatory response that can be difficult to differentiate from a nonallergic inflammation or low-grade toxicity (Fig. 8-6). Some materials, such as latex, cause allergy directly by activating antibodies to the material. These reactions (Type I, II, or III according to the Gell and Coombs classification of immune responses) tend to occur quickly and are modulated by eosinophils, mast cells, or B lymphocytes that produce antibodies. Other materials, such as metal ions, must first interact with a host molecule. These allergic reactions (Type IV) tend to be delayed and are modulated primarily by monocytes and T cells. Type I refers to an immediate atopic or anaphylactic reaction when an antigen interacts with mast cells or basophils. Type II is a cytotoxic **hypersensitivity** reaction. Type III is an immune complex hypersensitivity reaction. Type IV indicates a delayed or cell-mediated hypersensitivity. Type V is a stimulating-antibody reaction, and Type VI refers to an antibody-dependent, cell-mediated cytotoxicity reaction. (The reader is referred to a textbook on immunology for further details.)

A key difference between a nonallergic inflammatory response and an allergic response is the fact that in an allergic response, the individual's immune system recognizes a substance as foreign (see Fig. 8-6). Thus not all individuals will react to that substance. However, a general inflammatory response, such as the one seen in

Fig. 8-6 Example of nickel allergy around metal-ceramic crowns in a female patient. Significant inflammation is present in the lingual gingiva, especially around teeth numbers 6 (13), 7 (12), 10 (22), and 11 (23). The allergic reaction, which occurs even though the majority of the nickel alloy is covered with porcelain, is caused by release of nickel ions from the crowns into the adjacent tissues. Allergic reactions such as this are often very difficult to differentiate from gingivitis, periodontal disease, or general irritation from toxicity. See also color plate. (Photograph courtesy of Dr. Michael Myers, Medical College of Georgia School of Dentistry.)

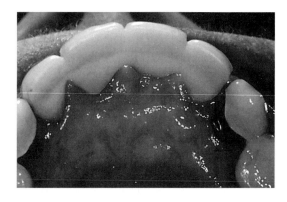

Figure 8-3 toward nickel, will occur for all individuals because it involves no specific recognition of the substance. Furthermore, allergic reactions tend to be dose-independent initially and disproportionate to the amount of the offending substance, whereas toxic or inflammatory reactions tend to be dose-dependent and proportional to the amount of the substance.

Mutagenic reactions result when the components of a material alter the base-pair sequences of the DNA in cells. These alterations are termed *mutations*. Mutations may be caused by direct interactions between a substance and DNA or indirectly by alterations in cellular processes that maintain DNA integrity. Mutations are common and are considered a natural occurrence in the DNA of all individuals. Thus the body dedicates much cellular energy and machinery to repairing these changes. Mutations may result from many factors, for example, radiation, chemicals, and errors in the DNA replication process. Several metal ions from dental materials such as nickel, copper, and beryllium are known mutagens, and some components of other materials such as root canal sealers have been shown to be mutagenic. Resin-based materials have also been identified as having some mutagenic potential. However, it must be clear that mutagenicity does not imply carcinogenicity (ability to cause tumors), because many mutations are repaired and others are irrelevant. Furthermore, the form of the material and its route of exposure are critically important to the mutagenic or carcinogenic response. Currently, no dental material has been shown to be carcinogenic in dental applications in patients. However, carcinogenesis is often exceedingly difficult to prove or disprove conclusively.

CRITICAL QUESTIONS

Why might the local response and systemic response to a dental material differ? What factors come into play to explain these differences?

Local and Systemic Effects of Materials

Any material used in the body may have local or systemic biological effects. These effects are modulated primarily by substances that are released from the material and the biological responses to those substances. The nature, severity, and location of these effects are determined by the distribution of released substances. For dental materials, local effects might occur in the pulp of the tooth, in the periodontium, at the root apex, or in nearby oral tissues such as the buccal mucosa or tongue (see Fig. 8-1). These local effects are a function of the ability of substances to be distributed to these sites, their concentrations, and exposure times that range from seconds to years. The allergic reaction of the gingiva to a nickel-containing crown seen in Figure 8-6 is one example of a local response.

Systemic effects from dental materials are also a function of the distribution of substances released from materials. These substances might gain access to the body via ingestion and absorption in the gut, inhaled vapor, release at the tooth apex, or absorption through the oral mucosa. Their distribution may occur by simple diffusion or transport via the lymphatic or blood vessels. The systemic biological response depends on (1) the duration and concentration of the exposure, (2) the excretion rate of the substance, and (3) the site of the exposure. Substances that have a long life in the body, such as mercury, may accumulate and reach critical levels more easily than other substances that are readily excreted. Furthermore, not all tissues react equally. Systemic reactions may also be influenced by organs such as the liver that alter substances in an attempt to digest or excrete them.

What is corrosion, and why is it important to biocompatibility?

Key Principles That Determine Adverse Effects from Materials

There are two key factors that appear to be paramount in determining a material's biocompatibility. The first factor involves the various types of metal corrosion or other types of material degradation. Corrosion results in the release of substances from a material into the host. Note that the definition used here is broad and may apply to any material. The release can take many forms and may be caused by many factors. For example, a metallic crown may release metal ions as a result of electrochemical forces, or it may release particles dislodged by mechanical forces, such as occlusion or tooth brushing. For some materials, such as resin composites, cyclical stresses contribute to the breakdown of the material and release of components. Still other materials such as sutures break down by design. The key point is that the biocompatibility of the material depends to a large degree on the degradation process. The biological response to the corrosion products depends on the amount, composition, and form of these products, as well as their location in tissues. Corrosion may be visible or invisible to the naked eye (Fig. 8-7), but it is ongoing for every dental material at some level.

Corrosion is determined not only by a material's composition but also by the biological environment in contact with a material. For example, salivary esterases have been shown to accelerate the breakdown of some dental resins, and ingestion of acidic substances may alter the corrosion of alloys or ceramics. The biological forces that influence corrosion may be specific to an individual (such as a person in diabetic ketoacidosis) or they may be common to all individuals (as with occlusal forces on materials). In any case, it is the biological interface that creates the conditions for corrosion. This interface is active and dynamic, with the material affecting the body and the body affecting the material.

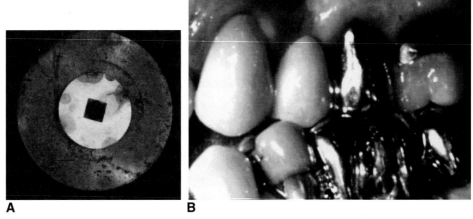

A   **B**

Fig. 8-7 **A,** Example of metal corrosion that is clearly visible to the naked eye. This corrosion resulted in release of metal ions and the formation of oxides on the surface of the metal. **B,** View of multiple types of prostheses (cast metal crowns, porcelain crown, and amalgam) in a patient's mouth. Although the surfaces of these materials may retain a high luster after years of service, corrosion from these materials is ongoing at a low rate. Therefore, corrosion is not always visible to the eye. (**B,** Courtesy of Dr. Steven Nelson, Medical College of Georgia School of Dentistry.)

The second key factor that affects the biocompatibility of a material is its surface characteristics. Research has shown that for all materials, the surface is quite different than the interior region of a material. For example, a dental casting alloy that has 70 wt% gold on average may have nearly 95% gold at its surface. Another example is the relatively unpolymerized state of a sealant at its surface relative to its interior because of oxygen inhibition of polymerization at the surface. Because the surface is the part of a material that the body "sees," the surface composition, roughness, mechanical properties, and chemical properties are critical to the biocompatibility of the material. The surface characteristics may affect the corrosion properties of a material, or they may influence biocompatibility in other ways. For example, research has shown that it is the chemical characteristics of titanium oxides that promote **osseointegration** of bone with many titanium alloys. The exact mechanisms are not clear, but the oxides probably promote the adsorption and adhesion of the appropriate elements in the extracellular matrix to encourage bone deposition and maturation. Similar responses have been seen with some ceramics (bioglasses). In this case, the surface not only allows osseointegration, but it also seems to promote bone formation through the dissolution of glass and corrosion of inorganic elements.

The surface may also negatively affect the biological response. For most materials, a rough surface promotes corrosion. If the corrosion products have adverse effects, then roughness is not desirable. Roughness may also promote the adherence of bacteria and promote periodontal inflammation or decay in teeth. The chemical properties of a surface may also hinder the biological response. Studies have shown that the surfaces of some materials chemically attract lipopolysaccharide more than others, even when the surface roughness is the same. Because lipopolysaccharide is a key agent in periodontal inflammation, the presence of this molecule is not desirable.

CRITICAL QUESTION

Is it possible for a material to have no obvious biological effects by itself but still alter body functions?

Immunotoxicity

The boundaries between toxic, inflammatory, allergic, and mutagenic reactions are disappearing as more is known about how materials and cells interact. One example is the concept of immunotoxicity. Immunotoxicity is based on the principle that small alterations in cells of the immune system by materials can have significant biological consequences. These significant consequences occur because of the amplifying nature of immune cells. For example, monocytes control and orchestrate much of the chronic inflammatory and immune response. To accomplish this role, monocytes secrete many substances that influence and direct other cells. Thus if a material were to alter a monocyte's ability to secrete these substances, the biological response would be significantly amplified. This concept combines the classic areas of toxicology and immunology, because the material causes nonlethal but toxic changes in the monocyte so that the immune system cannot function correctly.

Immunotoxicity may result from a material causing either an increase or decrease in cellular function. For example, mercury ions have been shown to increase the glutathione content of human monocytes in cell-culture, whereas palladium ions decrease it (Fig. 8-8). Glutathione is important in maintaining the oxidative stress in cells, and any change may, therefore, significantly alter cellular function. Mercury also

Fig. 8-8 A graph showing the response of human monocytes to palladium ions (**Pd^{2+}**) or mercury ions (**Hg^{2+}**). The cells were exposed to a range of concentrations of the metals (**x axis**). Total cellular glutathione was measured after 24 hr of exposure to the metal ions (**y axis**). The mercury ions caused a very large increase in glutathione at a level of about 8 μmol/L, followed by a drop as the mercury became toxic to the cell. For palladium content, the glutathione content dropped at a concentration 200-300 μmol/L, which is well below concentrations required to cause toxicity in these cells. Glutathione is an important cellular chemical defense against oxidative stress in cells. Thus both types of metal ions alter the monocytic stress response at subtoxic concentrations. These types of reactions are thought to play a role in immunotoxicity. Note the difference in the potency of the two types of metal ions.

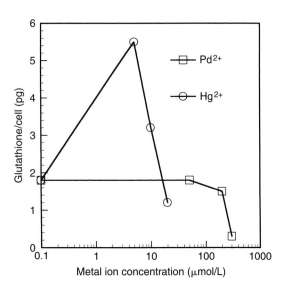

causes a decrease in glutathione at higher concentrations as the ions become toxic. However, the decreases found for palladium occur well below toxic levels. In immunotoxicity, the effect of the material may not be obvious until the cell is challenged in some manner. For example, hydroxyethylmethacrylate (HEMA), a common component of dentin-bonding agents, has no effect on secretion of the cytokine TNF-α from monocytes by itself, even at high concentrations (Fig. 8-9). However, TNF-α secretion is severely reduced when these monocytes are challenged. Therefore, although the HEMA does not alter TNF-α secretion by itself, it may change the ability of the monocyte to direct an immune response once challenged. Thus it may alter the ability of a monocyte to function properly if challenged by plaque or other agents.

Fig. 8-9 A graph showing that hydroxyethylmethacrylate (HEMA) reduces the ability of human monocytes to secrete TNF-alpha, a key cytokine in the inflammatory response to materials. Control monocytes (**x axis**) received no HEMA, but two other concentrations (both subtoxic) were used. The TNF-alpha secretion (**y axis**) was measured with and without subsequent stimulation by lipopolysaccharide (LPS), an important etiologic factor in periodontal disease. No concentration of HEMA caused TNF-alpha secretion by itself (**squares**), but the HEMA severely limited the ability of the monocytes to secrete TNF-alpha (**circles**). Results such as these demonstrate the concept of immunotoxicity because the monocyte is not killed by the HEMA, but it is significantly prevented from performing its normal function when challenged.

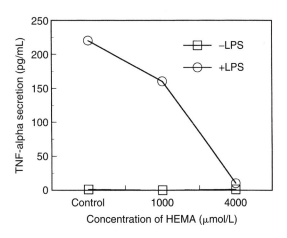

What special aspects of oral anatomy influence the biocompatibility of dental materials?

BIOLOGICAL RESPONSE IN THE DENTAL ENVIRONMENT
Oral Anatomy That Influences the Biological Response

Several aspects of oral anatomy influence the biocompatibility of dental restorative materials. The full effects of the oral anatomy on the biocompatibility of materials are not known, but these effects will be a major focus of biocompatibility research in coming years. The anatomy of the tooth, the periodontal attachment, and the periapical environment have profound influences on the biological response to materials, and all are sites of interface between materials and tissues in dentistry (see Fig. 8-1). The cursory discussion provided here is intended to give a general background in anatomical aspects important to dental materials. For more detailed information, refer to any of the numerous textbooks on dental histology, periodontology, endodontology, and anatomy.

The *enamel-dentin-pulp* environment (Fig. 8-10) represents a unique symbiosis of mineralized tissues and cells. The enamel of the tooth is virtually all inorganic material (96 wt%) arranged in a crystalline array called *enamel rods*. Although the enamel is permeable to some substances, such as the peroxides in bleaching agents, it is generally not permeable to material components, bacteria, or bacterial products.

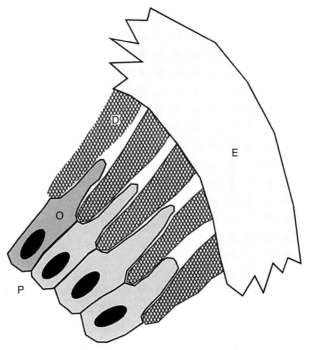

Fig. 8-10   Diagram of the enamel-pulpo-dentin complex. The enamel **(E)** is the external covering of the tooth and is impermeable to all but the smallest of molecules. The dentin **(D)** is a composite of collagen and mineralized tissue, and is permeated by numerous tubules running from the enamel to the pulp **(P)**. The tubule diameter gradually increases from the enamel to the pulp. Tubules permit diffusion of fluid and substances from the external environment into the pulp if enamel is not present. Odontoblasts **(O)** line the dentin on the pulpal side and have processes that extend into the dentinal tubules.

The dentin of a tooth, in contrast to enamel, is a mineralized matrix that embeds an organic network. The inorganic content of dentin is lower (70 wt%), and the organic portion (18 wt%) is primarily collagen but also contains other proteins and extracellular matrix components, the full role of which remains unclear. The composite nature of the dentin allows bonding to occur because acids may selectively dissolve the mineralized matrix, but not the collagenous network embedded in it. Therefore, most dentin bonding agents attempt to penetrate the undissolved collagen matrix. The dentin also has about 12 wt% water, which is important because many resin restorative materials are hydrophobic and must be designed to wet the dentin if they are to successfully bond to this structure.

Dentin is traversed by thousands of dentinal tubules, running from the enamel to the pulp. These tubules are about 0.5 μm in diameter near the enamel, but increase to 2.5 μm near the pulp of the tooth. The density of tubules is about 20,000/mm^2 near the enamel, but increases to more than 50,000/mm^2 near the pulp. If the enamel is violated by caries, other pathology, or by the dentist, the dentinal tubules may serve as conduits by which material components, bacteria, or bacterial products may reach and affect the pulp of the tooth. Because the tubule diameter and tubule density increase near the pulp, there is a greater risk of allowing substances to reach the pulpal tissues when deeper dental restorations are placed. When dentists cut the dentin, a "smear layer" of dentinal debris covers the dentin and inhibits diffusion of products through the tubules to some extent. However, the smear layer may be contaminated with bacterial products and it is not tenaciously bound to the uncut adjacent dentin. Thus many restorative procedures will take measures to remove the smear layer to both clean the tooth and promote stronger bonding of restorative materials. The diffusion of substances through the dentin is a complex topic, and further reading is available in the scientific literature, including the titles listed in the Selected Readings section of this chapter.

The pulpal side of the dentin is lined by odontoblasts (see Fig. 8-10) that formed the dentin during tooth development and maintain and form new dentin as the tooth ages or when triggered by noxious stimuli. The odontoblasts have odontoblastic processes that extend well into the dentinal tubules. The tubules are surrounded by an aqueous extracellular fluid that is continuous with the extracellular fluid of the pulp. The perception of pain in the pulp is believed to be related to the movement of this fluid and its influence on the odontoblastic processes as proposed in the so-called hydrodynamic theory (fluid model) of pulpal pain. This fluid pressure induced by the cardiovascular system may be as high as 24 mm Hg. Therefore, an outward pressure of fluid flows toward the enamel. When the enamel is removed during restoration of the tooth, fluid flows outward from the pulp chamber into the oral cavity. However, evidence indicates that this outward flow is not sufficient to eliminate the inward diffusion of bacteria, bacterial products, or material components into the pulp. The odontoblasts are sealed together with tight cellular junctions that limit the diffusion of substances past the odontoblastic layer. Caries and other noxious conditions may lead to infection and destruction of the odontoblasts, or they may stimulate deposition of additional dentin, depending on the relative rate of interaction with these cells. Restorative devices, such as burs and other cutting instruments, may destroy the odontoblasts if procedures are aggressive, but may leave the odontoblasts intact if conservative measures such as water cooling are used. Caries, restorative procedures, or material components may injure odontoblasts without destroying them. Recent studies have focused on the consequences of these sublethal effects.

The pulp of the tooth is a connective tissue containing normal elements such as fibroblasts, collagen, capillaries, and nerves. In addition, it has been shown that the pulp supplies the cells, which replace any odontoblasts destroyed during cavity preparation or material placement and allows the tooth to form secondary or reparative dentin. The biochemical factors regulating the formation of these secondary odontoblasts are not known. The diffusion of bacterial products or material components influence the ability of this repair process to occur, although details of these influences are also not well understood. Some materials, such as calcium hydroxide, seem to promote the formation of reparative dentin. The development of future biomaterials will almost certainly consider the permeability of the dentin and the ability of the material to induce formation of secondary odontoblasts as a basis for selection of restorative materials that are designed to treat or prevent pulpal disease.

The *periodontal attachment* to the tooth is an important junction between the outside of the body (oral cavity) and the inside of the body (Figs. 8-1 and 8-11). The dentin of the root of the tooth is covered by a thin layer of cementum that may seal the dentinal tubules. The cementum serves as the attachment point for the collagen fibers of the periodontal ligament (see Fig. 8-11). The gingiva normally extends above the level of the cementum and forms a potential space against the enamel called the *periodontal pocket*. The gingival epithelium is also attached to the cementum of the tooth by a specialized junctional epithelium. The periodontal pocket is the site of the development of periodontal disease, which can destroy the junctional epithelium, periodontal ligament and supporting alveolar bone.

Because many dental restorations are near or in the periodontal attachment area, the biocompatibility of these materials may influence the normal periodontal architecture, the periodontal disease process, or the body's ability to defend against bacteria that cause periodontal disease. Furthermore, the periodontal pocket is a unique microenvironment that may allow concentrations of components from materials to reach higher levels than are seen in the rest of the oral cavity. For example, some alloys used in South America and Eastern Europe, but not in the United States, release sufficient amounts of copper to cause inflammation in the

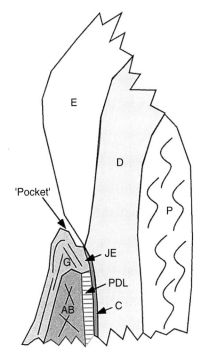

Fig. 8-11 Diagram showing the periodontal attachment area. The gingiva (**G**) attaches to the cementum (**C**) of the tooth with a specialized epithelium called the *junctional epithelium* (**JE**). The attachment occurs below the enamel (**E**). Some of the gingiva rises above the *JE* to form a potential space called the *periodontal pocket*. The cementum covers the dentin (**D**). Below the gingiva, the alveolar bone (**AB**) attaches to the cementum via specialized connective tissue called the *periodontal ligament* (**PDL**). The periodontal attachment site is very important in the biological response to materials, because many materials are in close contact with these tissues and may form a unique microenvironment in the pocket or attachment area.

periodontal tissues. In other cases, the influence of components released from materials on the periodontal architecture is suspected but not confirmed.

Defining the influence of dental materials on the periodontal structures is always complicated by inflammation that occurs in periodontal disease, and the biting (occlusal) forces that strain the periodontal ligament and supporting bone. It is often difficult to determine with certainty whether inflammation in this area is caused by periodontal disease, occlusal trauma, the material, or some combination of these factors. Therefore, definite evidence of inflammation in the periodontal attachment area caused by dental materials is scant. The periodontal pocket has also been used as a site to place materials that release therapeutic agents to combat periodontal disease. It is likely that this approach will expand as better drug delivery materials are developed.

The *periapical area* of the tooth is another interface between materials and the inside of the body (see Fig. 8-1). Normally, the apex of the tooth is the junction of the pulp of the tooth and the alveolar bone below it (Fig. 8-12). Nerves and blood vessels enter through the apical foramen (and sometimes via accessory foramina). However, when the pulp of the tooth is destroyed by infection or during restoration of a tooth, endodontic materials are placed in the pulpal space, and these materials interface with the body through the apex of the tooth. If the endodontic procedure is not performed correctly, the filling materials may be extruded from the apex into the periapical area and cause additional physical damage. The ability of the root canal material to seal against the migration of bacterial or bacterial products from the tooth crown toward the apex is also an important consideration. For endodontic procedures that use a retrograde approach to sealing the apical foramen, the

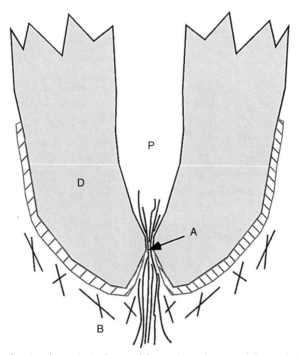

Fig. 8-12 Diagram showing the periapical area of the tooth. At the root of the tooth, the dentin **(D)** forms the apical foramen **(A)** that allows passage of nerves and blood vessels from the alveolar bone **(B)** to the pulp **(P)** of the tooth. When endodontic procedures replace the pulp with various sealers and filling materials, a biomaterial interface is created in the periapical area. This interface is unique because any release of substances from the filling materials gain access to the inside of the body.

filling materials will be in direct contact with the periapical tissues. Thus biological responses to these materials must be critically examined. As with the periodontal attachment area, the release of substances from root canal filling materials may cause adverse responses around the apex or may alter the body's reaction to bacterial products that have contaminated the area. The delineation between the bacterial and material threats are not clear, and the ability of materials to influence the body's immunological response in the periapical area has only recently been studied.

CRITICAL QUESTIONS

What is the difference between microleakage and nanoleakage? How can these processes influence the biological response to a material?

Special Biological Interfaces with Dental Materials

The use of materials to restore damaged or lost tooth structure creates specialized environments in which the biocompatibility of the material is of central importance to the long-term survival of the restoration. In the previous section, several areas of specialized oral anatomy were presented with information about their relevance to biocompatibility. In this section two specialized interfaces, the *dentin-resin interface* and the *implant-bone interface,* are explored in more detail as examples of how the biological interaction between materials and the body can influence both.

The *dentin-resin interface* is created when the clinician bonds resin-based restorative materials to dentin. The composite nature of the dentin allows the mineralized matrix to be dissolved away by acids while preserving the collagen network. If the network does not collapse, which may happen if the dentin is desiccated, it may be embedded by a resin-containing material, thereby mechanically bonding the resin material to the dentin. The dentin bonding process is complex and is discussed further elsewhere (see Chapter 14). However, the interface of the resin material with the collagenous network has a profound influence on the biocompatibility of the material.

If the resin material does not penetrate the collagenous network or debonds from it as the resin shrinks during polymerization, a gap will form between the resin and the dentin. This shrinkage may also occur with enamel. Although this gap is only a few microns wide, it is wide enough to permit bacteria and oral fluids to percolate from the pulp outward or from the oral cavity inward. This leakage has traditionally been termed *microleakage* (Fig. 8-13). The biocompatibility of a restoration is altered by the leakage process, which may cause a number of undesirable events. First, it may allow bacteria or bacterial products to reach the pulp and cause infection. Second, it may encourage the breakdown of the material. This breakdown then exposes the body to products of the material and increases the gap, thereby promoting more leakage. Finally, the leakage may discolor the margins of the restoration, making the tooth-restoration complex aesthetically unacceptable and possibly resulting in a decision to repair or replace the restorative material. Although it has also been hypothesized that bacterial contamination allows caries to reinitiate, recent evidence regarding amalgam restorations reported by Özer suggests that secondary caries are initiated at the outer surface of enamel in areas of plaque accumulation.

If the resin penetrates the collagen network of the dentin but does not penetrate it completely, a much smaller gap (<0.1 μm in most cases) will exist between the mineralized matrix of the dentin and the collagen-resin hybrid layer (see Fig. 8-13).

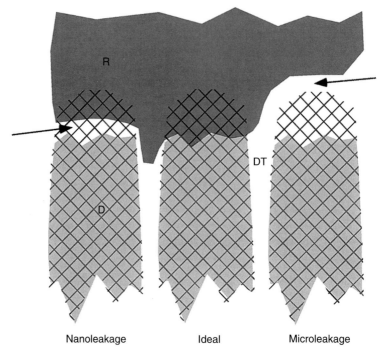

Nanoleakage   Ideal   Microleakage

Fig. 8-13 Diagram illustrating the concepts of microleakage **(right)** and nanoleakage **(left)** when bonding dental resins **(R)** to dentin **(D)**. The dentin has been acid-etched in preparation for the application of the resin, which leaves the collagenous matrix of the dentin exposed **(unshaded crosshatched area)**. If the resin does not completely penetrate the collagen network **(left)**, a small space of communication exists between the dentinal tubules **(DT)** and the external part of the tooth **(arrow, left)**. This situation is called *nanoleakage*. On the other hand, if the resin fails to penetrate the collagen network at all, or debonds from it, then the space is much larger **(arrow, right)**. This situation is called *microleakage*. In the ideal situation **(center)**, the resin penetrates the collagen network all the way to the mineralized dentin. Nanoleakage and microleakage are both important factors in the biocompatibility of dental resin materials.

This much smaller gap has been claimed to allow *nanoleakage*. Although nanoleakage probably does not allow bacteria or bacterial products to penetrate the marginal gaps of the restoration and the pulp, fluid exchange most likely occurs that can degrade the resin or the collagen network that has been incompletely embedded with resin, thereby reducing the longevity of the dentin-resin bond. This degradation process may also gradually increase the gap size until microleakage begins to occur. It is unclear what role nanoleakage plays, if any, in the biological response to materials, but most clinicians and researchers agree that it is better to completely embed an exposed dentin collagen network with the resin. Nanoleakage is not known to occur between restorations and enamel because enamel contains virtually no organic mass and therefore has no collagenous matrix into which a resin may be embedded. Although it is unclear whether leakage is a major factor in the biological response to dental materials, the clinician must also be concerned about immune responses in the pulp and periapical tissues that may occur independently of leakage phenomena.

CRITICAL QUESTION

What is the difference between osseointegration and biointegration?

Osseointegration

The use of endosseous dental implants has increased tremendously over the past decade. The success of these implants relies on the ability of the materials to promote osseointegration and allow a close approximation of bone with the material (Fig. 8-14). This interface must sustain the forces placed on it during the normal use of the implant (from biting, clenching, chewing, etc.). The ability of a material to allow osseointegration is closely related to its biocompatibility. In dentistry, relatively few materials allow osseointegration. These include (1) commercially pure titanium, (2) titanium-aluminum-vanadium alloy, (3) tantalum, and (4) several types of ceramics. Materials that allow osseointegration have very low degradation rates, and they tend to form surface oxides that promote bony approximation. The mechanisms by which these oxides encourage or allow bone formation without intervening fibrous tissue are not known. Some materials, such as the so-called bioglass ceramics, promote an integration between the bone and the material with no intervening space at all. When this integration occurs, the material is said to *biointegrate* with the bone. **Biointegration** appears to require a degradation of the ceramic to promote bone formation, although the specific reactions are not well understood. No known desirability of osseointegration over biointegration has been established. Like all biocompatibility phenomena, osseointegration and biointegration are dynamic processes that may be altered by changes in the host, fatigue of the materials, or function of the implant. It is also important to understand that neither osseointegration nor biointegration mimic the normal ligamentous connection between a tooth root and the alveolar bone (see Fig. 8-11).

The Oral Immune System

As has been noted previously, the immune system plays an important role in the biological response to any material. The immune system in the oral environment

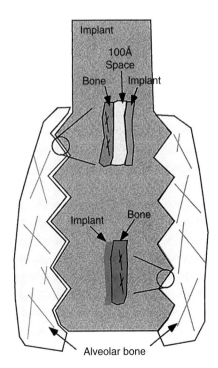

Fig. 8-14 Diagram illustrating the concepts of osseointegration and biointegration. If an endosseous implant is placed in the alveolar bone, the bony response may take one of three courses. It may not approximate the implant at all, and a connective tissue encapsulation of the implant occurs. In this case, the implant is a failure and must be removed. The bone may closely approximate the implant **(left side)**, in which case the implant is *osseointegrated*. A close examination **(left side, inset)** shows that the bone comes to within 100 Å of the bone without connective tissue between the bone and implant. Finally, the bone may fuse **(right side)** with the implant, in which case the implant is *biointegrated*. In this case, there is a gradient from material to bone **(right side, inset)** with no space. The outcome of implantation depends on the biocompatibility of the material used, the patient's anatomy and physiology, and the technique used to place the implant. The corrosion of the material is also critical to these biological responses. Additional information on implants is presented in Chapter 23.

appears to behave somewhat differently in oral epithelium and connective tissue than in the rest of the body, and the biological responses to materials in the mouth may not always parallel those seen in other locations. Studies performed on guinea pig models have shown that oral exposure to certain allergenic metals such as chromium or nickel may actually induce immunological tolerance to these metals. However, if the initial exposure occurs in other locations (including the gastrointestinal tract), allergy often develops. The mechanisms that control tolerance versus allergy to dental materials are not known, nor is the potential of these types of reactions to occur in humans. However, it is important to remember that the oral environment is not always equivalent in structure or function to other areas of the body and that these differences may alter the biological response to materials.

CRITICAL QUESTION

What factors might influence how you test the biocompatibility of a dental material?

MEASURING THE BIOCOMPATIBILITY OF MATERIALS
Defining the Use of a Material

The function or use of a material in the body has an important influence on the nature of the biological response it induces. There are several factors that must be considered when trying to measure the biological response. First, the location of a material is important to its overall biological response. Will the material be surrounded by soft or mineralized tissue, will it be external to the oral epithelium, or will it communicate through the epithelium like an endoesseous implant? Will the material be exposed directly to bone, tissue fluid, blood, and saliva, or will there be some sort of barrier, such as dentin or enamel between the material and living cells? These factors will play a major role in the biological response to a material. In general, materials that communicate through the epithelium or lie completely beneath it will need closer scrutiny when assessing the biological response than materials that do not penetrate the epithelium. Similarly, materials that penetrate tooth enamel will need more scrutiny than materials that do not.

The duration of the material in the body is important to the biological response. Materials such as impression materials, which are only present for 4 to 6 min in the mouth, may cause a different biological response than materials that will be present for 10 years. For example, an impression material that is present in the mouth for a few minutes may have time to cause an allergic reaction in an allergic individual, but the short duration in the mouth may limit any toxic or mutagenic effects. A copper band used as a matrix retainer for a large amalgam is unlikely to induce a detectable biological response when present for only 5 to 10 min but would elicit a severe gingival inflammatory response if allowed to remain in place for several weeks. The duration of the presence of a material is an important factor, because many interactive effects between the body and material take some time to develop. In general, the most stringent tests to measure biocompatibility are required for materials that are present for the longest times. Long durations give sufficient time for the material to affect the body and for the body to affect the material in many complex ways.

Finally, the stresses placed on the material are important to the biological response. These stresses may be physical, chemical, or thermal in nature. For example, a material may behave poorly if it is too weak and/or soft and it deforms or wears under the forces of occlusion. It may react unfavorably with salivary proteins, thereby degrading too much, or it may become too flexible at mouth temperature and experience failure or increased breakdown. Short-term, long-term, and fatigue stresses all need to be considered when assessing the effect of stress on the biological performance of material.

CRITICAL QUESTIONS

Is there a single test that can measure biocompatibility? Why or why not? What is considered the "gold standard"?

Types of Tests: Advantages and Disadvantages

There are three basic types of tests used to measure the biocompatibility of dental materials: the in vitro test, the animal test, and the usage test performed either in animals or in humans. Each of these tests has advantages and disadvantages, and each is used to some extent to evaluate a material before it may be sold to the public. Keep in mind that no single test can accurately estimate the biological response to a material and that considerable controversy exists about the appropriate mixture of the three basic types of tests. The remainder of this section will detail each of these fundamental types of tests.

In vitro tests are performed outside of an organism (see Fig. 8-2). Historically, in vitro tests have been used as the first screening test to evaluate a new material. These tests may be conducted in a test tube, cell-culture dish, flask, or other container, but they are performed separately from an intact organism. In any case, the material or an extract of a material is placed into contact with some biological system. The biological system may consist of mammalian cells, cellular organelles, tissues, bacteria, or some sort of enzyme. The contact between the biological system and the material may be direct or indirect. Direct contact involves the exposure of a material or an extract from a material directly with the biological system, whereas indirect contact occurs through a barrier of some sort, such as agar, a membrane filter, or dentin. In vitro tests can be subdivided into tests that measure cell growth or death, those that determine cellular function of some type, and those that evaluate the integrity of the genetic material of the cell. However, clear boundaries may not exist among these categories. For example, a material that suppresses cellular growth may do so by altering cellular DNA or by inhibiting some key enzyme required for division.

In vitro tests have several advantages over animal or usage tests. They are relatively fast, inexpensive, and easily standardized. Furthermore, they may be used for larger-scale screening than can either animal or usage tests. Conditions for these tests can be tightly controlled to provide the highest quality of scientific rigor. The greatest disadvantage of in vitro tests is their potential lack of relevance to the in vivo use of the material. For example, a test that measures the cytotoxicity of a material in an osteoblast cell-culture may not be relevant to the oral condition because the material never comes in contact with osteoblasts in vivo. The in vitro environment also lacks the complex coordination of systems that are present in an organism such as an immune system, an inflammatory system, and a circulatory system.

Animal tests place a material into an intact organism of some type (see Fig. 8-3). Common animals for this type of test are mice, rats, hamsters, ferrets, or guinea pigs, but many other types of animals have been used, including sheep, monkeys, baboons, pigs, cats, and dogs. Pulp studies and animal tests are distinct from in vitro tests. In the latter tests, an intact animal is used rather than cells or tissues from an animal. Animal tests are distinct from usage tests in that animal tests expose the animal to the material without regard to the material's final use. For example, the systemic toxicity of dental amalgam might be tested by grinding up set amalgam and feeding this to an animal, even though this type of exposure is less relevant to the clinical use of amalgam. Animal tests may also be subdivided into several types, including short-term or long-term systemic toxicity, exposure to intact or abraded membranes, and immune **sensitization** or bone response. There are also animal tests for mutagenicity, carcinogenicity and other specialized conditions.

Regardless of the type of test used, the advantage of an animal test is its ability to allow an intact biological system to respond to a material. The material may interact with the many complex biological systems within the animal and a more complete biological response is therefore measured. However, animal tests are expensive and difficult to control, and they may take many months or even years to complete, depending on the species used. These tests are also controversial because of ethical concerns about proper animal treatment. Furthermore, the relevance of an animal test is often questioned because of concerns about the ability of any animal species used to adequately represent the human species. Despite their disadvantages, animal tests provide an important bridge between the in vitro environment and the clinical use of the material, and these tests are likely to be used in some capacity for the foreseeable future.

Usage tests are performed in animals or humans. A usage test requires that the material be placed in an environment clinically relevant to the use of the material in clinical practice. If the test is performed in humans, it is called a *clinical trial* rather than a usage test. The choice of animals for a usage test will be more limited than for an animal test because not all species can be used for all clinical situations, often because of the size or anatomy of a given species. Thus usage tests are more likely to be performed on larger animals with anatomy that more closely resembles that of humans. The relevance of a usage test to clinical practice is potentially high by definition. However, the ultimate relevance of a usage test depends directly on the quality with which the test mimics the clinical use of the material in terms of time, area, clinical environment, and placement technique. The human clinical trial is therefore the "gold standard" of usage tests and is the standard by which in vitro and animal tests are judged.

Usage tests also have a number of disadvantages. These tests are extremely complex and difficult to perform in terms of experimental control and interpretation. The tests are exceptionally expensive; thousands of dollars may be needed for a single subject. If humans are to be used, approval for clinical trial must be obtained, by law, from an Institutional Review Board. The time required for these tests may stretch from months to years if data on the long-term performance of a material are desired. Finally, human usage tests may involve many legal liabilities and issues that are not factors for animal and in vitro tests.

CRITICAL QUESTION

If you were presented with a new material, never before used in a human being, how would you decide whether it was safe as a dental restorative material?

How Tests Are Used Together to Measure Biocompatibility

Generally, no single test is used to evaluate the biocompatibility of a new material. Rather, in vitro, animal, and usage tests are used together. However, the role of each of these basic tests in the overall testing scheme is controversial and is still evolving.

Three phases are generally recognized in the testing of a new biomaterial: *primary*, *secondary*, and *usage*. At first glance, these phases might appear to be redundant to the categories of in vitro, animal, and usage tests discussed in the previous section. However, there are differences, and these differences will increase in the future as better tests for biocompatibility are developed. *Primary tests* are performed initially in the testing of a new material; these tests are often in vitro in nature. For example, the first primary tests often conducted to evaluate a new casting alloy are in vitro cytotoxicity and mutagenicity tests. But primary tests might also include some animal tests to measure systemic toxicity. *Secondary tests* are almost always conducted in animals. For example, tests to measure dermal irritation, chronic toxicity, or response upon implantation are selected to observe the immune response. Secondary tests explore beyond toxicity or mutagenicity toward issues such as allergy, inflammation, and other sublethal and chronic biological responses. However, more sophisticated in vitro tests are being developed for inflammation, **estrogenicity**, surface effects, and osteoinduction that are also secondary in nature. The *usage phase* of testing is largely the same as described previously, because the material must be tested in a clinically relevant situation.

The testing of a new material is a linear progression from primary to secondary to usage tests (Fig. 8-15). Primary tests are conducted first, and only materials that "pass" these primary tests are tested in the secondary phase. Similarly, only materials that have favorable results in the secondary tests are subjected to usage tests. This paradigm for testing is depicted as a triangle, with the majority of materials (represented by the width of the bottom of the triangle) tested in the primary phase, fewer materials surviving to the secondary phase, and the fewest materials reaching the usage phase of testing. At its inception, this linear paradigm appears to be the most efficient and cost-effective way of bringing new materials safely to the public. To a large extent, this linear paradigm persists today in biocompatibility testing. However, questions about the accuracy of primary and secondary tests have challenged the wisdom of the linear paradigm over the past several decades.

In the late 1970s and early 1980s, several studies by Mjör et al (1977) were published comparing in vitro, animal, and usage tests for materials used clinically in dentistry for many years. The results (Table 8-1) showed that the in vitro and animal tests did not necessarily predict the results of usage tests or the successful

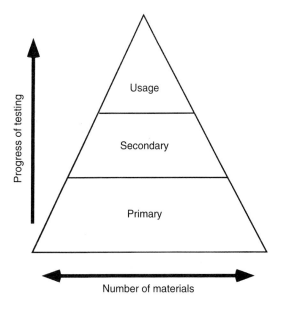

Fig. 8-15 Diagram showing the classical progression of biocompatibility tests in the assessment of a new material. The number of materials tested is represented by the width of the triangle. Thus all materials will be tested by primary tests, but many will not have responses favorable enough to be carried to secondary tests. Likewise, only materials that show favorable reactions in the secondary tests will be evaluated by the usage tests.

Table 8-1	Comparison of In Vitro and Animal Test Results with Usage Test Data for Three Dental Materials		
Restorative material	In vitro test	Animal test	Clinical trial
Silicate Cement	1+	1+	2+
Resin Composite	2+	2+	1+
ZOE Cement	3+	1+	0

0–3+ indicate degree of reaction to the material, with 0 indicating no adverse response and 3+ indicating a severe response.
Adapted from Mjör IA, Hensten-Pettersen A, and Skogedal O: Int Dent J 27: 127, 1977.

clinical experience with the material. The results from these studies also showed a rather poor correlation among in vitro tests. The authors of these studies questioned the usefulness of in vitro and animal tests for the primary and secondary phases of testing. One material used in these tests was a zinc oxide–eugenol (ZOE) cement. When tested in direct contact with a cell culture, ZOE reliably and completely kills every cell in the culture; yet in clinical practice, ZOE cements have been used successfully for many years, with no evidence of pulpal damage. This paradox spawned the concept of constructing in vitro tests to be as relevant as possible to their in vivo use. In the case of ZOE, the use of an in vitro dentin barrier between the cement and the cells showed that the dentin protected the cells from most of the toxic effects of the ZOE and better aligned the in vitro test results with the associated clinical experience. Until these studies by Hume, Hanks, and others, few attempts were made to ensure the clinical relevance of in vitro tests. Today, this relevance is a prerequisite for appropriate in vitro and, to some extent, animal tests.

The work by Mjör et al (1977) also challenged the linear testing paradigm itself. The linear paradigm relies heavily on the accuracy of the primary tests. If these tests are too severe, potentially good materials will be screened out. If they are too insensitive, materials with little clinical promise will be promoted to the next phase of testing, wasting time and money and placing animals and humans at unnecessary risk. Although the linear paradigm persists today within the standards and regulatory agencies, most researchers in the field have adopted other paradigms (Fig. 8-16). In these alternative paradigms, the basic linear paradigm is preserved, but the need to consider nonlinear thinking is also infused. For example, a new material may be tested first using classic primary tests followed by secondary and usage tests, but primary tests may be necessary at a later stage to answer a question that arose from an early clinical trial. This question may not have arisen until the clinical trial, and the in vitro environment may be the only environment with sufficient experimental controls to answer the question. Nonlinear paradigms such as those shown in Figure 8-16 will likely become standard, particularly as more is understood about material-cell reactions at the molecular levels.

Standards: Advantages and Disadvantages

Although the earliest attempts at formally developing standardized tests for the biocompatibility of materials came in 1933, it was not until 1972 that the Council on Dental Materials, Instruments, and Equipment (later called the Council on Scientific Affairs) of the American National Standards Institute/American Dental Association (ANSI/ADA) approved Document No. 41 for Recommended Standard Practices for Biological Evaluation of Dental Materials. To some extent this document was developed in response to a movement in the U.S. Congress to require biological testing of

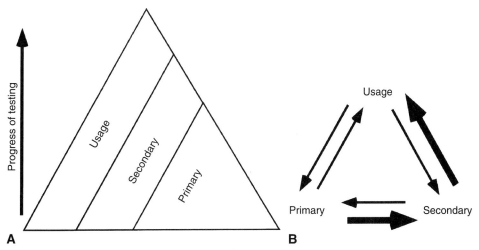

Fig. 8-16 Diagram showing several newer schemes for the progression of biocompatibility tests in the assessment of a new material. **A,** All three tests may be done initially, but as the testing progresses, the usage tests predominate. **B,** The most common progression is from primary to secondary to usage **(darker arrows)** tests, but any test may be performed at any time in the development of a material, depending on problems that are encountered. These alternative schemes recognize the complexities of biocompatibility testing and the need to avoid the rigid structure shown in Figure 8-15.

all medical devices, and this movement was formalized by the passage of the Medical Device Bill in 1976. An important point is that dental restorative materials are considered devices as opposed to drugs. In the view of the Food and Drug Administration (FDA) the rigor for devices is somewhat less than for drugs, which must show safety and efficacy. Devices are required to show safety only.

ANSI/ADA Document 41

The original ANSI/ADA Document No. 41 for biological testing of dental materials (released in 1972) was updated in 1982 to include tests for mutagenicity. This specification uses the linear paradigm for materials screening and divides testing into initial, secondary, and usage tests. The initial tests include in vitro assays for cytotoxicity, red blood cell membrane lysis, mutagenesis, and carcinogenesis, as well as animal tests for systemic toxicity by oral ingestion. Secondary tests include animal tests for inflammatory or immune responses. Usage tests include tests for pulpal and bone response. The required tests for a given material are not listed specifically. Rather, it is up to the manufacturer to select the tests and defend the selection to the ANSI/ADA and later to the FDA when applying for approval of the material. Document No. 41 is currently being revised, but the revision is not complete, so the 1982 version is still in force. The document is available from the Council on Scientific Affairs at the American Dental Association (www.ada.org), 211 E. Chicago Avenue, Chicago, IL 60611 or the American National Standards Institutes (www.ansi.org) 1819 L Street NW, Washington, DC 20036.

ISO Standard 10993

The ISO 10993 document is the international standard for testing the biocompatibility of materials. Unlike ANSI/ADA Document No. 41, the ISO 10993 standard is not restricted to dental materials. This document was first published in 1992, but modified versions are updated periodically. In 2002, ISO 10993 consisted of

16 parts, each addressing a different area of biological testing. For example, Part 3 governs tests for genotoxicity, carcinogenicity, and reproductive toxicity, whereas Part 4 covers tests for materials that interact with blood. Two types of tests are covered in the standard: initial tests for cytotoxicity, sensitization, and systemic toxicity, and supplementary tests for chronic toxicity, carcinogenicity, and biodegradation. In addition, some specialized tests for devices are addressed, such as the dentin barrier test for restorative dental materials. The initial tests may be in vitro or animal tests, whereas the supplementary tests are performed on animals or humans. In this standard, usage tests are part of the supplementary tests. As with the ANSI/ADA standard, the selection of tests is left to the manufacturer, who must then defend this selection upon application for approval. The document does give suggestions for test selection in Part 1 (Table 8-2); these suggestions are based on how long the material will be present, whether it will contact the body surface, blood, or bone, and whether it communicates externally once it is placed internally. The current working version is available from the International Organization for Standardization (www.iso.ch), Case Postate 56, CH-1211, Geneva 20, Switzerland, with reference to ISO10993-1:1992(E).

The standardization of biocompatibility testing of materials has done much to advance understanding of biocompatibility and to protect the public. Because the nature of biologic testing involves innumerable variables, standardization is critical to the unbiased comparison of results from different studies. In this sense, standards are very important. However, standards also have disadvantages. Most standards cannot keep pace with the development of new scientific information, such as the rapid advance of cellular and molecular biological techniques. By their nature, standards represent a compromise among manufacturers, academicians, and the lay public; therefore they tend to be developed slowly. Standards may also be arbitrary in nature because they must assign cut-off points for acceptability, and good scientific evidence to rationally select these cut-off points rarely exists. Individuals responsible for standards testing must recognize its economic impact on manufacturers and clinicians and must also be aware of the unavailability of certain techniques on a global scale. However, even with all these shortcomings, standards for biological testing are desirable and necessary for scientists, manufacturers, and patients alike.

CRITICAL QUESTION

Cite examples of how the biological properties of several materials used in dentistry require special consideration in use to ensure their biological safety.

CURRENT BIOCOMPATIBILITY ISSUES IN DENTISTRY
Latex

Exposure to latex comes from many sources, including toy balloons, condoms, swim goggles, dishwashing gloves, hairnet elastics, clothing elastics, footwear, cervical diaphragms, and hot water bottles. Of particular interest in dentistry is the use of the latex rubber dam, which exposes patients and dental personnel. In the early 1980s when the AIDS virus became known, dental personnel began to routinely wear gloves to reduce the risk of disease transmission. Since that time, the incidence of latex hypersensitivity reactions has increased dramatically. In 1991, the FDA estimated that about 6% to 7% of surgical personnel may be allergic to latex. Surveys of dental professionals have shown that 42% have adverse reactions to occupational

Table 8-2 Test Methods for Preclinical Evaluation of Medical Devices Used in Dentistry

Nature of Contact	Duration of Contact	Group I — Primary (initial) tests				Group II — Secondary tests							Group III — Preclinical usage tests		
		Cytotoxicity Test ISO XXXX Clauses 6, 7	Cytotoxicity Test ISO 10993-5	Cytotoxicity Test ISO XXXX Annex A	Genotoxicity Test ISO 10993-3 Clause 4	Acute Systemic Toxicity—Oral Application ISO 10993-11 Clause 6.5.1	Acute Systemic Toxicity—Application by Inhalation ISO 10993-11 Clause 6.5.3	Subchronic Systemic Toxicity—Oral Application ISO 10993-11 Clause 6.7.1	Skin Irritation and Intracutaneous Reactivity ISO 10993-10 Clauses 5.2, 5.4	Sensitization ISO 10993-10 Clauses 6.2, 6.3	Subchronic Systemic Toxicity—Application by Inhalation ISO 10993-11 Clause 6.7.3	Local Effects After Implantation ISO 10993-6 Clauses 4, 5, 6	Pulp and Dentine Usage Test ISO XXXX Clause 8	Pulp Capping and Pulpotomy Test ISO XXXX Clause 9	Endodontic Usage Test ISO XXXX Clause 10
Surface-contacting devices	≤24 hr	X	X				X		X	X					
	24 hr to 30 days	X	X				X	X	X	X	X	X			
	>30 days	X	X	X	X			X			X				
External communicating devices	≤24 hr	X	X	X			X		X	X					
	24 hr to 30 days	X	X	X	X		X	X	X	X	X	X	X	X	X
	>30 days	X	X	X	X	X	X	X	X	X	X	X	X	X	X
Implant devices	≤24 hr	X	X						X	X				X	X
	24 hr to 30 days	X	X	X	X			X	X	X		X	X	X	X
	>30 days	X	X	X	X			X	X		X	X	X	X	X

X in the columns indicates test that shall be considered for use. ISO XXXX in the column heading indicates that the official number will be designated when the ISO grants approval.

materials, most of which were related to dermatoses of the hands and fingers. Adverse reactions in 3.7% of adult patients and 5.7% of pediatric patients were associated with latex gloves. However, only 8.8% of the adult patients who experience hypersensitivity reactions used latex gloves at work. Thus latex hypersensitivity is a problem for both dental personnel and patients, and concerns about this problem are increasing.

Hypersensitivity to latex-containing products may represent a true latex allergy or a reaction to accelerators and antioxidants used in latex processing. Reactions to latex vary from localized rashes and swelling to more serious wheezing and anaphylaxis. Dermatitis of the hands (eczema) is the most common adverse reaction. A history of eczema and a familial history of allergies are predisposing factors, and repeated exposure and duration of exposure play a role in the degree of response. The most serious systemic allergic reactions occur when latex-containing products, such as gloves and rubber dams, contact the mucous membranes. Such exposures may result in angioneurotic edema, chest pain, and a rash on the neck and chest of severely allergic persons. Asthmatic reactions and other respiratory reactions have also been reported to components of the latex that are released into the air and carried by the powder coating on many latex products.

The processing of latex has made identification of specific protein allergens difficult. Natural latex products are made from a white, milky sap harvested from a tree that grows in tropical regions. Ammonia is added to the sap to preserve it, but at the same time the ammonia hydrolyzes and degrades the sap proteins to produce allergens. Vulcanization is the process by which liquid latex is hardened into rubber through the use of sulfur compounds and heat. These chemicals may be allergenic themselves, and are often present to some degree in the final product. The final manufacturing process leaches the allergens from the rubber products by soaking them in hot water. The leaching water is changed repeatedly to decrease the concentration of the allergens, but leaching brings other allergens to the surface and unfortunately places the highest concentrations near the skin of the wearer. Thus the allergenicity of a given batch of latex will be highly dependent on how the latex was collected, preserved, and processed. Synthetic latex is also available, but it suffers from similar problems, except that naturally occurring proteins and their degradation products are not present.

Nickel

Nickel is a common component of many dental alloys including those used for crowns, fixed partial dentures, removable partial dentures and some orthodontic appliances. Nickel is also used in many types of endodontic files, although the duration of exposure through this route is far shorter. The use of nickel-based alloys for fixed prosthodontics in the United States has increased dramatically over the past 20 years and currently accounts for somewhere between 30% and 50% of the market. The use of nickel in dental alloys has been controversial for many years because of the biological properties of nickel ions and nickel compounds.

Nickel is the most allergenic metal known, with an incidence of somewhere between 10% to 20%, depending on the study. Hypersensitivity to nickel is more common among women, presumably because of chronic exposure through jewelry, although the incidence among men is increasing. Reactions to nickel-containing dental alloys are well documented and can be quite severe in sensitive individuals. These reactions are probably underreported because the reactions are often subtle, and they resemble periodontal inflammation (see Fig. 8-6), but they may occur primarily outside the mouth.

Not all nickel-allergic individuals will react to intraoral nickel, and it is currently not possible to predict which individuals will react. Because the frequency of nickel allergy is high, it is possible that individuals will become sensitized to nickel after placement of nickel-containing alloys in the mouth. Some studies in guinea pigs have reported that oral exposure to nickel induces immunological tolerance, although this has not been shown in humans. There is a known cross-reactivity between nickel and palladium allergy. Virtually 100% of patients who are allergic to palladium will be allergic to nickel, whereas only about 33% of those allergic to nickel will be allergic to palladium. The mechanisms of the high allergy frequency to nickel are not known, but there is probably a genetic component. In addition, the tendency of nickel-containing alloys to release relatively large amounts of nickel ions probably contribute to their allergenicity. This release is particularly high in acidic conditions and for Ni-Cr alloys with less than 20 wt% chromium.

Nickel has other adverse biological effects in addition to allergy. Nickel subsulfide (Ni_2S_3) is a documented respiratory carcinogen in humans, but this compound is unknown in dentistry. Nickel ions (Ni^{2+}) are a documented mutagen in humans, but there is no evidence that nickel ions cause any carcinogenesis intraorally. Nickel carbonyl $[Ni(CO)_4]$ is an extremely toxic compound used industrially, but not in dentistry. Nickel ions also have been shown to be nonspecific inducers of inflammatory reactions (see Fig. 8-3) along with cobalt and mercury. Specifically, nickel ions appear to induce intercellular adhesion molecules in the endothelium and cause release of some cytokines from monocytes and other cells. It is not known to what extent these mechanisms contribute to any intraoral inflammation around nickel-containing crowns.

Beryllium

Beryllium is used in Ni-Cr alloys in concentrations of 1 wt% to 2 wt% (approximately 5.5 at% to 11 at%) to increase the castability of these alloys and lower their melting range. Beryllium also tends to form thin adherent oxides that are required to promote chemical bonding of porcelain. The use of beryllium in dental alloys is controversial because of its biological effects. First, beryllium is a documented carcinogen in either the metallic (Be^0) or ionic (Be^{2+}) state, although there are no studies showing that dental alloys containing beryllium cause cancer in humans. Any reaction is most probably mediated by beryllium released from the alloys, and although such release has been documented intraorally and in vitro, the release is not as prominent as for nickel. Acidic environments enhance beryllium release from Ni-Cr alloys.

Second, beryllium-containing particles that are inhaled and reach the alveoli of the lungs may cause a chronic inflammatory condition called *berylliosis*. In this condition, the alveoli of the lung are engorged with lymphocytes and macrophages. T cells in susceptible individuals proliferate locally in the lung tissue, presumably in a delayed hypersensitivity reaction to the beryllium metal. Berylliosis occurs only in individuals with a hypersensitivity to beryllium and may occur from inhalation of beryllium dusts (from grinding or polishing alloys), salts, or fumes, such as those encountered when casting beryllium-containing alloys.

Mercury and Amalgam

The controversy over the biocompatibility of amalgam has waxed and waned several times in the 170–plus-year history of its dental use in the United States. Most of the controversy stems from the known toxicity of mercury and the debate over whether mercury from amalgams has toxic effects. Mercury occurs in three forms: as the *metal* (Hg^0), as an *inorganic ion* (Hg^{2+}), or in one of several *organic forms,* such as methyl or ethyl mercury. Metallic mercury gains access to the body via the skin or as a vapor through the lungs. Ingested metallic mercury is poorly absorbed from the gut (0.01%), so the primary portal into the body is through inhalation of mercury vapor.

Numerous studies have shown that amalgams release sufficient vapor to cause between 1 and 3 μg of mercury absorption per day, depending on the number of amalgams present. The inhaled mercury gains access to the blood stream via the alveoli of the lungs. From the blood, mercury is distributed in the body, with preference for fat and nervous tissues. Mercury also is ingested through wear of amalgam restorations; about 45 μg/day of mercury may either reach the gut in the form of amalgam particulate or be dissolved and released as Hg^{2+} ions. The absorption of the ionic mercury is also poor (approximately 1% to 7%). Mercury trapped in amalgam particles is even more poorly absorbed. Methyl mercury is not produced from amalgams but is generally a product of bacteria or other biological systems acting on metallic mercury. Methyl mercury is the most toxic form of mercury and is also very efficiently absorbed from the gut (90% to 95%). The primary source of methyl mercury is in the diet, with fish (especially shark, swordfish, and tuna) contributing a significant portion.

Concerns about mercury stem from its toxicity and its relatively long half-life in the body. The toxicity of mercury is well known and the symptoms depend somewhat on the form. Acute symptoms are neurological or renal, ranging from paresthesia (at levels ≥500 μg/kg) to ataxia (≥1000 μg/kg), joint pain (≥2000 μg/kg) and death (≥4000 μg/kg). The lowest known level for any observable toxic effect is 3 μg/kg. This level translates to about 30 μg of mercury per gram of creatinine clearance in the urine. At chronic exposure levels, the symptoms are more subtle and include weakness, fatigue, anorexia, weight loss, insomnia, irritability, shyness, dizziness, and tremors in the extremities or the eyelids (hence the phrase "mad as a hatter," a reference to felt hat makers who used mercury and often showed signs of dementia). Although amalgams do not release anywhere near toxic levels of mercury, the long half-life of mercury in the body causes concern among some individuals. The half-life ranges from 20 to 90 days, depending on the form, with methyl mercury exhibiting the longest half-life and inorganic forms having the shortest half-life. Numerous tests for body burden of mercury have been developed, including analysis of blood, urine, and hair. Of these, the urine is the best long-term indicator of the total metallic mercury body burden, normalized to grams of creatinine clearance from the kidney.

Humans are exposed to mercury from a variety of sources in addition to dental amalgams. There are exquisitely sensitive methods for detecting mercury to the parts-per-trillion level, and these methods have made it possible to analyze the sources of mercury exposure for humans. Estimates of intake levels from air (in μg/day) are 0.12 for Hg^0, 0.04 for Hg^{2+}, and 0.03 for methyl mercury. Water probably contributes about 0.05 μg/day and food about 20.0 μg/day in the form of Hg^{2+}. Depending on a person's diet, consumption of fish contributes about 0.9 μg/day of Hg^0 and 3.8 μg/day of methyl mercury. These values help put the 1 to 3 μg/day of absorbed Hg^0 vapor from amalgams in perspective. Thus the intake of mercury is a complex issue with many sources and forms of exposure. Furthermore, intake amounts vary considerably among individuals, depending on diet, environment, and dental status. Despite the confirmed exposure of humans to these low levels of mercury, the biological effects of these levels are insignificant.

Many studies have attempted to determine whether mercury exposure from dental or other sources contributes to any documentable health problem. Several studies have estimated the number of amalgam surfaces that would be needed to expose an individual to mercury concentrations with a minimum observable effect (slight psychomotor performance, detectable tremor, and impaired nerve conduction velocity). Estimates are that 450 to 530 amalgam surfaces would be necessary to achieve these levels. Even if all 32 teeth were restored on all surfaces with amalgam, the total number of surfaces would be only 192. Other studies have measured renal function in patients in whom all amalgams were removed simultaneously (worst case). Despite markedly elevated blood, plasma, and urine levels of mercury, no renal impairment has been noted. Still other studies have investigated blood cell type and cell number in dentists, who are presumably exposed to higher levels of mercury because of daily occupational exposure. No effects of mercury have been noted. Other studies for neurological symptoms in various populations occupationally exposed have shown no effects. In summary, there are simply no data to show that mercury released from dental amalgams is harmful.

Estrogenicity

In 1996, a research group claimed that dental sealants released estrogenic substances in sufficient quantities to warrant concern. Since that time, the estrogenicity of dental composites has been questioned, particularly in children. Estrogenicity is the ability of a chemical to act as the hormone estrogen does in the body. If these chemicals are not indigenous to the body, the substance is called a **xenoestrogen**. The occurrence of xenoestrogens in the environment has been a concern for many years. Environmentalists fear that these substances will alter the reproductive cycles and developmental processes in wildlife, and there is evidence to support these concerns. The concern about estrogens in dentistry center around a chemical called *bisphenol A* (or *BPA*), which is a synthetic starting point for all Bis-GMA composites in dentistry, as well as many other plastics. The fear is that the release of these substances might alter normal cellular development or maintenance if the BPA has estrogenic effects.

There is fairly convincing evidence that BPA and BPA dimethacrylate (also known as *BAD*) may act on the estrogenic receptors in cells. Thus these chemicals are probably xenoestrogens. Evidence comes from molecular modeling studies and studies of estrogen receptor–BPA binding in vitro. However, these studies have also shown that BPA and BAD are probably 1000-fold less potent as estrogens than the native estrogen hormone.

One test commonly used to assess xenoestrogenic activity is called the *E-screen assay*. This in vitro test relies on the growth response of breast cancer cells that are estrogen sensitive to purported estrogenic compounds. Typically, the compound in question is applied to cells, and cell growth is measured over a period of 24 to 72 hr. A compound is deemed estrogenic if the growth rate of cells exceeds that of control compounds without the chemical. The E-screen test has several problems that make its accuracy doubtful. First, the test does not confirm that the chemical acts on the estrogenic receptor, a requirement for true estrogenicity. Second, the test uses cell growth to define estrogenicity, but many factors other than estrogenicity can cause such cell growth. Finally, several other problems exist with the test, such as reliability and sensitivity of the cell-lines used and difficulties in controlling variables. All of these factors cast doubt on the reliability of the E-screen assay as a predictor of estrogenicity.

Although the estrogenicity of BPA has been confirmed, no evidence exists that dental composites have estrogenic effects in vitro or in vivo. The original contentions of Olea et al in 1996 appear to have been overstated, because several errors in the method and interpretation have subsequently been reported in the literature. Studies have shown only trace amounts of BPA in dental composites, and elution of BPA from polymerized composites is low or not detectable. Coupled with the relative insensitivity of BPA as an estrogen and the likely dilution of any released BPA, the risks of estrogenic effects in vivo appear low. No studies have shown conclusive evidence of these effects from dental resin-containing materials.

Other Biological Effects of Resins

The explosion in the use of dental resins for restorative work has raised questions about the biological safety of these materials. The primary risk of these materials appears to be allergy, and the risk is highest for dental personnel because of frequent exposure to unpolymerized materials. The allergenicity of methylmethacrylate is well documented, and the use of gloves is not effective in preventing contact because most monomers pass easily through gloves. Also, allergic reactions to other methacrylates have been reported. The allergic reactions are primarily contact dermatitis, with the resins acting as haptens via delayed hypersensitivity (Type IV) mechanisms. In rare cases, anaphylactoid responses have been reported and dermatitis can be so severe as to be disabling. In the most severe cases, individuals must change work activities or select a different profession.

Resins also have significant toxic effects as demonstrated through the use of in vitro tests, often comparable and sometimes exceeding the potency of metals. There is ample evidence that resins release unpolymerized components into biological environments, although the release in vivo is not well documented either for resins or for metals. Resin components have also been shown to traverse the dentin, and newer techniques that advocate direct pulp capping with resins expose pulp tissue directly to these materials. The long-term, low-dose effect of released resin components is not well understood, and detecting adverse effects in vivo is difficult. Limited clinical evidence has linked the use of resins to oral inflammation. There is also limited in vivo evidence that resins potentiate the growth of some bacterial species. Other studies have advocated the use of special resins as antimicrobial agents to be incorporated into dental restorative materials.

CLINICAL GUIDELINES FOR SELECTING BIOCOMPATIBLE MATERIALS

Clinicians will likely be continually overwhelmed by marketing information on many new materials and claims of their clinical performance. Unconditional biocompatibility will often be claimed by manufacturers. It is difficult for clinicians to evaluate the biological safety of new materials and evaluate manufacturers' claims. However, with knowledge of biocompatibility issues and some common sense, clinicians can make reasonable judgments about biological safety. Several critical steps will ensure an informed decision. These steps are described in the following three sections.

Define the Use of the Material

An important consideration when evaluating biological safety is how the materials will be used. As discussed previously, the use of a material plays a crucial role in its biocompatibility. For example, even though a ceramic has enjoyed success as an anterior restorative material, it is not always successful as a posterior material. The clinician should consider whether the material's proposed use is new and whether it has been tested in its proposed use. If the material is to be used in a new way or in a new environment, more caution is advised.

A second consideration is the composition of the material. Studies have shown repeatedly that very small changes in composition or processing of a material can alter its biocompatibility. Clinicians should ask whether the material's composition is different from that of previous products or whether the processing of the material has changed. If so, caution is advised in applying previous biological data to the new situation.

CRITICAL QUESTION

A sales representative comes into your office presenting a new filling material. What should you learn about the material's biocompatibility tests?

Define How the Material Has Been Tested

Previous discussion has emphasized the difficulties in applying in vitro or animal tests to clinical applications. In some instances, the clinician will not have access to data on the clinical trials of a new material (or these data may not exist). In these cases, the clinician will have to rely on in vitro or animal tests. The first consideration is to understand which tests have been used. Clinicians should not be satisfied with nondescript statements such as "the material has been tested for biocompatibility with no problems." If clinical trials are available, make sure that the conditions and duration of the test are relevant. The quality of any usage test depends on the fidelity of reproducing the clinical use. If only animal or in vitro tests are available, the clinician should question the structure of these tests and the methods employed. Make sure that testing conditions were as relevant as possible, and look for multiple types of tests under different clinically relevant conditions. A well-controlled comparison with existing materials is always preferable to an isolated test on one material.

CRITICAL QUESTION

In the final analysis, who makes the choice about which materials are biologically safe for use in dentistry: the patient, the dentist, or the manufacturer?

Think in Terms of Risk and Benefit

In the end, no material can be shown to be 100% safe or risk-free. Furthermore, rarely will all data be available to adequately define the risks of using a material. Thus the clinician must rely on clinical judgment, common sense, and the data available to make a judgment. The clinician must always recognize that the use of materials in the body requires a risk-benefit analysis. The degree of risk assumed must be carefully weighed against possible benefits. Each clinician will have to adapt a philosophy about the degree of risk he or she is willing to assume on the patient's behalf. Furthermore, these risks must be communicated thoroughly and clearly to the patient so that he or she can decide whether the benefits outweigh the risks. This communication is the essence of *informed consent*, and nowhere in dentistry is this process more important than in evaluating the biological effects of materials.

SELECTED READINGS

American Dental Association: The dental team and latex hypersensitivity. ADA Council on Scientific Affairs. J Am Dent Assoc 130(2):257-264, 1999.

Amin A, Palenik CJ, Cheung SW, and Burke FJ: Latex exposure and allergy: A survey of general dental practitioners and dental students. Int Dent J 48(2):77-83, 1998.

Bergenholtz G: Evidence for bacterial causation of adverse pulpal responses in resin-based dental restorations. Crit Rev Oral Biol Med 11:467-480, 2000.

Bergman M: Side-effects of dental materials reported in Scandinavian countries. Dent Mater J 19(1):1-9, 2000.

Craig RG (ed): Restorative Dental Materials, 11th ed. St. Louis, Mosby, 2001.

Field EA: Dental surgeons with natural rubber latex allergy: A report of 20 cases. Occup Med (Lond) 49(2):103-107, 1999.

Garhammer P, Schmalz G, Hiller KA, Reitinger T, and Stolz W: Patients with local adverse effects from dental alloys: Frequency, complaints, symptoms, allergy. Clin Oral Investig 5(4):240-249, 2001.

Hamid A, and Hume WR: The effect of dentine thickness on diffusion of resin monomers in vitro. J Oral Rehabil 24(1):20-5, 1997.

Hensten-Pettersen A, and Jacobsen N: Perceived side effects of biomaterials in prosthetic dentistry. J Prosthet Dent 65(1):138-144, 1991.

Hume WR, and Gerzia TM: Bioavailability of components of resin-based materials which are applied to teeth. Crit Rev Oral Biol Med 7(2):172-179, 1996.

Kallus T, and Mjor IA: Incidence of adverse effects of dental materials. Scand J Dent Res 99(3):236-240, 1991.

Landrum LL: CE course for Human Research Subjects. www.mcg.edu/ce/research.htm.

Lonnroth EC, and Shahnavaz H: Adverse health reactions in skin, eyes, and respiratory tract among dental personnel in Sweden. Swed Dent J 22(1-2):33-45, 1998.

Mackert JR: Dental amalgam and mercury. J Am Dent Assoc 122:54-61, 1991.

Mackert JR, and Berglund A: Mercury exposure from dental amalgam fillings: absorbed dose and the potential for adverse health effects. Crit Rev Oral Biol Med 8:410-436, 1997.

Mackert JR, Leffell MS, Wagner DA, and Powell BJ: Lymphocyte levels in subjects with and without amalgam restorations. J Am Dent Assoc 122:49-53, 1991.

Mjör IA, Hensten-Pettersen A, and Skogedal O: Biologic evaluation of filling materials. A comparison of results using cell culture techniques, implantation tests and pulp studies. Int Dent J 27:124-129, 1977.

Noda M, Komatsu H, and Sano H: HPLC analysis of dental resin composite components. J Biomed Mater Res 47:374-378, 1999.

Olea N, Pulgar R, Perez P, et al: Estrogenicity of resin-based composites and sealants used in dentistry. Environ Health Perspect 104(3):298-305, 1996.

Örtengren U, Andreasson H, Karlsson S, Meding B, and Barregård L: Prevalence of self-reported hand eczema and skin symptoms associated with dental materials among Swedish dentists. Eur J Oral Sci 107:496-505, 1999.

Özer L: The relationship between gap size, microbial accumulation and the structural features of natural caries in extracted teeth with class I amalgam restorations: A stereo- and polarized microscopic study. Tandlaegebladet 102(NR6):318-319, 1998.

Pashley D: Dynamics of the pulpo-dentin complex. Crit Rev Oral Biol Med 7:104-133, 1996.

Pulgar R, Olea-Serrano MF, Novillo-Fertrell A, et al: Determination of bisphenol A and related aromatic compounds released from bis-GMA-based composites and sealants by high performance liquid chromatography. Environ Health Perspect 108(1):21-27, 2000.

Rankin KV, Jones DL, and Rees TD: Latex reactions in an adult dental population. Am J Dent 6(6):274-276, 1993.

Rankin KV, Jones DL, and Rees TD: Latex glove reactions found in a dental school. J Am Dent Assoc 124(5):67-71, 1993.

Rankin KV, Seale NS, Jones DL, and Rees TD: Reported latex sensitivity in pediatric dental patients from hospital- and dental school-based populations. Pediatr Dent 16(2):117-120, 1994.

Reichl FX, Durner J, Hickel R, et al: Distribution and excretion of TEGDMA in guinea pigs and mice. J Dent Res 80(5):1412-1415, 2001.

Schafer TE, Lapp CA, Hanes CM, Lewis JB, Wataha JC, and Schuster GS: Estrogenicity of bisphenol A and bisphenol A dimethacrylate in vitro. J Biomed Mater Res 45(3):192-197, 1999.

Vreeburg KJJ, VanHoogstraten IMW, VonBlomberg BME, and DeGroot K: Oral induction of immunological tolerance to chromium in the guinea pig. J Dent Res 69:1634-1639, 1990.

Walsh LJ, Lange P, and Savage NW: Factors influencing the wearing of protective gloves in general dental practice. Quintessence Int 26(3):203-209, 1995.

Wataha JC: Materials for endosseous dental implants. J Oral Rehabil 23:79-90, 1996.

Wataha JC: Biocompatibility of dental casting alloys: A review. J Prosthet Dent 83:223-234, 2000.

Wataha JC: Principles of biocompatibility for dental practitioners. J Prosthet Dent 86:203-209, 2001.

Wataha JC, and Hanks CT: Biological effects of palladium and risk of using palladium in dental casting alloys. J Oral Rehabil 23:309-320, 1996.

PART II
AUXILIARY DENTAL MATERIALS

9
Impression Materials
Chiayi Shen

OUTLINE

KEY TERMS

Accelerator—A compound that speeds up the reaction; also refers to the component called the *catalyst* in the reaction of impression materials.

Addition reaction—A polymerization reaction in which each polymer chain grows to a maximum length in sequence and no reaction by-product is formed.

Agar (reversible) hydrocolloid—An aqueous impression material used for recording maximum detail; for example, as required in the production of dies for fixed restorations.

Alginate (irreversible) hydrocolloid—An aqueous impression material used for recording minimal detail; for example, as required to produce study models.

Base paste/base putty—The component that forms the main three-dimensional structure of the final impression.

Cast—A dimensionally accurate reproduction of a part or parts of the oral cavity or extraoral facial structures produced in a durable hard material.

Catalyst paste/catalyst putty—A component of a polymerization reaction that decreases the energy required for the reaction to occur and usually does not become part of the final product; however, in the formulation of impression materials, the term *catalyst* refers to a structural component that initiates the polymerization reaction.

Colloid—A solid, liquid, or gaseous substance made up of large molecules or masses of smaller molecules that remain in suspension in a surrounding continuous medium of different matter.

Condensation reaction—A polymerization process in which the polymer chains grow simultaneously and a reaction by-product is formed with associated shrinkage.

KEY TERMS—cont'd

Cross-linking—Joining of polymer chains to form a three-dimensional network structure.

Cure—The reaction process that takes place primarily during the setting of a polymer but continues after setting.

Dashpot—An element of the viscoelastic model describing the viscous response of a polymer.

Dispersed phase/dispersed particles—Particles in a solution.

Dispersion phase/dispersed medium—A solution containing a suspension of particles.

Elastomer—A lightly cross-linked impression material that exhibits elastic behavior after setting.

Fusion temperature—The temperature below which a definite reduction in plasticity occurs during cooling of an impression compound.

Gel—A network of fibrils that forms a weak, slightly elastic brush-heap structure of hydrocolloid; also, the solid network structure that defines the cross-linked polymer.

Gelation—The transformation from a hydrocolloid sol to a gel.

Hydrocolloid (agar)—A colloid that contains water as the dispersion phase.

Hydrophilic—Tendency to demonstrate a strong affinity for water.

Hydrophobic—Tendency to demonstrate an aversion to water.

Imbibition—Process of water sorption.

Inelastic—Incapable of sustaining significant elastic deformation under stress.

Initiator—The component that starts a polymerization reaction; types include photo-initiators, chemical initiators, and heat initiators.

Irreversible hydrocolloid—Alginate impression material.

Micelle—An aggregate of surfactant molecules or ions in solution.

Model—A positive full-scale replica of teeth, soft tissues, and restored structures used as a diagnostic aid for construction of orthodontic and prosthetic appliances.

Monophase—See **single phase**.

Permanent deformation—Irreversible change in shape that occurs when the polymer responds as a viscous liquid under an applied pressure.

Polymerization—Chemical reaction that transforms small molecules into large polymer chains.

Pseudoplastic—Characteristic of a material to become more fluid when an applied force is increased; this behavior involves shear thinning and is strain rate–dependent.

Reversible hydrocolloid—Agar impression material.

Rheological—Pertaining to the science that describes the fluid or flow characteristic of materials.

Set—State of being sufficiently rigid or elastic to permit removal from the mouth without plastic deformation.

Setting time—The elapsed time from the start of mixing until the impression material becomes firm enough to resist permanent deformation; for an elastic impression material it represents the time at which the impression can be withdrawn from the mouth; for an inelastic impression material it is the time at which the impression is hard enough to resist penetration by a pointed object under an applied load.

Shear-thinning—Tendency for viscosity to decrease as shearing stress increases. (See **pseudoplastic**.)

Single phase—A single-component material that is viscous enough to serve as the tray material; it is also capable of shear-thinning and can serve as a syringe material.

Spring—An engineering mechanics element that mimics the elastic behavior of cross-linked polymers.

Strain in compression—The amount of deformation a material sustains under a constant load for 30 seconds; some permanent deformation may remain when the load is removed.

Syneresis—Expression of fluid onto the surface of gel structures; this process allows hydrocolloid impressions to achieve equilibrium through stress relaxation.

Thixotropic—Property of certain gels or other materials to become liquefied (less viscous) when shaken, stirred, patted, or vibrated. (See Chapter 3 for related properties.)

Undercuts—Recessed areas on oral structures, including teeth, edentulous ridges, prostheses, and restorations.

Viscoelastic—Ability of a polymer to behave as an elastic solid (spring) and as a viscous liquid (dashpot).

Working time—The total time from the start of mixing to the final time at which an impression tray can be fully seated without distortion.

CRITICAL QUESTIONS

*Which of the eight criteria that ensure accurate impression making are related to the time
the impression material is in the mouth? Which one is related primarily to the properties of
a set impression?*

IMPRESSION MATERIALS: PURPOSE AND REQUIREMENTS

Constructing a **model** or **cast** is an important step in numerous dental procedures.
Various types of casts and models can be made from gypsum products using an
impression mold or negative likeness of a dental structure. The dentist designs and
constructs both removable and fixed prostheses on a gypsum cast. Thus the cast
must be an accurate representation of oral structures, which requires that the
impression (mold) be accurate.

Materials used to produce accurate replicas of intraoral and extraoral tissues
should fulfill the following criteria to obtain an accurate impression: (1) They should
be fluid enough to adapt to the oral tissues; (2) they should be viscous enough to be
contained in the tray that is seated in the mouth; (3) while in the mouth, they should
transform **(set)** into a rubbery or rigid solid in a reasonable amount of time. Ideally
the total **setting time** should be less than 7 min; (4) the set impression should not
distort or tear when removed from the mouth; (5) the impressions made from these
materials should remain dimensionally stable at least until the cast can be poured;
(6) the impression should maintain its dimensional stability after removal of a cast
so that a second or third cast can be made from the same impression; (7) the materials should be biocompatible; and (8) the materials, associated processing equipment, and processing time should be cost-effective.

Environmental conditions and the characteristics of the tissue often dictate the
choice of materials, the quality of the impression, and the quality of the cast. This
chapter discusses the unique properties of currently used impression materials and
describes how these characteristics affect the quality of an impression and of the cast
or model that is constructed from the impression. Figure 9-1 shows typical impressions with associated gypsum casts.

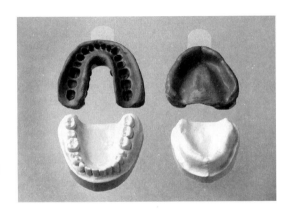

Fig. 9-1 Impressions of dentate **(left)** and
edentulous arches **(right)** with the
resulting respective gypsum casts.

MATERIALS USED FOR MAKING IMPRESSIONS

Historically, impression making was accomplished with **inelastic** materials for both soft and hard tissues. **Hydrocolloid** was initially introduced to make impressions of hard tissues in place of inelastic materials. After World War II, advances in polymer technology brought to the dental profession a group of synthetic rubbery materials called **elastomers**, which are capable of making impressions of both soft and hard tissues. These materials can be classified according to the mode through which the ingredients react (set or harden) to solids, their mechanical properties, and their uses. Table 9-1 shows the classification of the various dental impression materials based on the setting mechanism, dental applications, and mechanical deformation behavior. The mechanical behavior of the materials also dictates their primary applications in impression making.

Setting Mechanism

Impression materials can set by means of *reversible* or *irreversible* reactions. The term *irreversible* implies that chemical reactions have occurred and that the material cannot revert to its preset state in the dental office. For example, alginate, zinc oxide–eugenol (ZOE) impression paste, impression plaster, and elastomeric impression materials are hardened by chemical reactions. On the other hand, reversible materials soften under heat and solidify when they are cooled, with no chemical change taking place. **Reversible hydrocolloid** and impression compounds belong to this category.

Mechanical Properties

Some impression materials become rigid and cannot be removed past **undercuts** without fracturing or distorting the impression. They include ZOE impression paste, impression plaster, and impression compound. These impression materials are considered inelastic and were used for all impressions before the introduction of **agar hydrocolloid**. ZOE impression paste and impression plaster are called *mucostatic impression materials* because they do not compress the tissue during seating of the impression tray. They are ideal for making impressions of edentulous jaw structures.

Elastic impression materials make up the second use category. These materials can be stretched or compressed slightly, but they should rebound without **permanent deformation** when the impression tray is removed from the mouth. They include nonaqueous elastomers and hydrocolloids. Elastic impression materials are capable of accurately reproducing both the hard and soft structures of the mouth, including the undercuts and interproximal spaces.

Uses of Impression Materials

Impression materials can be used to capture the precise shape of edentulous ridge forms (soft tissues) and tooth forms (hard tissues). Elastomers are used extensively to prepare casts for fixed and removable partial dentures, as well as for single restorative units, such as crowns, onlays, and inlays. Very fluid, light-body elastomeric impression materials are also used for edentulous impressions.

CRITICAL QUESTION

What are the consequences of placing an impression material in the mouth when the working time has been exceeded?

Table 9-1 Classification of Dental Impression Materials

By setting mechanism	By elasticity and use				
	Inelastic or rigid		Elastic		
	Material	Use	Material	Use	

Chemical reaction (irreversible)	Plaster of Paris
	Zinc oxide–eugenol
		Edentulous ridge
		Interocclusal records
			Alginate hydrocolloid
			Nonaqueous elastomers
			  Polysulfide
			  Polyether
			  Condensation silicone
			  Addition silicone
				Teeth and soft tissues	

Thermally induced physical reaction (reversible)	Compound wax	Preliminary impression	Agar hydrocolloid	Teeth and soft tissues	

ELASTOMERIC IMPRESSION MATERIALS

Elastomers refer to a group of rubbery polymers, which are either chemically or physically cross-linked. They can be easily stretched and rapidly recover their original dimensions when the applied stress is released.

Chemically, there are four kinds of elastomers used as impression materials: *polysulfide, condensation-polymerizing silicone, addition-polymerizing silicone,* and *polyether.* Representative products are shown in Figure 9-2. All of these materials can replicate intraoral and extraoral structures with sufficient accuracy for use in the fabrication of fixed or removable prostheses. Most impression materials are two-component systems supplied in paste form. The different colored pastes are dispensed either through a spiral mixing tip or in equal lengths on a mixing pad and spatulated to a homogeneous color. Setting occurs through a combination of chain-lengthening **polymerization** and chemical **cross-linking** by either a **condensation reaction** or **addition reaction**. Impression materials of this type are called *nonaqueous elastomeric impression materials* in ANSI/ADA Specification No. 19. In this chapter, we will refer to them simply as *elastomeric impression materials.*

The current ANSI/ADA Specification No. 19 recognizes three types of elastomeric impression materials. Classification is based on selected elastic properties and the dimensional change of the set materials rather than on their chemistry. However, each type is further divided into four viscosity classes, including light-body, medium-body or regular-body, heavy-body, and putty. Viscosity is a material property that controls the flow characteristics of a material.

Characteristics

The **rheological** properties of the elastomeric impression materials play a major role in their successful application as high-accuracy impression materials. These materials are introduced into the mouth as viscous pastes with carefully adjusted flow properties. The setting reaction then converts them into **viscoelastic** solids. The appropriate flow behavior of the solid form is essential if an accurate impression is to be obtained. The viscosity and flow behavior of the unmixed components are also important, because these properties control the ease of mixing, the amount of air trapped during mixing, and the tendency for the trapped air to escape before the impression is made.

The **working time**, which begins at the start of mixing and ends just before the elastic properties have developed, must exceed the time required for mixing, filling the syringe and/or tray, injecting the material on tooth preparations, and seating the tray. Setting time can be described as the time elapsing from the beginning of mixing

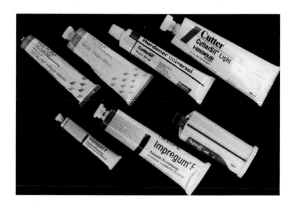

Fig. 9-2 Representative commercially available elastomeric impression materials: **Upper left pair,** polysulfide. **Upper right pair,** condensation silicone. **Lower left pair,** polyether. **Lower right,** addition silicone automixing cartridge.

until the curing process has advanced sufficiently so that the impression can be removed from the mouth with a minimum of distortion. If a material is not adequately "set," the material will not have sufficient elastic properties to respond to the strain of removing it from the mouth. Setting times posted by the manufacturers may be too short, and waiting an "extra minute" before removing the impression can ensure success. Remember, however, that polymerization may continue for a considerable time after setting.

Viscoelastic Properties

The ideal impression material should accurately record oral structure, be easily removable without distortion from the mouth, and remain dimensionally stable on the lab bench after pouring a gypsum product into the impression. The distortion produced during removal should be minimal if the clinician remembers to snap the tray away from the teeth after breaking the suction or the air seal. The borders of the tray should be pried loose parallel to the path of insertion until air leaks into the tray. Then the tray can be removed rapidly with minimal rotation or twisting.

Viscoelasticity describes the dependence of an impression material's response to the speed of removal (strain rate). Viscoelastic behavior is intermediate between that of an elastic solid and a viscous liquid. An elastic solid can be viewed as a **spring**, which deforms instantly to a certain extent when one applies a specific load. The deformation will be reversed completely when the load is removed. On the other hand, a viscous liquid is similar to an oil **dashpot**, which does not respond instantly to any sudden external load but deforms as the load is applied over time. The dashpot continues to deform at a rate proportional to the duration of loading until the load is removed. Compared with the reversible behavior of an elastic solid, the deformation exhibited by the dashpot is permanent.

The simplest model that demonstrates the viscoelastic behavior is a Maxwell-Voigt model (Fig. 9-3, A), which consists of a spring (S1) and a dashpot (D1) in series, and a second set (S2 and D2) in parallel. When one applies a force, either in a tensile or compressive mode, as shown by the arrow, spring S1 responds instantaneously with a definite amount of strain (deformation). At this instant, dashpot D1 does not show any deformation and dashpot D2 prevents spring S2 from deforming because of dashpot inertia (Fig. 9-3, B). If the same force is maintained on the model, both dashpots are activated and they continue to deform as long as loading is applied (Fig. 9-3, C). Meanwhile, spring S1 maintains the same magnitude of strain. At the moment the load is removed, the deformation exhibited by spring S1 recovers while the rest remains unchanged (Fig. 9-3, D). As time passes, spring S2 slowly overcomes the inertia of dashpot D2 and recovers along with D2 (Fig. 9-3, D). This process usually takes time, and the deformation will not recover completely. The deformation of dashpot D1 never recovers.

This viscoelastic behavior has considerable clinical importance. According to the model, the amount of permanent deformation attributed to either dashpot is dictated by the duration of tension or compression exerted on the material. A teasing or rocking method should not be used to remove the impression, but rather it should be removed suddenly in a direction as nearly parallel as possible to the long axes of the teeth. However, a slight teasing action will first be required to break the seal between the impression material and the hard and soft tissues.

The amount of permanent deformation exhibited by an elastomeric impression material should be clinically negligible, provided that: (1) the material has adequately gelled, (2) negligible pressure is applied to the tray during polymerization,

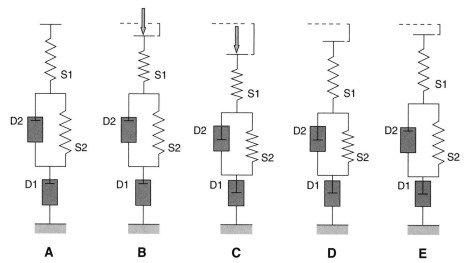

| A | B | C | D | E |

Fig. 9-3 A mechanical model showing the response of a viscoelastic material to external loading and unloading. **A,** Maxwell-Voigt viscoelastic model in a stress-free state. **B,** At the moment of loading, only spring S1 contracts in response to the load. **C,** When the loading continues, the piston in dashpot D1 and D2 move proportionally to the duration of loading. Spring S2 contracts along with dashpot D2. No change is expected for spring S1. **D,** The moment the load is released, spring S1 recovers instantly whereas the rest of elements remain unchanged. Spring S2 should also recover instantly, but it is retarded by the sluggishness of dashpot D2. **E,** As time passes, spring S2 recovers and extends dashpot D2 slowly to near its original position. Dashpot D1 remains unchanged. The right-hand bracket on the top of each model denotes the degree of deformation.

(3) the impression has been removed rapidly along the path of tray insertion, and (4) the undercuts present in the cavity preparation are minimal.

CRITICAL QUESTION

Which generic impression material type represents the most ideal material relative to dimensional accuracy, tear resistance, ability to be repoured two or more times without distortion, and hydrophilicity?

ELASTOMERIC IMPRESSION MATERIALS: CHEMISTRY AND COMPOSITION
Polysulfide

The main component of polysulfide materials is a multifunctional mercaptan (—SH) or polysulfide polymer. This linear polymer contains approximately 1 mole percent of pendant —SH groups. An oxidizing agent such as lead dioxide is used to initiate polymerization through chain lengthening between terminal —SH groups and cross-linking between the pendant —SH groups (Fig. 9-4). Lead dioxide is the component that gives polysulfide its characteristic brown color.

The reaction starts at the beginning of mixing and reaches its maximum rate soon after the spatulation is complete. At this stage a resilient network has started to form. During the final set, a material of adequate elasticity and strength is formed that can be removed past undercuts quite readily.

Moisture and temperature have a significant effect on the course of the reaction. In particular, hot and humid conditions will accelerate the setting of polysulfide impression material. The reaction yields water as a by-product. Loss of this small

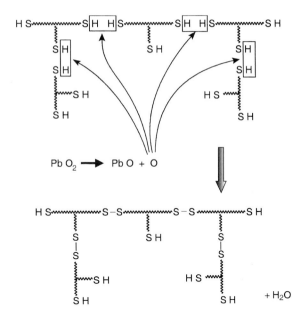

Fig. 9-4 Top, SH groups interact with oxygen from lead dioxide. **Bottom,** Completion of the condensation reaction results in water as a byproduct.

molecule from the set material has a significant effect on the dimensional stability of the impression.

The **base paste** contains the polysulfide polymer, a suitable filler (e.g., lithopone or titanium dioxide) to provide the required strength, a plasticizer (such as dibutyl phthalate) to confer the appropriate viscosity to the paste, and a small quantity of sulfur, approximately 0.5%, to accelerate the reaction.

The **catalyst** or **accelerator** paste contains lead dioxide. However, the terms *catalyst* and *accelerator* are really misnomers. *Reactor* is a more appropriate term for the polysulfide reaction. In addition, the same plasticizer and the same quantity of the filler used in the base paste are included in the reactor paste, along with oleic or stearic acid, which is added as a retarder to control the rate of the setting reactions.

Each paste is supplied in a dispensing tube with appropriately sized bore diameters at the tip so that equal lengths of each paste are extruded out of each tube to provide the correct ratio of polymer to cross-linking agent. Since the composition of the material in the tube is balanced with that of the accelerator, the matched tubes supplied by the manufacturer should always be used.

Condensation Silicone

The basic component in condensation impression materials is an α-ω-hydroxyl-terminated polydimethyl siloxane (Fig. 9-5, *Top*). The curing of this material involves a reaction of tri- and tetra-functional alkyl silicates, commonly tetraethyl orthosilicate, in the presence of stannous octoate. The average polymer chain consists of about 1000 units. The formation of the elastomer occurs through cross-linking between terminal groups of the silicone polymers and the alkyl silicate to form a three-dimensional network as shown in Figure 9-5, *Bottom*. Ethyl alcohol is a by-product of the condensation setting reaction. Its subsequent evaporation probably accounts for much of the contraction that takes place in a set silicone rubber impression.

The condensation silicone impression materials are supplied as a base paste and a low-viscosity liquid catalyst (or a paste catalyst). A high-viscosity material, commonly referred to as "putty," was developed to overcome the large polymerization shrinkage of the condensation silicone impression materials. These putties are

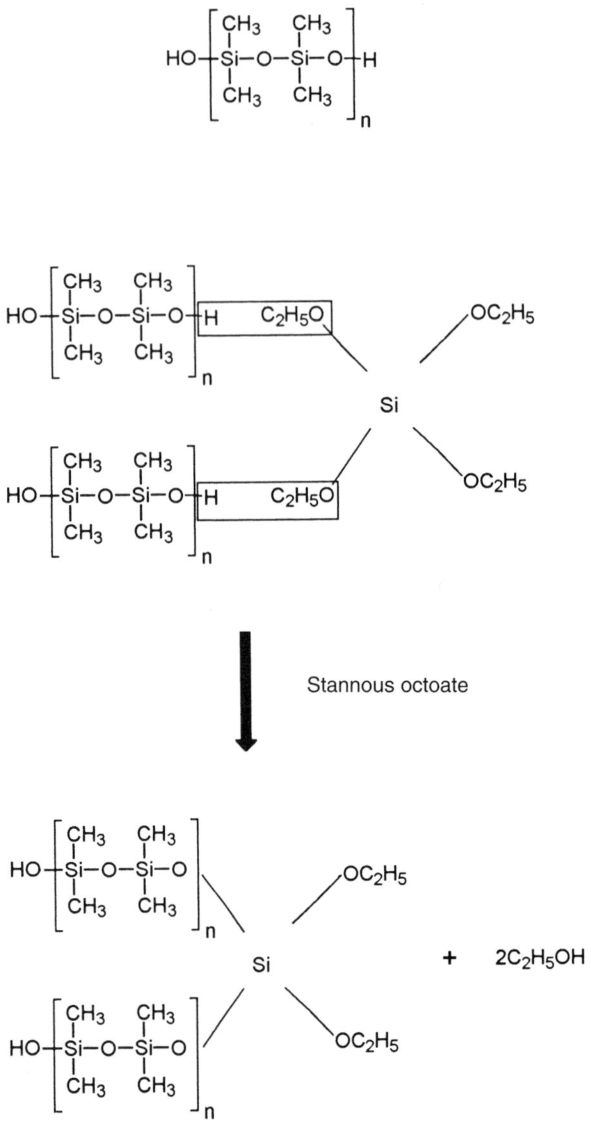

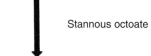

Fig. 9-5 **Top,** Structural formula of the molecules α-ω hydroxy-terminated poly (dimethyl siloxane). **Middle and bottom,** Condensation reaction between the OH terminal groups and tetraethyl orthosilicate in the presence of stannous octoate. The reaction results in the release of two ethanol molecules.

highly filled, so less polymer is present; hence there is less polymerization shrinkage. Putty is used as the tray material in conjunction with a low-viscosity silicone. This technique and details on the properties of these elastomers will be discussed later in this chapter. Each manufacturer supplies the material in several different colors corresponding to the viscosity. Pastel pinks, blues, greens, and purples are common.

Addition Silicone

The addition silicones are frequently called *polyvinyl siloxane* or *vinyl polysiloxane impression materials*. In contrast to the condensation silicones, the addition reaction polymer is terminated with vinyl groups and is cross-linked with hydride groups activated by a platinum salt catalyst. Figure 9-6 illustrates the addition polymerization reaction.

No reaction by-products develop as long as the correct proportions of vinyl silicone and hydride silicone are maintained and there are no impurities. However, a secondary reaction between moisture and residual hydrides of the base polymer can

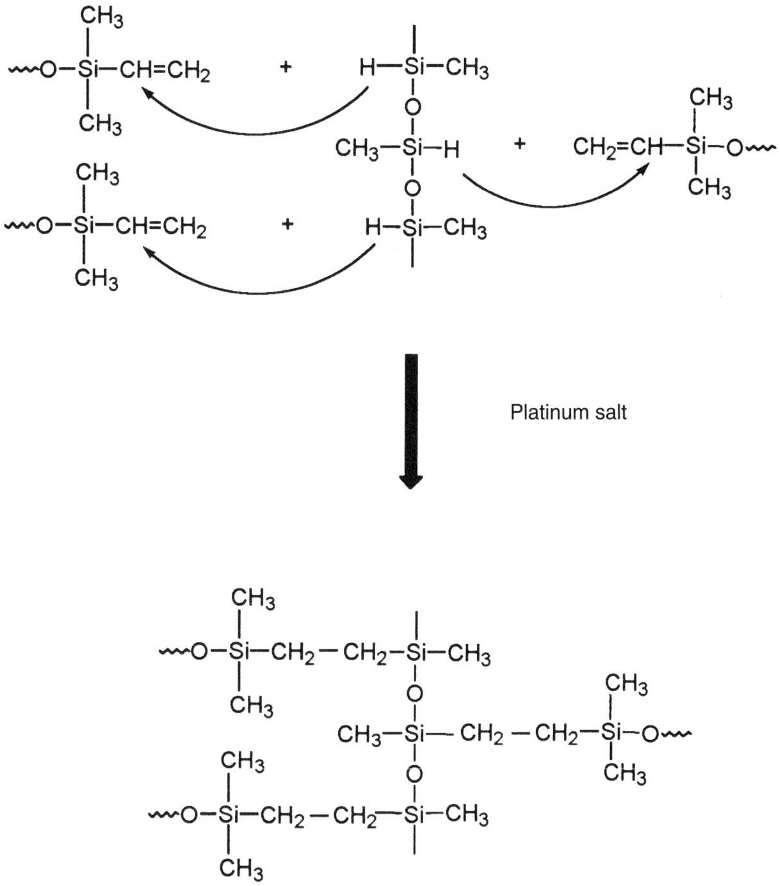

Fig. 9-6 **Top,** Hydrogen atoms along the backbone structure of the vinyl silicone chain move to the vinyl groups during addition polymerization. **Bottom,** Final structure after the platinum salt has initiated the addition polymerization reaction.

lead to the development of hydrogen gas. Although technically not a reaction by-product, the hydrogen gas that evolves from the set material can result in pinpoint voids in the gypsum casts that are poured soon after removing the impression from the mouth. Manufacturers often add a noble metal, such as platinum or palladium, to act as a scavenger for the released hydrogen gas. Another way to compensate for the hydrogen gas is to wait an hour or more before pouring the impression. This delay will not cause any clinically detectable dimensional change. Many current materials have been designed to eliminate or minimize this adverse effect.

The base paste contains polymethyl hydrogen siloxane, as well as other siloxane prepolymers. The **catalyst paste** contains divinyl polydimethyl siloxane and other siloxane prepolymers. If the "catalyst" paste contains the platinum salt activator, then the paste labeled "base" must contain the hybrid silicone. Retarder may also be present in the paste that contains the platinum catalyst. Both pastes contain fillers.

One of the disadvantages of the silicone impression materials is their inherent **hydrophobic** nature. Any distortion or loss of detail at the margins of the impression is probably caused by undetected moisture present in the area to be replicated. A nonionic surfactant is added to the paste to render the surface of the impression **hydrophilic**. This surfactant migrates toward the surface of the impression material and has its hydrophilic segment oriented toward the surface. This phenomenon allows the impression material to more readily wet soft tissue and enhance the ability of gypsum products to capture maximum detail when poured into an impression. These impression materials still require a dry field, but they reproduce the surface of soft tissue more accurately. Pouring the set impression with gypsum-forming slurry is easier, because the wet stone has a greater affinity for the hydrophilic surface. This is perhaps the greatest benefit of the hydrophilic additives incorporated in the vinyl polysiloxanes.

Sulfur contamination from natural latex gloves inhibits the setting of the addition silicone impression materials. Some vinyl gloves also may have the same effect because of the sulfur-containing stabilizer used in the manufacturing process. The contamination is so pervasive that touching the tooth with the glove before seating the impression can inhibit the setting of the critical surface next to the tooth. This inhibition of the polymerization reaction produces major distortion.

Polyether

Polyether elastomeric impression material was introduced in Germany in the late 1960s. It is a polyether-based polymer that is cured by a reaction between aziridine rings, which are at the end of branched polyether molecules (Fig. 9-7, *left*). The main chain is probably a copolymer of ethylene oxide and tetrahydrofuran. Cross-linking and setting are brought about by an **initiator**, an aromatic sulfonate ester (Fig. 9-7, *top*), where R is an alkyl group. This produces cross-linking by cationic polymerization via the imine end groups (Fig. 9-7). This material was the first elastomer to be developed primarily to function as an impression material. All of the other materials were adapted from other uses.

The polyether rubbers are supplied as two pastes. The base paste contains the polyether polymer, colloidal silica as filler, and a plasticizer such as a glycolether or phthalate. The accelerator paste contains an alkyl-aromatic sulfonate in addition to the filler and plasticizer.

ELASTOMERIC MATERIALS: MAKING AN IMPRESSION

The use of elastomeric impression material to fabricate gypsum models, casts, and dies involves five major steps: (1) preparing a tray, (2) preparing the material, (3) making an impression, (4) removing the impression, and (5) preparing stone casts and dies. All materials are supplied as a two-component system. The first step is to mix the two components properly to initiate the reaction. An acrylic custom tray may be required to minimize the effects of polymerization shrinkage, loss of reaction by-product, and deformation associated with tray seating and removal. Adhesion of the impression material to the tray is also essential. The next step involves the selection and use of the preferred viscosity for making an impression. These include a multiple mix or dual viscosity technique, a **monophase** technique, or a putty-wash technique. After setting, the impression is removed without unduly introducing stress. Finally, a gypsum-forming mass is poured into the impression within a reasonable period of time.

Preparation of Impression Materials

When the materials are provided in two paste tubes, the user should dispense the same length of materials onto a mixing pad or glass slab. The catalyst paste is first collected on a stainless steel spatula and then distributed over the base. The mixture is then spread out over the mixing pad. The mass is then scraped up with the spatula blade and spread uniformly back and forth on the mixing pad. The process is continued until the

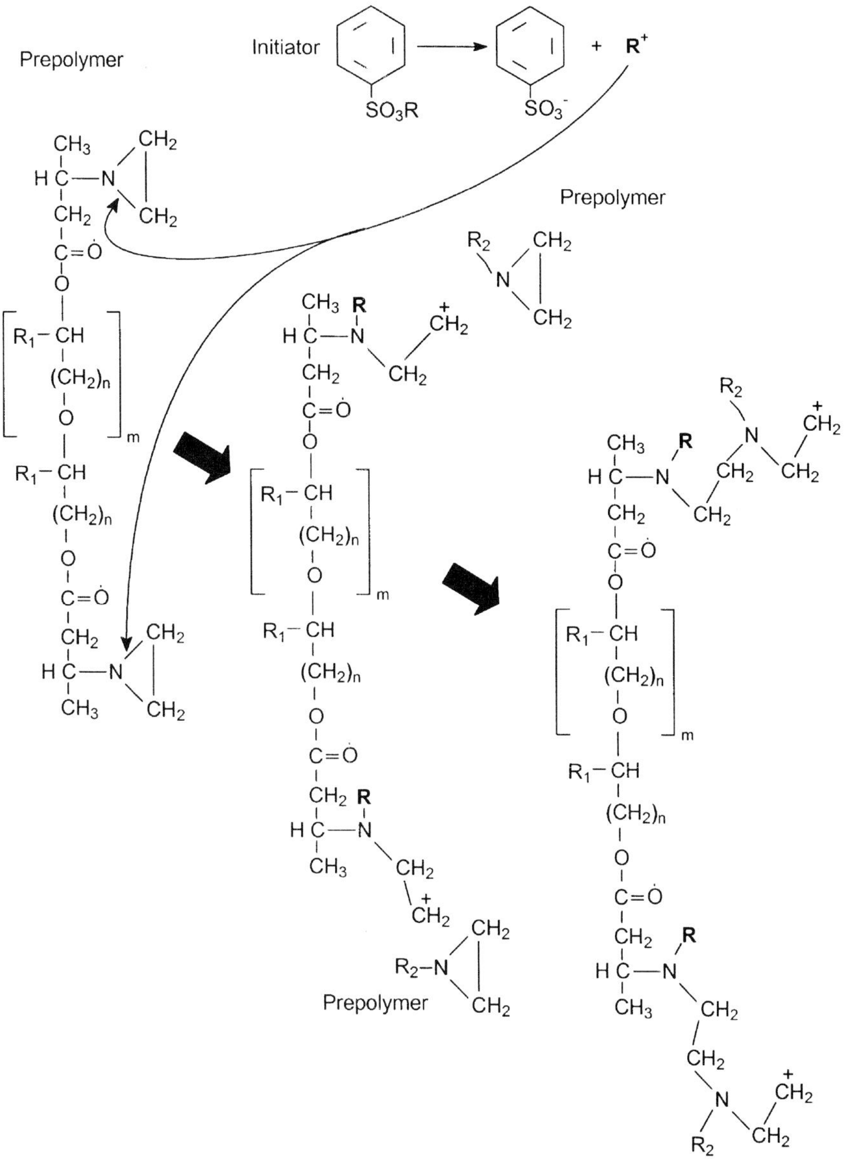

Fig. 9-7   Top, The initiator, aromatic sulfonate ester, dissociates and forms alkyl cations that bind the nitrogen atoms of the aziridine ring terminals of the prepolymer **(left).** The arrows indicate binding between the cations (R^+) with the nitrogen atoms. This action opens up the ring, and the reacted prepolymer **(center)** now has two charged ethylene imine terminals ($-NR–CH_2–C^+H_2$) that can react with the nitrogen atoms of adjacent unreacted prepolymers, shown as the R_2-aziridine ring. This chain propagation polymerization reaction yields a larger molecule **(right)** that continues growing by binding with aziridines rings of additional unreacted prepolymers. The polymerization reaction terminates when the growing chain combines with a counterion.

mixed paste is uniform in color, with no streaks of the base or catalyst appearing in the mixture. If the mixture is not homogeneous, curing will not be uniform, and a distorted impression will result. If one of the components is in liquid form, such as the catalyst for condensation silicones, a length of the base is dispensed from the tube onto a graduated mixing pad and one drop of the liquid catalyst is added for each unit length of base. These materials are somewhat difficult to mix because of the disparity in the viscosity of the two components.

The two-putty systems, which are available for condensation silicone and addition silicone, are dispensed by volume using an equal number of scoops of each putty. The best mixing technique is to knead the material with your fingers until a uniform color is obtained. When the catalyst is a liquid, such as in condensation silicones, the same kneading procedure with your fingers is adequate. However, some users prefer to incorporate the liquid by first mixing on a pad before completing the kneading procedure.

The similarity of the paste consistencies and the **shear-thinning** behavior of vinyl polysiloxanes make them suitable for an automatic dispensing and mixing device. An example of the device and several sizes of tips are shown in Figure 9-8. The basic automatic mixers sold by various manufacturers are interchangeable. They are generally used for light-and medium-viscosity materials, but heavy-body materials have been modified to accommodate the automatic mixing device. The mixing tips vary in diameter, length, and the size of the tip opening for specific consistency. Additionally, condensation silicones and polyethers are available with this delivery system.

The mixed impression material is injected directly into the adhesive-coated tray or onto the prepared teeth if the "syringe tip" is in place. This apparatus has certain advantages compared with hand dispensing and spatulation. For the mechanical device, there is greater uniformity in proportioning and in mixing, less air is incorporated into the mix, and the mixing time is reduced. Also, there are fewer possibilities for contamination of the material. One precaution that should be taken in using these automixing devices is to make sure that the openings of the tubes dispensing the pastes remain unclogged. Problems can be avoided if one expresses a small amount of material from the cartridge before attaching the mixing tip. The lack of a color difference between the base and catalyst material also makes it difficult to ensure that the mix is homogeneous. However, investigation of the automixing devices has demonstrated that the mix is adequate if the device is used properly. The device has also been adapted to mix and dispense temporary crown and bridge acrylic materials and ZOE temporary cement.

A recent development in the automatic dispensing and mixing device is a dynamic mechanical mixer. Instead of using a double-barrel cartridge, as just described, the materials are supplied in plastic bags housed in a cartridge. The device uses a motor to drive parallel plungers that force the materials into a mixing tip, and the spiral inside the mixing tip rotates as the materials are extruded through the tip. Using this device, thorough mixing of higher viscosity materials can be achieved

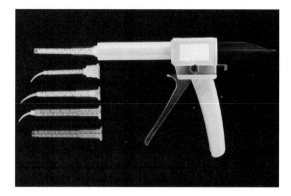

Fig. 9-8 Automixer and dispenser for addition silicone impression materials. When the trigger is pulled, the plunger is driven forward **(to the left),** so that the base and catalyst pastes are forced from the cartridge into the mixing tip **(extreme left)** containing a spiral mixing tip. The pastes pass through the bore and exit the nozzle as a uniform mixed paste. Four different sizes of mixing tips are shown on the left; they are designed for different consistencies of materials. The more viscous the material, the larger the mixing tip should be. Syringe tips can be fit to the nozzle to deliver the mixed paste directly to the prepared teeth.

with little effort. Both polyether and addition silicone impression materials of various viscosities are available with this dispensing system.

Impression Trays

The use of a custom tray is recommended to reduce the quantity of the materials used to make impressions; therefore, any dimensional changes attributed to the materials can be minimized. This is especially true for polysulfide impression material. To fabricate a custom tray, the clinician obtains an impression of intraoral structures using an alginate impression material. A stone cast is constructed. The important parts of the cast, such as the natural teeth and artificial teeth used for prosthetic devices, are covered with one or two layers of base plate wax to act as a spacer for the custom tray material, followed by adapting aluminum foil or painting a model-releasing agent for ease of tray removal. Chemical-curing or light-curing acrylic resin is placed over the foil-covered or painted wax surface to form the tray. After curing, the resin custom tray is separated from the cast, and the wax and aluminum foil are removed. The impression material is manipulated in the space previously occupied by the wax. A uniform thickness of tray adhesive is applied within the tray extending over the edge of the tray, and it is allowed to dry prior to the insertion of the impression material. The adhesive then forms a tenacious bond between the rubber impression material and the tray. A slightly roughened surface on the tray will increase adhesion. Tray adhesives furnished with the various types of elastomeric impression materials *are not interchangeable*.

The use of custom trays for polyether and addition silicone impressions is not critical since these materials are stiffer and have less polymerization shrinkage than the polysulfide material. These two materials do not require the custom tray support to avoid distortion and minimize setting shrinkage; disposable stock trays work satisfactorily. Tray adhesive is also needed for stock trays. Note that the use of less material in a custom tray reduces the compressibility of the impression, which can make the removal of the impression tray more difficult. When severe undercuts are present, the use of a custom tray should be avoided. Disposable stock trays are also used to support the putty when the putty-wash technique is used for making impressions.

A comparison of the different techniques shows that the use of a custom tray is the most accurate technique. However, if the material is used correctly, results that are clinically acceptable can be produced with any of these impression material techniques.

Steps Required to Make an Impression

Each material is available in several consistencies: (1) light-body, which is used with a syringe and placed directly on hard and soft tissues; (2) heavy-body, which is placed in the tray to support the light-body material; and (3) putty, which is useful for materials that exhibit significant polymerization shrinkage. The method of using the syringe and the tray materials is referred to as the *multiple mix technique* because two separate mixtures are required with two separate mixing pads and spatulas. Normally, the two groups of materials should be mixed simultaneously, each one by a different person. The tray is then filled with a uniform thickness of heavy material, whereas the syringe is loaded with lighter material. In actual practice, one person usually mixes the syringe material, fills the syringe, and hands it to the dentist or clinician. The lighter material is injected from the filled syringe within and around the tooth preparation. The filled tray is then inserted in the mouth and seated over the syringe material that has been extruded on hard or soft tissue. The tray material will force the syringe material to adapt to the prepared tissues. The two materials should bond together upon setting. If no dental assistant is present and only one dentist or clinician is available at the time of mixing, the dentist or clinician should mix and fill the tray material first. If either material has progressed past its working time when the two are brought together, the bond between them will be compromised. If a partially set material is seated, it will be compressed elastically. Once removed, the impression will "spring back" or relax, and the dies from this impression will be too narrow and too short, as illustrated in Figure 9-9.

In rare cases, a clinician may attempt to repair an impression that has small defects or that lacks sufficient details. This is usually performed by cutting away the interproximal and gingival areas of the impression. Even with proper relief of the initial impression, reseating the tray precisely is difficult. Entrapment of a minute fragment of impression material or debris will eliminate any chance of a successful repair. The impression material surface must be roughened to ensure that the new material bonds to the set impression. The safest method is to make a new impression when bubbles or similar defects are detected in critical areas.

Medium viscosities of polyether and addition silicone impression materials are often used for the monophase or single-viscosity technique. The procedure is similar to that of the multiple-mix technique, except that only one mix is made, part of the material is placed in the tray, and another portion is placed in the syringe for injection in the cavity preparation, on prepared teeth, or on soft tissue. The success of this technique depends on the **pseudoplastic** properties of these two materials. When a medium viscosity material is forced through the syringe tip, the viscosity is reduced and this allows the material to adapt well to the preparation. Meanwhile, the material in the tray retains its medium viscosity, and when seated, it can force the syringe material to flow past critical areas of the tooth preparation. Table 9-2 shows the effect of shear rate and time elapsed on some monophase addition silicones.

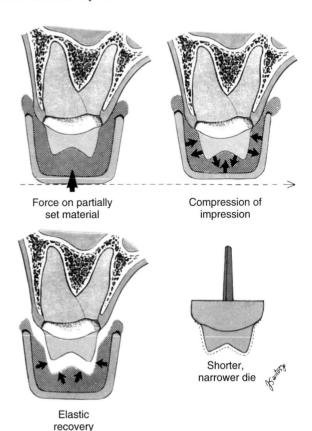

Force on partially set material

Compression of impression

Fig. 9-9   Top Left, Impression tray containing elastomeric impression material is seated too late as elasticity starts to develop. **Top right,** Increased seating pressure is applied to overcome the stiffness of impression material. **Lower left,** Distortion develops because of recovery of excessive elastic deformation. **Lower right,** The die produced in the inaccurate impression is too narrow and too short. See also color plate.

Elastic recovery

Shorter, narrower die

Table 9-2	Viscosity ($\times 10^4$ cp) of Single-Phase Vinyl Polysiloxanes at 37° C			
	Viscosity at 1 min		**Viscosity at 1.5 min**	
Material	**0.5 rpm**	**2.5 rpm**	**0.5 rpm**	**2.5 rpm**
Baysilex (Miles)	122.1 (2.8)	68.9 (2.5)	211.2 (14.7)	148.8 (1.2)
Green-Mouse (Parkell)	133.7 (8.9)	56.7 (2.9)	247.9 (14.9)	78.0 (2.8)
Hydrosil (Caulk)	194.2 (8.5)	129.4 (4.1)	398.1 (7.8)	153.5*
Imprint (3M)	106.5 (12.2)	79.7 (2.2)	245.1 (8.9)	146.2 (5.9)
Omnisil (Coe)	156.8 (11.5)	102.5 (1.9)	347.1 (5.2)	153.5†

From Kim K-N, Craig RG, and Koran A: Viscosity of monophase addition silicones as a function of shear rate. J Prosthet Dent 67:794, 1992.
*Value at 75 seconds after mixing
†Value at 77 seconds after mixing
()Standard deviation of the mean

The putty-wash technique was originally developed for condensation silicone to minimize the effect of polymerization shrinkage on the dimensional changes. The manufacturers of addition silicones also make putty materials for this technique. Two approaches can be used: a two-stage procedure and a single-stage procedure. For the former process, the thick putty material is placed in a stock tray and a preliminary impression is made. This procedure results in what is essentially an intraoral custom-made tray formed by the putty. Space for the light-body "wash" material is provided either by cutting away some of the "tray" putty or by using a thin polyethylene sheet as a spacer between the putty and the prepared teeth. A mix of the thin-consistency wash material is placed into the putty impression and then the putty-wash combination and tray are seated in the mouth to make the final impression. For reliable reproduction of sharp angles in cavity preparations, it is often necessary to use a syringe and inject the wash material within and onto the preparations. This method is referred to as the "two-stage putty-wash technique" or the "reline technique."

An alternative to the two-stage procedure is the single-stage procedure, in which the wash material is syringed into place, and then the unset putty is seated over the light-body material. One difficulty with combining the wash and putty steps is that the higher viscosity material may displace the more fluid wash material. If this occurs, critical areas of the preparation may be reproduced in putty rather than in the light-body material, but the putty is too viscous to replicate the required detail. Occlusal stops should be used in the tray to avoid pushing through the wash or syringe material when seating the plastic putty mass.

The putty-wash technique, when properly used, can produce impressions with accuracy comparable to that of the two-mix procedure. When the simultaneous technique is used, distortion or incomplete details can occur because of excessive pressure applied to the setting putty. These distortions can also occur with the set-putty used in the two-stage technique. After removing the impression from the mouth, the pressure is released and the putty recovers its "elastic deformation." The distortion that is produced with the stiff, compressible putty results in short, narrow dies (see Fig. 9-8). In addition to excessive pressure, some of the distortion in putty-wash impressions may be attributable to inadequate spacing for the wash material. The frequency of distortion associated with the stiffness of the putty material at the time the impression is seated has led some clinicians to abandon the use of putty-wash materials.

Removal of the Impression

Under no circumstances should the impression be removed until the curing has progressed sufficiently to provide adequate elasticity so that distortion will not occur. One method for determining the time of removal is to inject some of the syringe material onto a space not in the field of operation. This material can be probed with a blunt instrument from time to time; when it is firm and returns completely to its original contour, the impression is sufficiently elastic to be removed. When a multiple mix technique is used, it is advisable to test both the syringe and the tray materials in this manner. The curing times may vary for the two different consistencies.

From a practical standpoint, the curing rate of the rubber impression material should not be so slow that the time before removal from the mouth is unduly long. Typically, the impression should be ready for removal within at least 10 minutes from the time of mixing, allowing 6 to 8 minutes for the impression to remain in the mouth.

As discussed earlier, all elastomeric impression materials are viscoelastic, and it is necessary to use a quick snap to minimize plastic deformation of the impression during the final step of the removal process.

Preparation of Stone Casts and Dies

All nonaqueous elastomeric impression materials are compatible with all types of gypsum products during the setting of the gypsum products. However, the characteristics of each material also dictate how the pouring of the gypsum-forming product should be performed to ensure accurate and bubble-free casts and dies.

The excellent dimensional stability of addition silicone and polyether impression materials makes it possible to construct two or three casts or dies from these materials. It is also possible to construct successive stone dies or casts from polysulfide impressions when duplicate stone dies are needed. Note, however, that each successive die will be less accurate than the first die constructed from the material. The time interval between impression pours should not be greater than 30 minutes. To minimize tearing and gross distortion after the first pour, the clinician should remove the excess gypsum-forming mass from undercut areas along the periphery of the tray.

The hydrophobic characteristics of these vinyl polysiloxane impression materials make them compatible with epoxy resins used for more accurate casts and dies. These replica materials can be poured two or more times into the same impression with gypsum products. This hydrophobicity of the impression material makes it difficult to wet the surface by a gypsum-forming slurry, so it is difficult to pour a bubble-free stone cast from an addition silicone impression material. There are a number of surfactant sprays that can improve the ability of hydrophobic impression material surfaces to be wet by the stone slurry. Only a thin layer of surfactant should be applied to the impression surface; otherwise, bubbles may be created during vibration when pouring the gypsum product. A dilute solution of soap is also an effective surfactant. However, an alternative to the use of a surfactant is to select a hydrophilic addition silicone, which exhibits a contact angle with water in the range of 30° to 35° compared with 95° for many of the hydrophobic materials. Pouring the stone cast in a polyether impression is much easier than pouring it in one made from silicone materials. However, the stiffness of polyether polymer makes it difficult to remove the stone cast from the impression. A weak stone cast may fracture during removal.

CRITICAL QUESTION

Why are hydrophilic materials potentially more susceptible to distortion during disinfection prior to being poured with a gypsum-forming product?

ELASTOMERIC IMPRESSION MATERIALS: PROPERTIES
Working and Setting Times

Ordinarily, working time is measured at room temperature, whereas setting time is measured at mouth temperature. Penetrometer tests have been used to assess both working and setting times. For example, the end of working time might be defined as the time when a blunt needle of a certain diameter and weight fails to penetrate a volume of impression material to a specified depth. Setting time would not be reached until another flat-ended needle or other blunt instrument fails to permanently indent the set impression material. In the British Standards Test, a reciprocating rheometer is used to measure both setting and working times. The property being recorded is more closely related to viscosity and shear-thinning properties than it is to elasticity.

Table 9-3 lists working and setting times for the various kinds of elastomeric materials, as measured by an oscillating rheometer. An increase in temperature accelerates the curing rate of all these elastomeric impression materials and thus decreases both setting and working times. Cooling is a practical method of increasing the working time of elastomeric impression materials. This can be accomplished by storing the materials at room temperature (about 23° C) or by mixing on a chilled, dry glass slab. Then, when the impression material is carried to the mouth, the setting time is decreased at mouth temperature. The cooling process has little effect on viscosity.

Working time and setting time decrease as the viscosity increases. Altering the base/catalyst ratio will change the curing rate of these impression materials. If the base/catalyst ratio is altered by changing the relative amounts of materials used, it is necessary to test the setting time of the new ratio before material with the altered ratio is used for a patient. The curing rate of some, but not all, of the polysulfide impression materials is also sensitive to alterations in the base/accelerator ratio, which is affected by the relative amounts of base and catalyst pastes that are mixed. However, mechanical properties can be adversely affected when marked changes in the base/accelerator ratio occur. Altering the base/accelerator ratio to change the working or setting time is not economical, because a portion of the paste is not used. Moreover, since the accelerator paste contains a retarder, as well as a reactor, increasing the base/accelerator ratio may not produce a predictable change in the polymerization rate.

Table 9-3	Working and Setting Times of Nonaqueous Elastomeric Impression Materials			
	Mean working time (min)		Mean setting time (min)	
Impression material	23° C	37° C	23° C	37° C
Polysulfide	6.0	4.3	16.0	12.5
Condensation silicone	3.3	2.5	11.0	8.9
Addition silicone	3.1	1.8	8.9	5.9
Polyether	3.3	2.3	9.0	8.3

From Harcourt JK: A review of modern impression materials. Aust Dent J 23:178, 1978.

Dimensional Stability

There are five major sources of dimensional change: (1) polymerization shrinkage, (2) loss of a by-product (water or alcohol) during the condensation reaction, (3) thermal contraction from oral temperature to room temperature, (4) **imbibition** when exposed to water, disinfectant or a high humidity environment over a period of time, and (5) incomplete recovery of deformation because of viscoelastic behavior. Dimensional changes during curing have been measured directly and indirectly, using confined and freestanding specimens of the elastomers in various geometrical shapes. In ANSI/ADA Specification No. 19 for elastomeric impression materials, a disk of the impression material is placed on a talc-covered glass plate. At the end of 24 hours, the contraction should not exceed 0.5% for Types I and III materials or 1.0% for a Type II elastomer. Thus the measurement includes contraction associated with thermal change (37° C to 23° C), polymerization shrinkage, and loss of volatile components. For example, the linear coefficients of thermal expansion for the elastomeric impression materials range from 150 ppm/° C to 220 ppm/° C.

Figure 9-10 shows mean values for linear contraction for a number of nonaqueous elastomers, using the method just described. It is evident that all materials change dimensionally over time. The change is greater in magnitude for the polysulfide and condensation silicone materials than for the polyether and addition silicone elastomers. The result is expected because polysulfide and condensation silicone lose polymerization by-products, water and alcohol, respectively.

If maximal accuracy is to be maintained with polysulfide and condensation silicone materials, the slurry mix for a stone die or cast should be poured immediately into the impression after it is removed from the mouth. *Immediately* is defined as the period within the first 30 minutes, even when the putty-wash technique is used.

The stability exhibited by the addition silicone and polyether materials suggests that these impressions do not have to be poured with a gypsum product immediately. In fact, these impressions are often sent to the lab to be poured. Research has shown that a cast produced between 24 hours and 1 week was as accurate as a cast made in the first hour, assuming that there was no effect associated with the formation of hydrogen bubbles. These materials exhibit the least amount of distortion from the loads imposed on the set material. Thus pouring the impression and removing the cast several times will not alter the dimensional stability of the impression, even though a fairly substantial force is needed each time the cast is removed from the impression.

One property that has a negative effect on the polyether impression is the absorption of water or fluids and the simultaneous leaching of the water-soluble

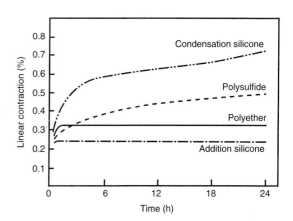

Fig. 9-10 Representative linear contraction of four elastomeric impression materials.

plasticizer. Thus the stored impression must be kept in a dry, cool environment to maintain its accuracy.

Reproduction of Oral Detail

The necessity for the impression material to reproduce the finest detail of the oral cavity is self-evident. Various tests have been employed by investigators to evaluate the ability of impression materials to reproduce surface detail. A surface reproduction test is a part of the specification for the elastic impression materials. There is no doubt that these elastomers and the reversible hydrocolloids record detail to a fine degree. When dental stone is poured on the surface of such test impressions, the finest detail is not always reproduced. In other words, the rubber impression materials are capable of reproducing detail more accurately than can be transferred to the stone die or cast.

The clinical significance of the surface reproduction tests is not entirely evident. It is possible that the detail obtained with the rubber impression materials on in vitro test specimens might be greater than that obtained in the mouth because of the hydrophobicity exhibited by some of these materials.

Disinfection

The need to disinfect impressions is well established. The duration and mode of applying the disinfectant depends on the potential of the impression material to absorb water and the time that has transpired since the impression was made.

Condensation silicones, addition silicones, and polysulfides can be disinfected with all EPA-registered* disinfectants without adverse dimensional changes, provided that the disinfection time is short. The impressions should be immersed for the time specified for the disinfectant used. After disinfection the impression should be removed, rinsed, and poured with the gypsum product as soon as possible. Be aware that a long immersion time may cause the surfactant in the hydrophilic vinyl polysiloxane to leach out and render the impression less hydrophilic.

The polyethers are also susceptible to dimensional change if immersed for a long time (>10 min), because of their pronounced hydrophilic nature. A satisfactory solution for most elastomers is 2% glutaraldehyde. The disinfectant should be sprayed on the impression until saturated. The impression should then be wrapped in a disinfectant-soaked paper towel and placed in a sealed plastic bag for 10 minutes. After removal of the paper towel, the impression must be rinsed, dried, and poured immediately with a gypsum product or other cast or model material.

Table 9-4 shows a guide for selection of appropriate disinfection methods for all types of impressions that are transferred to a dental laboratory.

CRITICAL QUESTION

Why is rapid seating of an impression tray not advisable for a pseudoplastic impression material?

---

* EPA: Environmental Protection Agency

Table 9-4	Guide for Selection of Appropriate Disinfection Methods for Impressions Transported to a Dental Laboratory		

Material	Method	Recommended disinfectant	Comments
Irreversible hydrocolloid (Alginate)	Immersion with caution Use only disinfectant with short-term exposure time (<10 min for alginate)	Chlorine compounds or iodophors	Short-term glutaraldehyde has been shown to be acceptable; but time is inadequate for disinfection.
Reversible hydrocolloid			Do not immerse in alkaline glutaraldehyde!
Polysulfide Silicone	Immersion	Glutaraldehydes, chlorine compounds, iodophors, phenolics	Disinfectants requiring more than 30-min exposure times are not recommended.
Polyether	Immerse with caution Use only disinfectant with a short exposure time (<10 min)	Chlorine compounds or iodophors	ADA recommends any of the disinfectant classes; however, short-term exposures are essential to avoid distortion.
ZOE impression paste	Immersion preferred; spraying can be used for bite registrations	Glutaraldehydes or iodophors	Not compatible with chlorine compounds! Phenolic spray can be used.
Impression compound		Iodophors or chlorine compounds	Phenolic spray can be used.

Rheological Properties

Polysulfide has the lowest viscosity and ranks as one of the least stiff of the elastomeric impression materials of a similar consistency. This flexibility allows the set material to be easily removed from undercut areas and from the mouth with a minimum of stress. The most common consistencies of the condensation materials are the putty and the wash materials. A light-body consistency with catalyst in paste form is also available.

Addition silicone and polyether are pseudoplastic impression materials. This property allows the manufacturer to formulate one-step materials. The significance of this property is that the clinician can use a high-viscosity material, which is more stable and resistant to distortion, to capture the details needed for fixed prostheses. The pseudoplastic (shear-thinning) behavior occurs only while the force is applied and does not alter the material permanently. A thinning agent is available for polyether materials to reduce the stiffness of the set material.

Another strain-dependant rheological behavior known as *thixotropy* is often confused with pseudoplasticity. A **thixotropic** material does not flow until sufficient energy in the form of impact force is applied to overcome its yield stress. Beyond this point, the material becomes very fluid.

Elasticity

The elastic properties of these elastomeric impression materials improve with an increase in curing time in the mouth. In other words, the longer the impression can remain in the mouth, the less distortion will occur during impression removal. The impression material must undergo some elastic distortion as it is removed from the mouth, but a sufficiently high elastic limit for the impression material minimizes permanent deformation. Setting time, as stated by a manufacturer or as determined by a rheometer, is not always adequate for the development of sufficient elasticity to prevent permanent deformation upon removal of the impression, especially with the polysulfide and addition silicone materials. For example, the setting times as measured by a rheometer are 1 or 2 min less than those required to produce an acceptable level of elasticity before removal of the impression.

The relative amount of permanent deformation following **strain in compression** increases in the following order: addition silicone, condensation silicone, polyether, and polysulfide. Recovery of elastic deformation following strain is less rapid for the polysulfide than for the other three types of impression material. However, even when strain is prolonged, as when an impression is removed slowly from the prepared teeth, recovery is sufficiently rapid that pouring of the impression need not be delayed.

Despite the possibility of a large dimensional change occurring when a polysulfide impression is removed from the mouth, there is no advantage to "bench curing" the materials. If the polymer chains have been stretched past their elastic limit, no amount of waiting will enable them to return to their original shape. Although the distortion is permanent, the chains may relax, but they have no "memory," so the relaxed state probably will not be the same as the undistorted shape no matter how long the impression is allowed to **cure**.

The vinyl polysiloxane impression materials are the most ideally elastic of the currently available materials. Distortion on removal from undercuts is virtually nonexistent, because these materials exhibit the lowest permanent distortion after strain in compression. The excellent elastic properties present a problem in that the heavy-body putty material begins to acquire elastic properties while still in the working time stage. If the material is at an advanced stage of elasticity and it is compressed excessively during the seating of the impression, distortion can occur when the material elastically rebounds.

Excluding the very high-viscosity putty class of elastomers, the stiffness (elastic modulus) of impression materials increases in the following order: polysulfide, condensation silicone, addition silicone, and polyether. The original polyether material was extremely difficult to remove from undercut areas because of the very high modulus of elasticity. It is approximately 27 times as stiff as light-body polysulfide impression material. Some of the new formulations of regular or medium-body materials are actually less stiff than the one-step hydrophilic vinyl polysiloxane impression materials.

Tear Strength

A tear strength test measures the resistance to fracture of an elastomeric material subjected to a tensile force acting perpendicular to a surface flaw. The test specimen usually is trouser-shaped. The maximum force needed to pull the specimen apart divided by the thickness of the specimen is the tear strength (in N/m or lb/in). This is an important property when dealing with impression materials used in interproximal and subgingival areas. High tear strength is essential also for maxillofacial materials and soft liners. The subgingival regions of an impression are often very thin. The material in this region can tear and leave a portion embedded within the gingival sulcus (Fig. 9-11). This residual segment is often difficult to detect, even with radiographs, because most materials are not radiopaque, except for polysulfide, which contains lead dioxide as the catalyst. The ranking of tear strength from the

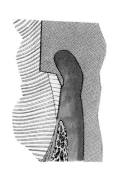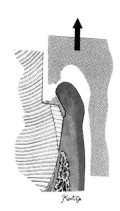

Fig. 9-11   Left, Impression material has polymerized within the gingival sulcus. **Right,** Impression material has torn during removal. See also color plate.

lowest to highest of all impression materials generally is as follows: hydrocolloids (agar and alginate), silicones (addition and condensation), polyether, and polysulfide. However, you may find in the literature that some polyethers or silicones have registered higher tear strength values than certain polysulfides. The tear strength values of hydrocolloids are about one-tenth of the values for the polysulfides.

In addition to the chemical composition of the materials, tear strength is influenced by the consistency and manner of removal of the materials. An increased consistency usually increases the tear strength of the material. The addition of thinner reduces tear strength slightly but increases the flexibility substantially. A rapid rate of force application during removal usually increases the tear strength. This means that after the air seal is released, the removal should be accomplished with a quick snap rather than by a slow motion.

The tear strength depicts only the stress associated with the tearing process during impression removal. However, the material is also under a certain strain before removal. For the same preparation, each impression material, regardless of its tear strength, will undergo the same amount of strain during the removal of the impression. The property that can delineate the combined behavior of the strength and the strain is the term energy (see Chapter 4), which includes the quantity of dimensional change of the material in the calculation. However, *tear strength* as defined carries the unit of N/m that can be converted to Nm/m^2 or joule $(J)/m^2$, which is the energy per unit area. You may find tear energy being used in the literature in place of tear strength. *Tear resistance* is used in this chapter to avoid the confusion.

Polysulfide has the highest resistance to tearing as measured by its dimensional change. Therefore, thin sections of polysulfide impression material are less likely to tear than polyether or silicone impression materials of a similar thickness. However, because of their susceptibility to permanent distortion, the polysulfide impressions may distort instead of tearing. This presents a problem since tearing can be seen immediately by carefully checking the impression, whereas distortion is not possible to detect by visual inspection. This distortion can result in a metal casting that does not seat completely. Because the strain rate influences tear resistance and permanent deformation, the impression should be strained rapidly for as short a time as possible to minimize adverse effects.

Biocompatibility

The ANSI/ADA specification for testing biocompatibility includes dental impression materials, despite the fact that the probability of allergic or toxic reactions from impression materials or their components is small. Comparing the cell cytotoxicity

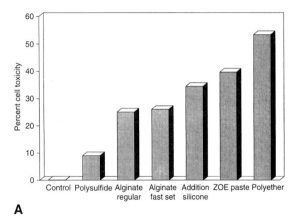

A

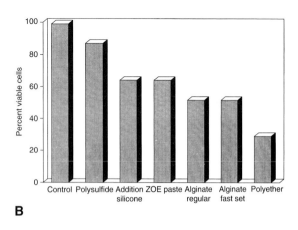

Fig. 9-12 **A,** Graph of cell cytotoxicity shows that, after 3 days of incubation with Vero cells, all of the impression materials were cytotoxic to varying degrees. The relative cytotoxicity of each material is shown relative to the control. **B,** The graph of cell viability exhibits the relative percent of viable cells after being exposed to the impression materials. (From Sydiskis RK, and Gerhardt DE: J Prosthet Dent 69:431, 1993.)

B

for different impression materials reveals that polysulfide results in the lowest cell death count and the set polyether impression material produces the highest cell cytotoxicity scores (Fig. 9-12). Similar results are also observed in multiple exposure tests.

Perhaps the most likely elastomer-induced biocompatibility problem occurs when a segment of impression material is lodged in a patient's gingival sulcus. A foreign body of impression material can cause severe gingival inflammation and may be misdiagnosed to have been caused by the tooth preparation or cementation. If evidence of tearing is detected during a careful visual inspection of the impression, it is important to examine the gingival sulcus immediately to remove any remnant of the impression or any other foreign body such as a piece of retraction cord. The radiopacity of polysulfide materials is an advantage in these situations.

Some concern exists about the hypersensitivity potential of the polyether catalyst system. Contact dermatitis from the polyether, especially to the dental assistant, has been reported. In contrast, no cytotoxic effects have been reported from exposure to polyether components, particularly the imine catalyst.

Shelf Life

Properly compounded impression material does not deteriorate appreciably in the tube or container when it is stored in a dry, cool environment. The tubes always should be kept tightly closed when they are not in use. It is also important to reseal the alginate container after dispensing the powder.

Effect of Mishandling

The failure to produce an acceptable epoxy or gypsum die or cast is more likely associated with an error in handling the impression material rather than a deficiency in the material properties. The common failures experienced with impression materials and their causes are summarized in Table 9-5. The comparative properties of elastomeric impression materials are listed in Table 9-6. A summary of the characteristics of the elastomeric impression materials is given in Table 9-7.

Table 9-5	**Common Failures That Occur with Use of Nonaqueous Elastomeric Impression Materials**
Type of failure	**Causes**
Rough or uneven surface on impression	Incomplete polymerization caused by premature removal from the mouth, improper ratio or mixing of components, or presence of oil or other organic material on the teeth. For addition silicone, agents that contaminate the material and inhibit polymerization
	Too rapid polymerization from high humidity or temperature
	Excessively high accelerator/base ratio with condensation silicone
Bubbles	Too rapid polymerization, preventing flow
	Air incorporated during mixing
Irregularly shaped voids	Moisture or debris on surface of teeth
Rough or chalky stone cast	Inadequate cleaning of impression
	Excess water left on surface of the impression
	Excess wetting agent left on impression
	Premature removal of cast. Improper manipulation of stone
	Failure to delay pour of addition silicone at least 20 min
Distortion	Resin tray not aged sufficiently; still undergoing polymerization shrinkage
	Lack of adhesion of rubber to the tray caused by not applying enough coats of adhesive, filling tray with material too soon after applying adhesive, or using wrong adhesive
	Lack of mechanical retention for those materials where adhesive is ineffective
	Development of elastic properties in the material before tray is seated
	Excessive bulk of material
	Insufficient relief for the reline material (if such technique is used)
	Continued pressure against impression material that has developed elastic properties
	Movement of tray during polymerization
	Premature removal from mouth
	Improper removal from mouth
	Delayed pouring of the polysulfide or condensation silicone impression

Table 9-6	Comparative Properties of Elastomeric Impression Materials			
Property	Polysulfide	Condensation silicone	Addition silicone	Polyether
Working time (min)	4–7	2.5–4	2–4	3
Setting time (min)	7–10	6–8	4–6.5	6
Tear strength (N/m)	2500–7000	2300–2600	1500–4300	1800–4800
Percent contraction (at 24 h)	0.40–0.45	0.38–0.60	0.14–0.17	0.19–0.24
Contact angle between set material and water (°)	82	98	98/53*	49
Hydrogen gas evolution (Y/N)	N	N	Y[†]	N
Automatic mixing (Y/N)	N	N	Y	Y
Custom tray (Y/N)	Y	N	N	N
Unpleasant odor (Y/N)	Y	N	N	N
Multiple casts (Y/N)	N	N	Y	Y
Stiffness (value of 1 indicates greatest stiffness)	3	2	2	1[‡]
Distortion on removal (value of 1 indicates greatest potential distortion)	1	2	4	3
Cost per unit volume (value of 1 indicates most costly material)	4	3	2	1

*The lower contact angle resulted from testing of a hydrophilic impression material.
[†]A hydrogen absorber is often included to eliminate hydrogen gas evolution.
[‡]The high stiffness (elastic modulus) may require blocking out of undercut areas.

CRITICAL QUESTION

How can distortion of a hydrocolloid impression be minimized during storage?

HYDROCOLLOIDS

Colloids are often classified as a fourth state of matter, the *colloidal state*. In a solution of sugar in water, the sugar molecules are uniformly dispersed in the water and there is no visible physical separation between the solute and the solvent molecules. If the sugar molecules are replaced with larger, visible insoluble particles, such as sand, the system is termed a *suspension*. If these particles are liquids, such as vegetable oil in water, the system is then called an *emulsion*. These suspended globules or oil droplets do not readily diffuse and tend to settle out of the suspending medium unless mechanically or chemically held in place. Somewhere between the extremes of the very small molecules in solution and the very large particles in suspension is the colloidal solution, or *sol*.

True solutions exist as a **single phase**. However, both the colloid and the suspension have two phases: the **dispersed phase** and the **dispersion phase**. In the colloid, the particles in the dispersed phase consist of molecules held together either by primary or secondary forces. The sizes of the colloid particles range from 1 to 200 nm.

Table 9-7 Characteristics of Elastomeric Impression Materials

Generic type	Brand names	Advantages	Disadvantages
Polysulfide	Coe-flex (GC-America)	Long working time	Requires custom tray
	Neo-plex (Heraeus Kulzer)	High tear resistance	Stretching leads to distortion
	Omniflex (GC-America)	Margins easily seen	Good with stone
	Permlastic (Kerr)	Modest cost	Stains clothing
			Obnoxious odor
			Pour within 1 hr
Condensation Silicone (Putty Wash)	Accoe (GC-America)	Putty for custom tray	High polymerization shrinkage
	Cuttersil (Heraeus Kulzer)	Clean and pleasant	Volatile by-product
	Silene (Bosworth)	Good working time	Low tear strength
	Speedex (Coltene/Whaledent)	Easily seen margins	Hydrophobic
	Xantopren (Heraeus Kulzer)		Pour immediately
Vinyl Polysiloxane	Aquasil/Reprosil/Hydrosil (Dentsply Caulk)	One material	Hydrophobic
	Cinch-Platinum (Parkell)	Putty for custom tray	No flow if sulcus is moist
	Dimension/Position (3M/ESPE)	Automix dispense	Low tear strength
	Exaflex/Examix/Exafast/Hydroflex (GC America)	Clean and pleasant	Putty displaces wash
	Express/Imprint/Imprint II (3M/ESPE)	Easily seen margins	Wash has low tear strength
	Extrude/Take 1 (Kerr)	Ideally elastic	Putty too stiff
	First QuarterFS/Star VPS (Danville Materials)	Pour repeatedly	Putty and wash separate
	Flexitime/Provil (Heraeus Kulzer)	Stable: delay pour	Difficult to pour cast
	Honigum (Zenith/DMG)		High cost
	Perfectim (J Morita)		
	Polysil (SciCan)		
	President/Rapid (Coltene)		
	Supersil (Bosworth)		

Material	Products	Advantages	Disadvantages
Polyether	Impregum F (3M/ESPE) Permadyne (3M/ESPE) Polyjel NF (Caulk)	Fast setting Clean Automix dispense Least hydrophobic Easily seen margins Good stability Delay pour Shelf life: 2 yr	Stiff, high modulus Bitter taste Needs to block undercuts Absorbs water Leaches components High cost
Reversible hydrocolloid (agar)	Acculoid/Cartriloids (Van R) Cohere/SuperBody/SuperSyringe (Ghingi-Pak) Indentic (Cadco)	Moist field OK Accurate and pleasant Hydrophilic Low cost Long shelf-life	Requires special equipment Thermal discomfort Tears easily Pour immediately Difficult to see margins and details
Irreversible hydrocolloid (alginate)	Coe Alginate (GC America) Integra (Kerr) Indentic/Kromafaze (Cadco) Jeltrate (Dentsply Caulk) Kromopan (Kromopan) Supergel (Bosworth) Xantalgin (Heraeus Kulzer)	Moist field OK Clean and pleasant Hydrophilic Low cost Long shelf-life	Not accurate/rough Tears easily Pour immediately Can retard setting of gypsum

Sol-Gel Transformation

If a hydrocolloid contains an adequate concentration of the dispersed phase, the sol under certain conditions may change to a semisolid material known as a **gel**. In the gel state, the dispersed phase agglomerates to form chains or fibrils, also called **micelles**. The fibrils may branch and intermesh to form a brush-heap structure, which can be envisioned as resembling the intermeshing of tree branches or twigs in a brush pile. The dispersion medium is held in the interstices between the fibrils by capillary attraction or adhesion. The colloidal materials used for impression making are either agar or alginate dissolved in water, and these solutions are called *hydrocolloids*.

For agar, secondary bonds hold the fibrils together. These bonds break at slightly elevated temperatures and become reestablished as the hydrocolloid cools to room temperature. The process is reversible. For alginate, the fibrils are formed by chemical action, and the transformation is not reversible.

Gel Strength

The gel can support considerable stress, particularly shear stress, without flow, provided the stress is applied rapidly. The stiffness and strength of the gel are directly related to the hydrocolloid concentration. The strength of reversible and **irreversible hydrocolloid** gels can be increased by the addition of certain modifiers, such as fillers and chemicals. However, the material will flow under sustained stresses. This flow will disturb the network relation between the dispersion medium and the fibrillar structure.

For the reversible gel, the lower the temperature, the stronger the gel (and vice versa). When the gel is heated, the kinetic energy of the fibrils increases, resulting in greater interfibrillar distances and a reduction in their cohesive interaction. As the temperature continues to rise, more of the fibrils dissociate until finally more fibrils are dissociating than are forming at the temperature at which the liquefaction to the sol state occurs.

On the other hand, the strength of the irreversible gel is not as greatly affected by normal temperature changes, because the fibrils are formed by chemical action and they do not revert to the sol condition upon heating.

Dimensional Effects

The gel may lose water by *evaporation* from its surface or by exuding fluid onto the surface by a process known as **syneresis**. The gel shrinks as the result of evaporation and syneresis. If a gel is placed in water, it absorbs water by a process known as *imbibition*. The gel swells during imbibition, thereby altering the original dimensions. Imbibition can cause just as much distortion as syneresis and evaporation.

The effects of syneresis, evaporation, and imbibition on the dimensional changes are of considerable importance in dentistry, since any change in dimension that occurs after the impressions are removed from the mouth will lead to inaccurate casts and models. The means of limiting these effects and ensuring the proper dimensions of the impression are discussed in the following sections.

AGAR (REVERSIBLE) HYDROCOLLOIDS

The setting of a reversible hydrocolloid, often called **gelation**, is a solidification process that involves phase changes from sol to gel states. The physical change from the sol to gel, and vice versa, is induced by a temperature change. The gel converts to the sol condition when it is heated to a certain temperature, known as the *liquefaction temperature* (70° to 100° C). When cooled from this temperature range, the sol transforms into a gel at a point known as the *gelation temperature* (between 37° and 50° C). The gelation temperature is critical for impression making. If the gelation temperature is too high, the heat from the sol may injure the oral tissues, or the sol transformation to a gel will be rapid and develop significant surface irregularities. Conversely, if the gelation temperature is too far below oral temperature, it will be difficult or even impossible to chill the material sufficiently to obtain a firm gel adjacent to the oral tissues.

Composition

One of the main constituents of the **hydrocolloid** impression materials is agar, but it is by no means the main constituent by weight (Table 9-8). Agar is an organic hydrophilic colloid (polysaccharide) extracted from certain types of seaweed. It is present in a concentration of 8% to 15%, depending on the desired properties of the material. The principal ingredient by weight in the set impression is water (>80%). A small percentage of borax is added to strengthen the gel. Since borax is an excellent retarder for the setting of gypsum, an accelerator such as potassium sulfate is added to counteract the effect of borax. Other fillers such as diatomaceous earth, clay, silica, wax, rubber, and similar inert powders are used to control strength, viscosity, and rigidity, as previously discussed. Thymol and glycerine may also be added as a bactericidal agent and plasticizer, respectively. Pigments and flavors are usually included as well.

The hydrocolloid is usually supplied in two forms: syringe material and tray material. Tubes are used to fill the water-cooled trays and cartridges for use with the syringes, as shown in Figure 9-13. The only differences between the syringe and tray material are the color and a greater fluidity of the syringe material.

Manipulation

The temperature lag between the gelation temperature and the liquefaction temperature of the gel makes it possible to use agar as a dental impression material. The manipulation includes liquefying the gel, placing it in the impression tray, tempering it to a lower temperature that the patient can tolerate, and maintaining it in its fluid state to capture the details of the oral structures. Once in the mouth, the material is cooled below mouth temperature to ensure gelation. Proper equipment to support the process is essential. Usually, there are at least three compartments in

Table 9-8	**Composition of Commercial Reversible Hydrocolloid Impression Materials**	
Component	**Function**	**Composition (%)**
Agar	Brush-heap structure	13-17
Borate	Strength	0.2-0.5
Sulfate	Gypsum hardener	1.0-2.0
Wax, hard	Filler	0.5-1.0
Thixotropic materials	Thickener	0.3-0.5
Water	Reaction medium	Balance

Courtesy of K. H. Strader.

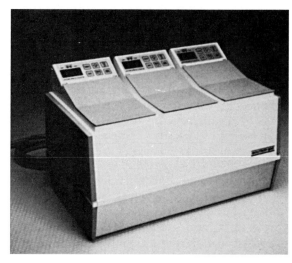

Fig. 9-13 Cartridge of agar hydrocolloid and syringes used for injecting onto the prepared tooth. Also shown is the holder for carrying the agar hydrocolloid into the conditioning unit.

the conditioning unit (such as the one shown in Fig. 9-14), making it possible to simultaneously liquefy, store, and temper the reversible hydrocolloid material. Temperatures required in each of the steps for preparing the hydrocolloid are critical, and equipment should be calibrated weekly.

Preparation and Conditioning of the Agar Material

The first step in material preparation is to liquefy the hydrocolloid gel in boiling water. The material must be held at this temperature for a minimum of 10 minutes. At high altitudes (e.g., in Denver, Colorado) the boiling point of water is too low to liquefy the gel. Propylene glycol can be added to the water to obtain a liquefaction temperature of 100° C. Otherwise, materials that have been formulated specifically to liquefy at lower temperatures should be used. It is possible to reliquefy a portion of an unused tube. Theoretically, one could reuse the material that was used to make

Fig. 9-14 Conditioning unit for agar hydrocolloid impression materials. The three compartments are used for liquefying the material, storing after boiling, and tempering the tray hydrocolloid. (Courtesy of Van R Dental Products, Inc. Los Angeles, Calif.)

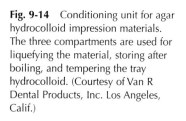

the impression. However, since disinfection would be a major problem, only unused portions should be reheated in the conditioning unit.

After the agar hydrocolloid material has been liquefied, it may be stored in the sol condition at 65° C until it is needed for injection into the cavity preparation or for filling a tray. Since the liquefaction process takes some time and the material can be stored for several days, it is a general practice to prepare a number of tubes and syringes for use throughout the week.

Tempering of the Material

Since 55° C is the maximum tolerable temperature, a storage temperature of 65° C would be too hot for the oral tissues, especially for the bulk of the tray material. Therefore, the material used to fill the tray must be *tempered*. For the immediate preparation step, a tube of hydrocolloid sol is removed from the storage bath, the tray is filled, a gauze pad is placed over the top of the tray material, and the tray is placed in the water-filled tempering container (~45° C) of the conditioning unit. The tempering time is short (3 to 10 min), just sufficient to ensure that all the material has reached a lower temperature (≤55° C). In any case, the loaded tray should never be left in this bath for more than 10 minutes, because gelation may have proceeded too far, thereby making the material unusable.

Tempering of tray material also increases the viscosity so that it will not flow out of the tray. The syringe material, on the other hand, is *never* tempered, since it must be maintained in a fluid state to enhance adaptation to the tissues. The effect of extruding the material out the small opening of the syringe lowers the temperature of the syringe material sufficiently so that it is comfortable for the patient.

Making the Agar Impression

Just before the tempering process for the tray material is completed, the syringe material is taken directly from the storage compartment and applied to the prepared teeth. It is first applied to the base of the preparation; then the remainder of the prepared tooth is covered. The point of the syringe is held close to the tooth, beneath the surface of the syringe material, to prevent entrapment of air bubbles. The water-soaked outer layer of tray hydrocolloid is removed from the container, and the gauze that was covering the tray impression material is also removed. If the outer surface of the hydrocolloid tray material is not removed, it may not firmly bond to the syringe hydrocolloid. The tray is immediately brought into position and seated with light pressure and held with a very light force. Too much pressure may displace the syringed agar sol on the tooth and distort the impression.

Gelation is accelerated by circulating cool water (approximately 18° to 21° C) through the tray for 3 to 5 min (Fig. 9-15). During the gelation process, the tray must be held in the mouth until gelation has proceeded to a point at which the gel strength is sufficient to resist deformation or fracture. Waiting an extra minute greatly increases the strength and tear resistance. Also, the lower the temperature, the more rapidly gelation occurs and, to a certain extent, the stronger the material will become.

As discussed in the section on elastomeric impression materials, hydrocolloid materials exhibit viscoelastic behavior; therefore, it is necessary to remove the impression suddenly, with a snap, rather than to tease it out. Any twisting or torquing should be avoided. Properly done, the resulting impression (Fig. 9-16) will accurately reproduce the dimensions and details of hard and soft tissues.

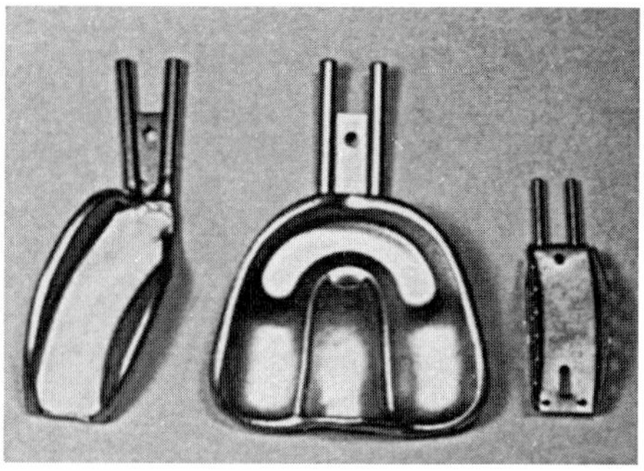

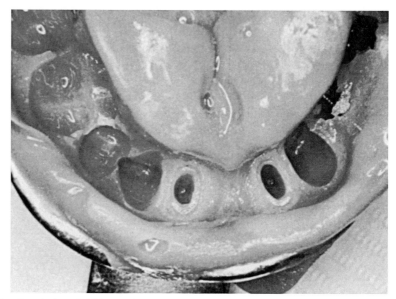

Fig. 9-15   Water-cooled trays used to accelerate gelation of agar hydrocolloids.

Fig. 9-16   Agar hydrocolloid impression.

Accuracy

Reversible hydrocolloid is among the most accurate of impression materials. It has a long history of successful use for single units and for fixed partial denture applications. To demonstrate the accuracy of an impression material, studies are designed to fabricate castings to fit standardized dies as shown in Figure 9-17. These standard preparations simulate an inlay, an onlay, and a full-coverage crown. Because of their blunt 90° axiogingival angles and a 6° to 8° taper, teeth requiring a mesial-occlusal-distal onlay preparation must be prepared with greater precision than most clinical cavity preparations. Therefore, any impression that accurately reproduces these dies will more than satisfy the conventional clinical requirements. To achieve this accuracy, the clinician must ensure that the following conditions are achieved.

Viscosity of the Sol

After the material has been liquefied, it must be sufficiently viscous so that it will not flow out of the tray even if the tray is inverted, such as when making a mandibular impression. On the other hand, its viscosity must not be so great that it will not readily penetrate every detail of the teeth and soft tissues.

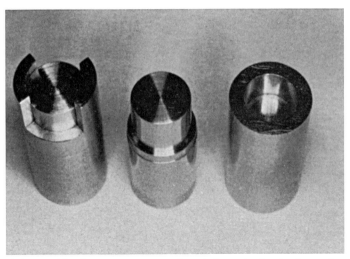

Fig. 9-17 Steel dies used for determining accuracy in techniques that involve impression materials and castings. **Left,** mesial-occlusal-distal preparation. **Center,** Full-crown preparation. **Right,** One-surface inlay preparation.

Even when the material has sufficient viscosity to be stabilized in a tray, it does not offer much resistance to seating. It is very easy for the patient to "bite through" the impression material. For this reason, the triple-tray is commonly used with reversible hydrocolloids. With a triple-tray technique, one impression records the oral structures of the maxillary and mandibular arches as well as the occlusal relationship. The procedure is somewhat technique-sensitive since the dentist must guide the patient into centric occlusion as the patient "bites" into the impression material. For this type of impression, the material must not resist the patient's efforts to articulate his or her teeth together. Most hydrocolloids have the optimal consistency to allow this technique to be used successfully.

Distortion During Gelation

Certain stresses are always introduced during gelation. Some contraction occurs because of the physical change in the hydrocolloid transformation from a sol to a gel. If the material is held rigidly in the tray, the impression material shrinks toward the center of its mass, thereby creating larger dies. Since the sol is a poor thermal conductor, rapid cooling may cause a concentration of stress near the tray where the gelation first takes place. Consequently, water at approximately 20° C is more suitable for cooling the impression than is ice water.

ALGINATE (IRREVERSIBLE) HYDROCOLLOIDS

The present **alginate hydrocolloid**, or irreversible impression material, was developed as a substitute for the agar impression material when its supply became scarce during World War II. This material is based on a natural substance extracted from certain brown seaweed. The substance is called anhydro-β-*d*-mannuronic acid or alginic acid and has the structural formula shown in Figure 9-18. The general use of irreversible hydrocolloid far exceeds that of other impression materials available today. The principal factors responsible for the success of this type of impression material are that it is easy to manipulate, comfortable for the patient, and relatively inexpensive since it does not require elaborate equipment.

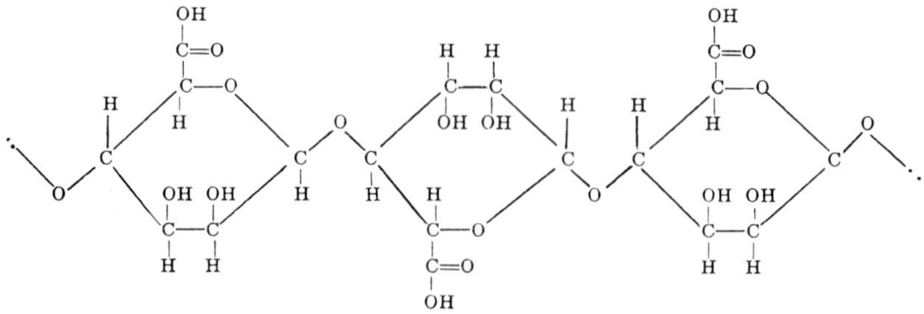

Fig. 9-18   Structural formula of alginic acid.

Composition

The chief active ingredient of the irreversible hydrocolloid impression materials is one of the soluble alginates, such as sodium, potassium, or triethanolamine alginate. When the soluble alginates are mixed with water, they form a sol quite readily. The sols are quite viscous even in low concentrations. The molecular weight of the alginate compounds may vary widely, depending on the manufacturing treatment. The greater the molecular weight, the more viscous is the sol. Table 9-9 shows a formula for the powder component of an alginate impression material.

The purpose of the diatomaceous earth is to act as filler to increase the strength and stiffness of the alginate gel, to produce a smooth texture, and to ensure the formation of a firm gel surface that is not tacky. It also aids in forming the sol by dispersing the alginate powder particles in the water. Zinc oxide also acts as a filler and has some influence on the physical properties and setting time of the gel. Calcium sulfate dihydrate is generally used as the reactor. A retarder is also added to control the setting time. A fluoride, such as potassium titanium fluoride, is added as an accelerator for the setting of the stone to be poured in the impression to ensure a hard, dense, cast surface.

When powder in the alginate can is fluffed to break loose the particles, fine silica particles will become airborne from the can when the lid is removed. The silica particles in the dust are of such a size and shape that long-term exposure through inhalation is a possible health hazard. In an effort to reduce the dust encountered after tumbling, manufacturers have introduced a "dustless" alginate in which they have incorporated glycerine on the alginate powder to agglomerate the particles. This causes the powder to become more dense than in the uncoated state. After tumbling, the powders no longer have a tendency to release fine particles as evidenced by the reduction in airborne particles as the canister lid is removed.

Table 9-9	Formula for the Powder Component of an Alginate Impression Material	
Component	**Function**	**Weight percentage**
Potassium alginate	Soluble alginate	15
Calcium sulfate	Reactor	16
Zinc oxide	Filler particles	4
Potassium titanium fluoride	Accelerator	3
Diatomaceous earth	Filler particles	60
Sodium phosphate	Retarder	2

Gelation Process

The typical sol-gel reaction can be described simply as a reaction of soluble alginate with calcium sulfate and the formation of an insoluble calcium alginate gel. Structurally, calcium ions replace the sodium or potassium ions of two adjacent molecules to produce a cross-linked complex or polymer network (Fig. 9-19). The production of the calcium alginate is so rapid that it does not allow sufficient working time. Therefore, in addition to soluble alginate and calcium sulfate, a third water-soluble salt (e.g., trisodium phosphate) is added to the solution to prolong the working time. The strategy is that the calcium sulfate will react with this salt in preference to the soluble alginate. Thus the rapid reaction between calcium sulfate and the soluble alginate is deferred as long as there is unreacted trisodium phosphate. For example, the following reaction will first take place:

$$2Na_3PO_4 + 3CaSO_4 \rightarrow Ca_3(PO_4)_2 + 3Na_2SO_4 \tag{1}$$

When the supply of trisodium phosphate is exhausted, the calcium ions begin to react with the potassium alginate to produce calcium alginate as follows:

$$K_{2n} Alg + n\ CaSO_4 \rightarrow n\ K_2SO_4 + Ca_n Alg \tag{2}$$

The third salt is known as a *retarder*. The amount of retarder is adjusted to provide the proper setting time.

In general, if approximately 16 g of the powder is mixed with 38 mL of water, gelation will occur in about 3 to 4 min at room temperature. The setting time must be sufficient to allow the dentist to mix the material, load the tray, and place it in the patient's mouth. The practical method of determining setting time for the dental

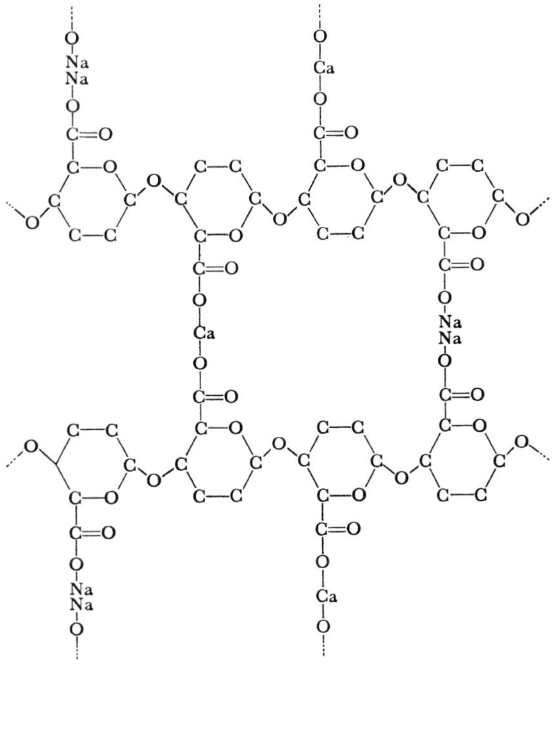

Fig. 9-19 Schematic illustration of sodium alginate cross-linked with calcium ions. The base molecules represent the sodium salt of alginic acid, in which hydrogen atoms of carboxyl groups are replaced by sodium atoms. With the exception of polar groups, all side chains have been omitted for simplification.

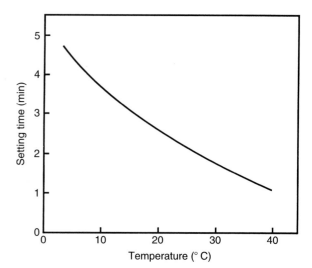

Fig. 9-20 Effect of water temperature on the setting time of an alginate impression material. (Courtesy of J. Cresson.)

practitioner is to observe the time from the start of mixing until the material is no longer tacky or sticky when it is touched with a clean, dry, gloved finger.

Controlling Setting Time

In the clinical setting, it is tempting to alter the setting time by changing the W/P ratio or the mixing time. This slight modification can have marked effects on the properties of the gel, the tear strength, and the elasticity. Thus the setting time is best regulated by the amount of retarder added during the manufacturing process. Normally, the manufacturers make both fast-setting alginate (1.5 to 3 min) and normal-setting alginate (3 to 4.5 min) to provide clinicians the opportunity to choose the materials that best suit their working style.

The clinician, however, can safely influence the setting time by altering the temperature of the water. It is evident from Figure 9-20 that the higher the temperature, the shorter is the setting time (i.e., a 1-min reduction in setting time occurs for each 10° C of temperature increase). Materials exhibit different degrees of sensitivity to temperature. In such a case, the temperature of the mixing water should be controlled carefully within a degree or two of a standard temperature, usually 20° C, so that a constant and reliable setting time can be obtained. It is better to select a product with the desired setting time and less sensitivity to temperature change rather than to resort to other modifications in the manipulation technique.

In hot weather, special precautions should be taken to provide cool water for mixing so that premature gelation does not occur. It may even be necessary to precool the mixing bowl and spatula, especially when small amounts of impression material are to be mixed. At higher temperatures, fast-setting materials should be used under carefully controlled conditions or the working time may be exceeded.

CRITICAL QUESTION

Why is it especially important to add water to the rubber mixing bowl before the powder when mixing a fast-setting alginate impression material?

Manipulation

Alginate impression materials are hydrophilic, so moist tissue surfaces are not a problem. Generally, alginates are used as a first preliminary impression to construct a custom tray for a more accurate second impression or to make study models to help with treatment planning and discussions with the patient. Unlike many of the other impression materials, alginate hydrocolloids are not available in a range of different viscosities.

The first step of manipulation is to prepare a proper mixture of water and powder. The measured powder is sifted into premeasured water that has already been poured into a clean rubber bowl. The powder is incorporated into the water by carefully mixing with a metal or plastic spatula that is sufficiently flexible to adapt well to the wall of the mixing bowl. The water is added first to wet the mixing bowl and to ensure complete wetting of powder particles. If the powder is placed first in the mixing bowl, penetration of the water to the bottom of the bowl is inhibited and greater mixing time may be required to ensure a homogeneous mix. Care should be taken to avoid incorporating air into the mix. A vigorous figure-8 motion is best, with the mix being swiped or stropped against the sides of the rubber-mixing bowl with intermittent rotations (180°) of the spatula to press out air bubbles. All of the powder must be dissolved.

The mixing time is particularly important; 45 sec to 1 min is generally sufficient, depending on the brand and type of alginate (fast-set or regular-set). Carefully read the instructions on the can listing the exact mixing time, working time, and setting time for the material you are using. The result should be a smooth, creamy mixture that does not readily drip off the spatula when it is raised from the bowl. A variety of mechanical devices are also available for mixing the alginate materials. Their principal benefits are convenience, speed, and elimination of human errors.

Clean equipment is important because many of the problems and related failures are attributed to dirty or contaminated mixing or handling devices. Contaminants, such as small amounts of gypsum left in the bowl from a previous mix of plaster or stone, can accelerate the set. It is best to use separate bowls for mixing alginate and stone.

Ideally, the powder should be weighed and not measured volumetrically by means of a scoop, as many manufacturers suggest. However, unless a grossly incorrect method is used for scooping the powder, the variations in individual mixes should have no measurable effect on the physical properties.

Making the Impression

Before seating the impression, the material should have developed sufficient body so that it will not flow out of the tray and gag the patient. The mixture is placed in a suitable tray, which is then placed in the mouth. It is imperative that the impression adhere and be retained to the tray so that the impression can be withdrawn from around the teeth. Therefore, a perforated tray is generally used. If a plastic tray or a metal rim-lock tray is selected, a thin layer of alginate tray adhesive should be applied and allowed to dry completely before mixing and loading the alginate in the tray. Alginate is very weak; therefore the tray must fit the patient's arch so that there is a sufficient bulk of material. The thickness of the alginate impression between the tray and the tissues should be at least 3 mm.

As can be noted from Table 9-10, the compressive strength in this case actually doubles during the first 4 min after gelation, but it did not increase appreciably after the first 4-min period. Most alginate materials improve in elasticity over time, which minimizes distortion of the material during impression removal, thus permitting

Table 9-10	Compressive Strength of an Alginate Gel as a Function of Gelation Time	
Time from gelation (min)		**Compressive strength (MPa)**
0		0.33
4		0.77
8		0.81
12		0.71
16		0.74

superior reproduction of undercut areas. Such data clearly indicate that the alginate impression should not be removed from the mouth for at least 3 min after gelation has occurred.

Although the more common problem is to remove the impression prematurely, it is possible to leave an alginate impression in the mouth too long. With certain alginates, it has been shown that if the impression is held for 6 to 7 min after gelation, rather than 3 min, significant distortion may result.

As with the reversible hydrocolloids, alginate hydrocolloid materials are strain-rate dependent. Thus the tear strength is increased when the impression is removed with a snap. The speed of removal must be a compromise between a rapid movement and a slower, more comfortable rate for the patient. Usually, an alginate impression does not adhere to the oral tissues as strongly as do some of the nonaqueous **elastomers**, so it is easier to remove the alginate impression rapidly. However, it is always best to avoid torquing or twisting the impression in an effort to remove it quickly. Specifically, the handle should be used minimally during breaking of the air seal ("suction") or removing the tray from the teeth.

Strength

Maximum gel strength is required to prevent fracture and to ensure elastic recovery of the impression upon its removal from the mouth. All manipulative factors under the control of the clinician affect the gel strength. For example, if too much or too little water is used in mixing, the final gel will be weakened, making it less elastic. The proper W/P ratio should be employed as specified by the manufacturer. Insufficient spatulation results in failure of the ingredients to dissolve sufficiently so that the chemical reactions can proceed uniformly throughout the mass. Overmixing breaks up the calcium alginate gel network as it is forming and reduces its strength. Manufacturers' directions supplied with the product should be followed in all respects.

Accuracy

Most alginate impression materials are not capable of reproducing the finer details that are observed in impressions with other elastomeric impression materials. Manufacturers have attempted to increase the concentration of alginate to make the material more accurate. However, this does not increase the dimensional stability of the material. The roughness of the impression surface is sufficient to cause distortion at the margins of prepared teeth. Nevertheless, alginate materials are sufficiently accurate that they can be used for making impressions for removable partial dentures.

OTHER APPLICATIONS AND HANDLING OF HYDROCOLLOIDS
Laminate Technique (Alginate-Agar Method)

A recent modification to the traditional agar procedure is the combined agar-alginate technique. The hydrocolloid in the tray is replaced with a mix of chilled alginate that bonds with the agar expressed from a syringe. The alginate gels by a chemical reaction, whereas the agar gels by means of contact with the cool alginate rather than with the water circulating through the tray. Since the agar, not the alginate, is in contact with the prepared teeth, maximum detail is reproduced. Because only the syringe material needs to be heated, equipment cost is lower and less preparation time is required. The main disadvantages to this technique are the following: the bond between the agar and the alginate is not always sound, the higher viscosity of the alginate material displaces the agar hydrocolloid during seating, and the dimensional inaccuracy of the alginate hydrocolloid limits its use to single units. Nevertheless, this laminate technique is the most cost-effective way of producing an impression with adequate detail.

Duplicating Materials

Both types of hydrocolloid are used in the dental laboratory to duplicate dental casts or models used in the construction of prosthetic appliances and orthodontic models. Reversible (agar) hydrocolloid is more popular because it can be used many times. Also, with intermittent stirring, agar hydrocolloid can be kept in a liquid form for 1 or 2 weeks at a constant pouring temperature. These factors make the cost of reversible impression materials quite reasonable.

The hydrocolloid-type duplicating materials have the same composition as the impression materials, but their water content is higher. Consequently, the agar or alginate content is lower, which influences their compressive strength and percent permanent set. These property requirements are identified in ANSI/ADA Specification No. 20.

Modified Alginates

Traditional alginate material is used as a two-component system of powder and water, in which no reaction occurs until the powder is added to the water to initiate the reaction. However, the alginate can also be purchased in the form of a sol, containing the water but no source of calcium ions. A reactor of plaster of Paris can then be added to the sol.

Yet another form of alginate is available: a two-component system in the form of two pastes, one containing the alginate sol and the second containing the calcium reactor. Impression materials of this type may also contain silicone and may be supplied both in a tray viscosity and in a syringe viscosity.

Biocompatibility

No known chemical or allergic reactions are associated with hydrocolloid impressions. The most likely side effect is thermal injury from reversible hydrocolloid as a result of improper tempering or faulty equipment during impression making. Inhaling fine airborne particles from alginate impression material can cause silicosis and pulmonary hypersensitivity. Dustless alginate is preferred to minimize this risk.

Disinfection

Since the hydrocolloid impression must be poured within a short time after removal from the mouth, the disinfection procedure should be relatively rapid to prevent dimensional change. Most manufacturers recommend a specific disinfectant, such as iodophor, bleach, or glutaraldehyde, which should be used according to the manufacturer's directions. Certain disinfectants may result in gypsum casts that have a lower surface hardness or diminished surface detail.

The current protocol for disinfecting hydrocolloid impressions recommended by the Center for Disease Control is to use household bleach (1 to 10 dilution), iodophors, or synthetic phenols as disinfectants. After the impression is rinsed thoroughly, the disinfectant can be sprayed liberally on the exposed surface. The impression is then wrapped immediately in a disinfectant-soaked paper towel and placed in a sealed plastic bag for 10 min. Finally, the wrapped impression is removed from the bag, unwrapped, rinsed, and shaken to remove excess water. The impression is then poured with the stone of choice. An alternative disinfection method is by immersion, but this should not exceed 10 min (see Table 9-4).

Dimensional Stability

Once the impression is removed from the mouth and exposed to air at room temperature, some shrinkage associated with syneresis and evaporation is bound to occur. Conversely, if the impression is immersed in water, swelling as the result of imbibition occurs. A typical example of the dimensional change that can occur during syneresis and imbibition of a hydrocolloid impression material is shown in Figure 9-21. This graph illustrates that the material has shrunk in air. During subsequent imbibition, excessive expansion may occur because of swelling by uptake of water.

It is clear that the impression should be exposed to the air for as short a time as possible if the best results are to be obtained. Various storage media, such as 2% potassium sulfate or 100% relative humidity, are suggested to reduce the dimensional change of agar impressions. Results obtained for impressions made from

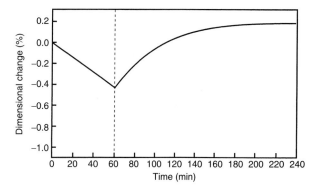

Fig. 9-21 Linear contraction of a representative reversible hydrocolloid in air (31% to 42% relative humidity) and subsequent expansion in water.

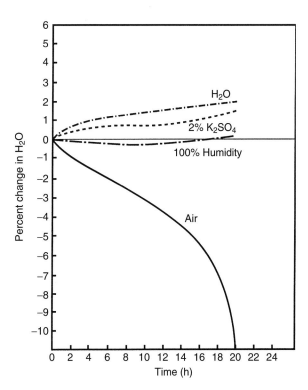

Fig. 9-22 Percentage of change in water content according to weight of an agar hydrocolloid impression material in various storage media. At 100% relative humidity, the percent change is minimal.

one agar hydrocolloid product stored in several media are given in Figure 9-22. These results are typical, and they indicate that 100% relative humidity is the best storage environment to preserve the normal water content of the impression.

Thermal changes also contribute to dimensional change. With alginates, impressions shrink slightly because of the thermal differential between mouth temperature (37° C) and room temperature (23° C). The agar hydrocolloid impression materials experience a temperature shift in the opposite direction, from the chilled water-cooled tray (15° C) to the warmer room temperature. Even this slight change can cause the impression to expand and become less accurate.

If pouring of the impression must be delayed, it should be rinsed in tap water, disinfected, wrapped in a surgical paper towel, saturated with water, and placed in a sealed plastic bag or a humidor.

Compatibility with Gypsum

The water content of the hydrocolloid impressions inhibits the setting of the gypsum at the surface. A known gypsum retarder, such as borax, is used as a filler in agar impression material, but it can cause the surfaces of gypsum casts prepared from an agar impression to be too soft for use as dies. The gelation process of alginate impression produces not only insoluble calcium alginate but also sodium sulfate. Sodium sulfate is a gypsum accelerator at low concentration, but it becomes a gypsum retarder at higher concentration. The amount of sodium salt used in the alginate impression material produces enough sodium sulfate to retard the setting of gypsum poured against the alginate. These deficiencies can be overcome in two ways: (1) by immersing the impression in a solution containing a gypsum accelerator, such as 2% potassium sulfate solution, prior to pouring the impression with the gypsum-forming product; or (2) by using products that incorporate a gypsum hardener or accelerator in the material. The sulfate in the formulation for agar (see Table 9-8) and the potassium titanium fluoride in alginate (see Table 9-9) satisfy the second condition.

A rough stone surface will result if excess rinsing water has collected on the surface of the impression at the time the stone mixture is poured. However, the surface of the impression should not be dried completely or the gel will adhere to the surface of the cast and possibly tear upon its removal. Excessive dehydration also causes syneresis and a distortion of the impression. The surface of the impression should be shiny but with no visible water film or droplets at the time the impression is poured with model or die material.

The pouring of a stone mixture to fill the impression should start from one end of the arch. After the impression has been filled with stone, somewhat superior stone surfaces may be obtained if the impression is placed in a humidor while the stone hardens. In any event, the filled impression should never be immersed in water while the stone sets.

The stone cast or die should be kept in contact with the impression for a minimum of 30 min, preferably for 60 min, before the impression is separated from the cast. The setting time of a more dilute gypsum-forming mixture in contact with the impression material will be longer, and sufficient time should be allowed for the stone to set. It is wise to separate the cast from the impression within a reasonable period of time so that desiccation of the hydrocolloid does not occur, thereby causing abrasion of the gypsum cast during its removal.

Shelf Life

Two major factors that affect the shelf life of alginate impression materials are storage temperature and moisture contamination from ambient air. The alginate impression powder may be purchased in individually sealed pouches, with sufficient powder preweighed for an individual impression, or in bulk form in a can. The individual pouches are preferred, since there is less chance for contamination during storage. In addition, the correct water/powder ratio is ensured, since calibrated plastic vials are provided for the measurement of the water. Nevertheless, the bulk form of packing is by far the most popular. If the bulk powder form of alginate is used, the lid should be firmly replaced on the container as soon as possible after dispensing the powder so that a minimal amount of moisture contamination occurs.

An expiration date under a stated condition of storage should be clearly identified by the manufacturer on each package. It is best not to stock more than 1 year's supply in the dental office. The material should be stored in a cool, dry environment.

Effects of Mishandling

Common causes for failures encountered with reversible and irreversible hydrocolloid impression materials are summarized in Table 9-11. See Table 9-7 for a summary of the characteristics of the hydrocolloids.

INELASTIC IMPRESSION MATERIALS

Inelastic impression materials exhibit an insignificant amount of elastic deformation when subjected to bending or tensile stresses. In addition, they tend

Table 9-11   Common Causes of Remaking Hydrocolloid Impressions

Effect	Cause	
	Agar	Alginate
Grainy material	Inadequate boiling	Improper mixing
	Storage temperature too low	Prolonged mixing
	Storage time too long	Excessive gelation
		Water/powder ratio too low
Separation of tray and syringe materials	Water-soaked tray material surface not removed	Not applicable
	Premature gelation of either material	
Tearing	Inadequate bulk	Inadequate bulk
	Premature removal from mouth	Moisture contamination
	Syringe material partially gelled when tray was seated	Premature removal from mouth
		Prolong mixing
External bubbles	Gelation of syringe material; prevents flow	Undue gelation preventing flow
		Air incorporated during mixing
Irregularly shaped voids	Material too cold	Moisture or debris on tissue
Rough or chalky stone model	Inadequate cleansing of impression	Inadequate cleaning of impression
	Excess water or hardening solution left in the impression	Excess water left in impression
	Premature removal of die	Premature removal of the impression
	Improper manipulation of stone	Model left in impression too long
	Air-drying the impression before pouring	Improper manipulation of stone
Distortion	Impression not poured immediately	Impression not poured immediately
	Movement of tray during gelation	Movement of tray during gelation
	Premature removal from mouth	Premature removal from mouth
	Improper removal from mouth	Improper removal from mouth
	Use of ice water during initial stages of gelation	

to fracture without exhibiting any plastic deformation if the stress from applied pressure exceeds their tensile, shear, or compressive strength values. These materials include impression plaster, impression compound, and ZOE impression paste. Because of these materials' inability to sustain a substantial amount of elastic deformation without fracture, their use in dental impression making is limited. In particular, impression plaster is rarely used today for impression making and will not be discussed further. However, some inelastic impression materials are used in other relevant dental applications such as interocclusal records.

IMPRESSION COMPOUND

Impression compound, also called *modeling plastic*, is supplied in the form of sheets and sticks (Fig. 9-23). This compound is softened by heat, inserted in an impression tray, and placed against tissue before it cools to a rigid mass. Its primary indication for use has been for making an impression of the edentulous ridge. A somewhat more viscous compound, called *tray compound*, can be used to form a tray for construction of dentures. An impression of soft tissue is obtained with tray compound. This impression is referred to as the *primary impression*. It is then used as a tray to support a thin layer of a second impression material, which is to be placed against the tissues. This impression is known as the *secondary impression*. Secondary impressions may also be made with a zinc oxide–eugenol paste, hydrocolloid, or a nonaqueous elastomer. The other common application of compound is for border molding of an acrylic custom tray during fitting of the tray.

Composition

In general, compounds are composed of a mixture of waxes, thermoplastic resins, filler, and a coloring agent. Shellac, stearic acid, and gutta percha are added to improve plasticity and workability. The waxes or resins in the impression compound are the principal ingredients that comprise the *matrix*. This structure is too fluid to handle and imparts a low strength even at room temperature. Consequently, a filler must be added. The filler increases the viscosity at temperatures above that of the mouth and increases the rigidity of the compound at room temperature.

CRITICAL QUESTION

What property of an impression compound material requires that the material be heated slowly to convert it to a totally plastic state?

Manipulation

Softening by heat is a prerequisite for the use of compounds. Their utilities are dictated by their responses to the temperature change in the surrounding environment. The **fusion temperature** of the compound indicates a definite reduction in plasticity of the material during cooling. Above this temperature, the softened material remains plastic while the impression is being made. Once the impression tray is seated, it should be held gently (passively) in position until the impression cools

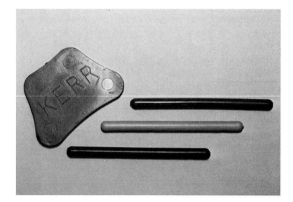

Fig. 9-23 Typical cake and stick configurations of commercial impression compound.

below the fusion temperature. Under no circumstances should the impression be disturbed or removed until it reaches oral temperature.

The thermal conductivity of these materials is very low, indicating the need for extended time to achieve thorough cooling and heating of the compound. The material should be uniformly soft at the time it is placed in the tray and thoroughly cooled in the tray before the impression is withdrawn from the mouth. Cold water can be sprayed on the tray while it is in the mouth until the compound is thoroughly hardened prior to removal of the impression tray from the mouth. Failure to attain a complete hardening of the material before withdrawing the impression can result in a serious distortion of the impression by relaxation.

Compound may be softened over a flame or by immersion in a warm water bath when a large amount is needed. When a direct flame is used, the compound should not be allowed to boil or ignite so that the constituents are volatilized. Prolonged immersion or overheating in the water bath is not indicated; the compound may become brittle and grainy if some of the low molecular weight ingredients leach out of the material. Softening of the compound in a warm water bath is the method recommended for separating the cast from a compound impression after the stone sets.

Dimensional Stability

Relaxation of impression compound can occur in a comparatively short period of time, especially with an increase in temperature. The result is warpage or distortion of the impression. The safest method of minimizing such distortion is to allow thorough cooling of the impression before removal from the mouth and to construct the cast or die as soon as possible after the impression has been obtained—at least within the first hr.

Disinfection

The recommended disinfectant solution for compound is 2% alkaline glutaraldehyde solution. The impressions should be immersed in this solution for the required amount of time, rinsed, and poured immediately (see Table 9-4).

ZINC OXIDE–EUGENOL (ZOE) IMPRESSION PASTES

Under proper conditions, the reaction between zinc oxide and eugenol yields a relatively hard mass that possesses certain medicinal advantages, as well as mechanical property benefits, for some dental operations. This type of material has been involved in a wide range of applications in dentistry, including use as an impression material for edentulous mouths, a surgical dressing, bite registration paste, temporary filling material, root canal filling material, cementing medium, and temporary relining material for dentures.

Composition

ZOE impression pastes are dispensed as two separate pastes (Fig. 9-24). A typical formula is shown in Table 9-12. One tube contains zinc oxide and vegetable or mineral oil; the other contains eugenol and rosin. The vegetable or mineral oil acts as a plasticizer and aids in offsetting the action of the eugenol as an irritant.

Oil of cloves, which contains 70% to 85% eugenol, is sometimes used in preference to eugenol because it produces less burning sensation for patients when it

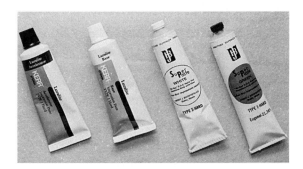

Fig. 9-24 Representative commercial products of zinc oxide–eugenol impression paste.

Table 9-12	Composition of a Zinc Oxide–Eugenol Impression Paste	
Components	**Percentage**	
TUBE NO. 1 (BASE)		
Zinc oxide (French-processed or U.S.P.)	87	
Fixed vegetable or mineral oil	13	
TUBE NO. 2 (ACCELERATOR)		
Oil of cloves or eugenol	12	
Gum or polymerized rosin	50	
Filler (silica type)	20	
Lanolin	3	
Resinous balsam	10	
Accelerator solution ($CaCl_2$) and color	5	

Courtesy of E.J. Molnar.

contacts the soft tissues. The addition of rosin to the paste in the second tube facilitates the speed of the reaction and yields a smoother, more homogeneous product. Canada balsam and Peru balsam are often used to increase flow and improve mixing properties. If the mixed paste is too thin or lacks body before it sets, a filler (such as a wax) or an inert powder (such as kaolin, talc, or diatomaceous earth) may be added to one or both of the original pastes.

Manipulation

The mixing of the two pastes is generally accomplished on an oil-impervious paper or a glass mixing slab. The proper proportion of the two pastes is generally obtained by squeezing two strips of paste of the same length, one from each tube, onto the mixing slab. A flexible stainless steel spatula is typically used for the mixing procedure. The two strips of contrasting colors are combined with the first stroke of the spatula, and the mixing is continued for approximately 1 min, or as directed by the manufacturer, until a uniform color is achieved.

These materials are classified as a hard paste (Type I) or as a soft paste (Type II). The final setting should occur within 10 min for a Type I paste (hard) and 15 min for a Type II paste (soft). When the final set occurs, the impression can be withdrawn from the mouth. The actual time will be shorter when setting occurs in the mouth, since humidity and temperature can accelerate the setting reaction.

Most factors for changing this setting time are solely under the control of the manufacturer. However, the clinician can still use a number of techniques to control the setting time. The setting time can be shortened by adding a small amount of accelerator, a drop of water, or extending the mixing time. To prolong the setting time, the operator can use a cool spatula and mixing slab, or a plasticizer, such as inert oil and wax, can be added.

A paste of a thick consistency or high viscosity can compress the tissues, whereas a thin, fluid material results in an impression that captures a negative replica of the tissues in a relaxed condition with little or no compression. In any event, the impression paste should be homogeneous. Pastes of varying consistencies are commercially available. An advantage of a heavier consistency material is its increased strength.

Dimensional Stability

The dimensional stability of the impression pastes is quite satisfactory. A negligible shrinkage (less than 0.1%) may occur during hardening. No significant dimensional change subsequent to hardening should occur with high-quality commercial products. The impressions can be preserved indefinitely without the change in shape that can result from relaxation or other causes of warpage. This condition can be satisfied only if the tray material is dimensionally stable.

Disinfection

The recommended disinfectant solution for ZOE impression paste is 2% alkaline glutaraldehyde solution. The impressions should be immersed in this solution for the required amount of time, rinsed, and poured immediately (see Table 9-4).

Noneugenol Pastes

One of the chief disadvantages of the ZOE pastes is the possible stinging or burning sensation caused by the eugenol that leaches out and contacts soft tissues. Zinc oxide can react with various carboxylic acids and form ZOE-like materials. Orthoethoxybenzoic acid, commonly abbreviated as EBA, is a valuable substitute for eugenol in this regard. The reaction is well understood, and it is not greatly affected by temperature or humidity. Bactericidal agents and other medicaments can be incorporated without interfering with the reaction.

Surgical Pastes

After a gingivectomy (i.e., the surgical removal of diseased or redundant gingival tissues), a zinc oxide–eugenol paste may be placed over the wound to aid in the retention of a medicament and to promote healing. These pastes are generally softer and slower in their setting reaction in comparison with impression pastes. The mixture should be capable of being formed into a rope that is packed into the gingival wounds and the interproximal spaces to provide retention of the dressing. The final product should be strong enough to resist displacement during mastication, but not so brittle that it shears readily under localized stresses.

Bite Registration Pastes

The materials used for recording the occlusal relationships between natural or artificial teeth include impression plaster, compound, wax, resin, and metal oxide paste. Zinc oxide–eugenol pastes are often used as recording materials in the construction of complete dentures and fixed or removable partial dentures. The ZOE impression paste offers almost no resistance to closing of the mandible, thus allowing a more accurate interocclusal relationship record to be formed. Furthermore, the ZOE interocclusal record is more stable than one made in wax.

SELECTED READINGS

Chai J., and Pang I-C: A study of the "thixotropic" property of elastomeric impression materials. Int J Prosthodont 7:155, 1994.

Chai JY, and Yeung T-C: Wettability of nonaqueous elastomeric impression materials. Int J Prosthodont 4:555, 1991.

Chee WWL, and Donovan TE: Polyvinyl siloxane impression materials: A review of properties and techniques. J Prosthet Dent 68:728, 1992.

Chew C-L, Chee WWL, and Donovan TE: The influence of temperature on the dimensional stability of poly (vinyl siloxane) impression materials. Int J Prosthodont 6:528, 1993.

Craig RG: Review of dental impression materials. Adv Dent Res 2:51, 1988.

Cullen DR, and Sandrik JL: Tensile strength of elastomeric impression materials, adhesive and cohesive bonding. J Prosthet Dent 62:141, 1989.

Davis BA, and Powers JM: Effect of immersion disinfection on properties of impression materials. J Prosthodont 3:31, 1994.

de Camargo LM, Chee WWL, and Donovan TE: Inhibition of polymerization of polyvinyl siloxanes by medicaments used on gingival retraction cords. J Prosthet Dent 70:114, 1993.

Hung SH, Purk JH, Tira DE, and Eick JD: Accuracy of one-step versus two-step putty wash addition silicone impression technique. J Prosthet Dent 67:583, 1992.

Johnson GH, and Craig RG: Accuracy of addition silicone as a function of technique. J Prosthet Dent 55:197, 1986.

Kim K-N, Craig RG, and Koran A: Viscosity of monophase addition silicones as a function of shear rate. J Prosthet Dent 67:794, 1992.

Klooster J, Logan GI, and Tjan AHL: Effects of strain rate on the behavior of elastomeric impressions. J Prosthet Dent 66:292, 1991.

Lim K-C, Chong Y-H, and Soh G: Effect of operator variability on void formation in impressions made with an automixed addition silicone. Aust Dent J 37:35, 1992.

McCormick JT, Antony SJ, Dial ML, et al: Wettability of elastomeric impression materials: Effect of selected surfactants. Int J Prosthodont 2:413, 1989.

Pratten DH, and Novetsky M: Detail reproduction of soft tissue: A comparison of impression materials. J Prosthet Dent 65:188, 1991.

Robinson PB, Dunne SM, and Millar BJ: An in vitro study of a surface wetting agent for addition reaction silicone impressions. J Prosthet Dent 71:390, 1994.

Salem NS, Combe EC, and Watts DC: Mechanical properties of elastomeric impression materials. J Oral Rehab 15:125, 1988.

Sydiskis RK, and Gerhardt DE: Cytotoxicity of impression materials. J Prosthet Dent 69:431, 1993.

Takahashi H, and Finger WJ: Effects of the setting stage on the accuracy of double-mix impressions made with addition-curing silicone. J Prosthet Dent 72:78, 1994.

Wassell RW, and Ibbetson RJ: The accuracy of polyvinyl siloxane impressions made with standard and reinforced stock trays. J Prosthet Dent 645:748, 1992.

10
Gypsum Products

Kenneth J. Anusavice

KEY TERMS

Cast—A reproduction of the shape and features of a surface made from an impression of the surface.

Dental plaster (plaster of Paris)—The beta form of calcium sulfate hemihydrate ($CaSO_4 \cdot \frac{1}{2} H_2O$).

Dental stone—The alpha form of calcium sulfate hemihydrate ($CaSO_4 \cdot \frac{1}{2} H_2O$).

Die—A reproduction of a prepared tooth made from a gypsum product, epoxy resin, a metal, or a refractory material.

Gypsum—Calcium sulfate dihydrate ($CaSO_4 \cdot 2H_2O$).

Gypsum dental investment—A refractory material, consisting of silica and gypsum as a binder, that is used for producing a mold for the metal casting process.

Hygroscopic expansion—The amount of setting expansion that occurs when a gypsum-bonded casting investment is immersed in water (usually heated to approximately 38° C [100° F]).

Model—A positive likeness of an object.

Normal setting expansion—The amount of setting expansion that occurs when a gypsum-bonded casting investment is allowed to set in air.

USES OF GYPSUM IN DENTISTRY

Gypsum ($CaSO_4 \cdot 2H_2O$) is a mineral mined in various parts of the world; however, it is also produced as a by-product of some chemical-processing operations.

Chemically, the gypsum produced for dental applications is nearly pure *calcium sulfate dihydrate* ($CaSO_4 \cdot 2H_2O$). Different crystalline forms of gypsum have been used for centuries for construction purposes and for making artifacts. For instance, it is believed that the alabaster used in the building of King Solomon's temple of biblical fame was a form of gypsum. Products made from gypsum are widely used in industry, and practically all homes and buildings have walls of plaster.

Gypsum products are used in dentistry for the preparation of study models for oral and maxillofacial structures and as important auxiliary materials for dental laboratory operations that are involved in the production of dental prostheses. Various types of **dental plaster** are produced, modified for specific property requirements, and used to form molds and casts on which dental prostheses and restorations are constructed. When plaster is mixed with fillers, such as different forms of silica, it is known as a **gypsum dental investment.** Such dental investments are used to form molds for the casting of dental restorations with molten metal; these are discussed at length in Chapter 12. The present discussion is confined to the relatively pure gypsum products, such as plaster and die stone, that harden when mixed with water.

The use of gypsum-based products in dentistry is widespread. Their use can be demonstrated through a description of the preparation of a cast for a denture. A mixture of **plaster of Paris** (Fig. 10-1) and water is placed in an impression tray and pressed against the tissues of, for example, a patient's edentulous jaw. The plaster is allowed to harden, or *set*, and the impression is withdrawn. The dentist now has a *negative* form of the tissues against which the impression tray was pressed within the oral cavity. If another variety of plaster known as **dental stone** is now mixed with water, poured into the impression, and allowed to set, the hardened plaster impression serves as a mold to form a positive **model,** master **cast,** or **die.** It is on a master cast that the denture is later constructed, without the patient present.

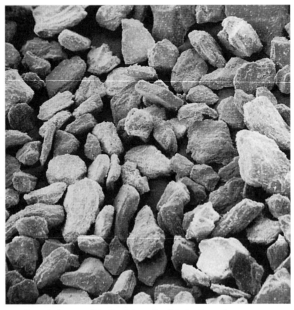

Fig. 10-1 Powder particles of plaster of Paris (β-hemihydrate). Crystals are spongy and irregular in shape. (×400.) (Courtesy of B. Giammara and R. Neiman.)

CRITICAL QUESTION

Why do some gypsum-forming products require more mixing water than others?

DENTAL PLASTER AND STONE
Production of Calcium Sulfate Hemihydrate

Plaster and stone products are produced by calcining calcium sulfate dihydrate, or gypsum. Commercially, the gypsum is ground and subjected to temperatures of 110° to 120° C (230° to 250° F) to drive off part of the water of crystallization that is the amount of water needed to convert $CaSO_4 \cdot 2H_2O$ to $CaSO_4 \cdot \frac{1}{2}H_2O$. This corresponds to the first step in reaction (1). As the temperature is further raised, the remaining water of crystallization is removed, and products are formed as indicated.

$$CaSO_4 \cdot 2H_2O \xrightarrow{110°-130° C} CaSO_4 \cdot \frac{1}{2}H_2O \xrightarrow{130°-200° C} CaSO_4 \xrightarrow{200°-1000° C} CaSO_4$$

| Gypsum (calcium sulfate dihydrate) | Plaster or stone (calcium sulfate hemihydrate) | Hexagonal anhydrite | Orthorhombic anhydrite |

$$(1)$$

The principal constituent of gypsum-based products such as dental plasters and stones is calcium sulfate hemihydrate, that is, $(CaSO_4)_2 \cdot H_2O$ or $CaSO_4 \cdot \frac{1}{2}H_2O$. Depending on the method of calcination, different forms of the hemihydrate can be obtained. These forms are referred to as α-hemihydrate, α-modified hemihydrate, and β-hemihydrate. The use of α and β prefixes seems to suggest two phases from the point of view of the phase rule, but this is not the case. The α and β designations are retained because of tradition and convenience. It should not be inferred that there are mineralogical differences between them. The differences between α- and β-hemihydrates are a result of differences in crystal size, surface area, and degree of lattice perfection. The β form, which is known as dental plaster, consists of large, irregularly shaped orthorhombic crystal particles with capillary pores, whereas the α form consists of smaller, regularly shaped crystalline particles in the form of rods or prisms. The α-modified hemihydrate is made by boiling gypsum in a 30% aqueous solution of calcium chloride and magnesium chloride. This process yields the smoothest, most dense powder particles of the three types, and the powder is used primarily for dies. The α-hemihydrate is called artificial stone, die stone, or improved stone.

If gypsum is heated to the temperatures indicated in the first step of reaction 1 in a vat or rotary kiln open to the air, a crystalline form of the hemihydrate is produced. As can be seen in Figure 10-1, the β-hemihydrate crystals are characterized by their "sponginess" and irregular shape. In contrast, the α-hemihydrate (stone) crystals are more dense and have a prismatic shape. Powder particles of dental stone (α-hemihydrate) are shown in Figure 10-2.

Different procedures can be employed to obtain the hemihydrate. The product of these processes is the principal constituent of the dental stones from which casts and models are made. When α-hemihydrate is mixed with water, reaction 1 is reversed, as described in the next section, and the product obtained is much stronger and harder than that resulting from β-hemihydrate. The chief reason for this difference is that the α-hemihydrate powder requires much less water when it is mixed

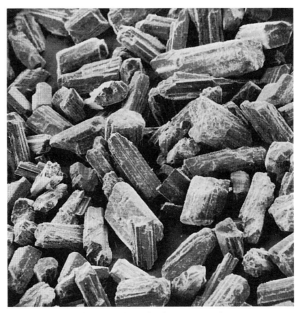

Fig. 10-2   Powder particles of dental stone (α-hemihydrate). Crystals are prismatic and more regular in shape than those of plaster. The very fine particles that are normally present have been removed, as was done for the plaster particles in Figure 10-1. (×400.) (Courtesy of B. Giammara and R. Neiman.)

than does the β-hemihydrate. The β-hemihydrate particles absorb more water, because the crystals are more irregular in shape and are porous in character.

Although particle size and the total surface area are the chief factors in gauging the amount of mixing water, the particle size distribution also plays an important role. Grinding the particles after the preparation of the hemihydrate can eliminate needlelike crystals and provide better packing characteristics, thereby lowering the amount of mixing water required.

Adhesion between the particles of hemihydrate is also a factor in determining the amount of water required to produce a product that can be poured. Small amounts of some surface-active materials, such as gum arabic plus calcium carbonate, added to the hemihydrate can markedly reduce the water requirements of both plaster and dental stone.

From the preceding description, it is clear that various gypsum products require different amounts of water and that these differences are accounted for principally by the shape and compactness of the crystals. These factors are regulated by the manufacturer.

Commercial Gypsum Products

The various commercially available plasters and stones consist mainly of one of the forms of hemihydrate. However, because they are processed products, they contain additional small amounts of impurities such as unconverted hexagonal or orthorhombic anhydrites. Additional gypsum and other salts may also be added to control the setting time and expansion, as discussed in later sections.

SETTING OF GYPSUM PRODUCTS

Reaction 1 described the process of calcining calcium sulfate dihydrate to form calcium sulfate hemihydrate, the starting material used for production of gypsum casts, models, certain casting investments, and impression plasters. The reverse of reaction 1 describes the reaction of calcium sulfate hemihydrate powder with water to produce gypsum:

$$(CaSO_4)_2 \cdot H_2O + 3H_2O \rightarrow 2\,CaSO_4 \cdot 2H_2O + \text{unreacted } (CaSO_4)_2 \cdot \tfrac{1}{2}\,H_2O + \text{Heat} \qquad (2)$$

The product of the reaction is gypsum, and the heat evolved in the exothermic reaction is equivalent to the heat used originally in calcination. Completely set material likely never attains 100% conversion to the dihydrate form unless exposed to high humidity for a long period of time.

The products formed during calcination all react with water to form gypsum, but at different rates. For example, hexagonal anhydrite reacts very rapidly, whereas the reaction may require hours when orthorhombic anhydrite is mixed with water, because the orthorhombic anhydrite has a more stable and closely packed crystal lattice.

Setting Reactions

Nature has provided us with a unique material in gypsum. The various dihydrates have a relatively low solubility, with a distinct difference between the greater solubility of the hemihydrate and that of the dihydrate. The dihydrate is too soluble for use in structures exposed to the atmosphere, which is probably fortunate, because such usage would long ago have exhausted our natural supply of gypsum for dental applications.

The setting reaction of gypsum occurs by dissolution of calcium sulfate hemihydrate, formation of a saturated solution of calcium sulfate, subsequent aggregation of less soluble calcium sulfate dihydrate, and precipitation of the dihydrate crystals. The crystallization of calcium sulfate dihydrate occurs while most of the remaining hemihydrate particles dissolve. Some x-ray diffraction data suggests that hemihydrate particles remain in the set product. Estimates from these data indicate that less than 50% gypsum is present in Type IV and Type V stones, about 60% in Type II die materials, and more than 90% in plasters. These results demonstrate a higher conversion in the weaker set material. Thus one must consider all of the proposed theories for explaining the setting reaction of calcium sulfate hemihydrate into gypsum when reacted with water.

The *colloidal theory* proposes that when mixed with water, plaster enters into the colloidal state through a sol-gel mechanism. In the sol state, hemihydrate particles are hydrated to form dihydrate, thereby entering into an active state. As the measured amount of water is consumed, the mass converts to a solid gel. The *hydration theory* suggests that rehydrated plaster particles join together through hydrogen bonding to the sulfate groups to form the set material. However, the most widely accepted mechanism is the *dissolution-precipitation theory* based on dissolution of plaster and instant recrystallization of gypsum, followed by interlocking of the crystals to form the set solid.

The hemihydrate is four times more soluble in water than is the dihydrate near room temperature (20° C). Thus the setting reactions can be understood as follows:

1. When the hemihydrate is mixed with water, a suspension is formed that is fluid and workable.
2. The hemihydrate dissolves until it forms a saturated solution.
3. This saturated hemihydrate solution, supersaturated in dihydrate, precipitates out dihydrate.

4. As the dihydrate precipitates, the solution is no longer saturated with the hemihydrate, so it continues to dissolve. Dissolution of the hemihydrate and precipitation of the dihydrate proceeds as either new crystals form or further growth occurs on the crystals already present. The reaction is continuous and continues until no further dihydrate precipitates out of solution. The anhydrite is not formed in aqueous media.

The curves in a plot of temperature during setting as a function of time are similar in shape to those shown in Figure 10-5 (discussed later) for compressive strength as a function of time. The peak is reached earlier or later, depending on the setting time. The mass will begin to cool in 5 to 15 min, but the reaction and strengthening process may continue slowly for hours.

The effect of varying the water/powder (W/P) ratio is best illustrated by measuring the compressive strength that develops. Figure 10-3 shows a plot of the strength values that have been measured for the five different types of gypsum products as a function of the W/P ratio. The products represented in Figure 10-3 cover the wide range of gypsum products that are used in dentistry. The figure includes data from many of the products on the market that meet American National Standards Institute/American Dental Association (ANSI/ADA) Specification No. 25 for dental gypsum products and the strength values represent the *wet strength* at 1 hr. The strength values increase as the specimens dry and may double in a week.

As the amount of gypsum increases during the setting period, the mass thickens because of the formation of needlelike crystals. When a lower W/P ratio is used, the crystals grow and, through intergrowth, they form a strong, solid mass. At a W/P ratio near the theoretical limit of 0.18, some of the hemihydrate crystals do not fully dissolve, but they hydrate and still tend to harden the structure.

CRITICAL QUESTION

During mixing of a calcium sulfate hemihydrate product with water, extra water may be added to facilitate the mixing and pouring processes. What three adverse changes may occur when the recommended W/P ratio has been exceeded?

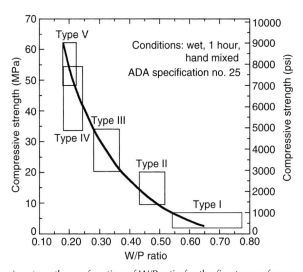

Fig. 10-3   Compressive strength as a function of W/P ratio for the five types of gypsum products.

W/P Ratio

The amounts of water and hemihydrate should be gauged accurately by weight. The ratio of the water to the hemihydrate powder is usually expressed as the W/P ratio, or the quotient obtained when the weight (or volume) of the water is divided by the weight of the powder. The ratio is usually abbreviated as W/P. For example, if 100 g of plaster is mixed with 60 mL of water, the W/P ratio is 0.6; if 100 g of dental stone is mixed with 28 mL of water, the W/P ratio is 0.28. The W/P ratio is an important factor in determining the physical and chemical properties of the final gypsum product. For example, as the W/P ratio increases, the setting time increases, the strength of the gypsum product decreases, and the setting expansion decreases. Although the W/P ratio varies for the particular brand of plaster or stone, the following are some typical recommended ranges: Type II plaster, 0.45 to 0.50; Type III stone, 0.28 to 0.30; and Type IV stone, 0.22 to 0.24. Using plaster or stone that is supplied in preweighed bags sometimes results in mixes that are too thick or too thin. Assuming that the correct amount of water was dispensed in either case, this variation may be caused by the normal variation of the powder mass, typically ± 2%.

TESTS FOR WORKING, SETTING, AND FINAL SETTING TIMES
Mixing Time (MT)

Mixing time is defined as the time from the addition of the powder to the water until the mixing is completed. Mechanical mixing of stones and plasters is usually completed in 20 to 30 sec. Hand-spatulation generally requires at least a minute to obtain a smooth mix.

Working Time (WT)

Working time is the time available to use a workable mix, one that maintains a uniform consistency to perform one or more tasks. It is measured from the start of mixing to the point where the consistency is no longer acceptable for the product's intended purpose. For example, sufficient working time might be needed to pour an impression, pour a spare impression, and clean the equipment before the gypsum fully sets. Generally, a 3-min working time is adequate.

Setting Time (ST)

Reaction 2 requires a definite time for completion. The powder is mixed with water, and the time that elapses from the beginning of mixing until the material hardens is known as the *setting time*. This is usually measured by some type of penetration test, using the instruments shown in Figure 10-4. A number of stages occur in the setting of a gypsum product, as illustrated by use of an actual strength test on a dental model plaster in Figure 10-5. In this figure, 1 min is indicated for the mixing time (MT), with an additional 3 min for the working time (WT), that is, pouring into an impression.

Loss of Gloss Test for Initial Set

As the reaction proceeds, some of the excess water is taken up in forming the dihydrate so that the mix loses its gloss. In Figure 10-5, this loss of gloss (LG) occurred at approximately 9 min, at which time the mass still had no measurable compressive strength. Therefore it could not be safely removed from the mold.

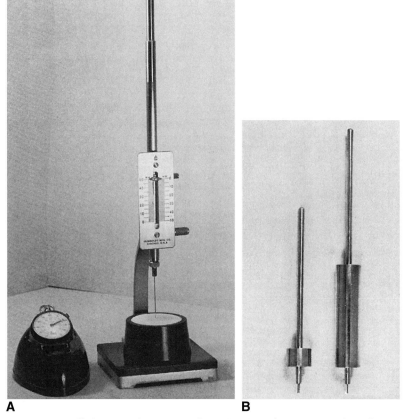

Fig. 10-4   A, Vicat needle being used to measure the setting time of a gypsum product. The setting time is the elapsed time from the start of mix until the needle no longer penetrates to the bottom. **B,** Set of Gillmore needles.

Initial Gillmore Test for Initial Set

On the right side of Figure 10-4 two Gillmore needles are shown. The smaller one is most frequently used for testing the setting time of dental cements, but it is sometimes used on gypsum products. The mixture is spread out, and the needle is lowered onto the surface. The time at which it no longer leaves an impression is called the *initial set*, noted as "Initial Gillmore" on the curve in Figure 10-5. This event is marked by a definite increase in strength. The initial set in the example shown in Figure 10-5 is 13 min.

Vicat Test for Setting Time

The next stage in the reaction is determined by use of another instrument, the Vicat penetrometer seen on the left in Figure 10-4. The needle with a weighted plunger rod is supported and held just in contact with the mix. Soon after the gloss is lost, the plunger is released. The time elapsed until the needle no longer penetrates to the bottom of the mix is known as the *setting time*. In some cases, the Vicat and initial Gillmore measurements occur at the same time, whereas in other instances, there is a small difference, as shown in Figure 10-5.

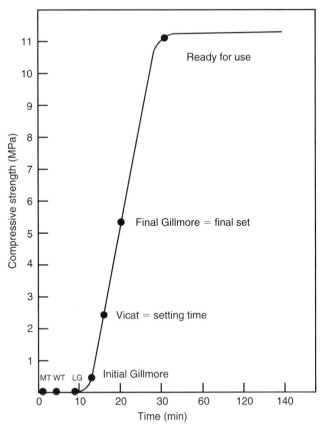

Fig. 10-5 Compressive strength of a Type-II model plaster during setting. The W/P ratio was 0.50. The various stages in the setting reaction are indicated by the particular instruments used in measuring the hardening of the mix. *MT,* mixing time; *WT,* working time; *LG,* loss of gloss from the surface of the mix.

Gillmore Test for Final Setting Time

The next stage in the setting process is measured by the use of the heavier Gillmore needle. The elapsed time at which this needle leaves only a barely perceptible mark on the surface is called the *final setting time.*

Ready-for-Use Criterion

The ready-for-use criterion is a subjective measure of the time at which the set material may be safely handled in the usual manner. The ready-for-use criterion is not determined by any designated test; the ability to judge readiness improves with experience. Technically, the set material may be considered ready for use at the time when the compressive strength is at least 80% of that which would be attained at 1 hr. Most modern products reach the ready-for-use state in approximately 30 min (see Fig. 10-5).

The preceding sections illustrate the stages in the setting of gypsum products. The figures provided apply to one typical model plaster, but the stages vary, depending on the particular product, the W/P ratio, and the time of mixing. Only the Vicat setting time is listed under tables of physical properties. Although manufacturers have developed their own tests for working time, the Vicat test is useful for controlling batch quality.

What are the recommended methods for the operator to accelerate or retard the setting time for a given gypsum-forming product?

CONTROL OF THE SETTING TIME

As previously noted, setting time must be controlled for different applications. Theoretically, at least three methods can achieve such control.

1. The solubility of the hemihydrate can be increased or decreased. For example, if the solubility of the hemihydrate is increased, supersaturation of the calcium sulfate increases, and the rate of crystalline deposition is also increased.

2. The number of nuclei of crystallization can be increased or decreased. The greater the number of nuclei of crystallization, the faster the gypsum crystals form and the sooner the hardening of the mass occurs because of crystalline intermeshing.

3. The setting time can be accelerated or retarded by increasing or decreasing the rate of crystal growth, respectively.

In practice, these methods have been incorporated into the commercial products available. Thus the operator can vary the setting time within reason by changing the W/P ratio and mixing time.

Impurities

If the calcination is not complete and gypsum particles remain, or if the manufacturer adds gypsum, the setting time is shortened because of the increase in potential nuclei of crystallization. If orthorhombic anhydrite is present, the induction period is increased; if hexagonal anhydrite is present, the induction period is decreased.

Fineness

The finer the particle size of the hemihydrate, the faster the mix hardens, particularly if the product has been ground during manufacture. Not only is the rate of the hemihydrate dissolution increased, but the gypsum nuclei are also more numerous. Therefore a more rapid rate of crystallization occurs.

W/P Ratio

The more water used for mixing, the fewer nuclei there are per unit volume. Consequently, the setting time is prolonged. This effect is evidenced by the results presented in Table 10-1.

Mixing

Within practical limits, the longer and the more rapidly the plaster is mixed, the shorter is the setting time. Some gypsum crystals form immediately when the plaster or stone is brought into contact with the water. As the mixing begins, the formation of these crystals increases. At the same time, the crystals are broken up by the mixing spatula and are distributed throughout the mixture, resulting in the formation of more nuclei of crystallization. Thus the setting time is decreased, as indicated in Table 10-1.

Table 10-1	Effect of Water/Powder (W/P) Ratio and Mixing Time on the Setting Time of Plaster of Paris	
W/P ratio	Mixing time (min)	Setting time (min)
0.45	0.5	5.25
0.45	1.0	3.25
0.60	1.0	7.25
0.60	2.0	4.50
0.80	1.0	10.50
0.80	2.0	7.75
0.80	3.0	5.75

From Gibson CS, and Johnson RN: J Soc Chem Ind 51:25T, 1932.

Temperature

An increase in water temperature would usually be expected to accelerate a chemical setting reaction. However, this is not the case for gypsum products. Although the effect of temperature on the setting time is likely to be erratic and may vary from one plaster (or stone) to another, little change occurs between 0° C (32° F) and 50° C (120° F). If the temperature of the plaster-water mixture exceeds 50° C (120° F), a gradual retardation occurs. As the temperature approaches 100° C (212° F), no reaction takes place. At the higher temperature range (50-100° C), reaction 2 is reversed, with the tendency for any gypsum crystals formed to be converted back to the hemihydrate form.

Retarders and Accelerators

Probably the most effective and practical method for controlling the setting time is the addition of certain chemical modifiers to the mixture of plaster or dental stone. If the chemical added decreases the setting time, it is known as an *accelerator*; if it increases the setting time, it is known as a *retarder*.

Retarders generally act by forming an adsorbed layer on the hemihydrate to reduce its solubility and on the gypsum crystals present to inhibit growth. Organic materials, such as glue, gelatin, and some gums, behave in this manner. Another type of retarder consists of salts that form a layer of a calcium salt that is less soluble than is the sulfate. These may include borax, potassium citrate, and sodium chloride (20%). In small concentrations, many inorganic salts (such as sodium chloride) act as accelerators, but when the concentration is increased, they can become retarders. Because the action of these chemical additions also affects other properties such as setting expansion, the behavior of accelerators and retarders will be discussed further in a subsequent section.

The operator should attempt to control the setting time by adding retarders or accelerators to the calcium sulfate hemihydrate powder. The setting time can be accelerated by adding gypsum (<20%), potassium sulfate, or sodium chloride (<28%). The gypsum is typically added by including a small percentage of slurry water in the mixing water. However, a significantly greater amount of powder should not be added to accelerate the reaction because it may be difficult to produce a product with optimal flow characteristics. If a substantially accelerated setting process is desired, the operator should instead purchase a fast-setting product. As an alternative, either the mixing time or the mixing rate may be increased slightly to accelerate the setting reaction; however, any increase in mixing time or mixing rate must be accommodated within the working time for the specific product.

To increase the setting time, select a product from the manufacturer's catalog that is designed with a longer setting time. The use of cooler water will not have a significant effect on the setting time. Thus, to ensure the longest working time, one should purchase a regular setting product and/or use minimum mixing times and slower rates of mixing.

SETTING EXPANSION

Regardless of the type of gypsum product employed, an expansion of the mass can be detected during the change from the hemihydrate to the dihydrate. Depending on the composition of the gypsum product, this observed linear expansion may be as low as 0.06% or as high as 0.5%.

On the other hand, if equivalent volumes of the hemihydrate, water, and the reaction product (dihydrate) are compared, the volume of the dihydrate formed will be less than the equivalent volumes of the hemihydrate and water. This represents a linear change in the gypsum object of approximately 2.4%. Thus, according to these calculations, a volumetric contraction should occur during the setting reaction. However, a setting expansion is observed instead; this phenomenon can be rationalized on the basis of the crystallization mechanism.

The calculations are as follows:

	$(CaSO_4)_2 \cdot H_2O$	+	$3H_2O$	→	$2CaSO_4 \cdot 2H_2O$	
Molecular mass	290.284		54.048		344.332	
Density (g/cm^3)	2.75		0.997		2.32	
Equivalent volume	*105.556*		*54.211*		*148.405*	
Total volume		159.767			148.405	(3)

The net change in volume is (148.405 − 159.767)/(159.767) 100, or −7.11%. This change can also be shown by the sol-gel theory in which a shrinkage should occur when the sol converts to a gel. However, this shrinkage cannot be measured, because it takes place while the mixture is in the fluid state.

As previously noted, the crystallization process is pictured as an outgrowth of crystals from nuclei of crystallization. On the basis of the entanglement of the dihydrate crystals, crystals growing from the nuclei can intermesh with and obstruct the growth of adjacent crystals.

If this process is repeated by thousands of the crystals during growth, an outward stress or thrust develops that produces an expansion of the entire mass. Thus a setting expansion will take place even though the *true volume* of the crystals alone will be less as calculated above. This crystal impingement and movement result in the production of micropores.

Because the product of the setting reaction for gypsum (see reaction 2) in practice is greater in external volume but less in *crystalline* volume, it follows that the set material must be porous. Therefore the structure immediately after setting is composed of interlocking crystals, between which are micropores and pores containing the excess water required for mixing. On drying, the excess water is lost, and the void space is increased.

As far as the technician or dentist is concerned, only the setting expansion that occurs after the initial set is of interest. Any expansion or contraction that occurs before this time can be overcome by friction between the mold surface against which the fluid mixture is poured. At the time of the initial set, the crystalline framework is sufficiently rigid that it can overcome, for the most part, such frictional retention. However, it cannot always overcome any confinement by the mold boundaries, such as the walls of a cylindrical metal ring. Furthermore, any initial contraction that occurs during the induction period does not affect the accuracy, because the mix is fluid at this stage and the contraction occurs at the free surface.

If a mixture of plaster and water is spread on a glass surface, the distance between any two surface reference points will not change appreciably during the induction period. The adhesion of the water-powder mix to the glass can prevent the linear contraction that is theoretically expected. Only when the crystalline framework is sufficiently rigid (after the initial set) is a visible setting expansion evident.

When sufficient crystals form to produce the outward thrust by impingement, setting expansion follows. The initial setting time occurs approximately at the minimal point of the curve, the point at which the expansion begins. According to the graph in Figure 10-6, the stone actually has shrunk during setting and it has not recovered its original dimensions. On the other hand, in the previous experiment on the glass plate, a setting expansion of approximately 0.12% would have been reported.

CRITICAL QUESTION

What is the most effective way to increase or decrease the setting expansion of gypsum?

Control of Setting Expansion

Sometimes a setting expansion is advantageous for a dental procedure; sometimes it is disadvantageous, because it may be a source of error. Consequently, setting expansion must be controlled to obtain the desired accuracy in dental applications.

As can be noted from the results presented in Table 10-2, a lower W/P ratio and a longer mixing time increases the setting expansion. Each of these factors increases the nuclei density. The effect of the W/P ratio on the setting expansion is to be expected on a theoretical basis. At higher W/P ratios, fewer nuclei of crystallization per unit volume are present than with the thicker mixes. Because it can be assumed

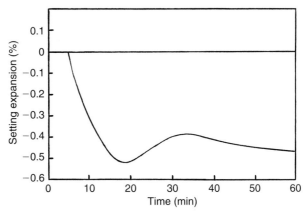

Fig. 10-6 Dimensional changes that occur during the setting of a gypsum product. (Courtesy of A.R. Docking.)

Table 10-2	Effect of Water/Powder (W/P) Ratio and Mixing Time on Setting Expansion of Plaster of Paris	
W/P ratio	Mixing time (min)	Setting expansion (%)
0.45	0.6	0.41
0.45	1.0	0.51
0.60	1.0	0.29
0.60	2.0	0.41
0.80	1.0	0.24

From Gibson CS, and Johnson RN: J Soc Chem Ind 51:25T, 1932.

that the space between the nuclei is greater in such a case, it follows that there is less growth interaction of the dihydrate crystals and less outward thrust. However, the most effective method for controlling the setting expansion is through the addition of chemicals by the manufacturer. The setting expansion can be reduced by adding either potassium sulfate, sodium chloride, or borax.

ACCELERATORS AND RETARDERS: PRACTICE AND THEORY

Why are accelerators and retarders used? In industry, the gypsum product requires a gradual set or hardening so that the object may be formed or shaped over time. However, its use in dentistry generally involves pouring or vibrating the mix into a mold, with careful control of flow requiring only a few minutes. At the end of the working time, the material should harden rapidly, and it should be ready for use within 30 min or less.

Figure 10-7 illustrates the interplay of accelerators and retarders on the strength (in MPa units) of plaster. The same effects hold true for other gypsum products, including investments used for casting or hot-pressing situations. The curve at the right shows the rate of hardening of a natural plaster, that is, β hemihydrate. It has only a few minutes of working time and then hardens gradually, usually too slowly for dental use. The addition of an accelerator (the curve at the left) produces a set that makes it possible to use the plaster within 30 min. However, the working time has been seriously reduced. Therefore, a retarder must be also added (the curve in the middle) to make a usable plaster. This increases the latent initial setting period so that the mix retains a reasonable plastic state that permits handling or working it into a useful shape. Then the mass hardens in time for use.

Not only do the chemical accelerators and retarders regulate the setting time of the gypsum products, but also they generally reduce the setting expansion. The theory of such effects is still not confirmed.

Accelerators

Because the rate of setting is influenced by the rate of hemihydrate dissolution, it is logical to assume that materials which increase the rate of dissolution also accelerate the setting reaction. However, the rate of precipitation of the dihydrate is also important. Therefore the accelerator must increase the solubility of the hemihydrate without also increasing the solubility of the dihydrate. Thus the acceleration caused by an additive depends on the amount and rate of solubility of the hemihydrate versus the same effect on the dihydrate.

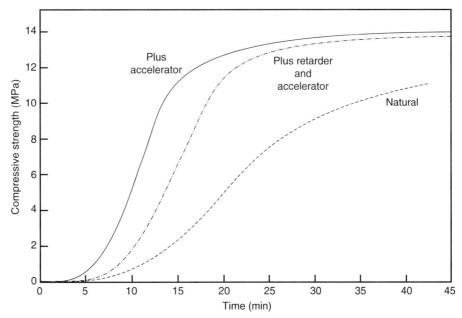

Fig. 10-7   Compressive strength of a model plaster plotted against time when accelerators and retarders are added to the plaster. The gain in strength is a measure of the rate of hardening or setting.

To further complicate matters, although inorganic salts are often accelerators, they can also become retarders when more than a certain amount is added. Sodium chloride is an accelerator up to about 2% of the hemihydrate, but at a higher concentration, it acts as a retarder. Sodium sulfate has its maximum acceleration effect at approximately 3.4%; at greater concentrations, it becomes a retarder.

The most commonly used accelerator is potassium sulfate. It is particularly effective in concentrations higher than 2%, since the reaction product, which seems to be syngenite ($K_2Ca[SO_4]_2 \cdot H_2O$), crystallizes rapidly. Many soluble sulfates act as accelerators, whereas powdered gypsum (calcium sulfate dihydrate) accelerates the setting rate, because the particles act as nuclei of crystallization. A slurry of ground gypsum casts (called slurry water) acts in this way, although the clear saturated liquid is hardly effective. It takes the crystals themselves to accelerate the setting. Thus the slurry water should be agitated before use. Another way of accomplishing this effect is to increase either or both the time and the speed of mixing, because this increases the formation of nuclei, thereby accelerating the mix. Decreasing the mixing time or adding more water will retard the reaction. However, the addition of excess water may adversely alter the properties of the gypsum.

Retarders

The behavior of retarders is even more complicated. The common belief is that certain chemicals form a coating on the hemihydrate particles and thus prevent the hemihydrate from going into solution in the normal manner.

Citrates, acetates, and borates generally retard the reaction. For a given anion, the particular cation employed appears to affect the retardation markedly. For example, with the acetates, the order of retardation in terms of the cation employed appears to be $Ca^+ < K^+ < H^+$, whereas potassium tartrate has a marked accelerating effect in contrast with the calcium salt, which has little effect on setting. The behavior of citrates is more complex.

Because the manufacturer has already added accelerators and retarders and other controlling agents, it is not wise to add other ingredients because they may counteract the effects already incorporated into the product.

HYGROSCOPIC SETTING EXPANSION

In the discussion thus far, the plaster or stone has been assumed to set in air. If the setting process is instead allowed to occur under water (usually at an elevated temperature), the setting expansion may more than double in magnitude. One possible reason for increased expansion is the expansion of the wax pattern during setting of the investment. The most well-accepted reason for the increased expansion when the hemihydrate reacts under water is the additional crystal growth permitted by allowing the crystals to grow freely, rather than being constrained by the surface tension when the crystals form in air.

This theory is illustrated diagrammatically in Figure 10-8. In Stage I, shown at the top of the figure, the initial mix is represented by the three round particles of hemihydrate surrounded by water.

In Stage II, the reaction has started and the crystals of the dihydrate are beginning to form. In the diagram on the left, the water around the particles is reduced by hydration and these particles are drawn more closely together by the surface tension of the water. In the right-hand diagram, because the setting is taking place under water, the water of hydration is replaced and the distance between the particles remains the same.

As the dihydrate crystals grow, they contact each other, and setting expansion begins. As indicated in Stage III, the water around the particles decreases in the example on the left. The particles with their attached crystals tend to be drawn together as before, but the contraction is opposed by the outward thrust of the growing crystals. On the other hand, the crystals in the diagram on the right are not as inhibited, because the water is again replenished from the outside. In fact, the orig-

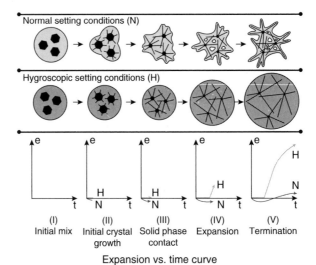

Fig. 10-8 Diagrammatic representation of the setting expansion of plaster. In the left column, the crystal growth is inhibited by the lack of excess water. As shown in the right column, water added during setting provides more room for longer crystal growth. *e*, expansion; *t*, time; *H*, hygroscopic setting expansion; *N*, normal setting expansion. (From Mahler DB, and Ady AB: Explanation for the hygroscopic setting expansion of dental gypsum products. J Dent Res 39:578, 1960.)

inal particles are now separated further as the crystals grow, and the setting expansion is definitely evident.

In Stages IV and V, the effect becomes more marked. The crystals that are inhibited on the left become intermeshed and entangled much sooner than those on the right, which grow much more freely during the early stages before the intermeshing finally prevents further expansion. Consequently, the observed setting expansion that occurs when the gypsum product sets under water may be greater than that which occurs during setting in air.

It follows, therefore, that the basic mechanism of crystal growth is the same in both instances, and both phenomena are true setting expansions. To distinguish between them, the setting expansion without water immersion is usually called **normal setting expansion** (see N in Fig. 10-8), whereas the expansion that occurs under water is known as **hygroscopic setting expansion** (see H in Fig. 10-8). The hygroscopic setting expansion is physical and is not caused by a chemical reaction any more than is the normal setting expansion. The reduction in the W/P ratio increases the hygroscopic setting expansion and the normal setting expansion in the same manner. Increased spatulation results in increased **hygroscopic expansion** as well.

Although the crystal interlocking theory represents a logical explanation of setting expansion, it is not the only theory. Setting expansion of gypsum may also be explained by simple hydrostatic pressure that develops in the water during setting.

The hygroscopic expansion obtained during the setting of dental stone or plaster is generally small in magnitude. For example, a dental stone used in making casts may exhibit a normal linear setting expansion of 0.15%, with a maximum hygroscopic expansion of not more than 0.30%. Nevertheless, this difference may be sufficient to cause the misfit of a denture or similar device made on the cast.

On the other hand, as explained in Chapter 12, the greater hygroscopic setting expansion of gypsum-bonded casting investments is sometimes used in the fabrication of cast restorations.

STRENGTH

The strength of gypsum products is generally expressed in terms of compressive strength, although tensile strength should also be considered in order to secure a satisfactory guide to the total strength characteristics.

As might be expected from the theory of setting, the strength of plaster or stone increases rapidly as the material hardens after the initial setting time. However, the free-water content of the set product definitely affects its strength. For this reason, two strength properties of gypsum are reported: the *wet strength* (also known as *green strength*) and the *dry strength*. The wet strength is the strength obtained when the water in excess of that required for hydration of the hemihydrate is left in the test specimen. When the excess water in the specimen has been driven off by drying, the strength obtained is the dry strength. The dry strength may be two or more times as high as the wet strength. Consequently, the distinction between the two is of considerable importance.

The effect of drying on the compressive strength of set plaster is shown in Table 10-3. Note the relatively slight gains in strength that occurred after 16 hr. Between an 8-hr and 24-hr period, only 0.6% of the excess water was lost, and yet the strength doubled. A somewhat similar change in surface hardness takes place during the drying process.

A good explanation of this effect is the fact that as the last traces of water leave, fine crystals of gypsum precipitate. These anchor the larger crystals. Then, if water is

Table 10-3	Effect of Drying on the Compressive Strength of Plaster of Paris		
	Compressive strength		
Drying period (hr)	(MPa)	(psi)	Loss in weight (%)
2	9.6	1400	5.1
4	11.7	1700	11.9
8	11.7	1700	17.4
16	13.0	1900	—
24	23.3	3400	18.0
48	23.3	3400	18.0
72	23.3	3400	—

From Gibson CS, and Johnson RN: J Soc Chem Ind 51:25T, 1932.

added or if excess water is present, these small crystals are the first to dissolve, and thus the reinforcing anchors are lost.

As previously noted, the set plaster or stone is porous in nature, and the greater the W/P ratio, the greater will be the porosity. As might be expected on such a basis, the greater the W/P ratio, the less is the dry strength of the set material, as shown by the data in Table 10-4, because the greater the porosity, the fewer crystals are available per unit volume for a given weight of hemihydrate.

The materials mixed at a high W/P ratio have tensile strengths as high as 25% of the corresponding compressive strength. When materials are mixed at low W/P ratios, the tensile strength is less than 10% of the corresponding compressive strength.

As shown in Table 10-4, the spatulation time also affects the strength of the plaster. In general, with an increase in mixing time, the strength is increased to a limit that is approximately equivalent to that of hand mixing for 1 min. If the mixture is overmixed, the gypsum crystals formed are broken up, and less crystalline interlocking results in the final product.

The addition of an accelerator or retarder lowers both the wet and the dry strengths of the gypsum product. Such a decrease in strength can be partially attributed to the salt added as an adulterant and to the reduction in intercrystalline cohesion.

Table 10-4	Effect of the Water/Powder (W/P) Ratio and Mixing Time on the Compressive Strength of Plaster of Paris		
	Compressive strength		
W/P ratio	Mixing time (min)	(MPa)	(psi)
0.45	0.5	23.4	3400
0.45	1.0	26.2	3800
0.60	1.0	17.9	2600
0.60	2.0	13.8	2000
0.80	1.0	11.0	1600

From Gibson CS, and Johnson, RN: J Soc Chem Ind 51:25T, 1932.

When relatively pure hemihydrate is mixed with minimal amounts of water, the working time is short and the setting expansion is unduly high. However, as just noted, dental gypsum products contain additives that reduce the setting expansion, increase the working time, and provide a rapid final set. The addition of more chemicals can upset the delicate balance of these properties. Thus if a change is desired in the setting time, it should be done by modest alterations in either or both the W/P ratio and the spatulation time.

TYPES OF GYPSUM PRODUCTS

Having discussed the basic principles of gypsum products, we turn our attention to the various types of dental gypsum and practical considerations in their use. The criteria for selection of any particular gypsum product depend on its use and the physical properties necessary for that particular use. For example, dental stone is a poor material for use as an impression material, because if teeth are present, the high strength of the stone (α hemihydrate) makes it impossible to remove the impression over the undercuts in the teeth without injury. On the other hand, if a strong cast is required on which to build a denture, a weak plaster (β-hemihydrate) should not be chosen. In other words, there is no all-purpose dental gypsum product.

The various types of gypsum products can be seen in Table 10-5. Listed are the five types identified by ANSI/ADA Specification No. 25 and the properties required for each.

Impression Plaster (Type I)

These impression materials are composed of plaster of Paris, to which modifiers have been added to regulate the setting time and the setting expansion. Impression plaster is rarely used anymore for dental impressions, because it has been replaced

| Table 10-5 | Typical Properties* of the Five Types of Gypsum Products |

Type	W/P ratio	Setting time (min)	2-Hr setting expansion (%)		1-Hr compressive strength[†]	
			Min	Max	(MPa)	(psi)
I. Plaster, impression	0.40–0.75	4±1	0.00	0.15	4.0	580
II. Plaster, model	0.45–0.50	12±4	0.00	0.30	9.0	1300
III. Dental stone[‡]	0.28–0.30	12±4	0.00	0.20	20.7	3000
IV. Dental stone, high strength[§]	0.22–0.24	12±4	0.00	0.10	34.5	5000
V. Dental stone, high strength, high expansion	0.18–0.22	12±4	0.10	0.30	48.3	7000

*Properties required in the five gypsum products covered by ANSI/ADA Specification No. 25.
[†]Minimum values.
[‡]Dental stone, sometimes designated as Class I stone or Hydrocal.
[§]Dental stone, high strength, sometimes designated as Class II stone, densite, or improved stone.

by less rigid materials, such as the hydrocolloids and elastomers (discussed in Chapter 9). Plaster is primarily restricted to use as a final impression (*wash impression*) in the construction of full dentures.

Model Plaster (Type II)

Model plaster, or laboratory Type II plaster, is now used principally to fill a flask in denture construction when setting expansion is not critical and the strength is adequate, according to the limits cited in the specification. It is usually marketed in the natural white color, thus contrasting with stones that are generally colored. Type II model plaster is relatively weak as evidenced by a compressive strength as low as 9 MPa and a tensile strength of 0.6 MPa.

Dental Stone (Type III)

In 1930 a major milestone was established when α-gypsum was discovered and introduced within dentistry. Combined with the advent of hydrocolloid impression material, the improved hardness of α-gypsum made stone dies workable, and the indirect pattern became possible.

Dentistry shared in the greatest improvement in plaster that has been made in all of history. A researcher at U.S. Gypsum Corporation learned that the plaster mold used for forming rubber denture bases in a vulcanizer under steam pressure became unusually hard overnight. Examination showed that the set gypsum, calcined under steam pressure, formed a much better quality of crystallized calcium sulfate hemihydrate. Because of this improvement, the product was soon thereafter patented as α-gypsum. Since this discovery, the process has been performed commercially in an autoclave.

Type III stone has a minimum 1-hr compressive strength of 20.7 MPa (3000 psi), but it does not exceed 34.5 MPa (5000 psi). It is intended for construction of *casts* in the fabrication of full dentures that fit soft tissues. Stone *dies* are reproductions of prepared teeth, on or within which prostheses are constructed. Because of the severe wear conditions that occur at the margins during carving of wax patterns and because of the higher stresses induced in stone dies during try-in and adjustments, greater strength and hardness are required of die materials. This type of stone is discussed in the following sections. In addition, a slight setting expansion can be tolerated in casts that reproduce soft tissues, but not when a tooth is involved. Type III stones are preferred for casts used to process dentures, because the stone has adequate strength for that purpose and the denture is easier to remove after processing.

Regardless of the type of stone used, there are at least two methods for the construction of the cast. In one method, a mold for the cast is constructed by wrapping soft, flat, wax strips around the impression so that they extend approximately 12 mm beyond the tissue side of the impression. A base for the cast is formed in this region. This process is called *boxing*. The mixture of stone and water is then poured into the impression under vibration. The mixture is allowed to flow slowly in a controlled pathway along the impression, so that it pushes the air ahead of itself as it fills all tooth impressions without entrapment of air bubbles.

Another method is to first fill the impression, as described, and then pour the remainder of the stone-water mixture on a glass plate. The filled impression is then inverted over the mound of stone, and the base is shaped with the spatula before the stone sets. Such a procedure is not indicated if an easily deformed impression material has been used or if the stone is "runny." The cast should not be separated from the impression until it has initially hardened. The minimum time allowed for setting varies from 30 to 60 minutes, depending on the setting rate of the stone or plaster and the type of impression material used. For a stiffer impression material like polyether, a minimum setting time of 60 minutes should be allowed to minimize the risk of fracturing teeth during removal of a cast.

CRITICAL QUESTION

Under what condition should a Type V gypsum die material be used rather than a Type IV material?

Dental Stone, High Strength (Type IV)

The principal requisites for a die material stone are strength, hardness, abrasion resistance, and minimum setting expansion. To obtain these properties, one should use an α-hemihydrate of the "Densite" type. The cuboidal-shaped particles (Fig. 10-9) and the reduced surface area produce such properties without undue thickening of the mix. Summarized in Table 10-5 are some of the physical properties of Type IV stones compared with those of Type III stones.

A hard surface is necessary for a die stone, because the cavity preparation is filled with wax that is carved flush with the margins of the die. A sharp instrument is used for this purpose; therefore, the stone must be resistant to abrasion. Gypsum-hardening solutions, silver-plating, and other methods of increasing the abrasion resistance are discussed in Chapter 12. Because the surface dries more rapidly, the surface hardness increases more rapidly than does the compressive strength. This is a real advantage in that the surface resists abrasion, whereas the core of the die is tough and less subject to accidental breakage. The average dry surface hardness of the Type IV stones ("die stones") is approximately 92 (Rockwell Hardness); that of Type III

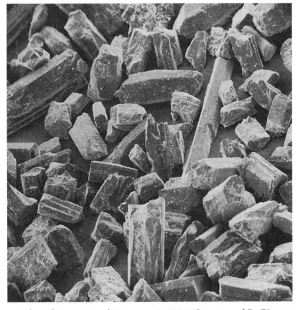

Fig. 10-9 Powder particles of Type IV and V stones. (×400.) (Courtesy of B. Giammara and R. Neiman.)

stone is 82. Even though the surface of the Type IV stone is harder, care should be observed when the pattern is being carved.

Dental Stone, High Strength, High Expansion (Type V)

The Type V dental stone gypsum product exhibits an even higher compressive strength than does the Type IV dental stone. The improved strength is attained by making it possible to lower the W/P ratio even further than that of Type IV stone. In addition, the setting expansion has been increased from a maximum of 0.10% to 0.30% (see Table 10-5). The rationale for the increase in setting expansion limits is that certain newer alloys, such as base metal, have a greater casting shrinkage than do the traditional noble metal alloys. Thus higher expansion is required in the stone used for the die to aid in compensating for the alloy solidification shrinkage. The use of a Type V stone may also be indicated when inadequate expansion may have been achieved during the fabrication of cast crowns. The use of Type V stones should be avoided in the production of dies for inlays, since the higher expansion may lead to unacceptably tight fits. Additional information on the use of Type IV and V stones, other die materials, and gypsum-bonded investments is provided in the discussion of die materials in Chapter 12.

Synthetic Gypsum

It is also possible to make α-hemihydrates and β-hemihydrates from the by-products or waste products of phosphoric acid production. The synthetic product is usually much more expensive than that made from natural gypsum, but when the product is properly made, its properties are equal to, or exceed those of, the latter. The processing problems are considerable, and few have succeeded. Because the methods employed are trade secrets, no further discussion is appropriate. For our purpose, the source of the hemihydrate is not as important as the nature and use of the final product, which is essentially the same regardless of the origin.

PROPORTIONING, MIXING, AND CARING FOR GYPSUM PRODUCTS
Proportioning

Because the strength of a stone is inversely proportional to the W/P ratio, it is important to keep the amount of water as low as possible. However, it should not be so low that the mix will not flow into every detail of the impression. Once the optimum W/P is determined (using the manufacturer's suggested W/P ratio as a guide) the same proportions should be used subsequently. The water and powder should be measured by using an accurate graduated cylinder for the water volume and a weighing balance for the powder. The powder should not be measured volume (use of a scoop), because powder varies from product to product and does not pack uniformly. Powder will pack harder as the container remains unused. If the container is shaken, the volume increases as a result of entrapment of air. Preweighed envelopes have become popular, because they promote accuracy, reduce waste, and save time.

Mixing

If mixing is performed by hand, the bowl should be parabolic in shape, smooth, and resistant to abrasion. The spatula should have a stiff blade and a handle that is convenient to hold. Entrapment of air in the mix must be avoided to prevent porosity, leading to weak spots and surface inaccuracies, as illustrated in Figure 10-10. The use of an automatic vibrator of high frequency and low amplitude is helpful. Place a measured amount of water in the bowl, and sift the weighed powder into the water as initial hand mixing is performed. Then stir the mixture vigorously, periodically wiping the inside of the bowl with the spatula to ensure the wetting of all of the powder and the breaking up of any agglomerates, or lumps. Continue mixing until a smooth mix is obtained, usually within a minute. A longer spatulation time drastically reduces the working time (see Table 10-1), particularly for pouring models.

The guesswork of repeatedly adding water and powder to achieve the proper consistency must be avoided, because this yields a lower strength and it may cause distortion, one of the main causes of inaccuracy in the use of gypsum products.

The preferred method of mixing is to add the measured water first, followed by gradual addition of the preweighed powder. The powder is incorporated during approximately 15 sec of mixing with a hand spatula, followed by 20 to 30 sec of mechanical mixing under vacuum. In this way, a properly mixed stone results in a solid cast (Fig. 10-11). The strength and hardness obtained in such mechanical vacuum mixing usually exceed that obtained by 1 min of hand mixing.

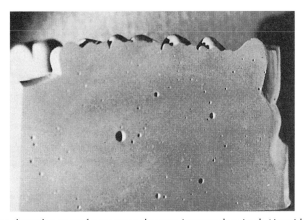

Fig. 10-10 Section through a cast of a set stone that was improperly mixed. Air voids weaken the stone and impair its appearance.

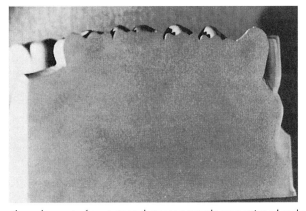

Fig. 10-11 Section through a cast of a set stone that was properly proportioned and mixed.

Caring for the Cast

If the surface of the cast is not hard and smooth when it is removed from the impression, its accuracy is questionable. The cast should be an accurate reproduction of the oral tissues, and any departure from the expected accuracy will probably result in a poorly fitting prosthesis. Therefore the cast should be handled carefully. Once the setting reactions in the cast have been completed, its dimensions will be relatively constant thereafter under ordinary conditions of room temperature and humidity. However, it is sometimes necessary to soak the gypsum cast in water, in preparation for other techniques. The gypsum cast is slightly soluble in water. When a dry cast is immersed in water, negligible expansion may occur, provided that the water is saturated with calcium sulfate. If it is not so saturated, gypsum may be dissolved. If the stone cast is immersed in running water, its linear dimension may decrease approximately 0.1% for every 20 min of immersion. The safest method for soaking the cast is to place it in a water bath made for the purpose, in which plaster debris is allowed to remain constantly on the bottom of the container to provide a saturated solution of calcium sulfate.

As previously noted, storage of either set plaster or stone at room temperature produces no significant dimensional change. However, if the storage temperature is raised to between 90° and 110° C (194° to 230° F), shrinkage occurs as the water of crystallization is removed and the dihydrate reverts to the hemihydrate. The contraction of plaster at high temperature is greater than that of the stone, and it also loses strength.

Such contractions may occur during storage in air above room temperature, such as when a stone cast is dried. It is not safe to store or heat a stone cast in air at a temperature higher than 55° C (130° F).

Special Gypsum Products

In addition to the standardized gypsum materials already described, there are some gypsum products that have been characterized for special purposes. For example, the orthodontist prefers a white stone or plaster for study models and may even treat the surface with soap for an added sheen. These products generally have a longer working time for ease of trimming.

The use of an articulator makes it necessary to mount the casts with a gypsum product, as shown in Figure 10-12. These materials are referred to as *mounting* stones or plasters. Both mounting stones and plasters are fast-setting and have low setting expansion. Mounting plaster, in particular, has low strength to permit easy trimming and to separate the cast readily from the articulator mounting plates.

Since 1991, a plethora of new dental stones have been introduced, mostly marketed as time savers. One type is extremely fast-setting and ready to use in 5 min, but it has little working time. Another product changes color to help denote when it is ready for use. Most recently, another trend is the addition of a small amount of plastic or resin, which reduces brittleness and improves resistance to abrasion during the carving of wax patterns.

Usually, in the production of new gypsum products, when one feature is improved, another feature is sacrificed. For instance, a faster set may be accepted in

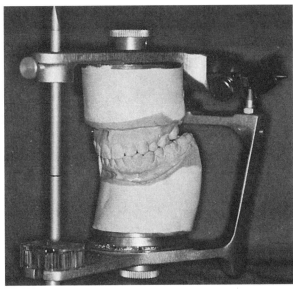

Fig. 10-12 Dental articulator, a device that incorporates artificial temporomandibular joints. This permits orientation of casts in a manner that simulates various positions of the mandible. (Courtesy of C. Munoz.)

return for less working time. An improved resistance to carving may be gained in return for greater difficulty in manipulation, a decrease in detail reproduction, or the need to box the impression because of excessive runniness. On the other hand, improvements in materials and testing equipment have made it possible to use silicone/stone combinations that can reproduce spaces between lines as fine as 10 μm or less. Current specifications require an accuracy of only 50 μm.

Currently, a wide choice of gypsum products is available to suit almost any desired individual requirements or combinations thereof.

Caring for Gypsum Products

Gypsum products are somewhat sensitive to changes in the relative humidity of their environment. Even the surface hardness of plaster and stone casts may fluctuate slightly with the relative humidity of the atmosphere. Gypsum surfaces made with thinner mixes appear to be affected more than those with a low W/P ratio.

The hemihydrate of gypsum takes up water from the air readily. For example, if the relative humidity exceeds 70%, the plaster takes up sufficient water vapor to start a setting reaction. The first hydration probably produces a few particles of gypsum on the surface of the hemihydrate crystal. These crystals act as nuclei of crystallization, and the first manifestation of the plaster deterioration is a decrease in the setting time.

As the hygroscopic action continues, more particles of gypsum form until the entire hemihydrate crystal is covered. Under these conditions, the water penetrates the dihydrate coating with difficulty, and the setting time is unduly prolonged. Therefore it is important that all types of gypsum products be stored in a dry atmosphere. The best means of storage is to seal the product in a moisture-proof metal container. When gypsum products are stored in closed containers, the setting time is generally retarded only slightly, approximately 1 or 2 min per year. This may be counteracted by a slight increase in the mixing time if necessary.

CRITICAL QUESTION

What procedure should be followed if it is unknown whether the impression or the gyp-sum cast has been disinfected?

INFECTION CONTROL

As noted elsewhere in this textbook, there is increased interest in expanding infection control measures to the dental laboratory. Concern over possible cross-contamination to dental office personnel by microorganisms, including hepatitis B virus and human immunodeficiency virus, via dental impressions has prompted study of the effect of spray and immersion-disinfecting techniques on impression materials, as discussed in Chapter 9. The effect of such agents on the surface quality and accuracy of the resulting gypsum casts is an important consideration.

If an impression has not been disinfected (see Chapter 9), or if the laboratory has no assurance that an appropriate disinfection protocol was followed, it is necessary to disinfect the stone cast. Disinfection solutions can be used that do not adversely affect the quality of the gypsum cast. Alternatively, a dental stone containing a disinfectant may also be employed. Although the addition of a disinfectant may have a slight effect on some physical properties of certain products, the disinfected stones apparently compare favorably with the nondisinfected controls.

The widespread availability of a spectrum of disinfecting dental stones (Types II to V) with proven efficacy and unimpaired physical properties would undoubtedly strengthen the barrier system of infection control in the dental laboratory. When patients with known cases of infection are being treated, overnight gas sterilization is an option. However, this procedure is impractical for routine use by practitioners and dental laboratory personnel. Useful disinfectants for stone casts include spray disinfectants, hypochlorites, and iodophors. Proper disinfection conditions provided by the manufacturer should be followed whenever possible.

In the United States, the incorporation of disinfectants in dental stones has been delayed by failure to obtain approval by the U.S. Food and Drug Administration.

SELECTED READINGS

Bailey JH, Donovan TE, and Preston JD: The dimensional accuracy of improved dental stone, silver-plated, and epoxy resin die materials. J Prosthet Dent 59:307, 1988.
Silver-plated and epoxy resin die systems were found to be acceptable alternative systems to the improved dental stones.

Dilts WE, Duncanson MG Jr, and Collard EW: Comparative stability of cast mounting materials. J Okla Dent Assoc 68:11, 1978.
Certain properties of mounting gypsum products are cited, particularly their low setting expansion.

Donovan T, and Chee WWL: Preliminary investigation of a disinfected gypsum die stone. Int J Prosthodont 2:245, 1989.
Two such die materials were found comparable with existing products in almost all physical properties tested. One of the new materials was weaker in compressive and tensile strength and deficient in detail reproduction.

Jørgensen KD: Studies on the setting of plaster of Paris. Odont T 61:305, 1953.
Porosity of set gypsum was calculated, as influenced by the W/P ratio. The higher the ratio, the greater the porosity.

Kuntze RA: The Chemistry and Technology of Gypsum. Philadelphia, American Society for Testing and Materials, STP 861, 1984.
This is an excellent reference on the basic chemistry and technological aspects of gypsum.

Lautenschlager EP, Harcourt JK, Ploszaj LC. Setting reactions of gypsum materials investigated by x-ray diffraction. J Dent Res 48:43-8, 1969.
This article demonstrates the conversion of the hemihydrate to the dihydrate of calcium sulfate, but suggests the presence of residual hemihydrate in the set material.

Mahler DB, and Ady AB: Explanation for the hygroscopic setting expansion of dental gypsum products. J Dent Res 39:578, 1960.
This is a classic study that best defines the mechanics of hygroscopic expansion.

Schelb E, Cavozos E, Kaiser DA, and Troendle K: Compatibility of Type IV dental stones with polyether impression materials. J Prosthet Dent 60:540, 1988.
A further study on impression material–stone compatibility using polyethers. A plea is made to manufacturers to identify stones that are compatible with their impression materials.

Schelb E, Mazzocco CV, Jones JD, and Prihoda T: Compatibility of Type IV dental stones with polyvinyl siloxane impression materials. J Prosthet Dent 58:19, 1987.

Before a dental stone is used with an impression material, the compatibility of the two components should be determined. Differences in surface reproduction are noted between various combinations.

11

Dental Waxes

Kenneth J. Anusavice

OUTLINE

Types of Inlay Wax

Composition

Desirable Properties

Flow

Thermal Properties

Wax Distortion

Manipulation of Inlay Wax

Other Dental Waxes

KEY TERMS

Baseplate wax—Dental wax provided in sheet form that is used to establish the initial arch form in the construction of complete dentures.

Bite wax—A wax form used to record the occlusal surfaces of teeth as an aid to establish maxillomandibular relationships.

Boxing wax—A sheet wax used as a border at the perimeter of an impression to provide an enclosed boundary for the base of the cast to be made from a poured material such as gypsum or resin.

Corrective wax—A thermoplastic wax used to make a type of dental impression; also called *dental impression wax.*

Dental wax—A low–molecular-weight ester of fatty acids derived from natural and synthetic components such as petroleum derivatives that soften to a plastic state at a relatively low temperature.

Direct wax technique—Method by which a wax pattern is made directly on the prepared tooth in the mouth.

Elastic memory—Tendency of a solid wax form to partially return to its original shape when it is stored at a temperature higher than that to which it was cooled.

Flow—The relative ability of wax to plastically deform when it is heated slightly above mouth temperature.

Indirect wax technique—Method by which a wax pattern is prepared on a die.

Inlay wax—A specialized dental wax that can be applied to dies to form direct or indirect patterns for the lost-wax technique used for casting metals or hot pressing of ceramics.

Sticky wax—A variety of dental wax that exhibits relatively good adhesion to dry, clean surfaces when it is heated to a plastic condition.

CRITICAL QUESTION

Why does a wax pattern of an inlay made using the direct technique result in a looser-fitting inlay than one made using the indirect technique?

TYPES OF INLAY WAX

Dental waxes are supplied in a variety of colors, including blue, green, yellow, red, and ivory. The colors are useful to provide a suitable contrast against a die that is an accurate replica of a prepared tooth or arch form. Ivory-colored wax is useful for aesthetic case presentations. If the wax is applied as a veneer in a sufficient thickness, its opacity may be sufficient to mask colored die stone.

Inlay waxes may be softened over a flame or in water at 54°–60° C (130°–140° F) to enable their **flow** in the liquid state and adaptation to the prepared tooth or die. These waxes are designed to maintain uniform workability over a wide temperature range, thereby facilitating accurate adaptation under pressure. Additive layers and corrections may be applied to produce a homogeneous pattern. Inlay waxes can be carved easily without chipping or flaking. A regular or soft type is used for indirect work at room temperature or in cool weather. A harder or medium type that has a low flow property is indicated for use in warm weather.

The first procedure in the casting of an inlay or crown for the lost-wax process is the preparation of a dental wax pattern. The cavity is prepared in the tooth, and the pattern is carved either directly in the tooth or on a die that is a reproduction of the tooth and the prepared cavity. If the pattern is made within the tooth, it prepared by the **direct wax technique.** If it is prepared within a die, the procedure is called the **indirect wax technique.** Because the thermal expansion coefficient of wax is extremely high compared with the values for other dental materials, a wax pattern made in the mouth (direct method) will shrink appreciably as it is cooled to room temperature. A pattern made using the indirect method may not shrink as much, although the amount depends on whether the pattern was allowed to reach room temperature before it was removed from the die. Modifications of these two techniques may be used, but these two classifications are sufficient for the present discussion.

The American National Standards Institute/American Dental Association (ANSI/ADA) Specification No. 4 for Dental Inlay Casting Wax covers two types of inlay wax: Type I is the classification for *medium wax* used in direct techniques; Type II is for *soft waxes* used in the indirect techniques. Somewhat different properties are required for the various types (as discussed in more detail later).

However the pattern is prepared, it should be an accurate reproduction of the missing tooth structure. The wax pattern forms the outline of the mold into which the molten alloy is cast. Consequently, the casting can be no more accurate than the wax pattern, regardless of the care observed in subsequent procedures. Therefore the pattern should be well adapted to the prepared cavity and properly carved, and distortion should be minimized. Before the adaptation of the wax pattern within a tooth or a die, a separating medium must be used to ensure the complete separation of the wax pattern without distortion. After the pattern is removed from the prepared cavity, it is surrounded by a gypsum-containing material or other type of refractory material known as an *investment.* This process is referred to as *investing the pattern.* Investments and investing procedures are discussed in Chapter 12.

Wax patterns are used in the casting of many complex restorations other than inlays and crowns, but the present discussion is limited primarily to the construction of restorations employed in operative dentistry.

COMPOSITION

A number of formulas for inlay wax have been reported, some of which are quite complex. The essential ingredients of a typical inlay wax are natural waxes (hydrocarbons of the paraffin and microcrystalline wax series, carnauba wax, candelilla wax, and resins) and/or synthetic waxes. Natural waxes are derived from mineral, vegetable, or animal origins. Synthetic waxes are chemically synthesized analogs of natural wax molecules. Normally, the synthetic waxes are relatively more homogeneous and pure than natural waxes. Coloring agents are added for aesthetic purposes. Some formulations contain a compatible filler to control expansion and shrinkage of the wax product.

Paraffin wax is generally the main ingredient of inlay waxes, usually in a concentration of 40 to 60 wt%. Paraffin is derived from the high-boiling fractions of petroleum. It is composed mainly of a complex mixture of hydrocarbons of the methane series, together with a minor amount of amorphous or microcrystalline phases. The wax can be obtained in a wide melting or softening range, depending on the molecular weight and distribution of the constituents. The melting range can be determined by a temperature-time cooling curve, as shown in Figure 11-1 for a paraffin-based inlay wax. The temperature-time relationship during cooling indicates the successive solidification of progressively lower–molecular-weight fractions. Such a condition is desirable from a dental standpoint, because it imparts a moldability to the wax below the temperature of liquefaction. Paraffin can be produced with a range of melting points. For example, paraffin used for Type I wax is required to have a higher melting point than does the paraffin used for Type II waxes.

Paraffin wax is likely to flake when it is trimmed, and it does not present a smooth, glossy surface, which is a desirable requisite for an inlay wax. Consequently, other waxes and natural resins are added as modifying agents.

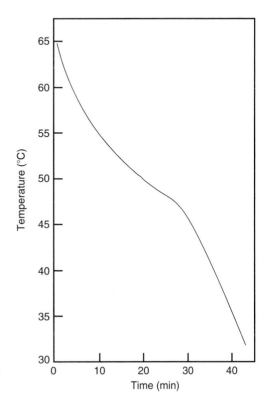

Fig. 11-1 Time-temperature cooling curve for Type I inlay wax.

Gum dammar, or dammar resin, is a natural resin added to paraffin to improve its smoothness in molding and to render it more resistant to cracking and flaking. Dammar resin also increases the toughness of the wax and enhances the smoothness and luster of the surface.

Carnauba wax occurs as a fine powder on the leaves of certain tropical palms. This wax is quite hard, and it has a relatively high melting point. It is combined with paraffin to decrease the flow at mouth temperature. Carnauba wax has an agreeable odor, and it contributes to the glossiness of the wax surface even more than does dammar resin.

Candelilla wax can also be added to the paraffin to partially or entirely replace the carnauba wax. The candelilla wax provides the same general qualities as the carnauba wax, but its melting point is lower, and it is not as hard as carnauba wax. Ceresin may replace part of the paraffin to modify the toughness and carving characteristics of the wax.

In modern inlay waxes, carnauba wax is often replaced in part with certain synthetic waxes that are compatible with paraffin wax. At least two waxes of this type can be used. One is a complex nitrogen derivative of the higher fatty acids; the other is composed of esters of acids derived from montan wax, a petroleum derivative. For an impression compound, a synthetic wax is preferable to a natural wax, because it has greater uniformity. Because of the high melting point of the synthetic waxes, more paraffin can be incorporated and the general working qualities of the product are improved.

Control of the properties of the inlay wax is accomplished by a combination of factors, including the amount of carnauba wax used, the melting range of the hydrocarbon wax, and the presence of resin.

DESIRABLE PROPERTIES

The following is a summary of some of the properties that are desirable in an inlay wax:

1. When softened, the wax should be uniform. In other words, it should be compounded with ingredients that blend with one another so that there are no grainy areas or hard spots when the wax is softened.
2. The color should be such that it contrasts with the die material or prepared tooth. It is necessary to carve the wax margins close to the die. Therefore a definite contrast in color facilitates proper finishing of the margins.
3. There should be no flakiness or similar surface roughening when the wax is bent and molded after softening. Such flakiness is likely to be present in paraffin wax; this is one of the reasons modifiers are added.
4. After the wax pattern has solidified, it is necessary to carve the original tooth anatomy in the wax and to carve the wax at the margins so that the pattern conforms exactly to the surface of the die. The latter procedure sometimes requires that the wax be carved to a very thin layer. If the wax pulls away with the carving instrument or if it chips as it is carved, such precision cannot be attained.
5. After the mold has been formed, the wax is eliminated from the mold. Elimination is usually accomplished by heating the mold to ignite the wax. If, after burning, the wax leaves a residue that might provide an impervious coating on the walls of the mold, the final cast inlay may be adversely affected. Consequently, the wax should burn out, forming carbon, which is later eliminated by oxidation to volatile gases. ANSI/ADA Specification No. 4 requires that the melted wax, when vaporized at 500° C (932° F),

leave no solid residue in excess of 0.10% of the original weight of the specimen.

6. The wax pattern should be completely rigid and dimensionally stable at all times until it is eliminated. The wax pattern is subject to flow unless it is handled carefully. It is also subject to relaxation, a factor that must be taken into consideration in its manipulation.

Expansion and shrinkage of casting wax is very sensitive to temperature. Normally, soft wax shrinks more than hard wax. High-shrinking wax may cause significant pattern distortion when it solidifies. Excessive shrinkage and expansion due to temperature change must be avoided. For this reason, organic filler is added sometimes to the wax formulation. Such fillers should be completely miscible with the components of the inlay wax during manufacture, and they should not leave an undesirable residue after burnout.

FLOW

Ideally, Type I inlay wax should exhibit a marked plasticity, or flow, at a temperature slightly above that of the mouth. The temperatures at which the wax is plastic are indicated by the time-temperature cooling curve for a typical Type I wax shown in Figure 11-1. The interpretation of this curve is the same as that for a typical time-temperature cooling curve for a solid solution alloy. The wax begins to harden at approximately 58° C (136° F), the point at which the curve first departs from a straight line, and it is solid below approximately 40° C (104° F), when it again cools at a constant rate.

Each type of casting wax exhibits a characteristic flow curve as a function of temperature. Each wax also exhibits a sharp transition point (temperature) at which it loses its plasticity. Soft wax exhibits this transition point at a lower temperature, and hard wax exhibits it at a relatively higher temperature.

Inlay waxes do not solidify with a space lattice, as does a metal. Instead the structure is more likely to consist of crystalline and amorphous structural regions, displaying limited ordering of the molecules. The wax lacks rigidity and may flow under stress even at room temperature.

ANSI/ADA Specification No. 4 provides certain requirements for the flow properties of inlay waxes at specific temperatures, as indicated in Table 11-1. The flow is measured by subjecting cylindrical specimens to a designated load at the stated temperature and measuring the percentage of reduction in length. The maximum flow permitted for Type I waxes at 37° C (98° F) is 1%. The low flow at this temperature permits carving and removal of the pattern from the prepared cavity at oral temperature without distortion. In addition, both Type I and Type II waxes must have a minimal flow of 70% and a maximum flow of 90% at 45° C (113° F). At approximately this temperature, the wax is inserted into the prepared cavity. If the wax does not have sufficient plasticity, it will not flow into all of the areas in the preparation and reproduce the required detail.

Table 11-1 Inlay Wax Flow (%) Requirements for ANSI/ADA Specification No. 4

Type of Wax	T = 30° C (Maximum)	T = 37° C (Maximum)	T = 40° C (Minimum)	T = 40° C (Maximum)	T = 45° C (Minimum)	T = 45° C (Maximum)
I	—	1.0	—	20	70	90
II	1.0	—	50	—	70	90

THERMAL PROPERTIES

As previously noted, the inlay waxes are softened with heat, forced into the prepared cavity in either the tooth or the die, and cooled. The thermal conductivity of the waxes is low, and time is required both to heat them uniformly throughout and to cool them to body or room temperature.

Another thermal characteristic of inlay waxes is their high coefficient of thermal expansion. As shown in Figure 11-2, the wax may expand as much as 0.7% with an increase in temperature of 20° C (36° F), or it may contract as much as 0.35% when it is cooled from 37° to 25° C (99° to 77° F). The average linear coefficient of thermal expansion over such a temperature range is $350 \times 10^{-6}/°$ C.

A comparison of the coefficients of thermal expansion of dental materials (see Chapter 3) indicates that inlay wax thermally expands and contracts more per degree of temperature change than any other dental material. This is one of the inherent disadvantages of waxes when they are used in the direct technique. This property is less significant when the wax is used in the indirect technique, because the pattern is not subjected to a change from mouth to room temperature.

The thermal dimensional change may be affected by the previous treatment of the wax. Curve A in Figure 11-2 represents the thermal expansion of an inlay wax that has been previously cooled under pressure. As shown, the expansion rate increases abruptly above approximately 35° C (95° F). The temperature at which the change in rate occurs is known as the *glass transition temperature*. Some constituents of the wax probably change crystalline form at this temperature, and the wax is more plastic at higher temperatures. Not all waxes exhibit glass transition temperatures. The transition point shown in Figure 11-2 is characteristic of a paraffin wax.

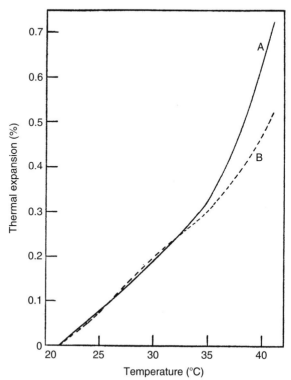

Fig. 11-2 Thermal expansion of inlay wax. **Curve A** represents the thermal expansion when the wax is held under pressure while it is cooling from the liquid state. When the same wax is allowed to cool without pressure and again heated, **curve B** results.

If the wax is allowed to cool without being placed under pressure, the transition temperature is not so pronounced when it is reheated, nor is the change in the thermal expansion so great, as shown in curve B of Figure 11-2. Another possible explanation exists for the difference in behavior, on reheating, of a wax cooled under pressure and the same wax cooled without applied pressure. This explanation is related to the behavior of dissolved or occluded air or solvents. Certain waxes have a phenomenal capacity for gas and solvent retention, which may often remain undetected. The gas trapped within the wax expands on reheating, causing a pronounced expansion as the wax becomes sufficiently plastic to flow.

Other factors, such as the temperature of the die and the method used for applying pressure to the wax as it solidifies, also influence the amount of thermal expansion. However, the thermal dimensional change of inlay waxes is probably not a serious problem when the indirect technique is used, provided no marked variation in temperature occurs after the removal of the pattern from the die.

CRITICAL QUESTION

How can the potential distortion effects associated with elastic memory and temperature changes be minimized?

WAX DISTORTION

Wax distortion is probably the most serious problem that can occur during forming and removal of the pattern from the mouth or die. This distortion results from thermal changes and the relaxation of stresses that are caused by contraction on cooling, occluded air, molding, carving, removal, and the time and temperature of storage.

A freshly made wax pattern tends to change its shape and size over a period of time. Upon cooling it contracts, and after it attains equilibrium, the pattern reaches a state of dimensional stability. It is imperative that the wax pattern be retained on the die for several hours to avoid distortion and to ensure that equilibrium conditions are established.

Waxes, like other thermoplastics, tend to return partially to their original shape after manipulation. The property responsible for this phenomenon is commonly known as **elastic memory**. A stick of inlay wax can be softened over a Bunsen burner, bent into a horseshoe shape, and chilled in this position. If it is then floated in room-temperature water for a number of hours, the horseshoe will open, as shown in Figure 11-3, *A* and *B*. This tendency is more critical in inlay waxes than other impression materials, because the resulting metallic or hot-pressed ceramic restorations made from the wax must fit onto unyielding, hard tooth tissue.

The elastic memory of waxes is further illustrated during the measurement of the thermal expansion of a wax held under pressure during cooling. The expansion increases above the glass transition temperature, more so than when it is cooled without pressure, as shown in Figure 11-1. Again, this result illustrates the nature of wax to attempt to return to its normal, stress-free state. In Figure 11-3, *A*, when the wax was bent into a horseshoe, the inner molecules were under compression and the outer ones were under tension. Once the stresses were gradually relieved at room temperature, the wax tended to straighten. The possible effect of storing the wax pattern is shown in Figure 11-4. Note that the casting fits best when the pattern is invested immediately after its removal from the preparation (see Fig 11-4, *A*).

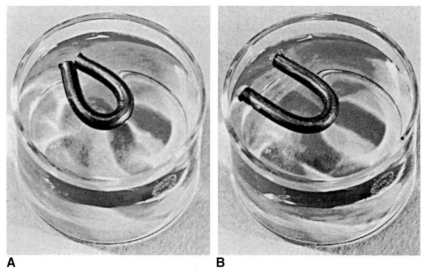

Fig. 11-3 A, A stick of inlay wax is bent into the shape of a horseshoe and floated on water at room temperature. **B,** After 24 hr the same stick of wax tends to relax and distortion occurs.

A pattern made of hard wax is less sensitive to temperature conditions than one made of soft wax. The exothermic heat generated during the setting of investment affects the pattern selectively. A soft wax pattern may result in a slightly larger and relatively rougher casting than a hard wax pattern.

MANIPULATION OF INLAY WAX

In the process of manipulating inlay wax, dry heat is generally preferred to the use of a water bath. The latter can result in the inclusion of droplets of water, which could splatter on flaming, smear the wax surface during polishing, and distort the pattern during thermal changes.

When stick wax is softened over a flame, care should be taken not to overheat it. The wax should be twirled until it becomes shiny and then removed from the flame. The process is repeated until the wax is warm throughout. It is then kneaded together and shaped to the prepared cavity. Type I wax has adequate plasticity in a

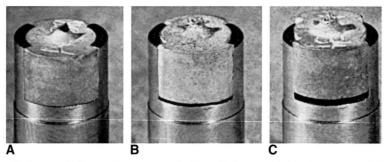

Fig. 11-4 Castings made from patterns prepared with melted wax cooled under pressure. **A,** Pattern invested immediately. **B,** Pattern stored for 2 hours before investing. **C,** Pattern stored for 12 hr before investing.

temperature range safely tolerated by the pulp. Pressure should be applied by the clinician's finger or by the patient biting on the wax. The wax should be cooled gradually at mouth temperature, not by cold water.

Care should be exercised in removing the pattern. It should be hooked with an explorer point and carefully removed from the cavity. A mesial-occlusal-distal (MOD) pattern can best be removed by luting a staple or loop of thread so that each prong is fastened above a corresponding proximal box portion. The pattern can then be removed with minimum distortion by passing dental floss through the staple and withdrawing it in a direction parallel to the axial walls. After removal, avoid touching the wax pattern with the fingers as much as possible to prevent any temperature changes.

For fabricating indirect patterns, the die should be lubricated, preferably with a lubricant containing a wetting agent. Any excess must be avoided, because it would prevent intimate adaptation to the die. The melted wax may be added in layers with a spatula or a waxing instrument, or it may be painted on with a brush. The prepared cavity is overfilled, and the wax is then carved to the proper contour. When the margins are being carved, extreme care should be taken to avoid abrading any surface of the stone die. A silk or other fine cloth may be used for a final polishing of the pattern, rubbing toward the margins. Theoretically, applying pressure is undesirable (see Fig. 11-2). However, many clinicians prefer to apply finger pressure as the wax cools to help fill the cavity and to prevent distortion during cooling. The fingers also accelerate cooling. Again, although temperature changes should be avoided, some technicians prefer to repeatedly remelt tiny portions around the margins while carving and examine them under a low-power microscope.

Regardless of the method chosen, the most practical method for avoiding any possible delayed distortion is to invest the pattern immediately after removal from the mouth or the die, as noted previously. Once the investment hardens, there will be no more distortion of the pattern.

Softer waxes, having higher flow, produce larger castings than do harder waxes, because softer waxes expand more as the investment warms during setting. They also offer less resistance to the expanding investment during setting.

As economy concerns continue to increase, faster waxing procedures are emphasized. Some dental laboratories virtually operate an assembly line process. To meet this demand, laboratories sometimes use "dipping" waxes that are kept molten for constant usage. Although standard types of inlay waxes may be used, the trend has included newer types of waxes that are more "rubbery," tending toward a more amorphous rather than crystalline nature. Wax pots that can be set to different temperatures are also used. The properties of these dipping waxes have not been characterized, nor do they fall into any present specification. As these waxes become more popular and better understood, their standardization will eventually follow.

Waxes oxidize on heating, and on prolonged heating some evaporate. There will also be a darkening and a precipitation of gummy deposits. Therefore care should be exercised to use the lowest temperature possible and to clean the pot and replace the wax periodically.

CRITICAL QUESTION

Under what conditions should medium and hard waxes be used?

OTHER DENTAL WAXES

A number of other types of waxes are used for purposes somewhat different than those of the inlay waxes described. The composition of each type of wax is adjusted to meet the particular requirements for each purpose. One of the most common of these alternatives is **baseplate wax.**

As its name suggests, baseplate wax is used principally to establish the initial arch form in the construction of complete dentures. Supplied in red or pink sheets 1 mm to 2 mm thick, the wax is approximately 75% paraffin or ceresin, with additions of beeswax and other resins or waxes. ANSI/ADA Specification No. 24 includes Types I, II, and III, also designated as soft, medium, and hard, respectively. Differentiation of one type from another is by the percentage of flow of each type of wax at room temperature, at mouth temperature, and at 45° C (113° F). The harder the wax, the less the flow at a given temperature. These differences in flow offer advantages for particular applications. Type I, a soft wax, is used for building veneers; Type II, a medium wax, is designed for patterns to be tried in the mouth in normal climatic conditions; and Type III, a hard wax, is for trial fitting in the mouth in tropical climates. Because residual stress is present within the wax as a result of contouring and manipulation, the finished denture pattern should be invested as soon as possible after completion.

Another alternative group is composed of the impression waxes, also referred to as **bite waxes** or **corrective waxes.** These waxes distort if they are withdrawn from undercut areas. Therefore they are limited to use in edentulous portions of the mouth or in occlusal surface areas. Although corrective waxes are quite soft at mouth temperature, they do have sufficient body to register the detail of soft tissue, and they are rigid at room temperature.

Other waxes include **sticky wax,** which is quite tacky when melted, but firm and brittle when cooled. Sticky wax is used to join and temporarily stabilize the components of a bridge before soldering the pieces of a broken denture before the repair. **Boxing wax** is yet another useful material for enclosing an impression before the plaster or stone cast is poured. *Carving wax* and *presentation wax* are used for demonstration purposes. Such waxes contain synthetic and polymeric materials and additives such as fillers and coloring agents.

SELECTED READINGS

Baum L, Phillips RW, and Lund MR: Textbook of Operative Dentistry, 2nd ed. Philadelphia, WB Saunders, 1985.
Techniques for manipulating wax and forming the pattern are described.

Craig RG, Eick JD, and Peyton FA: Strength properties of waxes at various temperatures and their practical application. J Dent Res 46:300, 1967.
Properties of waxes are controlled by the composition and melting range of certain components.

Ito M, Yamagishi T, Oshida Y, and Munoz CA: Effect of selected physical properties of waxes on investments and casting shrinkage. J Prosthet Dent 75(2):211-216, 1996.
This study evaluated the properties of flow, bending strength, and softening temperature of paraffin and dental inlay waxes and their relationship to casting shrinkage when patterns were invested with a phosphate-bonded investment. Casting shrinkage decreased as the flow of the wax pattern increased. If a low-flow wax or thick-pattern is to be used, the size of the casting ring should be increased.

Ito M, Kuroiwa A, Nagasawa S, Yoshida T, Yagasaki H, and Oshida Y: Effect of wax melting range and investment liquid concentration on the accuracy of a three-quarter crown casting. J Prosthet Dent 87:57-56, 2002.
The relationship between wax characteristics and the casting accuracy of a three-quarter crown was investigated using four different wax materials: paraffin 135, a wax with a softening temperature of 37.5° C (P38), paraffin 1080, a wax with a softening temperature of 63.5° C, another wax with a softening temperature of 41.5° C, and a hard wax with a softening temperature of 51° C. Two mixtures of phosphate-bonded investment were prepared, one with 100% special liquid and another with 75% special liquid plus 25% distilled water. P38 demonstrated the best results. Casting shrinkage was reduced with the use of 100% special liquid. Casting shrinkage was affected by the type of wax used and was sensitive to the site at which dimensional measurements were performed. The casting shrinkage increased when waxes with a higher softening temperature were used.

Jorgensen KD, and Ono T: Distortion of wax crowns. Scand J Dent Res 92(3):253-256, 1984.

Distortion of wax crowns is sufficient to reduce the fit of the final restoration to a degree that is clinically unacceptable. This study suggests that wax pattern distortion can be minimized simply by the use of a pattern/die investing technique. However, an investment for this technique is not yet available.

Kotsiomiti E, and McCabe JF: Stability of dental waxes following repeated heatings. J Oral Rehabil 22(2):135-143, 1995.

The flow and strength properties of dental waxes were examined following excessive and repeated heatings of the materials. Reductions in flow and elastic modulus were observed in some cases after the heating temperature was increased to 300 ˚C. Repeated exposure of dental waxes to temperatures higher than 200˚ C may affect the composition and properties, resulting in inferior materials.

McMillan LC, and Darvell BW: Rheology of dental waxes. Dent Mater 16(5):337-350, 2000.

The rheological properties of waxes were evaluated using a modified Stokes' falling ball method. Waxes were shown to be pseudoplastic and did not display a yield point. The pseudoplasticity followed a power law whose exponent was temperature-dependent in a. A standardized viscosity number was defined to characterize the flow behavior of dental waxes. The reciprocal of the pseudoplasticity parameter provides a similarly convenient measure of the stress-sensitivity of the wax.

Steinbock AF: An overview of dental waxes. Dental Lab News July:50, 1989.

An excellent review of the various types of waxes, their composition, and their properties.

Zeltser C, Lewinstein I, and Grajower R: Fit of crown wax patterns after removal from the die. J Prosthet Dent 53(3):344-346, 1985.

The effects of loading wax patterns before investment was determined. Repetitive loading revealed that the plastic deformation in wax was less after the second loading than after the first cycle for a specific load.

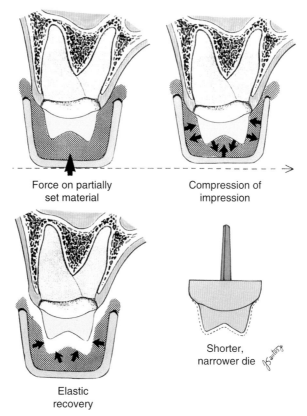

Force on partially
set material

Compression of
impression

Elastic
recovery

Shorter,
narrower die

10 **Top Left,** Impression tray containing elastomeric impression material is seated too late as elasticity starts to develop. **Top right,** Increased seating pressure is applied to overcome the stiffness of impression material. **Lower left,** Distortion develops because of recovery of excessive elastic deformation. **Lower right,** The die produced in the inaccurate impression is too narrow and too short.

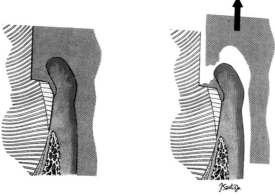

11 **Left,** Impression material has polymerized within the gingival sulcus. **Right,** Impression material has torn during removal.

12

Casting Investments and Procedures

Kenneth J. Anusavice

OUTLINE

Gypsum-Bonded Investment

Phosphate-Bonded Investment

Ethyl Silicate–Bonded Investment

Clinical Evaluation of Casting Fit

Compensation for Solidification Shrinkage

Preparation of the Master Die

Variables and Principles of Optimal Sprue Design

Casting Ring Liner

Investing Procedure

Casting Procedure

Technical Considerations for Phosphate-Bonded Investment

Causes of Defective Castings

KEY TERMS

Burnout—Process of heating an invested mold to eliminate the embedded wax or plastic pattern.

Divesting—Process of removing the investment from a casting or hot-pressed ceramic.

Hygroscopic expansion—The amount of setting expansion that occurs when a gypsum-bonded casting investment is immersed in water (usually heated to approximately 38° C [100° F]).

Refractory—Capable of sustaining exposure to a high temperature without significant degradation.

Sprue—The mold channel through which molten metal or ceramic flows into the mold cavity.

Sprued wax pattern—Wax form consisting of the prosthesis pattern with attached sprue network.

CRITICAL QUESTION

Why should gypsum-bonded investment not be heated above 700° C?

GYPSUM-BONDED INVESTMENT

The principal laboratory method used to form metal inlays, onlays, crowns, and bridges is to cast molten alloys by centrifugal force, under pressure, or under vacuum and pressure, into a mold cavity. The mold cavity is produced by elimination of a wax or resin pattern by a **burnout** process. To provide a pathway to the mold cavity for molten metal, the wax or resin pattern has one or more cylindrical wax segments attached at the desired point(s) of metal entry, and this arrangement is termed a **sprued wax pattern**. A **sprue** is the channel in a **refractory** investment mold through which molten metal flows. After the wax pattern has been made, either directly on a prepared tooth or on a die replica of the tooth, a *sprue former base* is attached to the sprued wax pattern, and it is surrounded with investment. This process is described later in the casting section, using Figure 12-12 to illustrate examples of sprued wax patterns on a sprue former base. The investment material is mixed in the same manner as plaster or dental stone, placed around the pattern, and allowed to set. After the investment hardens, the sprue former base is removed. The wax may be eliminated by boiling in water or by burning it out in an oven. This latter process is called *burnout*. The molten metal is then forced into the mold cavity left by the wax, through the *sprue* or *ingate* created by the sprue former base.

This chapter deals with the investments and casting methods used for the fabrication of small dental crown and bridge castings or ceramic **copings** produced by hot-pressing. Generally, two types of investment—gypsum-bonded and phosphate-bonded—are employed, depending on the melting range of the alloy and the preference of the clinician. The gypsum-based materials represent the type traditionally used for conventional casting of gold alloy inlays, onlays, crowns, and fixed partial dentures (FPDs). Phosphate-based investments are designed primarily for alloys used to produce copings or frameworks for metal-ceramic prostheses (see Chapter 21) and for some base metal alloys. It can also be used for pressable ceramics. A third type is the ethyl silicate–bonded investment, which is used principally in the casting of removable partial dentures with base metal alloy (cobalt-based or nickel-based alloy).

American National Standards Institute/American Dental Association (ANSI/ADA) Specification No. 2 for casting investments for dental gold alloys encompasses three types of investments. The type used depends on whether the appliance to be fabricated is fixed or removable and on the method of obtaining the expansion required to compensate for the contraction of the molten gold alloy during solidification. Type I investments are those employed for the casting of inlays or crowns when the alloy casting shrinkage compensation is accomplished principally by thermal expansion of the investment. Type II investments are also used for casting inlays, onlays, or crowns, but the major mode of compensation for alloy shrinkage during solidification is by the **hygroscopic expansion** of the investment generated by immersing the invested ring in a water bath. Burnout of the investment is performed at a lower temperature than that used for the high-heat burnout technique. Type III investments are used in the construction of partial dentures with gold alloys. This chapter focuses only on Type I and Type II investments.

Composition

As already noted, the essential ingredients of the dental inlay investment employed with the conventional gold casting alloys are α-hemihydrate of gypsum, quartz, or cristobalite, which are allotropic forms of silica. Most investments now contain the α-hemihydrate of gypsum because greater strength is obtained. This gypsum product serves as a binder to hold the other ingredients together and to provide rigidity. The strength of the investment is dependent on the amount of binder present. The investment may contain 25% to 45% of the calcium sulfate hemihydrate. The remainder consists of silica allotropes and controlling chemicals.

Gypsum

The α-hemihydrate form of gypsum is generally the binder for investments used in casting gold-containing alloys with melting ranges below 1000° C (1800° F). When this material is heated to the temperatures required for complete dehydration and sufficiently high to ensure complete castings, it shrinks considerably and occasionally fractures.

The thermal expansion curves of the three common forms of gypsum products are shown in Figure 12-1. All forms shrink considerably after dehydration between 200° C and 400° C (392° F to 752° F). A slight expansion takes place between 400° C and approximately 700° C (1292° F), and a large contraction then occurs. This latter shrinkage is most likely caused by decomposition and the release of sulfur gases, such as sulfur dioxide. This decomposition not only causes shrinkage but also contaminates the castings with the sulfides of the non-noble alloying elements, such as silver and copper. Thus it is imperative that gypsum investments not be heated above 700° C (1292° F). However, for gypsum products containing carbon, the maximum temperature should be 650° C (1202° F). In this way, proper fit and uncontaminated alloys are obtained.

Usually, castings that are made in pure gypsum molds are extremely undersized. The α-hemihydrate, which requires less mixing water and shrinks less, is now the optimum choice as a binder.

Silica

Silica (SiO_2) is added to provide a refractory component during the heating of the investment and to regulate the thermal expansion. Usually, the wax pattern is eliminated from the mold by heat. During the heating, the investment is expected to expand thermally to compensate partially or totally for the casting shrinkage of the gold alloy. As shown in Figure 12-1, gypsum shrinks considerably when it is heated, regardless of whether it is set plaster or stone. If the proper forms of silica are employed in the investment, this contraction during heating can be eliminated and changed to an expansion. Silica exists in at least four allotropic forms: quartz, tridymite, cristobalite, and fused quartz. Quartz and cristobalite forms are of particular dental interest.

When quartz, tridymite, or cristobalite is heated, a change in crystalline form occurs at a transition temperature characteristic of the particular form of silica. For example, when quartz is heated, it inverts from a "low" form, known as α-quartz, to a "high" form, called β-quartz, at a temperature of 575° C (1067° F). In a similar manner, cristobalite undergoes an analogous transition between 200° C (392° F) and 270° C (518° F) from "low" (α-cristobalite) to "high" (β-cristobalite). Two inversions of tridymite occur at 117° C (243° F) and 163° C (325° F), respectively. The β-allotropic forms are stable only above the transition temperature noted, and an inversion to the lower α form occurs on cooling in each case. In powdered form, the inversions occur over a range of temperature rather than instantaneously at a specific temperature.

The density decreases as the α form changes to the β form, with a resulting increase in volume that is exhibited by a rapid increase in the linear expansion as indicated in Figure 12-2. Consequently, the shrinkage of gypsum shown in

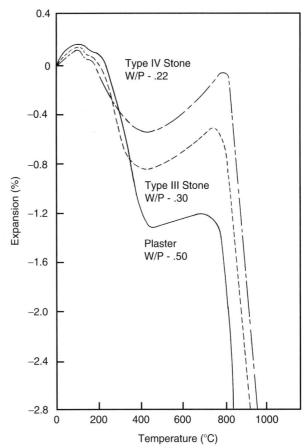

Fig. 12-1 Dimensional change of three forms of gypsum when heated. (Courtesy of R. Neiman, Whip-Mix Corporation, Louisville, KY.)

Figure 12-1 can be counterbalanced by the inclusion of one or more of the crystalline silicas.

Fused quartz is amorphous and glasslike in character, and it exhibits no inversion at any temperature below its fusion point. It has an extremely low linear coefficient of thermal expansion and is of little use in dental investments. Quartz, cristobalite, or a combination of the two forms may be used in a dental investment. Both are now available in pure form. Tridymite is no longer an expected impurity in cristobalite. On the basis of the type of silica principally employed, dental investments are often classified as *quartz* or *cristobalite investments.*

Modifiers

In addition to silica, certain modifying agents, coloring matter, and reducing agents, such as carbon and powdered copper, are present. The reducing agents are used in some investments to provide a nonoxidizing atmosphere in the mold when the gold alloy is cast.

Unlike the dental stones, a setting expansion is usually desirable to assist in compensating for the contraction of the alloy. Some of the added modifiers, such as boric acid and sodium chloride, not only regulate the setting expansion and the setting time, but also prevent most of the shrinkage of gypsum when it is heated above 300° C (572° F), as discussed subsequently. In some instances, the modifiers are lim-

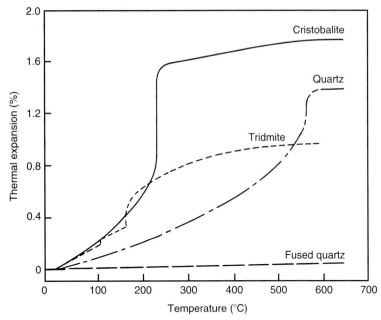

Fig. 12-2 Thermal expansion of four forms of silica. (Courtesy of R. Neiman, Whip-Mix Corporation, Louisville, KY.)

ited to the usual *balancing agents* to regulate the setting time and setting expansion, as described for the dental stones. The microstructure of a set gypsum-bonded investment can be seen in Figure 12-3.

Setting Time

The setting time of an investment can be measured in the same manner as plaster. Furthermore, it can be controlled in the same manner. According to ANSI/ADA

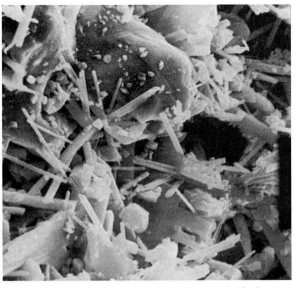

Fig. 12-3 Microstructure of the surface of a set cristobalite investment. The large, irregular particles are silica, and the rodlike particles are cristobalite. (×3000.) (Courtesy of R. Earnshaw.)

Specification No. 2 for dental inlay casting investment, the setting time should not be shorter than 5 min or longer than 25 min. Usually, the modern inlay investments set initially in 9 to 18 min. Sufficient time should be allowed for mixing and investing the pattern before the investment sets.

Normal Setting Expansion

A mixture of silica and calcinated gypsum (calcium sulfate hemihydrate) results in setting expansion greater than that of the gypsum product used alone. The silica particles probably interfere with the intermeshing and interlocking of the crystals as they form. Thus the thrust of the crystals is outward during growth, and they increase expansion. Generally, the resulting setting expansion in such a case is high. ANSI/ADA Specification No. 2 for Type I investment permits a maximum setting expansion in air of only 0.6%. The setting expansion of such modern investments is approximately 0.4%. It can be regulated by retarders and accelerators, as described previously.

The purpose of the setting expansion is to aid in enlarging the mold to compensate partially for the casting shrinkage of the gold. There is some doubt as to whether all of the setting expansion is effective in expanding the mold cavity formed by the wax pattern. The normal setting expansion of investment has traditionally been determined in a manner similar to that for dental plaster, in which the expansion is measured as the linear dimensional change that occurs as the investment sets in a V-shaped trough. Thus the normal setting expansion can occur essentially unrestricted. However, the trough technique does not accurately measure the actual or effective expansion of the investment while it is setting under the conditions of practical usage. For example, the effectiveness of the setting expansion in enlarging the mold containing the wax pattern may be related to the thermal expansion of the pattern caused by the heat of reaction that occurs coincidentally with the setting of the investment. It follows from such a theory that the setting expansion is effective only to the extent that the exothermic heat is transmitted to the pattern. The amount of heat present depends on the gypsum content of the investment; therefore the setting expansion of an investment with a comparatively high gypsum content is more effective in enlarging the mold than is a product with a lower gypsum content. Likewise, manipulative conditions that increase the exothermic heat increase the effective setting expansion as well; for example, the lower the water/powder ratio, or the drier the mix for the investment, the greater the effective setting expansion.

Variables other than the exothermic heat of reaction also influence the effective setting expansion. As the investment sets, it eventually gains sufficient strength to produce a dimensional change in the wax pattern and mold cavity as setting expansion occurs. The inner core of the investment adjacent to a mesial-occlusal-distal (MOD) wax pattern can actually force the proximal walls outward to a certain extent. If the pattern has a thin wall, the effective setting expansion is somewhat greater than for a pattern with thicker walls, because the investment can move the thinner wall more readily. Also, the softer the wax, the greater the effective setting expansion, because the softer wax is more readily moved by the expanding investment. If a wax softer than a Type II inlay wax is used, the setting expansion may cause a serious distortion of the pattern.

Hygroscopic Setting Expansion

The theory of the hygroscopic setting expansion was previously described in connection with the setting of dental plaster and stone. Hygroscopic setting expansion, which is greater in magnitude than normal setting expansion, differs from the normal setting expansion in that it occurs when the gypsum product is allowed to set when placed in contact with water.

The hygroscopic setting expansion was first discovered in connection with an investigation of the dimensional changes of a dental investment during setting. As illustrated in Figure 12-4, the hygroscopic setting expansion may be six or more times the normal setting expansion of a dental investment. In fact, it may be as high as 5 linear percent. The hygroscopic setting expansion is one of the methods for expanding the casting mold to compensate for the casting shrinkage of the gold alloy.

Commercial investments exhibit different amounts of hygroscopic expansion. Although all investments appear to be subject to hygroscopic expansion, the expansion in some instances is not as great as in others. For this reason, certain investments are specially formulated to provide a substantial hygroscopic expansion when the investment is permitted to set in contact with water. ANSI/ADA Specification No. 2 for such Type II investments requires a minimum setting expansion in water of 1.2%; the maximum expansion permitted is 2.2%. As discussed in the following sections, a number of factors are important in the control of the hygroscopic expansion.

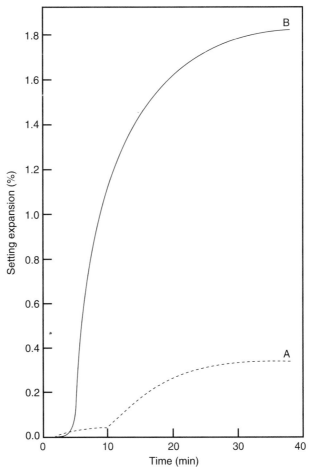

Fig. 12-4 **Curve A,** Normal setting expansion of dental investment. **Curve B,** Hygroscopic setting expansion. Water was added 5 min after the beginning of mixing; the water/powder ratio is 0.30.

Effect of Composition

The magnitude of the hygroscopic setting expansion of a dental investment is generally proportional to the silica content of the investment, other factors being equal. The finer the particle size of the silica, the greater the hygroscopic expansion. In general, α-hemihydrate is apt to produce a greater hygroscopic expansion in the presence of silica than is the β-hemihydrate, particularly when the expansion is unrestricted. As previously stated in Chapter 10, the hygroscopic expansion of the stone or plaster alone is slight.

A dental investment should have enough hemihydrate binder with the silica to provide sufficient strength after hygroscopic expansion. Otherwise, a shrinkage occurs during the subsequent drying of the set investment. At least 15% of binder is necessary to prevent a drying shrinkage.

Effect of Water/Powder Ratio

The higher the water/powder ratio of the original investment water mixture, the less the hygroscopic setting expansion. This effect is more marked in some commercially available investments than in others.

Effect of Spatulation

With most investments, as the mixing time is reduced, the hygroscopic expansion is decreased. This factor is also important in the control of the effective setting expansion.

Shelf Life of the Investment

The older the investment, the lower its hygroscopic expansion. Consequently, the amount of investment purchased at one time should be limited.

Effect of Time of Immersion

The greatest amount of hygroscopic setting expansion is observed if the immersion takes place before the initial set. The longer that the immersion of the investment in the water bath is delayed beyond the time of the initial set of the investment, the lower is the hygroscopic expansion.

Effect of Confinement

Both the normal and the hygroscopic setting expansions are confined by opposing forces, such as the walls of the container in which the investment is poured or the walls of a wax pattern. However, the confining effect on hygroscopic expansion is more pronounced than the similar effect on the normal setting expansion. Therefore the effective hygroscopic setting expansion is likely to be less relative to the expected expansion than is the normal setting expansion.

When the dimensional change in the wax pattern itself is measured after investing, the increase in the effective setting expansion during immersion of investment in a 37.7° C (100° F) water bath is apparently not only the result of hygroscopic expansion. Rather, it may be caused mainly by heating and expanding the wax pattern and softening the pattern at the water temperature, permitting an increase in effective setting expansion. The latter results from a combination of thermal expansion of the wax pattern plus the softened condition of the wax, reducing its confining effect on the expansion of the setting investment. This is substantiated by the fact that immersion in water at room temperature reduces the effective expansion.

Effect of Added Water

In the previous discussions, it has been assumed that the investment was immersed in a water bath to absorb as much water as necessary to control the expansion. However, the magnitude of the hygroscopic setting expansion can be controlled by the amount of water that is added to the setting investment. It has been proved that the magnitude of the hygroscopic expansion is in direct proportion to the amount of water added during the setting period until a maximum expansion occurs. No further expansion is evident regardless of any amount of water added.

The effect of some of the factors previously discussed (water/powder ratio, mixing, and shelf life) on the maximum hygroscopic setting expansion is illustrated in Figure 12-5 relative to the amount of water added. As shown in Figure 12-5, the magnitude of the hygroscopic setting expansion below the maximum expansion value is dependent only on the amount of water added and is independent of the water/powder ratio, the amount of mixing, and the age or shelf life of the investment. This finding is the basis for a mold expansion technique.

As discussed in connection with the hygroscopic expansion of gypsum products (see Chapter 10), the hygroscopic setting expansion is a continuation of the ordinary setting expansion, because the immersion water replaces the water of hydration, thus preventing the confinement of the growing crystals by the surface tension of the excess water. Because of the dilution effect of the quartz particles, the hygroscopic setting expansion in these investments is greater than that of the gypsum binder when used alone. This effect is the same as previously described for normal setting expansion.

The phenomenon is purely physical. The hemihydrate binder is not necessary for the hygroscopic expansion, because investments with other binders exhibit a similar expansion when they are allowed to set under water. As a matter of fact, expansion can be detected when water is poured into a vessel containing only small,

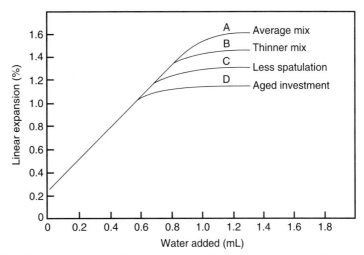

Fig. 12-5 Graphical representation of the relationship of the linear hygroscopic setting expansion and the amount of water added, as influenced by certain manipulative factors. (From Asgar K, Mahler DB, and Peyton FA: Hygroscopic technique for inlay casting using controlled water additions. J Prosthet Dent 5:711, 1955.)

smooth quartz particles. The water is drawn between the particles by capillary action and thus causes the particles to separate, creating an expansion. The effect is not permanent after the water is evaporated, unless a binder is present.

Any water-insoluble powder that is wettable can be mixed with the gypsum hemihydrate, and hygroscopic expansion results. Consequently, the quartz is not a factor. The influence of all the factors previously described can be related to the theory presented. The greater the amount of the silica or the inert filler, the more easily the added water can diffuse through the setting material and the greater the expansion, for the same reason as described for the normal setting expansion of investment. The water/powder ratio affects the hygroscopic expansion for the same reason that it affects the normal setting expansion. Once setting starts, the later water is added to the investment, the less is the hygroscopic setting expansion, because part of the crystallization has already started in a "normal" fashion. Some of the crystals have intermeshed, inhibiting further crystal growth after the water is added. On the same basis, the less water added, the lower the expansion; that is, there is less counteraction of the surface tension.

Finally, the term *hygroscopic* in a strict sense is a misnomer. Although the added water may be drawn into the setting material by capillary action, the effect is not related to hygroscopy. Furthermore, on the basis of the theory, the hygroscopic setting expansion is as normal a phenomenon as that which occurs during normal setting expansion. However, the term has gained general acceptance by usage even though it may be inaccurate on the basis of theoretical considerations.

Thermal Expansion

As noted in a previous section, the thermal expansion of a gypsum-bonded investment is directly related to the amount of silica present and to the type of silica employed. A considerable amount of quartz is necessary to counterbalance the contraction of the gypsum during heating. Even when the quartz content of the investment is increased to 60%, with the balance being hemihydrate binder, the initial contraction of the gypsum is not eliminated.

The contraction of the gypsum is entirely balanced when the quartz content is increased to 75% (Fig. 12-6). If a sufficient amount of setting expansion had been present, the casting made at 700° C (1292° F) would probably have fit the die reasonably well. The thermal expansion curves of quartz investments are influenced by the particle size of the quartz, the type of gypsum binder, and the resultant water/powder ratio necessary to provide a workable mix.

The effect of cristobalite compared with that of quartz is strikingly demonstrated in Figure 12-7. Because of the much greater expansion that occurs during the inversion of the cristobalite, the normal contraction of the gypsum during heating is easily eliminated. Furthermore, the expansion occurs at a lower temperature because of the lower inversion temperature of the cristobalite in comparison with that of quartz. As can be noted in Figure 12-7, a reasonably good fit of the castings is obtained when the gold alloy is cast into the mold at temperatures of 500° C (932° F) and higher. The thermal expansion curves of an investment provide some idea of the form of the silica that is present. As can be seen from Figures 12-6 and 12-7, the investments containing cristobalite expand earlier and to a greater extent than those containing quartz. Some of the modern investments are likely to contain both quartz and cristobalite.

The desirable magnitude of the thermal expansion of a dental investment depends on its use. If the hygroscopic expansion is to be used to compensate for the contraction of the gold alloy, as for the Type II investments, ANSI/ADA Specification

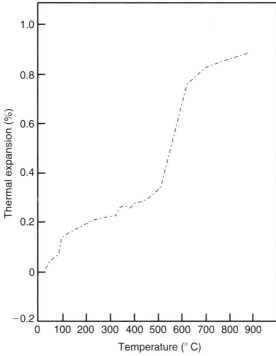

Fig. 12-6 Thermal expansion of an investment that contains 25% plaster of Paris and 75% quartz. (Courtesy of G.C. Paffenbarger.)

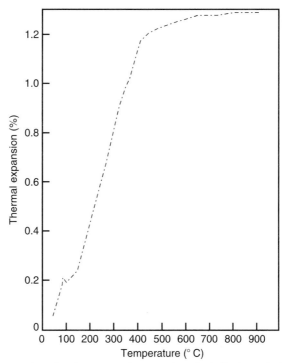

Fig. 12-7 Thermal expansion of an investment that contains cristobalite instead of quartz. (Courtesy of G.C. Paffenbarger.)

No. 2 requires that the thermal expansion be between 0% and 0.6% at 500° C (932° F). However, for the Type I investments, which rely principally on thermal expansion for compensation, the thermal expansion must be not less than 1% nor greater than 1.6%. In addition, the specification establishes minimum and maximum values for the combined setting or hygroscopic expansion, whichever the case may be, and the respective thermal expansion.

Another desirable feature of an inlay investment is that its maximum thermal expansion be attained at a temperature not higher than 700° C (1292° F). Thus when a thermal expansion technique is employed, the maximum mold temperature for the casting of gold alloy should be less than 700° C. As noted earlier and as shown later, the gold alloys can become contaminated at a mold temperature higher than this.

Effect of the Water/Powder Ratio

The magnitude of thermal expansion is related to the amount of solids present. Therefore it is apparent that the more water that is used in mixing the investment, the less the thermal expansion achieved during subsequent heating. This effect is demonstrated by the curves shown in Figure 12-8. Although the variations in the water/powder ratios shown are rather extreme, the curves indicate that it is imperative to measure the water and powder accurately if the proper compensation is to be realized.

Effect of Chemical Modifiers

A disadvantage of an investment that contains sufficient silica to prevent any contraction during heating is that the weakening effect of the silica in such quantities is likely to be too great. The addition of small amounts of sodium, potassium, or lithium chlorides to the investment eliminates the contraction caused by the gypsum and increases the expansion without the presence of an excessive amount of silica.

Boric acid has a similar effect. It also hardens the set investment. However, it apparently disintegrates during the heating of the investment and a roughened surface on the casting may result. Silicas do not prevent gypsum shrinkage but counterbalance it, whereas chlorides actually reduce gypsum shrinkage below temperatures of approximately 700° C (1292° F).

Thermal Contraction

When an investment is cooled from 700° C, its contraction curve follows the expansion curve during the inversion of the β-quartz or β-cristobalite to its stable α form at room temperature. Actually, the investment contracts to less than its original dimension. This contraction below the original dimension is unrelated to any property of the silica; it occurs because of the shrinkage of gypsum when it is first heated.

If the investment is reheated, it expands thermally to the same maximum reached when it was first heated. However, in practice the investment should not be heated a second time, because internal cracks may develop.

Strength

The strength of the investment must be adequate to prevent fracture or chipping of the mold during heating and casting of the gold alloy. Although a certain minimum

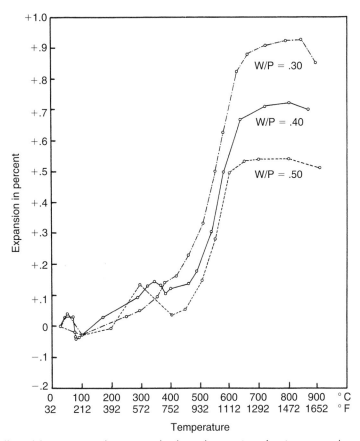

Fig. 12-8   Effect of the water/powder ratio on the thermal expansion of an investment that contains 20% plaster of Paris and 80% quartz. (Courtesy of G.C. Paffenbarger.)

strength is necessary to prevent fracture of the investment mold during casting, it has been suggested that the compressive strength should not be unduly high. In several studies on the fit of castings made by various techniques, it has been found that all castings for the National Institute of Standards and Technology MOD die showed a constant pattern of distortion. The distortion apparently results from a directional restraint by the investment to the thermal contraction of the casting as the alloy cools to room temperature.

Although the total thermal contraction of the investment is similar to that of the gold alloy from the casting temperature to room temperature, the contraction of the investment is fairly constant until it cools to below 550° C (1022° F). Thus when the alloy is still quite hot and weak, the investment can resist alloy shrinkage by virtue of its strength and constant dimension. This can cause distortion and even fracture in the casting if the hot strength of the alloy is low. Although this is rarely a factor with gypsum-bonded investments, it can be important with other types of investments (see later discussion).

Thus it is theorized that the compressive strength of the investment mold can be a primary factor to be considered, in addition to the expansion, when evaluating the dimensional accuracy of dental castings. Ideally, the investment should have sufficient expansion to compensate for all of the thermal contraction of the alloy. However, after burnout of the mold, the strength need be no greater than that required to resist the impact of the metal entering the mold.

The strength of an investment is usually measured under compressive stress. The compressive strength is increased according to the amount and the type of the gypsum binder present. For example, the use of α-hemihydrate instead of plaster definitely increases the compressive strength of the investment. The use of chemical modifiers as described in the previous section also aids in increasing the strength, because more of the binder can be used without a marked reduction in the thermal expansion.

According to ANSI/ADA Specification No. 2, the compressive strength for the inlay investments should not be less than 2.4 MPa (350 psi) when tested 2 hr after setting. Any investment that meets this requirement should possess adequate strength for the casting of an inlay. However, when larger, complicated castings are made, a greater strength is necessary, as required for Type III partial denture investment.

The strength of the investment is affected by the water/powder ratio in the same manner as any other gypsum product; the more water that is employed in mixing, the lower the compressive strength. Heating the investment to 700° C (1292° F) may increase or decrease the strength as much as 65%, depending on the composition. The greatest reduction in strength on heating is found in investments containing sodium chloride. After the investment has cooled to room temperature, its strength decreases considerably, presumably because of fine cracks that form during cooling.

Other Gypsum Investment Considerations

Fineness. The fineness of the investment may affect its setting time, the surface roughness of the casting, and other properties. It was previously noted that a fine silica results in a higher hygroscopic expansion than does a coarser silica. A fine particle size is preferable to a coarse one, because the finer the investment, the smaller the surface irregularities on the casting.

CRITICAL QUESTION

What are two measures that may be taken to minimize porosity in dental castings?

Porosity

During the casting process, the molten metal is forced into the mold under pressure. As the molten metal enters the mold, the air must be forced out ahead of it. If the air is not completely eliminated, a backpressure builds up to prevent the gold alloy from completely filling the mold. The common method for venting the mold is through the pores of the investment. Thus it is important that the extremity of a wax pattern not be covered by more than approximately 6 mm of investment to allow sufficient interconnectivity of the porous network, which will permit gas within the mold cavity to escape during filling of the mold with molten metal.

Generally, the more gypsum crystals that are present in the set investment, the less its porosity. It follows, therefore, that the lower the hemihydrate content and the greater the amount of gauging water used to mix the investment, the more porous it becomes.

The particle size of the investment is also a factor. The more uniform the particle size, the greater its porosity. This factor is of greater importance than is the actual particle size. A mixture of coarse and fine particles exhibits less porosity than an investment composed of a uniform particle size.

Storage

The same precautions for storage of plaster or dental stone apply to the storage of an investment. Under conditions of high relative humidity, the setting time may change. Under such conditions, the setting expansion and the hygroscopic expansion may be altered so that the entire casting procedure may be adversely affected. Therefore the investments should be stored in airtight and moisture-proof containers. During use, the containers should be opened for as short a time as possible. All investments are composed of a number of ingredients, each of which possesses a different specific gravity. There is a tendency for these components to separate as they settle, according to their specific gravity, under the normal vibration that occurs in the dental laboratory. Under certain conditions this separation may influence the setting time and other properties of the investment. For this reason, and because of the danger of accidental moisture contamination, it is advisable to purchase prepackaged investments in relatively small quantities.

The selection of an investment is largely a matter of preference. Some investments are formulated for casting inlays and crowns employing thermal expansion as the main factor for casting shrinkage compensation, and some are designed for use with hygroscopic setting expansion. Consequently, the choice is dependent partly on the specific techniques for which the investment is designed. Acceptable castings for the range of typical dental cavity preparations can be made with a number of investments and techniques.

As previously noted, the investment should be weighed and the water should be measured according to the proportion of the investment mix. Only in this manner can one expect to control the setting or the thermal expansion in relation to the compensation needed for the casting shrinkage and other important properties. Some dental manufacturers supply their investment in preweighed packages so that one need only measure the gauging water.

PHOSPHATE-BONDED INVESTMENT

The rapid growth in use of metal-ceramic and hot-pressed ceramic prostheses has resulted in an increased use of phosphate or silicate-bonded investments. Although these investments are somewhat more difficult to remove from castings than are gypsum investments, that problem has been reduced recently, and the phosphate-bonded investments produce satisfactory results with conventional gold alloys.

The phosphate investments now enjoy a popularity even greater than that of the gypsum-bonded investments. The tremendous increase in the use of metal-ceramic prostheses necessitates the use of higher melting gold alloys that do not cast well into gypsum investments. Likewise, the present trend is toward the use of the less expensive base metal alloys, most of which require phosphate investments. Commercially pure titanium and titanium alloys require specially formulated investments to minimize the interaction of the molten metal with the investment.

Composition

These investments, like the gypsum investments, consist of refractory fillers and a binder. The filler is silica, in the form of cristobalite, quartz, or a mixture of the two and in a concentration of approximately 80%. The purpose of the filler is to provide high-temperature thermal shock resistance (refractoriness) and a high thermal expansion. The particle size varies from a submicron level to that of a fine sand. The sandy feel of the investment does not necessarily relate to casting smoothness or affect the ease of removing the casting from the investment.

The binder consists of magnesium oxide (basic) and a phosphate that is acid in nature. Originally phosphoric acid was used, but monoammonium phosphate has replaced it, because it can be incorporated into the investment powder.

Because the newer gold-containing alloys and other alloys used for metal-ceramic restorations have higher melting temperature ranges than traditional gold alloys, it usually follows that their contraction during solidification is also greater. This necessitates a greater expansion of the investment. It is fortunate that the colloidal silica suspensions are available for use with the phosphate investments in place of water.

Because colloidal silica liquid suspensions can freeze and become unusable, these suspensions and their investment powder should be stored in a frost-free environment. Some suspensions are available as freeze-stable products. Although they freeze solid at low temperatures, they become useful again after they have been thawed out and shaken. Some phosphate investments are made to be used with water for the casting of many alloys. For predominantly base metal alloys, a 33% dilution of the colloidal silica is required.

Carbon is often added to the powder to produce clean castings and facilitate the **divesting** of the casting from the mold. This addition is appropriate when the casting alloy is gold, but there is disagreement regarding the effects of carbon in phosphate investments used for casting silver-palladium alloys, palladium-silver alloys, or base metal alloys. It is believed that carbon embrittles the alloys, even though the investment is heated to temperatures that burn out the carbon. The latest evidence indicates that palladium reacts with carbon at temperatures above 1504° C (2740° F). Thus if the casting temperature of a high palladium alloy exceeds this critical point, a phosphate investment without carbon should be used. Also, a carbon crucible should not be employed for melting the alloy. Generally even gold alloys used with porcelain should not be premelted or fluxed on charcoal blocks because trace elements that provide high strength are removed or are reduced below the desired level.

Setting Reactions

The chemical reaction for the binder system that causes the investment to set and harden is generally written as follows:

$$NH_4H_2PO_4 + MgO + 5H_2O \rightarrow NH_4MgPO_4 \cdot 6H_2O \tag{1}$$

However, phosphates are quite complex, and the reaction is not as simple as indicated here. One version is that the magnesium ammonium phosphate formed is polymeric. Although the stoichiometric quantities are equal molecules of magnesia and monoammonium phosphate, an excess of magnesia is usually present, and some of it is never fully reacted. What is thus formed is a predominantly colloidal multimolecular $(NH_4MgPO_4 \cdot 6H_2O)_n$ aggregate around excess MgO and fillers.

On heating, the binder of the set investment undergoes thermal reactions as suggested in the following sequence:

$$MgO + NH_4H_2PO_4 + H_2O$$

Room temperature

$$(NH_4MgPO_4 \cdot 6H_2O)_n$$
$$MgO$$
$$NH_4H_2PO_4$$
$$H_2O$$

Colloidal-type particles

Prolonged setting at 25° C
or dehydration at 50° C

$$(NH_4MgPO_4 \cdot 6H_2O)_n$$

Dehydrated at 160° C

$$(NH_4MgPO_4 \cdot H_2O)_n$$

Heated from 300-650° C

$$(Mg_2P_2O_7)_{n'}$$

Noncrystalline polymeric phase

$$Mg_2P_2O_7$$

Heated above 1040° C

$$Mg_3(P_2O_4)_2 \tag{2}$$

The final products are crystalline $Mg_2P_2O_7$ and some excess MgO, along with essentially unchanged quartz, cristobalite, or both. Some $Mg_3(P_2O_4)_2$ may be formed if the investment is grossly overheated or when the molten metal contacts the mold cavity surfaces.

Setting and Thermal Expansion

Theoretically, the reaction should entail a shrinkage, as in gypsum products, but in practice there is a slight expansion, and this can be increased considerably by using a colloidal silica solution instead of water. This latter substitution gives phosphate investments an unusual advantage in that the expansions can be controlled from a shrinkage to a significant expansion. Figure 12-9 shows the effect of the concentration of a typical liquid, essentially colloidal silica in aqueous suspension, on increasing the setting and thermal expansion.

Figure 12-10 illustrates the thermal expansion of a typical phosphate investment when mixed with water, as compared with the same investment when mixed with its accompanying special liquid. When phosphate investments are mixed with water, they exhibit a shrinkage within essentially the same temperature range as gypsum-bonded investments (200° C to 400° C [392° F to 752° F]). This contraction is practically eliminated when a colloidal silica solution replaces the water. Some users of phosphate-bonded investment prefer to decrease expansion by increasing the liquid/powder (L/P) ratio rather than by decreasing the concentration of the special liquid, or they may use a combination of these methods.

The early thermal shrinkage of phosphate investments is associated with the decomposition of the binder, magnesium ammonium phosphate, and is accompanied by evolution of ammonia, which is readily apparent by its odor. For gypsum investments the shrinkage is caused by the transformation of the calcium sulfate from the hexagonal to the rhombic configuration. However, some of the shrinkage is masked because of the expansion of the refractory filler, especially in the case of cristobalite.

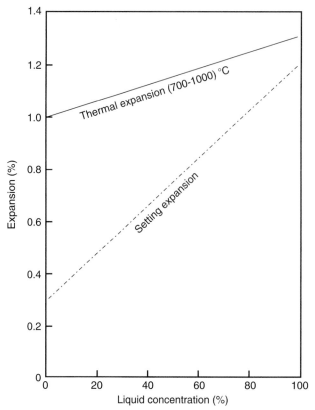

Fig. 12-9   The influence of liquid concentration on the setting and thermal expansion of a phosphate-bonded investment. (Courtesy of R. Neiman, Whip-Mix Corporation, Louisville, KY.)

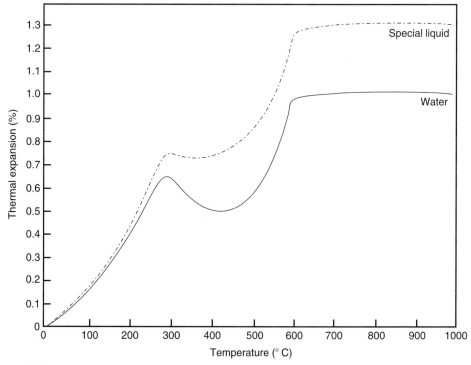

Fig. 12-10   Thermal expansion of a phosphate-bonded investment mixed with water as compared with the special liquid. (Courtesy of R. Neiman, Whip-Mix Corporation, Louisville, KY.)

Working and Setting Time

Unlike gypsum investments, phosphate investments are markedly affected by temperature. The warmer the mix, the faster it sets. The setting reaction itself gives off heat, and this further accelerates the rate of setting. Increased mixing time and mixing efficiency, as determined by the type of mixer and speed of mixing, result in a faster set and a greater rise in temperature. In general, the more efficient the mixing, the better the casting in terms of smoothness and accuracy. The ideal technique is to mix as long as possible yet have just enough time for investing. Mechanical mixing under vacuum is preferred.

A third variable that has a considerable effect on the working and setting time is the L/P ratio, which is often varied considerably depending on user preference. An increase in the L/P ratio increases the working time, which can be very short (2 min or less) when the investment is mixed at the manufacturer's recommended L/P ratio, at high speed (1750 rpm) for the recommended time, and if the laboratory is warm and the liquid has not been chilled.

Miscellaneous Properties

At one time, detail reproduction and surface smoothness of a metal-ceramic gold alloy restoration cast in a phosphate-bonded investment were generally considered inferior to those characteristic of a conventional gold alloy that had been cast in a gypsum-bonded investment. Increasing the special liquid/water ratio used for the mix markedly enhances casting surface smoothness, but it can lead to oversized extracoronal castings. However, improvement in the technique, and also perhaps the investment, now makes it possible to fabricate castings having few surface imperfections when the phosphate-bonded investment is used with either a low-fusing gold alloy, a high-fusing gold alloy, or a base-metal alloy. The phosphate investment now approaches that of the gypsum investments in fineness. However, their ability to improve the smoothness is dependent on the alloy and casting procedure employed.

ETHYL SILICATE–BONDED INVESTMENT

Ethyl silicate–bonded investment is losing popularity because of the more complicated and time-consuming procedures involved with its use; however, it is still used in the construction of the high-fusing base metal partial denture alloys. In this case, the binder is a silica gel that reverts to silica (cristobalite) on heating. Several methods may be used to produce the silica or silicic acid gel binders. When the pH of sodium silicate is lowered by the addition of an acid or an acid salt, a bonding silicic acid gel forms. The addition of magnesium oxide strengthens the gel. An aqueous suspension of colloidal silica can also be converted to a gel by the addition of an accelerator, such as ammonium chloride.

Another system for binder formation is based on ethyl silicate. A colloidal silicic acid is first formed by hydrolyzing ethyl silicate in the presence of hydrochloric acid, ethyl alcohol, and water. In its simplest form, the reaction can be expressed as:

$$Si(OC_2H_5)_4 + 4H_2O \rightarrow Si(OH)_4 + 4C_2H_5OH \qquad (3)$$

Because a polymerized form of ethyl silicate is used, a colloidal sol of polysilicic acids is expected instead of the simpler silicic acid sol shown in the reaction.

The sol is then mixed with the quartz or cristobalite, to which is added a small amount of finely powdered magnesium oxide to render the mixture alkaline. A coherent gel of polysilicic acid then forms, accompanied by a setting shrinkage. This soft gel is dried at a temperature below 168° C (334° F). During the drying process, the gel loses alcohol and water to form a concentrated, hard gel. As might be expected, a volumetric contraction accompanies the drying, which reduces the size of the mold. This contraction is known as *green shrinkage*, and it occurs in addition to the setting shrinkage.

This gelation process is likely to be slow and time-consuming. An alternative and faster method for the production of the silica gel can be used. Certain types of amines can be added to the solution of ethyl silicate so that hydrolysis and gelation occur simultaneously. It follows that with an investment of this type, the mold enlargement before casting must compensate not only for the casting shrinkage of the metal but also for the green shrinkage and the setting shrinkage of the investment.

Investments of this type are designed to reduce the layer of silica gel around the particles. They have a special particle-size gradation and are handled in a different manner. The powder is added to the hydrolyzed ethyl silicate liquid, mixed quickly, and vibrated into a mold that has an extra collar to increase the height. The mold is placed on the platform of a special type of vibrator that provides a so-called tamping action. This allows the heavier particles to settle quickly while the excess liquid and some of the fine particles rise to the top. In about 30 min, the accelerator in the powder hardens the settled part, and the excess at the top is poured off. Thus the L/P ratio in the settled part is greatly reduced, and the setting shrinkage is reduced to 0.1%.

The remaining cast is somewhat fragile because the amount of binder is quite low and is essentially composed of silica. The wax pattern is formed on the cast and invested in a manner similar to other investments. However, the process for an ethyl silicate–bonded investment is a little more complicated than that for the phosphate type in that care must be exercised during handling and burnout because flammable alcohol is given off. If the ethyl silicate–bonded investment is heated to a sufficiently high temperature, some silica converts to quartz and provides added expansion. This type of investment can be heated between 1090° C and 1180° C (2000° F and 2150° F) and is compatible with the higher fusing alloys. Its low setting expansion minimizes distortion.

CRITICAL QUESTION

Why is the marginal fit of cast crowns on a prepared tooth essential to the long-term clinical success of metal prostheses?

CLINICAL EVALUATION OF CASTING FIT

Although dental castings of any size (from a denture base to the smallest inlay) can be made, the procedures employed for the construction of a small restoration, such as an inlay, onlay, crown, and endodontic post, are emphasized in this chapter. The fundamental principles are the same, regardless of the size of the casting, and the techniques differ only in sprue design, type of investment, and method of melting the alloy.

The objective of the casting process is to provide a metallic duplication of missing tooth structure with as much accuracy as possible. The tolerance limits for the fit and marginal adaptation of a cast restoration are not known. In a clinical study, 10 experienced dentists were asked to evaluate the marginal adaptation of a group of inlays, using an explorer and radiographs. After the cemented restorations were graded, they were microscopically measured at the marginal openings of various areas. For "acceptable" restorations, the mean opening was 21 μm at the occlusal surface and 74 μm at the gingival region, which is not as accessible visually. There was little agreement among these 10 dentists on the acceptability of the marginal openings in some areas when evaluated by either explorers or radiographs. The difficulty in detecting small discrepancies at the margins of cemented restorations is associated with the use of explorers that have a relatively large radius of curvature at the tip compared with the width of margin gaps that are being evaluated. As shown in Figure 12-11, the tip of this unused explorer may not "catch" a 60-μm margin gap, whose width is represented by the diameter of a human hair, as it traverses along a path perpendicular to the gap. If this explorer tip substantially penetrates into a gap during probing, the fit of a crown, inlay, or onlay will not be clinically acceptable. The illustration poses the question of how readily a hairline gap can be detected by running an explorer over the margins of the restoration, especially in interdental areas that must often be probed at a small angle to the surface.

Therefore it is obvious that the accuracy of the inlay or crown should be greater than can be detected by the eye or by the conventional methods of clinical testing. At the margins of the cemented restoration, a thin line of cement is always present, even though it may not be readily visible. With the exception of resin-based luting materials, the present dental cements are somewhat soluble and can deteriorate in the oral cavity. Thus the less accurate the casting fit and the greater the amount of cement exposed, the more likely the cement will degrade. Certainly, a high degree of accuracy in margin adaptation of 25 μm or less cannot be guaranteed for all cast restorations. It stands to reason, however, that the more accurate the fit of the casting, the less the likelihood of leakage and secondary caries.

Assuming that the wax pattern is satisfactory, the procedure then becomes a matter of enlarging the mold uniformly and sufficiently to compensate for the casting shrinkage of the gold alloy. Theoretically, if the shrinkage of the wax and the gold alloy are known, the mold can be expanded an amount equal to such shrinkage, and the problem is solved. Unfortunately, there are variables in the behavior of the materials involved, especially the wax, which cannot be rigidly controlled. The overall dimensional accuracy possible with current techniques has never been clearly defined. Thus neither the allowable tolerance of accuracy in the fit of the casting nor that obtainable during the casting procedure is known. In the final analysis, the

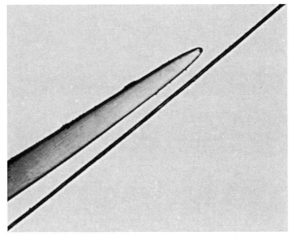

Fig. 12-11 Cross-section of an unused explorer tip **(top)** and a 60-μm hair. (×25.) (From McLean JW, and Van Fraunhofer JA: The estimation of cement film thickness by an in vivo technique. Br Dent J 131:107, 1971.)

casting procedure is partly empirical and a matter of routine procedure. Routine procedures should be rigidly followed.

There are many steps in the procedure for which a considerable number of facts are known. In addition, certain variations in the techniques described here produce equally satisfactory results. However, any technique involves strict adherence to certain fundamental principles that are common to all. These are the fundamentals emphasized in this chapter.

COMPENSATION FOR SOLIDIFICATION SHRINKAGE

The compensation for the shrinkages inherent in the dental casting procedure may be obtained by either one or both of the following two methods:

- Setting or hygroscopic expansion of the investment
- Thermal expansion of the investment

Both of these techniques are currently in use and are commonly termed the *hygroscopic expansion* (low-heat) *method* and the *thermal expansion* (high-heat) *method*, respectively. As their names alone might indicate, the high-heat method requires thermal expansion of the investment to occur between room temperature and a high temperature (650° to 700° C for gypsum-bonded investments and up to 1050° C for phosphate-bonded investments).

Despite these differences, the overall procedures involved in investing and casting are quite similar, and therefore they are described simultaneously. If not stated to the contrary, the reader can assume that the procedures mentioned are common to both the high-heat and the low-heat techniques. For best results, the manufacturer's recommendations for the specific alloy used should be followed.

Ringless Casting System

A ringless system that provides maximum expansion of investment is available commercially. The system, called the *PowerCast Ringless System* (Whip-Mix Corporation, Louisville, KY), consists of three sizes of rings and formers, preformed wax sprues and shapes, investment powder, and a special investment liquid. The tapered plastic rings allow for removal of the investment mold after the material has set. This system is suited for the casting of alloys that require greater mold expansion than traditional gold-based alloys.

CRITICAL QUESTION

What methods may be used to increase the abrasion resistance of master dies?

PREPARATION OF THE MASTER DIE

The most commonly used die materials are Type IV (dental stone, high strength) and Type V (dental stone, high strength, high expansion) improved stones. These materials are relatively inexpensive, easy to use, and generally compatible with all impression materials. Certified Type IV stones have a setting expansion of 0.1% or less, whereas the harder Type V stones expand as much as 0.3% in accordance with ANSI/ADA Specification No. 25. This greater expansion is useful for compensation of the relatively large solidification shrinkage of base metal alloys.

The chief disadvantage of the Type IV gypsum die is its susceptibility to abrasion during carving of the wax pattern. Gypsum dies are sometimes modified (1) to make them more abrasion-resistant, (2) to change the dimensions of the dies, (3) to increase the refractoriness of the dies, or (4) to produce a combination of these effects. Several means are used to increase the abrasion resistance, including silver plating, coating the surface with cyanoacrylate, and adding a die hardener to the gypsum. However, each of these methods may also increase the die dimensions slightly, thus reducing accuracy (Table 12-1).

Methods of Altering Die Dimensions

Additional accelerator (potassium sulfate) and retarder (borax) can be added to the gauging water to reduce the setting expansion of the Type IV die stone to less than 0.1% and, therefore, to reduce the diameter of the die. To produce relief space for cement, clinicians commonly use a *die spacer* with a stone die. The most common die spacers are resins. Although proprietary paint-on liquids are sold for this purpose, model paint, colored nail polish, and thermoplastic polymers dissolved in volatile solvents are also used. Such spacers are applied in several coats to within 0.5 mm of the preparation finish line to provide relief for the cement luting agent and to ensure complete seating of an otherwise precisely fitting casting or coping.

Die Stone-Investment Combination

Another technique employs a die material and the investing medium with a comparable composition. A commercial gypsum-bonded material called *Divestment* (Whip-Mix Corporation, Louisville, KY) is mixed with a colloidal silica liquid. The die is made from this mix, and the wax pattern is then constructed on it. Then the entire assembly (die and pattern) is invested in a mixture of Divestment and water, thereby eliminating the possibility of distortion of the pattern on removal from the die or during the setting of the investment. When it is heated to 677° C, the setting expansion of the material is 0.9% and the thermal expansion is 0.6%. Because Divestment is a gypsum-bonded material, it is not recommended for high-fusing alloys that are used for metal-ceramic restorations. However, it is a highly accurate technique for use with conventional gold alloys, especially for extracoronal preparations. The phosphate-bonded investment for Divestment is used in the same manner as the Divestment material, and it is suitable for use with high-fusing alloys.

| Table 12-1 | Dimensional Change in Dies Made from a Silicone Impression Compared with a Standardized Die |

Material	Dimensional change (%)	
	Occlusal	Cervical
Type IV stone	0.06	0.00
Type IV stone plus gypsum hardener A	0.16	0.08
Type IV stone plus gypsum hardener B	0.10	0.10
Silica-filled epoxy resin	−0.15	−0.26
Aluminum-filled epoxy resin	−0.14	−0.19
Electroformed silver die	−0.10	−0.20

With permission from Toreskog S, Phillips RW, and Schnell RJ: J Prosthet Dent 16:119, 1966.

Phosphate-bonded die-investment materials formulated for use in making ceramic prostheses can also be used when casting high-fusing alloys.

Other Die Materials

With inelastic impression material, such as compound, amalgam may be condensed into the impression to form the die. Other nongypsum die materials are also available, such as acrylic, polyester, and epoxy resins. These materials are limited in their compatibility with impression materials, which would ordinarily be nonaqueous elastomers rather than hydrocolloid or compound. Compatibility is specific and germane only to the particular brand rather than to chemical types of impression materials. Moreover, in the case of filled autopolymerizing acrylic resins, the curing contraction is excessive (0.6 linear percent for one material). Therefore acrylic resin cannot be used when an accurate die is required. The same is true for polyester resin materials.

Various epoxy die materials are reliable with respect to the 0.1% to 0.2% dimensional change on polymerization (see Table 12-1). Even though epoxy dies are generally undersized in comparison with the prepared tooth, especially in the axial direction, they are used successfully by some commercial dental laboratories, presumably because of their superior abrasion resistance.

In some cases the resin die should be no more undersized than the stone die is oversized. However, this issue must be taken into consideration, because it may be necessary to adjust the investing and casting technique accordingly. A cast crown that is fabricated on a slightly undersized resin die may not seat completely on the tooth compared with one made on a slightly large stone die.

The high-strength stones (Types IV and V) appear to be the most successful die materials available. With care, abrasion during carving of the wax pattern can be avoided. However, in the construction of a metal-ceramic crown that is made with a metal foil coping (such as Captek), the metal is burnished on the die. This process requires the application of high localized pressure to adapt the metal foil intimately to the die surface. Gypsum dies may be readily damaged, so a less brittle material, such as resin or metal, is sometimes preferred.

In the last few years, several gypsum die stones have been compounded with resins to provide the advantages of both materials. These modified die stones maintain the low expansion of stone, but they also have the increased toughness and resistance to carving imparted by the resins.

Electroformed Dies

Metal dies produced from electroplated impression material have moderately high strength, adequate hardness, and excellent abrasion resistance. Detail reproduction of a line 4 μm or less in width is readily attainable on an electroplated die when a nonaqueous elastomeric impression material is used.

The popularity of copper-plated compound dies began in the early 1930s, and silver-plated dies became more popular in later years. Several modifications of the fabrication technique are used, but the following description is typical.

The first step in the procedure is to treat the surface of the impression material so that it conducts electricity. This process is referred to as *metallizing*. In this process, a thin layer of metal, such as silver powder, is deposited on the surface of the impression material. This metal layer determines to a large extent the surface character of the finished die. Various metallizing agents are available, including bronzing powder and aqueous suspensions of silver powder and powdered graphite. These agents can be deposited on the surface of the impression with a camel-hair brush.

The electroplating bath itself is primarily a solution of silver cyanide. Care must be taken to avoid the addition of acids to the cyanide solution, which can cause the release of cyanide vapor, a "death chamber" gas. Chemical deposition of silver from a silver nitrate solution can be used if greater surface detail reproduction is desired.

In the silver-plating process, the greater the concentration of silver in the bath, the faster the silver is deposited. The acid content increases the *throwing power*, a term that refers to the penetration of current into a concave structure, such as an impression for a full crown. Impressions of teeth generally have walls with significant depth relative to the location of the occlusal area. Therefore a considerable amount of throwing power is desirable. An electrical contact is made with the metallized surface of the impression, which is the cathode in the electroplating bath. A plate of silver is used as the anode. A direct current is applied for approximately 10 hr.

Hydrocolloid impressions are extremely difficult to electroplate, and the process is not feasible for dental use. Electroformed dies made from polysulfide rubber impressions are clinically acceptable when a silver cyanide bath is used, although they are generally slightly less accurate than a properly constructed stone die.

Polysulfide rubber impressions are cleaned thoroughly and dried. They are then metallized with a fine silver powder. Although other metallizing agents can be used, the silver powder results in a superior surface on the electroformed die. An anode of pure silver, at least twice the size of the area to be plated, is employed, and the electroplating is carried out as before for approximately 10 hr, using 5 to 10 mA/cm^2 of cathode surface.

An impression that contains the electroformed die surface is then filled with dental stone. When the stone hardens, it is mechanically locked into the rough interior of the electroformed metal shell. The impression material is then removed to provide a die with greater surface hardness and resistance to abrasion than one of gypsum. The model and die are prepared in the normal manner, and margins of the die are trimmed with a finishing disk.

CRITICAL QUESTION

What casting deficiencies may result when: (1) the sprue former is too small in diameter, (2) the sprue former is attached without flaring to thinner areas, (3) the sprues are oriented toward thin areas of a wax pattern, or (4) the sprues are of inadequate length to position the wax pattern within 6 mm of the end of the invested ring?

VARIABLES AND PRINCIPLES OF OPTIMAL SPRUE DESIGN

The purpose of a *sprue former*, or sprue pin, is to provide a channel through which molten alloy can reach the mold in an invested ring after the wax has been eliminated. With large restorations or prostheses, such as removable partial denture frameworks and fixed partial dentures, the sprue formers are made of wax.

The diameter and length of the sprue former (also referred to simply as sprue) depend to a large extent on the type and size of the pattern, the type of casting machine to be used, and the dimensions of the flask or ring in which the casting will be made. Prefabricated sprue formers are available in a wide range of gauges or diameters (Table 12-2).

Wax Pattern Removal

The sprue former should be attached to the wax pattern with the pattern on the master die, provided the pattern can be removed directly in line with its path of

Table 12-2	American (Brown & Sharpe) Wire Gauge Numbers and Wire Diameter	
Brown & Sharpe gauge number	**Diameter**	
	Millimeters	**Inches**
6	4.115	0.1620
8	3.264	0.1285
10	2.588	0.1019
12	2.053	0.0808
14	1.628	0.0641
16	1.291	0.0508
18	1.024	0.0403

Reprinted with permission from Handbook of Chemistry and Physics, 58th ed. Boca Raton, FL, Copyright CRC Press, Inc, 1977-1978, p F-16.

withdrawal from the die. Any motion that might distort the wax pattern should be avoided during removal.

The gauge selection and design for the sprue former are often empirical, but optimal performance during the casting process is based on the following five general principles.

Sprue Diameter

Select a sprue former with a diameter that is approximately the same size as the thickest area of the wax pattern. If the pattern is small, the sprue former must also be small, because attaching a large sprue former to a thin, delicate pattern could cause distortion. On the other hand, if the sprue former diameter is too small, this area will solidify before the casting itself and localized shrinkage porosity ("suck-back" porosity) may develop. Reservoir sprues are used to help overcome this problem (Fig. 12-12).

Sprue Position

The position of the sprue former attachment is often a matter of individual judgment, based on the shape and form of the wax pattern. Some clinicians prefer placement at the occlusal surface, whereas others choose sites such as a proximal wall or just below a nonfunctional cusp to minimize subsequent grinding of occlusal anatomy and contact areas. As indicated earlier, the ideal area for the sprue former is the point of greatest bulk in the pattern to avoid distorting thin areas of wax during attachment to the pattern and to permit complete flow of the alloy into the mold cavity.

Sprue Attachment

The sprue former connection to the wax pattern is generally flared for high-density gold alloys, but it is often restricted for lower-density alloys. Flaring of the sprue former may act in much the same way as a reservoir, facilitating the entry of the fluid alloy into the pattern area. If possible, the sprue former should be attached to the portion of the pattern with the largest cross-sectional areas. It is best for the molten alloy to flow from a thick section to surrounding thin areas (e.g., the margins) rather than the reverse. This design minimizes the risk for turbulence. Also, the sprue former orientation should minimize the risk for metal flow onto flat areas of the investment or onto small areas such as line angles.

The length of the sprue former should be long enough to position the pattern properly in the casting ring within 6 mm of the trailing end and yet short enough so that the molten alloy does not solidify before it fills the mold. The type of sprue former selected influences the burnout technique used. Wax sprue formers are more common than plastic. It is advisable to use a two-stage burnout technique whenever plastic sprue formers or patterns are involved to ensure complete carbon elimination, because plastic sprues soften at temperatures above the melting point of inlay waxes. Patterns may be sprued either *directly* or *indirectly*. For direct spruing, the sprue former provides a direct connection between the pattern area and the sprue base or *crucible former* area (Fig. 12-12). With indirect spruing, a connector or *reservoir bar* is positioned between the pattern and the crucible former (see right side of Fig. 12-12). It is common to use indirect spruing for multiple single units and fixed partial dentures, although several single units can be sprued with multiple direct sprue formers.

A *reservoir* should be added to a sprue network to prevent localized shrinkage porosity (Fig. 12-13). When the molten alloy fills the heated casting ring, the pattern area should solidify first and the reservoir last. Because of its large mass of alloy and position in the heat center of the ring, the reservoir remains molten to furnish liquid alloy into the mold as it solidifies. The resulting solidification shrinkage occurs in the reservoir bar and not in the prosthesis, assuming that the reservoir bar is larger in volume than that of the patterns and that the sprue formers attached to those patterns were of the correct diameter and were placed in the appropriate position.

Sprue Direction

The sprue former should be directed away from any thin or delicate parts of the pattern, because the molten metal may abrade or fracture investment in this area and result in a casting failure. The sprue former should not be attached at a right angle to a broad flat surface. Such an orientation leads to turbulence within the mold cavity and severe porosity in this region (Fig. 12-14, *A*). When this same pattern is sprued at a 45-degree angle to the proximal area, a satisfactory casting is obtained (Fig. 12-14, *B*).

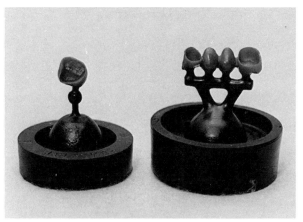

Fig. 12-12 **Left,** Primary sprue oriented directly toward the wax pattern. Note the spherical reservoir on the vertical sprue. **Right,** Indirect sprue design showing a horizontal reservoir runner bar that is positioned near the heat center of the invested ring.

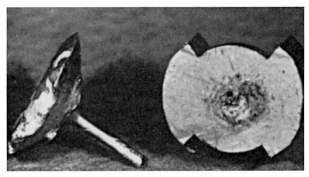

Fig. 12-13 Localized shrinkage caused by using a sprue of improper diameter.

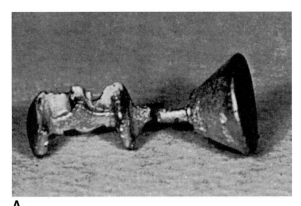

A

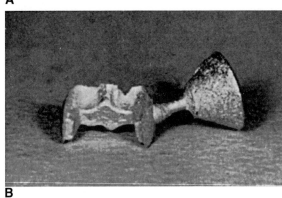

B

Fig. 12-14 **A,** Detached sprue indicates severe porosity at the point of attachment because of turbulence caused by an improper sprue angle. **B,** Sound casting results with sprue at approximately 45 degrees to the proximal wall.

Sprue Length

The length of the sprue former depends on the length of the casting ring. If the sprue is too short, the wax pattern may be so far removed from the end of the casting ring that gases cannot be adequately vented to permit the molten alloy to fill the ring completely. When these gases are not completely eliminated, porosity may result. Therefore the sprue length should be adjusted so that the top of the wax pattern is within 6 mm of the open end of the ring for gypsum-bonded investments (Fig. 12-15). With the higher-strength phosphate-bonded investments, it may be possible to position the wax pattern within 3 to 4 mm of the top of the investment. For reproducibility of casting accuracy, the pattern should be placed as close as possible to the

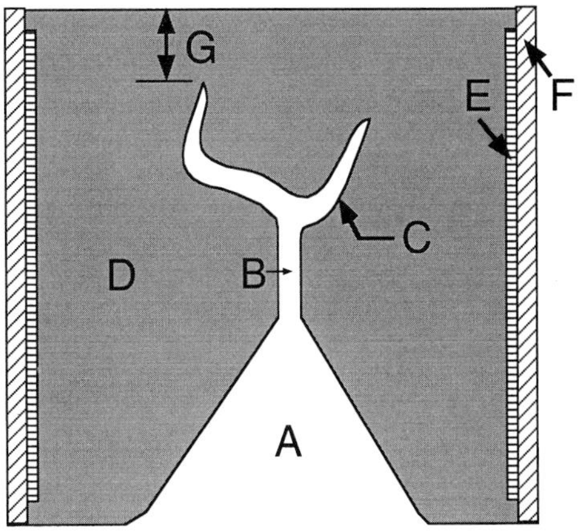

Fig. 12-15 Diagrammatic representation of a dental casting mold: **A,** crucible former; **B,** sprue; **C,** cavity formed by wax pattern after burnout; **D,** investment; **E,** liner; **F,** casting ring; **G,** recommended maximum investment thickness of approximately 6 mm between the end of the mold cavity and the end of the invested ring to provide pathways for sufficient gas escape during casting.

center of the ring. However, the wax pattern position for vacuum pressure casting may be different.

CRITICAL QUESTIONS

How does nonuniform investment expansion occur? How can excessive longitudinal expansion be minimized?

CASTING RING LINER

With the use of solid metal rings or casting flasks, provision must be made to permit investment expansion. The mold may actually become smaller rather than larger because of the reverse pressure resulting from the confinement of the setting expansion. This effect can be overcome by using a split ring or flexible rubber ring that permits the setting expansion of the investment.

However, the most commonly used technique to provide investment expansion is to line the walls of the ring with a ring liner. Traditionally, asbestos was the material of choice, but it can no longer be used because its carcinogenic potential makes it a biohazard. Two types of nonasbestos ring liner materials have been produced: an aluminosilicate ceramic liner and a cellulose (paper) liner.

To ensure uniform expansion, the clinician or technician cuts the liner to fit the inside diameter of the casting ring with no overlap. The dry liner is tacked in position with sticky wax, and it is then used either dry or wet. With a wet liner technique, the lined ring is immersed in water for a time, and the excess water is shaken away. Squeezing the liner should be avoided, because this leads to variable amounts of water removal and nonuniform expansion. Although a ceramic liner may not absorb water like a cellulose liner, its network of fibers can retain water on the surface.

Not only does the liner afford greater normal setting expansion in the investment, but also the absorbed water causes a semi-hygroscopic expansion as it is drawn into the investment during setting, as shown for gypsum investments in Figure 12-16. The use of one liner *(C)* increases the normal setting expansion compared with no liner. Using a thicker liner material or two layers of liner *(D)* provides even greater semihygroscopic expansion and also affords a more unrestricted normal setting expansion of the investment. As shown in Fig. 12-16, two layers of liner can be used to increase the expansion slightly compared with that obtained from one liner. In any case, the thickness of the liner should not be less than approximately 1 mm.

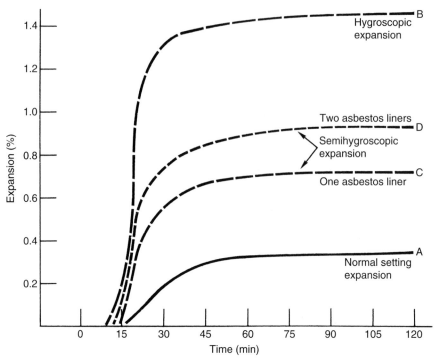

Fig. 12-16   Normal setting **(A)** and hygroscopic expansion **(B)** of an investment as compared with the somewhat restricted expansion that occurs in an inlay ring containing one liner **(C)** and two liners **(D)**. (Courtesy of R. Neiman, Whip-Mix Corporation, Louisville, KY.)

Because cellulose liners are paper products, they are burned away during the burnout procedure and a technique must be found to secure the investment in the ring. However, the desired length of the liner remains a matter of controversy. If the length of the liner is somewhat shorter than the ring itself, the investment is confined at one or both ends of the ring. The longitudinal setting and hygroscopic expansion are thereby restricted, as compared with an end where the liner is flush with the ends of the ring.

The expansion of the investment is always greater in the unrestricted longitudinal direction than in the radical direction, that is, toward the ring. Therefore it is desirable to reduce the expansion in the longitudinal direction. Placing the liner somewhat short (3.25 mm) of the ends of the ring tends to produce a more uniform expansion; thus there is less chance for distortion of the wax pattern and the mold.

INVESTING PROCEDURE

The wax pattern should be cleaned of any debris, grease, or oils. A commercial wax pattern cleaner or a diluted synthetic detergent is used. Any excess liquid is shaken off, and the pattern is left to air-dry while the investment is being prepared. The thin film of cleanser left on the pattern reduces the surface tension of the wax and permits better "wetting" of the investment to ensure complete coverage of the intricate portions of the pattern.

While the wax pattern cleaner is air-drying, the appropriate amount of distilled water (gypsum investments) or colloidal silica special liquid (phosphate investments) is dispensed. The liquid is added to a clean, dry mixing bowl, and the powder is gradually added to the liquid, using the same care and caution to minimize air entrapment as was discussed for the mixing of dental stones. Mixing is performed gently until all the powder has been wet; otherwise, the unmixed powder may inadvertently be pushed out of the bowl. Although hand-mixing is an option, it is far more common to mix all casting investments mechanically under vacuum.

Vacuum Mixing

Mechanical mixing under vacuum removes air bubbles created during mixing and evacuates any potentially harmful gases produced by the chemical reaction of the high-heat investments. Once mixing is completed, the pattern may be hand-invested or vacuum invested. For investing by hand, the entire pattern is painted (inside and out) with a thin layer of investment. The casting ring is positioned on the crucible former, and the remainder of the investment is vibrated slowly into the ring. With vacuum investing, the same equipment used to mix the investment is employed to invest the pattern under vacuum.

As noted, the amount of porosity in the investment is reduced by vacuum investing. As a result, the texture of the cast surface is somewhat smoother with better detail reproduction. The tensile strength of vacuum-mixed investment is also increased. In one study, it was found that 95% of vacuum-invested castings were free of nodules, whereas only 17% of castings made in hand-invested molds were entirely free of defects. Freedom of any surface imperfections is highly important, because even a small nodule on a casting may damage a fragile enamel margin when the casting is evaluated for fit in the prepared cavity. The finished casting should always be checked under magnification for such defects before fitting it on the die.

Air bubbles that remain in the mix, even with vacuum mixing, can be entrapped on flat or concave surfaces that are not oriented suitably for air evacuation. Tilting the ring slightly aids in releasing these bubbles so that they can rise to the surface. Excessive vibration should be avoided, because it can cause solids in the investment to settle and may lead to free-water accumulation adjacent to the wax pattern, resulting in surface roughness. Excessive vibration may also dislodge small patterns from the sprue former, resulting in a miscast.

If the hygroscopic technique is employed, the filled casting ring is immediately placed in a 37° C water bath with the crucible former side-down. For the thermal expansion or high-heat technique, the invested ring is allowed to bench set undisturbed for the time recommended by the manufacturer.

Compensation for Shrinkage

Occasionally, it may be desirable to alter the mold dimensions of a full cast crown compared with a small inlay. A number of factors influence the mold size. As previously discussed, two liners allow a greater setting and thermal expansion than does a single liner. Also, the setting, hygroscopic, and thermal expansions of investments can be controlled to a certain extent by varying the L/P ratio of the investment. The lower the L/P ratio, the greater the potential for investment expansion. Conversely, thinner mixes reduce the expansion. With some investments, however, the effect of minor adjustments to the L/P ratio is insignificant.

There is a limit to which the L/P ratio can be altered. If the mix is too thick, it cannot be applied to the pattern without a likelihood of distorting the pattern and producing air voids during investing. On the other hand, if the mixture is too thin, a rough surface may result on the casting.

Another possible problem is too much expansion of the mold when using the thermal expansion technique with a cristobalite investment. As was discussed in Chapter 11, a thermal expansion of 1.3% may take place. If an effective setting expansion of 0.3% to 0.4% is added to such a thermal expansion, a total linear expansion as high as 1.7% may be obtained, higher than the average casting shrinkage of a gold alloy. As a result, a cast crown may be too large.

In addition to controlling the hygroscopic expansion by the L/P ratio, the clinician can regulate expansion by reducing the time of immersion of the setting investment or by controlling the amount of water to be added during the setting process. The longer the delay before the investment is immersed in the water bath, the less the hygroscopic expansion.

The modern hygroscopic investment technique generally provides correct expansion for most types of patterns. However, some patterns may require a variation in expansion. Increasing the burnout temperature and the water bath temperature increases the expansion and vice versa.

In one technique, the shrinkage compensation is controlled by the addition of water during the setting of the investment. This method is usually referred to as the *controlled water-added technique*.

Controlled Water-Added Technique

The linear hygroscopic expansion increases directly with the amount of water added until maximum expansion is attained. The compositions of investments for use with the water-added hygroscopic casting technique ensure maximal expansion during immersion in water. The amount of hygroscopic expansion needed for compensation is then obtained by adding only enough water to provide the desired expansion.

A soft, flexible rubber ring is used instead of the usual asbestos-lined metal ring. The pattern is invested as usual. A specified amount of water is then added on the top of the investment in the rubber ring, and the investment is allowed to set, usually at room temperature. The controlled water-added technique is rarely used, however, because the hygroscopic expansion method described earlier provides adequate expansion in most cases.

CASTING PROCEDURE

Once the investment has set for an appropriate period—approximately 1 hr for most gypsum-and phosphate-bonded investments—it is ready for burnout. The procedures for the two types of investment are similar, so the following discussion focuses on gypsum investments. The crucible former and any metal sprue former are carefully removed. Any debris from the ingate area (funneled opening at end of the ring) is cleaned with a brush. If the burnout procedure does not immediately follow the investing procedure, the invested ring is placed in a humidor at 100% humidity. If possible, the investment should not be permitted to dry out. Rehydration of set investment that has been stored for an extended period may not replenish all of the lost water.

Wax Elimination and Heating

The invested rings are placed in a room-temperature furnace and heated to the prescribed maximum temperature. For gypsum-bonded investments, this temperature can be either 500° C for the *hygroscopic technique* or 700° C for the *thermal expansion technique*. With phosphate-bonded investments, the maximum temperature setting may range from 700° to 1030° C, depending on the type of alloy selected. The temperature setting is more critical with gypsum-bonded investments than with the phosphate type, because the gypsum investments are more prone to investment decomposition. During burnout, some of the melted wax is absorbed by the investment, and residual carbon produced by ignition of the liquid wax becomes trapped in the porous investment. It is also advisable to begin the burnout procedure while the mold is still wet. Water trapped in the pores of the investment reduces the absorption of wax, and as the water vaporizes, it flushes wax from the mold. This process is facilitated by placing the ring with the sprue hole down over a slot in a ceramic tray in the burnout furnace. When the high-heat technique is used, the mold temperature generates enough heat to convert carbon to either carbon monoxide or carbon dioxide. These gases can then escape through the pores in the heated investment.

Hygroscopic Low-Heat Technique

This technique obtains its compensation expansion from three sources: (1) the 37° C water bath expands the wax pattern; (2) the warm water entering the investment mold from the top adds some hygroscopic expansion; and (3) the thermal expansion at 500° C provides the needed thermal expansion. This low-heat technique offers the advantages of less investment degradation, a cooler surface for smoother castings, and the convenience of placing the molds directly in the 500° C furnace. The last benefit makes it possible to keep one or more furnaces at the burnout temperature so that molds may be put in as they are ready. This is particularly useful in large laboratories, where molds are ready for burnout at various times. Care must nevertheless be taken to allow sufficient burnout time, because the wax is more slowly oxidized (eliminated) at the low temperature. The molds should remain in the furnace for at least 60 min, and they may be held up to 5 hr longer with little damage. Since the temperature of the furnace is lowered each time a mold is placed, extra time should be allowed to ensure complete wax elimination when molds are placed at intervals. Even though the mold is usually held at this temperature for 60 to 90 min, sufficient residual fine carbon may be retained to reduce the venting of the mold. Because of this potential for reduced venting, back-pressure porosity is a greater hazard in the low-heat technique than in the high-heat technique, since the investments generally employed with the low-heat technique may be more dense.

The standardized hygroscopic technique was developed for alloys with a high gold content; the newer noble alloys may require slightly more expansion. This added expansion may be obtained by making one or more of the following changes:

1. Increasing the water bath temperature to 40° C
2. Using two layers of liner
3. Increasing the burnout temperature to a range of 600° to 650° C.

High-Heat Thermal Expansion Technique

This approach depends almost entirely on using a high-heat burnout to obtain the required expansion, while at the same time eliminating the wax pattern. Additional expansion results from the slight heating of gypsum investments on setting, thus expanding the wax pattern, and the water entering the investment from the wet liner adds a small amount of hygroscopic expansion to the normal setting expansion.

Gypsum Investments

These casting investments are relatively fragile and require the use of a metal ring for protection during heating. The molds are usually placed in a furnace at room temperature, slowly heated to 650° C to 700° C in 60 min, and held for 15 to 30 min at the upper temperature.

The rate of heating has some influence on the smoothness and, in some instances, on the overall dimensions of the investment. Initially, the rapid heating can generate steam, which can cause flaking or spalling of the mold walls. Too many patterns in the same plane within the investment often cause separation of a whole section of investment, because the expanding wax creates excessive pressure over a large area.

Too rapid a heating rate may also cause cracking of the investment. In such a case, the outside layer of the investment expands much more than the center sections. Consequently, the outside layer starts to expand thermally, resulting in compressive stress in the outside layer, which counteracts tensile stresses in the middle regions of the mold. Such a stress distribution causes the brittle investment to crack from the interior outwardly in the form of radial cracks. These cracks, in turn, produce a casting with fins or spines similar to those shown in Figure 12-17. This condition is especially likely to be present with a cristobalite investment. The comparatively low inversion temperature of the cristobalite, and the rapid rate of expansion during the inversion, makes it especially important to heat the investment slowly.

Breakdown of the dental investment and the resulting contamination and brittleness of the gold alloy casting probably occur more frequently than is generally realized. The mechanism of this investment decomposition and alloy contamination is related to a chemical reaction between the residual carbon and calcium sulfate binder. Calcium sulfate per se does not decompose unless it is heated above 1000° C. However, the reduction of calcium sulfate by carbon takes place rapidly above 700° C in accordance with the following reactions:

$$CaSO_4 + 4C \rightarrow CaS + 4CO$$

$$3CaSO_4 + CaS \rightarrow 4CaO + 4SO_2 \tag{4}$$

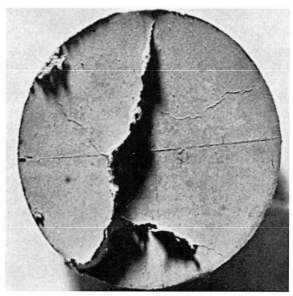

Fig. 12-17 Fins on the surface of a casting that formed as a result of cracks in the investment before casting of the metal.

This reaction takes place whenever gypsum investments are heated above 700° C in the presence of carbon. The sulfur dioxide as a product of this reaction contaminates gold castings and makes them extremely brittle. This fact emphasizes the need for completely eliminating the wax and avoiding burnout temperatures above 700° C, particularly if the investment contains carbon. Furthermore, sulfur gases are generated by the gypsum investment when it is heated above 700° C.

After the casting temperature has been reached, the casting should be made immediately. Maintaining a high temperature for any considerable length of time may result in sulfur contamination of the casting and also in a rough surface on the casting because of the disintegration of the investment. To avoid this problem, some technicians use furnaces with heating elements on all four sides, thereby reducing the burnout time.

Notwithstanding all of the these precautions and reasons for using a slow burnout technique, the desire for rapid results has led to improved investment formulations. A few gypsum investments, some with a considerable amount of cristobalite, are now offered for use with a much more rapid burnout procedure. Some suggest placing the mold in a furnace at 315° C for 30 min and following with very rapid heating to the final burnout temperature. In addition, a few investments may be placed directly into a furnace at the final burnout temperature, held for 30 min, and cast. Because the design of the furnace, the proximity of the mold to the heating element, and the availability of air in the muffle may affect size and smoothness, it is advisable to examine these factors carefully before a casting is made in this manner.

Phosphate Investments

Many of the earlier statements about gypsum investments also apply to phosphate investments. There are several differences, however, because the setting mechanism and reactions on heating are quite different.

Phosphate investments obtain their expansion from the following sources:
1. Expansion of the wax pattern—this is considerable because the setting reaction raises the mold temperature substantially.
2. Setting expansion—this is usually higher than in gypsum investments, especially because special liquids are used to enhance such expansion.
3. Thermal expansion—this is greater when taken to temperatures higher than those used for gypsum-bonded investments.

A total expansion of 2% or more is required for alloys used to produce metal-ceramic prostheses, since these gold-based, palladium-based, and base metal alloys have higher melting and solidification temperatures.

Although phosphate investments are usually much harder and stronger than gypsum investments, they are nevertheless quite brittle and are subject to the same unequal expansion of adjacent sections as phase changes occur during heating.

The usual burnout temperatures for phosphate-bonded investments range from 750° to 1030° C. The highest temperatures are required for base metal alloys. The heating rate is usually slow to 315° C and is quite rapid thereafter, reaching completion after a hold at the upper temperature for 30 min. Most burnout furnaces are now capable of being programmed for heating rates and holding times.

Because the entire process involving phosphate investments takes a long time, the demand for time-saving changes is strong. Again, investment manufacturers have attempted to answer this demand, resulting in the availability of some investments that can be subjected to two-stage heating more rapidly, placed directly in the furnace at the top temperature, held for 20 to 30 min, and then cast. To save more time, manufacturers have also eliminated the use of a metal ring and liner, the metal ring being replaced with a plastic ring that is tapered so that once the investment has set, it can be pushed out of the ring, held for a specified time to ensure complete setting, and then placed directly into the hot furnace. Obviously, the expansion on setting with this method is different from that when a lined ring is used, and changes in overall fit must be considered. The required expansion may be adjusted by varying the liquid concentration.

Time Allowable for Casting

The investment contracts thermally as it cools. When the thermal expansion or high-heat technique is used, the investment loses heat after the heated ring is removed from the furnace, and the mold contracts. Because of the liner and the low thermal conductivity of the investment, a short period can elapse before the temperature of the mold is appreciably affected. Under average conditions of casting, approximately 1 min can pass without a noticeable loss in dimension.

In the low-heat casting technique, the temperature gradient between the investment mold and the room is not as great as that employed with the high-heat technique. Also, the thermal expansion of the investment is not as important to the shrinkage compensation. However, the burnout temperature lies on a fairly steep portion of the thermal expansion curve rather than on a plateau portion, as in the high-heat technique. Therefore, in the low-heat casting technique, the alloy should also be cast soon after removal of the ring from the oven; otherwise a significant variation from the desired casting dimensions may occur.

Casting Machines

Alloys are melted in one of the four following ways, depending on the available types of casting machines:
1. The alloy is melted in a separate crucible by a torch flame and is cast into the mold by centrifugal force (Fig. 12-18).
2. The alloy is melted electrically by a resistance heating or induction furnace, then cast into the mold centrifugally by motor or spring action. A representative casting machine of this type is shown in Figure 12-19.
3. The alloy is melted by induction heating, then cast into the mold centrifugally by motor or spring action. A representative casting machine of this type is shown in Figure 12-20.
4. The alloy is vacuum arc melted and cast by pressure in an argon atmosphere.
In addition to these three melting methods, the molten metal may be cast by air pressure, by vacuum, or both. The general procedure for each is described in the following sections, with certain advantages and disadvantages cited. However, it is important to follow the manufacturer's directions precisely for any of these devices.

Torch Melting/Centrifugal Casting Machine

The casting machine spring is first wound from two to five turns (depending on the particular machine and the speed of casting rotation desired). The alloy is melted by a torch flame in a glazed ceramic crucible attached to the "broken arm" of the casting machine. The torch flame is generated from a gas mixture of propane and air, natural gas and air, acetylene and air, or acetylene and oxygen. The broken-arm feature accelerates the initial rotational speed of the crucible and casting ring, thus increasing the linear speed of the liquid casting alloy as it moves into and through

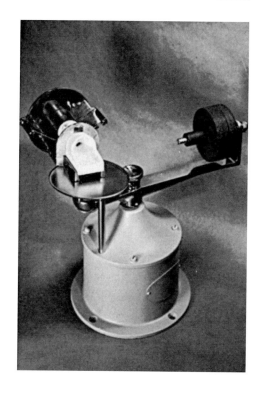

Fig. 12-18 Centrifugal casting machine, spring-wound.

the mold. Once the metal has reached the casting temperature and the heated casting ring is in position, the machine is released and the spring triggers the rotational motion.

As the metal fills the mold, a hydrostatic pressure gradient develops along the length of the casting. The pressure gradient from the tip of the casting to the bottom

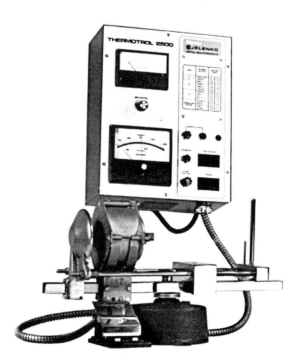

Fig. 12-19 Spring-wound casting machine with electrical resistance melting furnace.

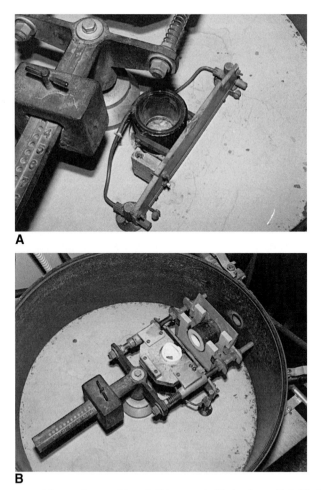

Fig. 12-20 Induction melting casting machine. **A,** Water-cooled induction coil. **B,** Vertical crucible **(white area)** positioned within the induction coil.

surface is quite sharp and parabolic in form, reaching zero at the button surface. Ordinarily, the pressure gradient at the moment before solidification reaches about 0.21 to 0.28 MPa (30 to 40 psi) at the tip of the casting. Because of this pressure gradient, there is also a gradient in the heat transfer rate such that the greatest rate of heat transfer to the mold is at the high pressure end of the gradient (i.e., the tip of the casting). Because this end also is frequently the sharp edge of the margin of a crown, there is further assurance that the solidification progresses from the thin margin edge to the button surface.

Electrical Resistance–Heated Casting Machine

In this device, current is passed through a resistance heating conductor, and automatic melting of the alloy occurs in a graphite or ceramic crucible. This is an advantage, especially for alloys such as those used for metal-ceramic prostheses, which are alloyed with base metals in trace amounts that tend to oxidize on overheating. Another advantage is that the crucible in the furnace is located flush against the casting ring. Therefore the alloy button remains molten slightly longer, again ensuring that solidification progresses completely from the tip of the casting to the button surface. A carbon crucible should not be used in the melting of high-palladium alloys, palladium-silver alloys, nickel-chromium alloys, or cobalt-chromium base metal alloys. An example of the electrical resistance casting machine is shown in Figure 12-19.

Induction Melting Machine

With this unit, the alloy is melted by an induction field that develops within a crucible surrounded by water-cooled metal tubing (see Fig. 12-20). The electric induction furnace is a transformer in which an alternating current flows through the primary winding coil and generates a variable magnetic field in the location of the alloy to be melted in a crucible. Once the alloy reaches the casting temperature in air or in vacuum, it is forced into the mold by centrifugal force, by air pressure, or by vacuum. The device has become popular in the casting of jewelry, but it has not been used as much as the other two techniques for noble alloy castings. It is more commonly used for melting base metal alloys.

There is little practical difference in the properties or accuracy of castings made with any of the three types of casting machines. The choice is a matter of access to specialized equipment and personal preference.

Direct-Current Arc Melting Machine

The direct-current arc is produced between two electrodes: the alloy and the water-cooled tungsten electrode. The temperature within the arc exceeds 4000° C, and the alloy melts very quickly. This method has a high risk for overheating the alloy, and damage may result after only a few seconds of prolonged heating.

Vacuum- or Pressure-Assisted Casting Machine

For this method, the molten alloy is heated to the casting temperature, drawn into the evacuated mold by gravity or vacuum, and subjected to additional pressure to force the alloy into the mold. For titanium and titanium alloys, vacuum arc heated-argon pressure casting machines are required.

Casting Crucibles

Generally, four types of casting crucibles are available: clay, carbon, quartz, and zirconia-alumina. Clay crucibles are appropriate for many of the crown and bridge alloys, such as the high noble and noble types. Carbon crucibles can be used not only for high noble crown and bridge alloys but also for the higher-fusing, gold-based metal-ceramic alloys.

Crucibles made from alumina, quartz, or silica are recommended for high-fusing alloys of any type. These are especially suited for alloys that have a high melting temperature or those that are sensitive to carbon contamination. Crown and bridge alloys with a high palladium content, such as palladium-silver alloys for metal-ceramic copings, and any of the nickel-based or cobalt-based alloys are included in this category.

Torch Melting of Noble Metal Alloy

This type of alloy is best melted by placing it on the inner sidewall of the crucible. In this position, the operator can better observe the progress of the melting, and there is a greater opportunity for any gases in the flame to be reflected from the surface of the alloy rather than being absorbed.

The fuel used in most instances is a mixture of natural or artificial gas and air, although oxygen-air and acetylene can also be used. The temperature of the gas-air flame is greatly influenced by the nature of the gas and the proportions of gas and air in the mixture. Considerable care should be taken to obtain a nonluminous brush flame, with the different combustion zones clearly differentiated. Two types of flame can be obtained with a casting torch, as shown in Figure 12-21. The air supply for the lower flame (see Fig. 12-21) is excessive, and incomplete combustion and a lower temperature will result. This type of flame is likely to be favored by the beginner, because the roaring sound that accompanies this flame adjustment "sounds" hot. The upper brush flame indicates the proper adjustment for maximal efficiency and temperature.

The parts of the flame can be identified by the conical areas in Figure 12-21. The first long cone emanating directly from the nozzle is the zone in which the air and gas are mixed before combustion. No heat is present in this zone. The next cone, which is green and immediately surrounding the inner cone, is known as the combustion zone. Here, the gas and air are partially burned. This zone is definitely oxidizing, and it should always be kept away from the molten alloy during fusion.

The next zone, dimly blue and located just beyond the tip of the green combustion zone, is the *reducing zone*. This is the hottest part of the flame, and it should be kept constantly on the alloy during melting. The outer cone (*oxidizing zone*) is the area in which combustion occurs with the oxygen in the air. Under no circumstances should this portion of the flame be used to melt the alloy. Not only is its temperature lower than that of the reducing zone, but it also oxidizes the alloy.

With a little practice, the clinician can readily detect whether the proper zone of the flame is in contact with the metal by observing the condition of the alloy surface. When the reducing zone is in contact, the surface of the gold alloy is bright and mirrorlike, as indicated in Figure 12-22, *A*. When the oxidizing portion of the flame is in contact with the alloy, there is a dull film of "dross" developed over the surface, as seen in Figure 12-22, *B*. Although care should be taken not to overheat the alloy, there is generally more likelihood of underheating when the gas-air flame is used. The alloy first appears to be spongy, and then small globules of fused alloy appear. The molten alloy soon assumes a spheroidal shape, as indicated in Figure 12-22, *A*. At the proper casting temperature, the molten alloy is light orange and tends to spin or follow the flame when the latter is moved slightly. At this point, the alloy should be approximately 38° to 66° C above its liquidus temperature. The casting should be made

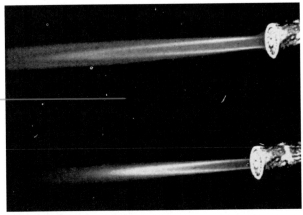

Fig. 12-21 Two types of nonluminous flame showing combustion areas. The upper flame should be employed for fusing the noble metal alloy. The lower flame results from too much air in the mixture.

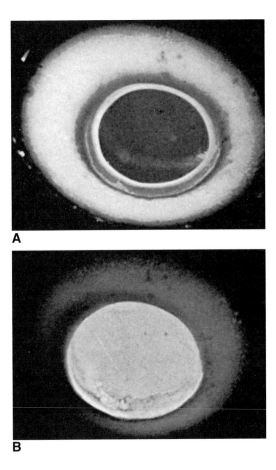

Fig. 12-22 **A,** Mirrorlike surface of the metal indicates proper fusion. **B,** Cloudy surface indicates surface oxidation by improper positioning of the torch flame.

immediately when the proper temperature is reached. As previously discussed, there are also various devices available for melting the alloy electrically.

It is desirable to use a flux for gold crown and bridge alloys to aid in minimizing porosity. When properly used, the flux increases the fluidity of the alloy, and the film of flux formed on the surface of the molten alloy helps prevent oxidation. Reducing fluxes containing powdered charcoal are often used, but small bits of carbon may be carried into the mold and cause a deficiency at a critical margin. Although such reducing fluxes are excellent for cleaning old alloy, a better flux for the casting procedure may be made from equal parts of fused borax powder ground with boric acid powder. The boric acid aids in retaining the borax on the surface of the alloy. The flux is added when the alloy is completely melted and should be used with both old and new alloy. Old sprues and buttons from the same alloy may be recast if they are not contaminated.

Cleaning the Casting

Let us first consider the gold crown and bridge alloys. After the casting has solidified, the ring is removed and quenched in water as soon as the button exhibits a dull-red glow. Two advantages are gained in quenching: (1) the noble metal alloy is left in an annealed condition for burnishing, polishing, and similar procedures, and (2) when the water contacts the hot investment, a violent reaction ensues, resulting in a soft, granular investment that is easily removed.

Often the surface of the casting appears dark with oxides and tarnish. Such a surface film can be removed by a process known as *pickling*, which consists of heating the discolored casting in an acid. One of the best pickling solutions for gypsum-bonded investments is a 50% hydrochloric acid solution. The hydrochloric acid aids in the removal of any residual investment, as well as of the oxide coating. The disadvantage of hydrochloric acid is that the fumes from the acid are likely to corrode laboratory metal furnishings. In addition, these fumes are a health hazard and should be vented via a fume hood. However, the pickling process can be performed ultrasonically while the prosthesis is sealed in a Teflon container. A solution of sulfuric acid may also be more advantageous in this respect. Ultrasonic devices are useful for cleaning the casting, as are commercial pickling solutions made of acid salts. Abrasive blasting devices are also useful for cleaning the surface of castings.

The best method for pickling is to place the casting in a test tube or dish and to pour the acid over it. It may be necessary to heat the acid, but boiling should be avoided because of the considerable amount of acid fumes involved. After pickling, the acid is poured off and the casting is removed. The pickling solution should be renewed frequently, because it is likely to become contaminated after reusing the solution several times.

In no case should the casting be held with steel tongs so that both the casting and the tongs come into contact with the pickling solution, because this may contaminate the casting. The pickling solution usually contains small amounts of copper dissolved from previous castings. When the steel tongs contact this electrolyte, a small galvanic cell is created and copper is deposited on the casting at the point where the tongs grip it. This copper deposition extends into the alloy and is a future source for discoloration in the area.

It is a common practice to heat the casting and then drop it into the pickling solution. The disadvantage of this method is that a delicate margin may be melted in the flame or the casting may be distorted by the sudden thermal shock when plunged into the acid.

Gold-based and palladium-based metal-ceramic alloys and base metal alloys are bench-cooled to room temperature before the casting is removed from the investment. Castings from these alloys are generally not pickled, and when pickling is recommended for certain metal-ceramic alloys, it is only to selectively remove specific surface oxides.

Melting of Base Metals

Although torch melting can be used in some cases, most base metals of Ni-Cr, Ni-Cr-Be, Co-Cr, Co-Ni-Cr, commercially pure Ti, and Ti-Al-V require special melting equipment, such as induction melting machines, vacuum melting devices, or arc-melting units. The procedures required are designed to minimize the risk for excessive oxidation or an interaction of the molten alloys with the recommended casting investments. It is beyond the scope of this book to discuss these methods; the reader is referred to specialized instruction manuals developed by the manufacturers of these products.

TECHNICAL CONSIDERATIONS FOR PHOSPHATE-BONDED INVESTMENT

The procedure for investing a wax pattern in a phosphate-bonded investment is essentially the same as that for a gypsum-bonded investment. As previously mentioned, the working time can vary depending on the L/P ratio, special liquid concentration, temperature, mixing time, mixing rate, and operator skill and experience.

As with any investment that has a high thermal expansion, especially when marked changes in expansion or contraction occur, it is necessary to use a slow heating rate during burnout to prevent possible cracking or spalling. Some furnaces provide slow rates of heating. For those that do not, it is advisable to use a two-stage burnout, holding at 200° to 300° C for at least 30 min before completing the burnout. Recommendations for the rate of heating vary, so it is wise to follow the instructions for the specific investment used.

Although phosphate investments appear strong, they are still subject to a number of disrupting influences during burnout. At first the wax softens and then expands much more than does the investment. When investing, it is desirable to leave 3 to 6 mm of investment around each pattern and to stagger the patterns if several are placed in the same ring. A number of patterns positioned along a plane can exert tremendous pressure and fracture almost any investment, but particularly the phosphate-bonded materials. The rapid expansion of cristobalite investment at approximately 300° C requires slow heating to prevent fracture. After the temperature reaches 400° C, the rate of heating can be safely increased. After burnout, usually at a final temperature of 700° to 1030° C depending on the alloy melting range, the casting is made. As previously mentioned, the permeability of the phosphate investment is low compared with that of a gypsum-bonded investment. Therefore the required casting pressure should be greater than for a gypsum mold.

Recovery and cleaning of the casting are more difficult when a phosphate-bonded investment is used because such materials do not contain the soft gypsum products. Also, the particles usually include large grains of quartz. In some instances, such as with gold-containing alloys, the investment adheres rather tenaciously, usually requiring cleansing in an ultrasonic cleaner. Neither the phosphate binder nor the silica refractory is soluble in hydrochloric or sulfuric acid. Cold hydrofluoric acid dissolves the silica refractory quite well without damage to a gold-based or a palladium-silver alloy, but this must be used carefully with other alloys. In fact, even dilute hydrofluoric acid should not be used unless the necessary neutralizing solutions are immediately at hand and the clinician is familiar with the correct handling techniques. However, once tissue injury has occurred, it cannot be reversed with such solutions. Alternative solutions such as No-San can be used with greater safety.

Base metal alloys require a light sandblasting, usually with fine alumina. Chromium-based partial dentures are usually sandblasted to remove the investment. Acid should not be used for cleaning base metal alloys.

The selection of the appropriate phosphate-bonded investment must be made on the basis of the composition of the alloy to be used. Carbon-containing investments are well suited for gold-based crown and bridge casting alloys and metal-ceramic alloys. However, if the alloy is carbon-sensitive (such as in silver-palladium, high palladium, palladium-silver, nickel-chromium-beryllium, nickel-chromium, and cobalt-chromium alloys), a noncarbon investment should be used.

CAUSES OF DEFECTIVE CASTINGS

An unsuccessful casting results in considerable trouble and loss of time. In almost all instances, defects in castings can be avoided by strict observance of procedures governed by certain fundamental rules and principles. Seldom is a defect in a casting attributable to factors other than the carelessness or ignorance of the operator. With present techniques, casting failures should be the exception, not the rule.

Defects in castings can be classified under four headings: (1) distortion; (2) surface roughness and irregularities; (3) porosity; and (4) incomplete or missing detail. Some of these factors have been discussed in connection with certain phases of the casting techniques. The subject is summarized and analyzed in some detail in the following sections.

Distortion

Any marked distortion of the casting is probably related to a distortion of the wax pattern, as described in the chapter on inlay wax. This type of distortion can be minimized or prevented by proper manipulation of the wax and handling of the pattern.

Unquestionably, some distortion of the wax pattern occurs as the investment hardens around it. The setting and hygroscopic expansions of the investment may produce a nonuniform expansion of the walls of the pattern. This type of distortion occurs in part from the nonuniform outward movement of the proximal walls. The gingival margins are forced apart by the mold expansion, whereas the solid occlusal bar of wax resists expansion during the early stages of setting. The configuration of the pattern, the type of wax, and the thickness influence the distortion that occurs, as has been discussed. For example, distortion increases as the thickness of the pattern decreases. As would be expected, the less the setting expansion of the investment, the less the distortion. Generally, this is not a serious problem, except that it accounts for some of the unexplained inaccuracies that may occur in small castings. Nevertheless, not a great deal can be done to control this phenomenon.

Surface Roughness, Irregularities, and Discoloration

The surface of a dental casting should be an accurate reproduction of the surface of the wax pattern from which it is made. Excessive roughness or irregularities on the outer surface of the casting necessitate additional finishing and polishing, whereas irregularities on the cavity surface prevent a proper seating of an otherwise accurate casting.

Surface roughness should not be confused with surface irregularities. Surface roughness is defined as relatively finely spaced surface imperfections whose height, width, and direction establish the predominant surface pattern. Surface irregularities are isolated imperfections, such as nodules, that are not characteristic of the entire surface area.

Even under optimal conditions, the surface roughness of the dental casting is invariably somewhat greater than that of the wax pattern from which it is made. The difference is probably related to the particle size of the investment and its ability to reproduce the wax pattern in microscopic detail. With proper manipulative techniques, the normal increased roughness in the casting should not be a major factor in dimensional accuracy. However, improper technique can lead to a marked increase in surface roughness, as well as to the formation of surface irregularities.

Air Bubbles

Small nodules on a casting are caused by air bubbles that become attached to the pattern during or subsequent to the investing procedure. Such nodules can sometimes be removed if they are not in a critical area. However, for nodules on margins or on internal surfaces, as shown in Figure 12-23, A, removal of these irregularities might alter the fit of the casting. As previously noted, the best method to avoid air bubbles is to use the vacuum investing technique.

If a manual method is used, various precautions can be observed to eliminate air from the investment mix before the investing. As previously outlined, the use of a

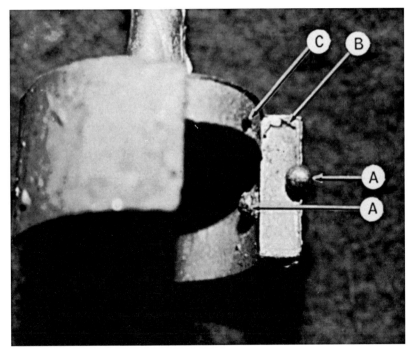

Fig. 12-23 Surface irregularities on an experimental casting caused by air bubbles **(A),** water film **(B),** and inclusion of foreign body **(C).** (Courtesy of D. Veira.)

mechanical mixer with vibration both before and after mixing should be practiced routinely. A wetting agent may be helpful in preventing the collection of air bubbles on the surface of the pattern, but it is by no means a certain remedy. As previously discussed, it is important that the wetting agent be applied in a thin layer. It is best to air-dry the wetting agent, because any excess liquid dilutes the investment, possibly producing surface irregularities on the casting.

Water Films

Wax is repellent to water, and if the investment becomes separated from the wax pattern in some manner, a water film may form irregularly over the surface. Occasionally, this type of surface irregularity appears as minute ridges or veins on the surface, as shown in Figure 12-23, *B*. If the pattern is slightly moved, jarred, or vibrated after investing, or if the painting procedure does not result in an intimate contact of the investment with the pattern, such a condition may result. A wetting agent is of aid in the prevention of such irregularities. Too high an L/P ratio may also produce these surface irregularities.

Rapid Heating Rates

This factor, which has been discussed in a previous section, may result in fins or spines on the casting, similar to those shown in Figure 12-17. Also, a characteristic surface roughness may be evident because of flaking of the investment when the water or steam pours into the mold. Furthermore, such a surge of steam or water may carry some of the salts used as modifiers into the mold, and these salts are left as deposits on the walls after the water evaporates. As previously mentioned, the mold should be heated gradually; at least 60 min should elapse during the heating of the investment-filled ring from room temperature to 700° C. The greater the bulk of the investment, the more slowly it should be heated.

Underheating

Incomplete elimination of wax residues may occur if the heating time is too short or if insufficient air is available in the furnace. These factors are particularly important with the low-temperature investment techniques. Voids or porosity may occur in the casting from the gases formed when the hot alloy comes in contact with the carbon residues. Occasionally, the casting may be covered with a tenacious carbon coating that is virtually impossible to remove by pickling.

Liquid/Powder Ratio

The amount of water and investment should be measured accurately. The higher the L/P ratio, the rougher the casting. However, if too little water is used, the investment may be unmanageably thick and cannot be properly applied to the pattern. In vacuum investing, the air may not be sufficiently removed. In either instance, a rough surface on the casting may result.

Prolonged Heating

When the high-heat casting technique is used, a prolonged heating of the mold at the casting temperature is likely to cause a disintegration of the gypsum-bonded investment, and the walls of the mold are roughened as a result. Furthermore, the products of decomposition are sulfur compounds that may contaminate the alloy to the extent that the surface texture is affected. Such contamination may be the reason that the surface of the casting sometimes does not respond to pickling. When the thermal expansion technique is employed, the mold should be heated to the casting temperature—never higher—and the casting should be made immediately.

Temperature of the Alloy

If an alloy is heated to too high a temperature before casting, the surface of the investment is likely to be attacked, and a surface roughness of the type described in the previous section may result. In all probability, the alloy will not be overheated with a gas-air torch when used with the gas supplied in most localities. If other fuel is used, special care should be observed that the color emitted by the molten gold alloy, for example, is no lighter than a light orange.

Casting Pressure

Too high a pressure during casting can produce a rough surface on the casting. A gauge pressure of 0.10 to 0.14 MPa in an air pressure casting machine or three to four turns of the spring in an average type of centrifugal casting machine is sufficient for small castings.

Composition of the Investment

The ratio of the binder to the quartz influences the surface texture of the casting. In addition, a coarse silica causes a surface roughness. If the investment meets

ANSI/ADA Specification No. 2, the composition is probably not a factor in the surface roughness.

Foreign Bodies

When foreign substances get into the mold, a surface roughness may be produced. For example, a rough crucible former with investment clinging to it may roughen the investment on its removal so that bits of investment are carried into the mold with the molten alloy. Carelessness in the removal of the sprue former may also be a cause.

Usually, contamination results not only in surface roughness but also in incomplete areas or surface voids. An example of this may be seen in Figure 12-23, C. Any casting that shows sharp, well-defined deficiencies indicates the presence of some foreign particles in the mold, such as pieces of investment and bits of carbon from a flux. Bright-appearing concavities may be the result of flux being carried into the mold with the metal.

Surface discoloration and roughness can result from sulfur contamination, either from investment breakdown at elevated temperatures or from a high sulfur content of the torch flame. The interaction of the molten alloy with sulfur produces a black or grey layer on the surface of gold alloys that is brittle and does not clean readily during pickling.

Impact of Molten Alloy

The direction of the sprue former should be such that the molten gold alloy does not strike a weak portion of the mold surface. Occasionally, the molten alloy may fracture or abrade the mold surface on impact, regardless of its bulk. It is unfortunate that sometimes the abraded area is smooth so that it cannot be detected on the surface of the casting. Such a depression in the mold is reflected as a raised area on the casting, often too slight to be noticed yet sufficiently large to prevent complete seating of the casting. This type of surface roughness or irregularity can be avoided by proper spruing so as to prevent the direct impact of the molten metal at an angle of 90 degrees to the investment surface. A glancing impact is likely to be less damaging, and at the same time an undesirable turbulence is avoided.

Pattern Position

If several patterns are invested in the same ring, they should not be placed too close together. Likewise, positioning too many patterns in the same plane in the mold should be avoided. The expansion of wax is much greater than that of the investment, causing breakdown or cracking of the investment if the spacing between patterns is less than 3 mm.

Carbon Inclusions

Carbon, as from a crucible, an improperly adjusted torch, or a carbon-containing investment, can be absorbed by the alloy during casting. These particles may lead to the formation of carbides or even create visible carbon inclusions.

Other Causes

Certain surface discolorations and roughness may not be evident when the casting is completed but may appear during service. For example, various gold alloys, such as solders, bits of wire, and mixtures of different casting alloys should never be melted together and reused. The resulting mixture would not possess the proper physical properties and might form a eutectic phase with low corrosion resistance. Discoloration and corrosion may also occur.

A source of discoloration often overlooked is the surface contamination of a gold alloy restoration by mercury. Mercury penetrates rapidly into the alloy and causes a marked loss in ductility and a greater susceptibility to corrosion. Thus it is not a good practice to place a new amalgam restoration adjacent to a high noble alloy restoration. In addition, these dissimilar metals form a galvanic cell that can lead to breakdown of the anode (amalgam) relative to the cathode (noble alloy).

CRITICAL QUESTION

How can the risk for porosity and incomplete castings be minimized?

Porosity

Porosity may occur both within the interior region of a casting and on the external surface. The latter is a factor in surface roughness, but also it is generally a manifestation of internal porosity. Not only does the internal porosity weaken the casting, but if it also extends to the surface, it may be a cause for discoloration. If severe, it can cause plaque accumulation at the tooth-restoration interface, and secondary caries may result. Although the porosity in a casting cannot be prevented entirely, it can be minimized by use of proper techniques.

Porosities in noble metal alloy castings may be classified as follows:
    I. Solidification defects
        A. Localized shrinkage porosity
        B. Microporosity
    II. Trapped gases
        A. Pinhole porosity
        B. Gas inclusions
        C. Subsurface porosity
    III. Residual air

Localized shrinkage is generally caused by premature termination of the flow of molten metal during solidification. The linear contraction of noble metal alloys in changing from a liquid to a solid is at least 1.25%. Therefore continual feeding of molten metal through the sprue must occur to make up for the shrinkage of metal volume during solidification. If the sprue freezes in its cross-section before this feeding is completed to the casting proper, a localized shrinkage void will occur in the last portion of the casting that solidifies. Four types of porosity are shown in Figure 12-24, *A* and *B*: (a) localized shrinkage porosity, (b) microporosity, (c) pinhole porosity, and (d) subsurface porosity. Localized shrinkage porosity is also shown in Figure 12-24, *C*. The porosity in the pontic area is caused by the ability of the pontic to retain heat because of its bulk and because it was located in the heat center of the ring. This problem can be solved simply by attaching one or more small-gauge sprues (e.g., 18-gauge) at the surface most distant from the main sprue attachment and extending the sprue(s) laterally within 5 mm of the edge of the ring. These small chill-set sprues ensure that solidification begins within the sprues, and they act as cooling pins to carry heat away from the pontic.

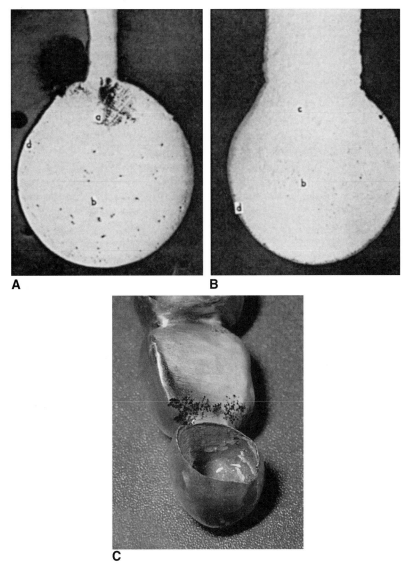

Fig. 12-24 **A** and **B,** Spherical gold alloy casting showing localized shrinkage microporosity **(a),** microporosity **(b),** pinhole porosity **(c),** and subsurface porosity **(d).** **C,** Localized shrinkage porosity in pontic of three-unit bridge caused by delayed solidification and lack of a chill-set sprue. (**A** and **B** from Ryge G, Kozok SF, and Fairhurst CW: Porosities in dental gold casting. J Am Dent Assoc 54:746, 1957.)

Localized shrinkage generally occurs near the sprue-casting junction, but it may occur anywhere between dendrites, as shown in Figure 12-25, C, where the last part of the casting to solidify was in the low melting metal that remains as the dendrite branches develop.

This type of void may also occur externally, usually in the interior of a crown near the area of the sprue, if a hot spot has been created by the hot metal impinging from the sprue channel on a point of the mold wall. This hot spot causes the local region to freeze last and results in what is called *suck-back porosity*, as shown in Figure 12-26 (*left*). Suck-back porosity often occurs at an occlusoaxial line angle or incisoaxial line angle that is not well rounded. The entering metal impinges onto the mold surface at this point and creates a higher localized mold temperature in this region, known as a *hot spot*. A hot spot may retain a localized pool of molten metal after

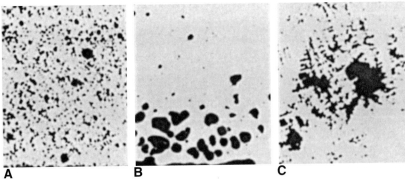

Fig. 12-25   A, Microporosity, pinhole porosity, and gas inclusions. Microporosity voids are irregular in shape, whereas the two other types tend to be spherical; the largest spherical voids are gas inclusions. **B,** Subsurface porosity. **C,** Localized shrinkage porosity. (Courtesy of G. Ryge.)

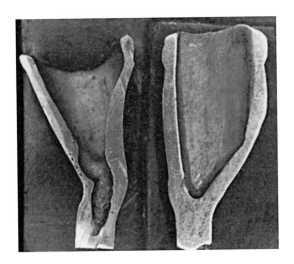

Fig. 12-26   Example of suck-back porosity. **Left,** The coping was cast at 1370° C (2500° F). **Right,** This coping was cast at 1340° C (2450° F). (Courtesy of J. Nielsen.)

other areas of the casting have solidified. This in turn creates a shrinkage void, or suck-back porosity. Suck-back porosity can be eliminated by flaring the point of sprue attachment and reducing the mold-melt temperature differential, that is, lowering the casting temperature by about 30° C.

Microporosity also occurs from solidification shrinkage but is generally present in fine-grain alloy castings when the solidification is too rapid for the microvoids to segregate to the liquid pool. This premature solidification causes the porosity shown in Figure 12-24, *C,* and portions of Figure 12-26 in the form of small, irregular voids.

Such phenomena can occur from rapid solidification if the mold or casting temperature is too low. Unfortunately, this type of defect is not detectable unless the casting is sectioned. In any case, it is generally not a serious defect. The effects of various factors involved in formation of microporosity, and other types of porosity, are summarized in Table 12-3.

Both *pinhole* and the *gas inclusion porosities* are related to the entrapment of gas during solidification. Both are characterized by a spherical contour, but they are decidedly different in size. The gas inclusion porosities are usually much larger than pinhole porosity, as indicated in Figure 12-25, *A.* Many metals dissolve or occlude gases while they are molten. For example, both copper and silver dissolve oxygen in large amounts in the liquid state. Molten platinum and palladium have a strong affinity for hydrogen as well as oxygen. On solidification, the absorbed gases are

Table 12-3	Effects of Technical Factors on the Porosity Resulting from Metal Solidification			
Type of porosity	Increase in sprue thickness	Increase in sprue length	Increase in melt temperature	Increase in mold temperature
Localized shrinkage	Reduced	Increased	Reduced	Reduced
Subsurface porosity	Increased	Reduced	Increased	Increased
Microporosity	No effect	No effect	Reduced	Reduced

With permission from Ryge G, Kozak SF, and Fairhurst CW: J Am Dent Assoc 54:746, 1957.

expelled and pinhole porosity results. The larger voids (see Fig. 12-25, *A*) may also result from the same cause, but it is more logical to assume that such voids are caused by gas that is mechanically trapped by the molten metal in the mold or by gas that is incorporated during the casting procedure. All castings probably contain a certain amount of porosity, as exemplified by the photomicrographs shown in Figure 12-27. However, the porosity should be kept to a minimum because it may adversely affect the physical properties of the casting.

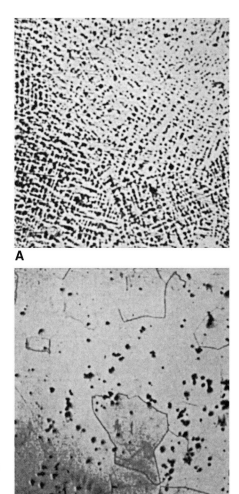

Fig. 12-27 **A,** Grain structure of an as-cast Type III noble metal alloy. **B,** Same alloy after a homogenization heat treatment at 725° C (1337° F) for 70 min. Pinhole porosity is visible. (Courtesy of B. Hedegard.)

Oxygen is dissolved by some of the metals, such as silver, in the alloy while they are in the molten state. During solidification, the gas is expelled to form blebs and pores in the metal. As was pointed out earlier, this type of porosity may be attributed to abuse of the metal. Castings that are severely contaminated with gases are usually black when they are removed from the investment and do not clean easily on pickling (Fig. 12-28). The porosity that extends to the surface is usually in the form of small pinpoint holes (see Fig. 12-25, *A*). When the surface is polished, other pinholes appear.

Larger spherical porosities can be caused by gas occluded from a poorly adjusted torch flame, or by use of the mixing or oxidizing zones of the flame rather than the reducing zone (see Fig. 12-25, *A*). These types of porosity can be minimized by premelting the gold alloy on a graphite crucible or a graphite block, if the alloy has been used before, and by correctly adjusting and positioning the torch flame during melting.

Subsurface porosity occurs on occasion, as is shown in Figures 12-24, *B*, and 12-25, *B*. At other times, it may be particularly evident. The reasons for such voids have not been completely established. They may be caused by the simultaneous nucleation of solid grains and gas bubbles at the first moment that the alloy freezes at the mold walls. As has been explained, this type of porosity can be diminished by controlling the rate at which the molten metal enters the mold.

Entrapped-air porosity on the inner surface of the casting, sometimes referred to as *back-pressure porosity*, can produce large concave depressions such as those seen in Figure 12-29. This is caused by the inability of the air in the mold to escape through the pores in the investment or by the pressure gradient that displaces the air pocket toward the end of the investment via the molten sprue and button. The entrapment is frequently found in a "pocket" at the cavity surface of a crown or mesio-occlusal-distal casting (see Fig. 12-29). Occasionally, it is found even on the outside surface of the casting when the casting temperature or mold temperature is so low that solidification occurs before the entrapped air can escape. The incidence of entrapped air can be increased by use of the dense modern investments, by an increase in mold density produced by vacuum investing, and by the tendency for the mold to clog with residual carbon when the low-heat technique is used. Each of these factors tends to slow the venting of gases from the mold during casting.

Proper burnout, an adequate mold and casting temperature, a sufficiently high casting pressure, and proper L/P ratio can help to eliminate entrapped-air porosity. It is good practice to make sure that the thickness of investment between the tip of the pattern and the end of the ring not be greater than 6 mm.

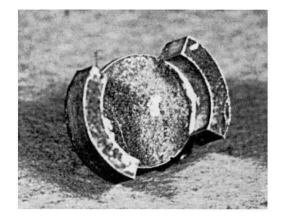

Fig. 12-28 A black-coated noble metal alloy casting resulting from sulfur contamination or oxidation during melting of the alloy.

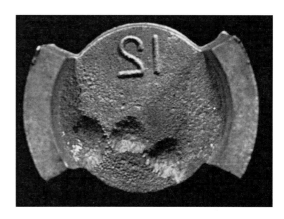

Fig. 12-29 Surface irregularity on cavity side of casting caused by back-pressure porosity.

Incomplete Casting

Occasionally, only a partially complete casting, or perhaps no casting at all, is found. The obvious cause is that the molten alloy has been prevented, in some manner, from completely filling the mold. At least two factors that may inhibit the ingress of the liquefied alloy are insufficient venting of the mold and high viscosity of the fused metal.

The first consideration, insufficient venting, is directly related to the back pressure exerted by the air in the mold. If the air cannot be vented quickly, the molten alloy does not fill the mold before it solidifies. In such a case, the magnitude of the casting pressure should be suspected. If insufficient casting pressure is used, the back pressure cannot be overcome. Furthermore, the pressure should be applied for at least 4 sec. The mold is filled and the alloy is solidified in 1 sec or less; yet it is quite soft during the early stages. Therefore the pressure should be maintained for a few seconds beyond this point. An example of an incomplete casting because of insufficient casting pressure is shown in Figure 12-30. These failures are usually exemplified in rounded, incomplete margins.

A second common cause for an incomplete casting is incomplete elimination of wax residues from the mold. If too many products of combustion remain in the mold, the pores in the investment may become filled so that the air cannot be vented completely. If moisture or particles of wax remain, the contact of the molten alloy with these foreign substances produces an explosion that may produce sufficient back pressure to prevent the mold from being filled. An example of a casting failure caused by incomplete wax elimination can be seen Figure 12-31 and is shown

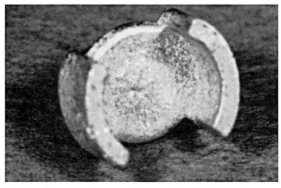

Fig. 12-30 Rounded, incomplete margins are evidence of insufficient casting pressure.

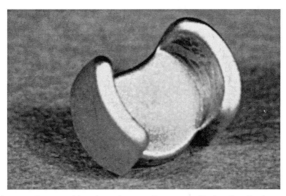

Fig. 12-31 Incomplete casting resulting from incomplete wax elimination is characterized by rounded margins and shiny appearance.

schematically in Figure 12-32. Although similar to the incomplete casting in Figure 12-30, the rounded margins in Figure 12-31 are quite shiny rather than dull. This shiny condition of the metal is caused by the strong reducing atmosphere created by carbon monoxide left by the residual wax.

The possible influence of the L/P ratio of the investment has already been discussed. A lower L/P ratio is associated with less porosity of the investment. An increase in casting pressure during casting solves this problem.

Different alloy compositions probably exhibit varying viscosities in the molten state, depending on composition and temperature. However, both the surface tension and the viscosity of a molten alloy are decreased with an increase in temperature. An incomplete casting resulting from too great a viscosity can be attributed to insufficient heating. The temperature of the alloy should be raised higher than its liquidus temperature so that its viscosity and surface tension are lowered and so that

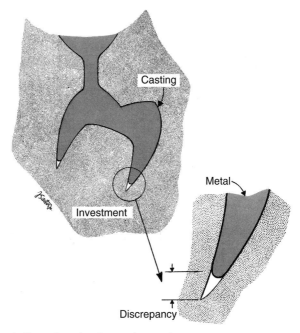

Fig. 12-32 Schematic illustration of an incomplete casting.

it does not solidify prematurely as it enters the mold. Such premature solidification may account for the greater susceptibility of the white gold alloys to porosity because their liquidus temperatures are higher. Thus they are more difficult to melt with a gas-air torch flame.

SELECTED READINGS

Christensen GJ: Marginal fit of gold inlay castings. J Prosthet Dent 16:297-305, 1966.

In this laboratory study, 10 dentists accepted cemented gold inlays with a mean occlusal margin opening of 21 μm (range of 2 to 51 μm), a mean proximal margin opening of 26 μm (range of 9 to 34 μm), and a gingival margin opening of 74 μm (range of 34 to 119 μm). Explorer examination of visually accessible areas was superior to either explorer or radiographic examination of visually inaccessible areas.

Cooney JP, and Caputo AA: Type III gold alloy complete crowns cast in a phosphate-bonded investment. J Prosthet Dent 46:414-419, 1981.

Marginal fit was superior for castings made in phosphate-bonded investment; surface roughness was less when cast in the gypsum-bonded investment.

Dootz ER, and Asgar K: Solidification patterns of single crowns and three-unit bridge castings. Quint Dent Technol 10:299-305, 1986.

Solidification rates and patterns differed for Type III gold alloy and a palladium-silver alloy. The gold alloy solidified or random pattern, whereas the palladium-silver metal-ceramic alloy solidified in a unidirectional manner.

Eames WB, O'Neal SJ, Monteiro J, et al: Techniques to improve the seating of castings. J Am Dent Assoc 96:432-437, 1978.

Die spacing was the most suitable method to compensate for casting variables and to ensure improved marginal adaptation while also increasing retention by 25%.

Earnshaw R: The effect of casting ring liners on the potential expansion of a gypsum-bonded investment. J Dent Res 67:1366-1370, 1988.

Total expansion, setting expansion, and thermal expansion, of the investment setting against a smooth, dry surface was 1.7%; against a dry ceramic liner, 1.6% to 1.7%; and against wet cellulose or wet asbestos, 2.2% to 2.3%. The ceramic liner can be used wet if it is treated with a surfactant instead of water.

Finger W: Effect of the setting expansion of dental stone upon the die precision. Scand J Dent Res 88:159-160, 1980.

The addition of potassium sulfate and borax to Type IV gypsums reduced setting expansion without affecting the physical properties.

Finger W, and Ohsawa M: Accuracy of cast restorations produced by a refractory die-investing technique. J Prosthet Dent 52:800-803, 1984.

By minimizing distortion of the wax pattern, the refractory die-investing procedure can produce consistently accurate cast gold alloy restorations.

Jorgensen KD, and Okamoto A: Restraining factors affecting setting expansion of phosphate-bonded investments. Scand J Dent Res 94:178-81, 1986.

The authors suggest that setting expansion is a highly unreliable means to compensate partially for the thermal contraction of casting alloys.

Junner RE, and Stevens L: Anisotropic setting expansion of phosphate-bonded investment. Aust Dent J 31:434-439, 1986.

The vertical setting expansion was significantly greater than the horizontal expansion in a rigid ring with liners. A flexible ring offered little restriction to horizontal expansion, reducing mold distortion.

Kaplan J, and Newman SM: Accuracy of the divestment casting technique. Oper Dent 8:82-87, 1983.

Castings made using the divestment procedure fit more accurately than did castings made using a conventional stone-die and gypsum-bonded refractory investment technique.

Lautenschlager EP, Harcourt JK, and Ploszaj LC: Setting reaction of gypsum materials investigated by x-ray diffraction. J Dent Res 48:43-48, 1969.

An early study of the conversion from calcium sulfate hemihydrate to calcium sulfate dihydrate.

Mackert JR Jr: An expert system for analysis of casting failures. Int J Prosthodont 1:268-280, 1988.

An expert system is proposed for the diagnosis of common lost-wax casting problems, based on an interactive consultation session at a PC station, during which the user answers questions about defective castings. The computer responds with conclusions on the most likely cause of each problem.

Mahler DB, and Ady AB: An explanation for the hygroscopic setting expansion of dental gypsum products. J Dent Res 39:578, 1960.

A classic publication on the theory of hygroscopic setting expansion. Excellent reference for those interested in the mechanics of this phenomenon.

Martin KH: An investigation of the effect of the water/powder ratio on the accuracy of the fit of gold alloy castings. Aust Dent J 1:202, 1956.

Use of the correct water/powder ratio with a gypsum investment is essential to obtaining a good fit of castings, especially when using the low-heat technique.

Matsuya S, and Yamane M: Decomposition of gypsum-bonded investments. J Dent Res 60:1418-1423, 1981.

At 900° C decomposition of gypsum-bonded investments occurred, leading to the formation of $CaSiO_3$ and Ca_2SiO_4.

Mueller HJ, Reyes W, and McGill S: Surfactant-containing phosphate investment. Dent Mater 2:42-44, 1986.

The addition of surfactants in a phosphate-bonded casting investment can increase the hygroscopic setting expansion. The surfactant also makes the unset investment more viscous and reduces the compressive strength.

Naylor WP, Moore BK, and Phillips RW: A topographical assessment of casting ring liners using scanning electron microscopy (SEM). Quint Dent Technol 11:413-420, 1987.

Three types of nonasbestos ring liners exist: ceramic, cellulose, and a ceramic-cellulose combination. A liner containing an aluminosilicate component has the potential to produce respirable-size ceramic particles.

Neiman R, and Sarma AC: Setting and thermal reactions of phosphate investments. J Dent Res:1478-1485, 1980.

An explanation of the chemical reaction involved in the setting of phosphate-bonded investments.

Nielsen JP: Pressure distribution in centrifugal dental casting. J Dent Res 57:261-269, 1978.

This article discusses the factors contributing to the pressure gradient that develops along the length of a casting when cast in a centrifugal casting machine.

Nielsen JP, and Ollerman R: Suck-back porosity. Quint Dent Technol 1:61-65, 1976.

Using a gold-palladium-silver alloy with different sprue former lengths, diameters, and angles of attachment, lower casting temperature and flaring of the sprue former reduced suck-back porosity. The authors postulated that a "hot spot" is created in the mold that causes this type of porosity.

Nomura GT, Reisbick MH, and Preston JD: An investigation of epoxy resin dies. J Prosthet Dent 44:45-50, 1980.

In a comparison of three epoxy die materials with a Type IV stone, full crown epoxy dies were undersized, MOD onlay resin dies were accurate, and detail reproduction was found to be comparable to the Type IV gypsum. However, only one epoxy material had a hardness approaching that of the dental stone.

Santos JF, and Ballester RY: Delayed hygroscopic expansion of phosphate-bonded investments. Dent Mater 3:165-7, 1987.

Delayed hygroscopic expansion occurs when the investment is immersed in water after setting. Increased time of immersion and an increase in the special liquid concentration increased the hygroscopic setting expansion.

Stevens L: The effect of early heating on the expansion of a phosphate-bonded investment. Aust Dent J 28:366-369, 1983.

The thermal expansion of a phosphate-bonded investment decreased as heating was delayed from 1 to 6 hr after mixing. The setting expansion increased as the special liquid replaced water for mixing.

Taggart WH: A new and accurate method of making gold inlays. Dent Cosmos 49:1117, 1907.

The dental "lost wax" process was developed by Taggart, opening up the opportunity to cast accurate restorations in an investment mold.

Vaidyanathan TK, Schulman A, Nielsen JP, and Shalita S: Correlation between macroscopic porosity location and liquid metal pressure in centrifugal casting technique. J Dent Res 60:59-66, 1981.

Radiographic analysis of uniform cylindrical castings revealed that the porosity is dependent on the location at which the sprue is attached to the casting. The location of the macroscopic porosity, at portions of the casting close to the free surface of the button, is dependent on the pressure gradient and, therefore, different heat transfer rates in different portions of the casting.

Verrett RG, and Duke ES: The effect of sprue attachment design on castability and porosity. J Prosthet Dent 61:418-24, 1989.

Flared and straight sprue attachments optimized castability and minimized porosity.

13

Finishing and Polishing Materials

Kenneth J. Anusavice and Sibel A. Antonson

OUTLINE

Benefits of Finishing and Polishing Restorative Materials

Principles of Cutting, Grinding, Finishing, and Polishing

Abrasion and Erosion

Abrasive Instrument Design

Types of Abrasives

Finishing and Polishing Procedures

Dentifrices

KEY TERMS

Abrasive—A hard substance used for grinding, finishing, or polishing a less-hard surface.

Buffing—Process of producing a lustrous surface through the abrading action of fine abrasives bound to a nonabrasive binder medium.

Bulk reduction—Process of removing excess material by cutting or grinding a material with rotary instruments to provide a desired anatomic form.

Contouring—Process of producing a desired anatomical form by cutting or grinding away excess material.

Cutting—Process of removing material from the substrate by use of a bladed bur or an abrasive embedded in a binding matrix on a bur or disk.

Finished and polished restoration—A prosthesis or direct restoration whose outer surface has been progressively refined to a desired state of surface finish.

Finishing—Process of removing surface defects or scratches created during the contouring process through the use of cutting or grinding instruments or both.

Glaze ceramic—A specially formulated ceramic powder that, when mixed with a liquid, applied to a ceramic surface, and heated to an appropriate temperature for a sufficient time, forms a smooth glassy layer on a dental ceramic surface (see **natural glaze**).

Grinding—Process of removing material from a substrate by abrasion with relatively coarse particles.

Natural glaze—A vitrified layer that forms on the surface of a dental ceramic containing a glass phase when the ceramic is heated to a glazing temperature for a specified time.

Overglaze—Thin surface coating of glass formed by fusing a thin layer of glass powder that matures at a lower temperature than that associated with the ceramic substrate.

Polish—Luster or gloss produced on a finished surface.

Polishing—Process of providing luster or gloss on a material surface.

What are the advantages of polishing the surface of restorative materials?

BENEFITS OF FINISHING AND POLISHING RESTORATIVE MATERIALS

Finished and polished restorations provide three benefits of dental care: oral health, function, and aesthetics. A well-contoured and polished restoration promotes oral health by resisting the accumulation of food debris and pathogenic bacteria. This is accomplished through a reduction in total surface area and reduced roughness of the restoration surface. Smoother surfaces have less retention areas and are easier to maintain in a hygienic state when preventive oral home care is practiced because dental floss and the toothbrush bristles can gain more complete access to all surfaces and marginal areas. Tarnish and corrosion activity of some dental materials can be significantly reduced if the entire restoration is highly polished. Oral function is enhanced with a well-polished restoration because food glides more freely over occlusal and embrasure surfaces during mastication. More important, smooth restoration surfaces minimize wear rates on opposing and adjacent teeth. This is particularly true for restorative materials such as ceramics, which contain phases that are harder than tooth enamel and dentin.

Rough material surfaces lead to the development of high-contact stresses that can cause the loss of functional and stabilizing contacts between teeth. Rough surfaces on ceramics also act as stress concentration points. **Finishing** and **polishing** these surfaces can improve the strength of the restoration, especially in areas that are under tension. Finally, aesthetic demands may require the dentist to handle highly visible surfaces of restorations differently than those that are not accessible. Although a high mirror-like **polish** is preferred for the previously mentioned reasons, this type of surface may not be aesthetically compatible with adjacent teeth in highly visible areas, such as the facial surfaces of the maxillary anterior teeth. Fortunately, these surfaces are not subject to high-contact stresses, and they are easily accessible for cleaning. Subtle anatomical features and textures may be added to these areas without affecting oral health or function.

How does the clinician achieve the smoothest polished surface when severe scratches and gouges are present initially?

PRINCIPLES OF CUTTING, GRINDING, FINISHING, AND POLISHING

Even though there are distinct differences in function of cutting, grinding, finishing, and polishing, at times they overlap, depending on the hardness, shape, and size of the **abrasive** particle used and the speed of the handpiece. Higher speeds provide more rapid removal of surface material. Higher pressures also increase the rate of material removal. **Grinding**, finishing, and polishing systems vary considerably. They consist of abrasive-coated paper or plastic disks, abrasive impregnated rubber-tipped mandrels, diamond-bonded burs, and abrasive pastes. The concentration, size, and type of abrasive particles affect the rate of material removal (**cutting** efficiency) and the relative roughness of the abraded or cut surfaces.

The goals of finishing and polishing procedures are to obtain the desired anatomy, proper occlusion, and the reduction of roughness, gouges, and scratches that were produced by the contouring and finishing instruments. The instruments available for finishing and polishing restorations include fluted carbide burs, diamond burs, stones, coated abrasive disks and strips, polishing pastes, and soft and hard polymeric cups, points, and wheels impregnated with specific types and sizes of abrasive particles. The polished surface should be smooth enough to be well tolerated by oral soft tissues and to resist bacterial adhesion and excessive plaque accumulation. When plaque deposits exist, they should be easily removable by toothbrushing and flossing.

Particles of a substrate material (workpiece) are removed by the action of a harder material that comes into frictional contact with the substrate. This contact must generate sufficient tensile and shear stresses to break atomic bonds and release a particle from the substrate. With rotary instrumentation, the blades of a carbide bur or the tips of abrasive particles transfer the force to the substrate. These tensile and shear stresses are induced within both the substrate and the rotary instrument. The instrument will fail to cut, grind, or polish if the stress that develops in any part of the cutting or grinding surface exceeds its strength compared with the strength of the substrate (workpiece). Blade edges will become dull, and abrasive particles will fracture or tear away from their binder. Such degradation of finishing instruments is discussed in more detail in a later section.

Subtle differences distinguish the cutting, grinding, and polishing processes. A *cutting operation* usually refers to the use of a bladed instrument or the use of any instrument in a bladelike fashion. Substrates may be divided into large separate segments, or they may sustain deep notches and grooves by the cutting operation. High-speed tungsten carbide burs have numerous regularly arranged blades that remove small shavings of the substrate as the bur rotates. As shown in Figure 13-1, *A*, the unidirectional cutting pattern reflects the action of the regularly arranged blades

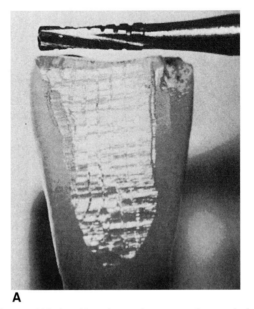

A

Fig. 13-1 A, Tooth cut by a carbide bur. Note the regular pattern of removal of tooth structure that corresponds to the regular arrangement of blades on the bur.

Continued

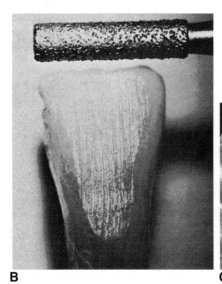

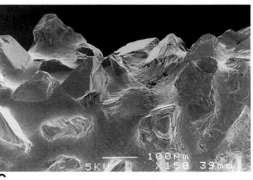

B   **C**

Fig. 13-1, Cont'd   B, Tooth ground by a diamond bur. Note the multiple scratches formed by the random arrangement of abrasive particles on the diamond bur. **C,** Photomicrograph of the bonded diamond particles on a coarse diamond bur. (×150.)

on a carbide bur. The pattern produced by a diamond bur is shown in Figure 13-1, *B.* When 30-fluted finishing burs have been used on a surface, the regular pattern of the cutting blades is only discernible if the surface is magnified for inspection. A separating wheel is an example of an instrument that can be used in a bladelike fashion. A separating wheel does not contain individual blades, but its thin blade design allows it to be used in a rotating fashion to slice through cast metal sprues and die stone materials.

A *grinding operation* removes small particles of a substrate through the action of bonded or coated abrasive instruments. Grinding instruments contain many randomly arranged abrasive particles. Each particle may contain several sharp points that run along the substrate surface and remove particles of material. For example, a diamond-coated rotary instrument may contain many sharp diamond particles that pass over a tooth during each revolution of the instrument. Because these particles are randomly arranged, innumerable unidirectional scratches are produced within the material surface, as illustrated in Figure 13-1, *B,* which shows a tooth surface ground by a diamond bur. Cutting and grinding are both considered to be predominantly *unidirectional* in their course of action. This means that a cut or ground surface exhibits cuts and scratches oriented in one predominant direction.

Different types of burs have unique effects on surfaces. The 16-flute carbide bur produces a smoother finish than the 8-flute carbide bur, but the latter removes material more rapidly. Similarly, the coarsest diamond bur removes material more quickly but leaves a rougher surface. (See Figure 13-2 for SEM images of carbide and diamond burs.)

Polishing procedures, the most refined of the finishing processes, remove the finest surface particles. Each type of polishing abrasive acts on an extremely thin region of the substrate surface. Polishing progresses from the finest abrasive that can remove scratches from the previous grinding procedure and is completed when the desired level of surface smoothness is achieved. Each step is followed by the use of progressively finer polishing media until no further improvement in surface finish is observed. The final stage produces scratches so fine that they are not visible unless

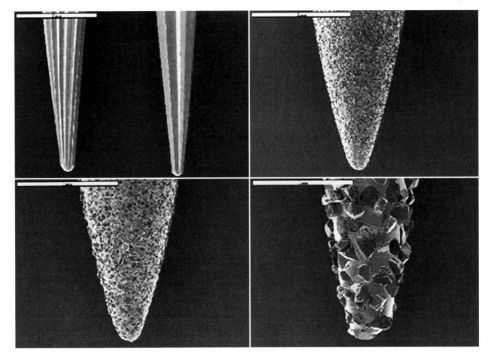

Fig. 13-2 SEM images. **Upper left,** 16-fluted **(left)** and 8-fluted **(right)** tungsten carbide finishing burs. **Upper right,** Fine diamond bur. **Bottom left,** Medium-grit diamond bur. **Bottom right,** Coarse-grit diamond bur.

greatly magnified. Examples of polishing instruments are rubber abrasive points, fine-particle disks and strips, and fine-particle polishing pastes. Polishing pastes are applied with soft felt points, muslin (woven cotton fabric) wheels, prophylaxis rubber cups, or **buffing** wheels. A nonabrasive material should be used as an applicator while using polishing pastes. Felt, leather, rubber, and synthetic foam are popular applicator materials for buffing. A common feature of some of these materials is their porous texture that allows fine abrasive particles to be retained during the buffing procedure. Polishing is considered to be *multidirectional* in its course of action. This means that the final surface scratches are oriented in many directions. Some examples of ground and polished surfaces are shown in Figure 13-3. Note that the differences in surface appearance are subtle because of the transitional nature of the grinding and polishing processes. If there were larger differences in the size of particles removed, the surface change would be more easily detected.

Bulk Reduction Process

Bulk reduction can be achieved through the use of instruments such as diamond, carbide, and steel burs, abrasive-coated disks, or separating disks. Whereas diamond burs and abrasive-coated disks provide this action by grinding, steel and carbide burs remove materials through a cutting action of the hard blades. Abrasive-coated disks are popular instruments for bulk reduction of resin-based composite restorations. For bulk reduction, the clinician should choose 8- to 12-fluted carbide burs or abrasives with a particle size of 100 μm or larger with sufficient hardness (9 to 10 Mohs hardness). SEM images of the surface finishes produced on a resin-based composite by a coarse diamond, a 12-flute carbide bur, a 16-flute carbide bur, and two types of finishing/polishing systems are shown in Figure 13-3.

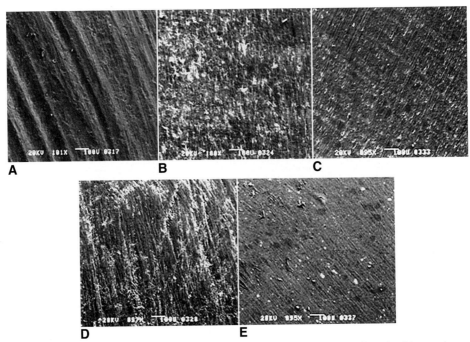

Fig. 13-3   SEM images of the surface of a resin-based composite after the grinding, finishing, and polishing processes using five instruments: **A,** a coarse diamond, **B,** a 12-flute carbide bur, **C,** a 16-flute carbide bur, **D,** an abrasive impregnated finishing disk, and, **E,** an abrasive impregnated polishing disk.

Contouring

Even though **contouring** can be achieved during bulk reduction, in some cases it requires finer cutting instruments or abrasives to provide better control of contouring and surface details. At the end of this process, the desired anatomy and margins should be established. The smoothness of the surface at this stage depends on the instrument used and may require extra steps to establish a smoother surface. Usually, 12- to 16-fluted carbide burs, or abrasives ranging in size from 30 to 100 μm, provide the fine contouring action.

CRITICAL QUESTION

One observes new fine scratches on a metal partial denture framework when an additional increment of the same abrasive paste is applied with a buffing wheel that was used previously. What is the cause of the new scratches?

Finishing

In general, finishing and polishing processes require a stepwise approach, introducing finer scratches to the surface of the substrate in order to methodically remove the deeper scratches. This process may require several steps to reach the desired surface smoothness. Surface imperfections can be an integral part of the internal structure, or they can be created by the instruments that are used for gross removal because of the size of the abrasives or the flute geometry. Finishing provides a relatively blemish-free, smooth surface. The finishing action is usually accomplished using 18- to 30-flute carbide burs, fine and superfine diamond burs, or abrasives between 8 and 20 μm in size.

Polishing

The purpose of polishing is to provide an enamel-like luster to the restoration. Smaller particles provide smoother and shinier surfaces. The speed of achieving a luster, however, depends on the hardness and size of the abrasive particles and the method of abrasion (e.g., two-body abrasion or three-body abrasion). Ideally, abrasive particles ranging up to 20 μm provide luster at a low magnification. At the end of this process, there should be no visible scratches. However, there will always be scratches that are detectable at higher magnification. The surface must be cleaned between steps, because an abrasive particle left on the surface from the previous step can cause deep scratches.

The quality of the surface finish and polish can be characterized by the measurement of the surface roughness using a profilometer, an optical microscope, or a scanning electron microscope (SEM). In clinical practice, the surface luster is usually judged without magnification. Even though, most of the time surface smoothness is correlated with the luster, as in cases such as resin-based composite restorations, the smoothest surface does not necessarily provide the most lustrous surface. For industrial applications, reflectometers are used to measure the luster. However, it is difficult to use them successfully for dental applications because of the irregular contour and small size of dental restorations.

Heat generation during cutting, contouring, finishing, and polishing processes of direct restorations is a major concern. To avoid adverse effects to the pulp, the clinician must cool the surface with a lubricant, such as an air-water spray, and avoid continuous contact of high-speed rotary instruments with the substrate. Intermittent contact during operation is necessary, not only to cool the surface but also to remove debris that was formed between the substrate and the instrument. The effectiveness and the speed of the contouring, finishing, and polishing procedures will be greatly improved by removal of debris.

CRITICAL QUESTIONS

What precautions should be taken to minimize the generation of aerosols? What precautions should be taken to minimize the exposure to and inhalation of aerosols?

Biological Hazards of the Finishing Process

Dispersions of solid particles are generated and released into the breathing space of laboratories and dental clinics whenever finishing operations are performed. These airborne particles may contain tooth structure, dental materials, and microorganisms. Such aerosols have been identified as potential sources of infectious and chronic diseases of the eyes and lungs and present a hazard to dental personnel and their patients. *Silicosis*, also called *grinder's disease*, is a major aerosol hazard in dentistry because a number of silica-based materials are used in the processing and finishing of dental restorations. Silicosis is a fibrotic pulmonary disease that severely debilitates the lungs and doubles the risk for lung cancer. The risk for silicosis is substantial because 95% of generated aerosol particles are smaller than 5 μm in diameter and can readily reach the pulmonary alveoli during normal respiration. Additionally, 75% of airborne particles are potentially contaminated with infectious microorganisms. Furthermore, aerosols can remain airborne for more than 24 hr before settling and are therefore capable of cross-contaminating other areas of the treatment facility. Aerosol sources, in both the dental operatory and laboratory environments, must be controlled whenever finishing procedures are performed. A concise and informative source of information on aerosol hazards has been written by Cooley (1984).

Aerosols produced during finishing procedures may be controlled in three ways: First, they may be controlled at the source through the use of adequate infection control procedures, water spray, and high-volume suction. Second, personal protection, such as safety glasses and disposable facemasks, can protect the eyes and respiratory tract from aerosols. Masks should be chosen to provide the best filtration along with ease of breathing for the wearer. Third, the entire facility should have an adequate ventilation system that efficiently removes any residual particulates from the air. Many systems are also capable of controlling chemical contaminants such as mercury vapor from amalgam scrap and monomer vapor from acrylic resin.

ABRASION AND EROSION
Abrasion

Wear is a material-removal process that can occur whenever surfaces slide against each other. The process of finishing a restoration involves abrasive wear through the use of hard particles. In dentistry, the outermost particles or surface material of an abrading instrument is referred to as the *abrasive*. The material being finished is called the *substrate*. In the case of a diamond bur abrading a tooth surface, such as that illustrated in Figure 13-4, the diamond particles bonded to the bur represent the abrasive, and the tooth is the substrate. Also notice that the bur in the high-speed handpiece rotates in a *clockwise* direction as observed from the head of the handpiece. The rotational direction of a rotary abrasive instrument is an important factor in controlling the instrument's action on the substrate surface. When a handpiece and bur are translated in a direction opposite to the rotational direction of the bur at the surface being abraded, a smoother grinding action is achieved. However, when the handpiece and bur are translated in the same direction as the rotational direction of the bur at the surface, the bur tends to "run away" from the substrate, thereby producing a more uncontrolled grinding action and a rougher surface.

Abrasion is further divided into the processes of two-body and three-body wear. *Two-body abrasion* occurs when abrasive particles are firmly bonded to the surface of the abrasive instrument and no other abrasive particles are used. A diamond bur abrading a tooth represents an example of two-body wear. *Three-body abrasion* occurs when abrasive particles are free to translate and rotate between two surfaces. An example of three-body abrasion involves the use of nonbonded abrasives, such as exist in dental prophylaxis pastes. These nonbonded abrasives are placed in a rubber cup, which is rotated against a tooth or material surface. These two processes are not mutually exclusive. Diamond particles may debond from a diamond bur and cause three-body wear. Likewise, some abrasive particles in the abrasive paste can become trapped in the surface of a rubber cup and cause two-body wear. Lubricants are often used to minimize the risk for these unintentional shifts from two-body to three-body wear and vice versa. Thus the efficiency of cutting and grinding will be improved with lubricants. Water, glycerin, or silicone can be used as lubricants. Intraorally, a water-soluble lubricant is preferred. Excessive amounts of lubricant may reduce the cutting efficiency by reducing the contact between the substrate and the abrasive.

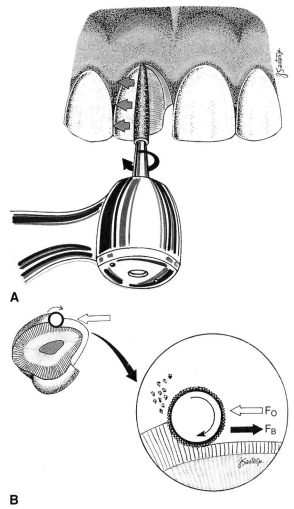

Fig. 13-4 The mechanics of high-speed rotary instrumentation. **A,** The *black arrow* indicates that the high speed diamond bur rotates in a clockwise direction when viewed from the head of the handpiece. The *gray arrows* indicate the direction that the instrument should be drawn to counteract the rotational force of the bur and to achieve optimal control of the abrasive action of the bur. **B,** Incisal view of the forces generated during high-speed rotary tooth preparation. As the bur rotates in a clockwise direction, it generates a rotational force at the tooth surface, F_B (represented by the *large black arrow*). The operator of the instrument must generate an opposing force, F_O (*open white arrow*), which will exceed the rotational force of the bur, F_B, and carry the instrument against the tooth surface where the surface will be abraded.

Erosion

Erosive wear is caused by hard particles impacting a substrate surface, carried by either a stream of liquid or a stream of air, such as occurs when sandblasting a surface. Figure 13-5 illustrates schematically two-body abrasion, three-body abrasion, and hard-particle erosion. Most dental laboratories have air-driven grit-blasting units that employ *hard-particle erosion* to remove surface material. A distinction must be made between this type of erosion and *chemical erosion*, which involves chemicals such as acids and alkalis instead of hard particles to remove substrate material. Chemical erosion, more commonly called *acid etching*, is not used as a method of finishing dental materials. It is used primarily to prepare surfaces to enhance bonding or coating.

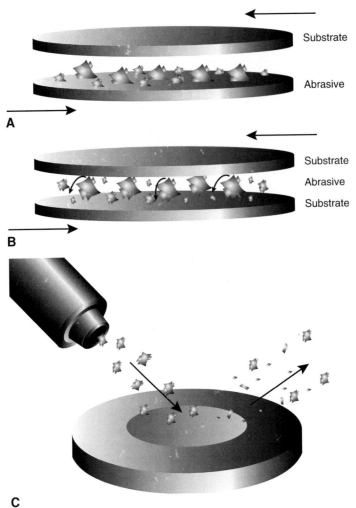

Fig. 13-5   Illustrations of two-body abrasion, three-body abrasion, and hard particle erosion. **A,** Two-body abrasion occurs when abrasive particles are tightly bonded to the abrasive instrument that is removing material from the substrate surface. **B,** Three-body abrasion occurs when abrasive particles are free to translate and rotate between two surfaces. **C,** Hard particle erosion is produced when abrasive particles are propelled against a substrate by air pressure. (Illustrations courtesy of Joel Anusavice.)

Hardness of Abrasives

As stated previously, the inherent strength of cutting blades or abrasive particles on a dental instrument must be great enough to remove particles of substrate material without becoming dull or fracturing too rapidly. The durability of an abrasive is related to the *hardness* of its particles or surface material. Hardness is a surface measurement of the resistance of one material to be plastically deformed by indenting or scratching another material. The first ranking of hardness was published in 1820 by Friedrich Mohs, a German mineralogist. He ranked 10 minerals to one another by their relative scratch resistance. The least scratch-resistant mineral, talc, received a score of 1 and the most scratch-resistant mineral, diamond, received a score of 10. Mohs' scale was later expanded in the 1930s to accommodate several new abrasive materials that received scores in the 9 to 10 range. Knoop and Vickers hardness tests are based on indentation methods that quantify the hardness of materials. The tip of a Knoop diamond indenter has an elongated pyramid shape, whereas the Vickers diamond indenter has an equilateral pyramid design. Both tests involve the application of the indenter to a test surface under a known load (usually 100 N). The depth of surface penetration is reported as hardness in units of force per unit area. Although a number of other factors affect a material's abrasivity, the farther apart a substrate and an abrasive are in hardness, the more efficient is the abrasion process. Based on a comparison of hardness values for several dental materials in Table 13-1, it is expected that silicon carbide and diamond abrasives will abrade dental porcelain more readily than does garnet, even though the abrasive particles for all three materials have very sharp edge characteristics.

CRITICAL QUESTION

Why is it sometimes inappropriate to select the hardest abrasive to reduce the time required for finishing and polishing a prosthesis?

ABRASIVE INSTRUMENT DESIGN
Abrasive Grits

Abrasive grits are derived from materials that have been crushed and passed through a series of mesh screens to obtain different particle-size ranges. Table 13-2 lists grit and particle sizes for commonly used dental abrasives. Dental abrasive grits are classified as coarse, medium coarse, medium, fine, and superfine according to particle size ranges. Experience generally indicates which grades of an abrasive give the best results in finishing a given material. Keep in mind that the rate of material removal is not the only important factor. The surface finish obtained with each abrasive is just as important. If too hard an abrasive is used, or if the grain size is too coarse for use on a given material, deep scratches result in the substrate that cannot be removed easily in subsequent finishing operations. Additionally, if an abrasive does not have the proper particle shape or does not break down in a manner that creates or exposes new sharp-edged particles, it will tend to *gouge* the substrate.

Bonded Abrasives

Bonded abrasives consist of abrasive particles that are incorporated through a binder to form grinding tools such as *points, wheels, separating disks, coated thin disks,* and a wide variety of other abrasive shapes. Particles are bonded by four general methods: (1) *sintering*, (2) *vitreous bonding* (glass or ceramic), (3) *resinoid bonding* (usually phenolic resin), and (4) *rubber bonding* (latex-based or silicone-based rubber). Because most of the rubber wheels, cups, and points contain latex, a known allergen, all residues must be removed from polished surfaces.

Abrasive disks are used for gross reduction, contouring, finishing, and polishing of restoration surfaces. Most types of disks are coated with aluminum oxide abrasive. *Abrasive strips* with either a plastic or metal backing are also available to smooth and polish the proximal surfaces of all direct and indirect bonded restorations. Metal strips are usually limited to situations in which very tight proximal contacts are involved. They are particularly useful for ceramic restorations, but are also used for composites and amalgams. However, care must be taken to avoid lacerating the gingival tissues. The metal-backed strips are more costly, but they can be autoclaved and

Table 13-1	Hardness Values of Dental Materials, Tooth Structure, and Abrasives		
Material	Moh's hardness	Knoop hardness (kg/mm^2)	Vickers hardness (kg/mm^2)
Talc	1	—	—
Gypsum	2	—	12
Denture base resin	2–3	20	—
Cementum	—	40	—
Calcite	3	135	—
Metal-reinforced glass ionomer		14–24	40
Dentin	3–4	70	57–60
Type III gold alloy	3	—	122–180 (softened)
			155–250 (hardened)
Type IV gold alloy	4	220	150–194 (softened)
			248–280 (hardened)
Amalgam	4–5	90	120 (Ag$_2$Hg$_3$ phase)
Enamel (apatite)	5	340–431	294–408
Rouge	5–6	—	—
Glass (glass-ceramics)	5–6	360	—
Microfilled composite	5–7	30	37–160
Hybrid composite	5–7	55	61–159
Titanium	—	—	210
Ti-6Al-4V	—	—	320
Ni-Cr alloy (as-cast)	—	153–328	200–395
Co-Cr alloy (as-cast)	—	—	280–380
Layered gold alloy (for PFM)	—	—	35
Pressed lithia disilicate core	—	—	640
Tripoli	6	—	—
Pumice	6–7	460–560	—
Porcelain	6–7	560	430
Tin oxide	6–7	—	—
Sand	7	—	—
Cuttle	7	800	—
Quartz	7	820	—
Zirconium silicate	7.5	—	—
Garnet	8–9	1350	—
Emery	7–9	2000	—
Corundum	9	2000	—
Aluminum oxide	9	2100	1200
Tungsten carbide	9.8	1900	—
Silicon carbide	9–10	2500	—
Diamond	10	7000–10000	—

Note: Shading indicates tooth structure values.

Table 13-2	Abrasive Particle Sizes*			
Grit/Mesh (USA)	Aluminum oxide, silicon carbide, and garnet (μm)	Coated disk grade†	Diamond (μm)	Diamond bur grade and diamond polishing paste
120	142	Coarse	142	Supercoarse–coarse
150	122		122	Coarse–regular
180	70–86		86	Coarse–regular
240	54–63		60	Fine
320	29–32	Medium	52	Fine
400	20–23		40	Fine–Superfine–Coarse Finishing
600	12–17	Fine	14	Superfine–Medium Finishing
800	9–12		8	Ultrafine–Fine Finishing
1200	2–5	Superfine	6	Milling Pastes
1500	1–2		4	Polishing Pastes (2–5μm)
2000	1		2	Polishing Pastes (2–5μm)

*Average particle sizes. Grades vary among manufacturers.
†Popular brand of aluminum oxide–coated disks. SiC and garnet may vary among manufacturers.

used several times if they are not damaged. Plastic-backed strips are used primarily for composites, compomers, hybrid ionomers, and resin cements.

Sintered abrasives are the strongest type because the abrasive particles are fused together. Vitreous-bonded abrasives are mixed with a glassy or ceramic matrix material, cold-pressed to the instrument shape, and fired to fuse the binder. Resin-bonded abrasives are cold-pressed or hot-pressed and then heated to cure the resin. Hot pressing yields an abrasive binder with extremely low porosity. Rubber-bonded abrasives are made in a manner similar to that for resin-bonded abrasives.

The type of bonding method employed for the abrasive greatly affects the grinding behavior of the tool on the substrate. Bonded abrasives that tend to disintegrate rapidly against a substrate are too weak and result in increased abrasive costs because of the reduced instrument life. Those that tend to degrade too slowly clog with grinding debris and result in the loss of abrasive efficiency, increased heat generation, and increased finishing time. An ideal binder holds the abrasive particles in the tool sufficiently long enough to cut, grind, or polish the substrate, yet releases the particles either before cutting efficiency is lost or before heat build-up causes thermal damage to the substrate. Binders are specifically formulated for substrate specific applications. Several examples of bonded abrasives are illustrated in Figure 13-6.

A bonded abrasive instrument should always be trued and dressed before its use. *Truing* is a procedure through which the abrasive instrument is run against a harder abrasive block until the abrasive instrument rotates in the handpiece without eccentricity or runout when placed on the substrate. The *dressing procedure,* like truing, is used to shape the instrument, but it accomplishes two different purposes as well. First, the dressing procedure reduces the instrument to its correct working size and shape. Second, it is used to remove clogged debris from the abrasive instrument to

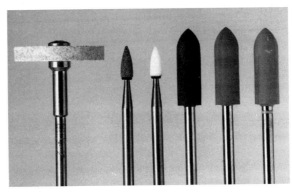

Fig. 13-6 Typical bonded abrasive instruments used in the dental laboratory include vitreous bonded abrasive wheels and points (*three instruments on left*) and rubber-bonded abrasive bullets (*three instruments on right*).

restore grinding efficiency during the finishing operation. The clogging of the abrasive instrument with debris is called *abrasive blinding*. Abrasive blinding occurs when the debris generated from grinding or polishing occludes the small spaces between the abrasive particles on the tool and reduces the depth that particles can penetrate into the substrate. As a result, abrasive efficiency is lost and greater heat is generated. A blinded abrasive appears to have a coating of the substrate material on its surface. Frequent dressing of the abrasive instrument during the finishing operation on a truing instrument, such as that illustrated in Figure 13-7, maintains the efficiency of the abrasive in removing the substrate material.

Binders for diamond abrasives are manufactured specifically to resist abrasive particle loss rather than to degrade at a certain point and release particles. One reason for this is that diamond is the hardest material known—so hard that diamond abrasive particles do not lose their cutting efficiency against substrates. There is no need for new abrasive particles to be exposed during the grinding process. Another reason is that diamond grits are expensive and must be used in limited quantities for instrument manufacture. Special bonding processes have been designed to allow for extended instrument life by keeping the abrasive particles firmly bound to the instrument shank with maximal particle exposure.

Diamond particles are bonded to metal wheels and bur blanks with special heat-resistant resins such as polyimides. The super-coarse through fine grades are then plated with a refractory metal film such as nickel. The nickel plating provides improved particle retention and acts as a heat sink during grinding. Titanium nitride coatings are used as an additional layer on some of the recent diamond abrasive instruments to further extend their longevity. *Finishing diamonds* used for resin-based composites contain diamond particles 40 µm or less in diameter, and many are not nickel-plated. Therefore they are highly susceptible to debonding and should always be used with light force and copious water spray to ensure retention of the very-fine diamond particles. Diamond burs should always be used with water spray and at rotational speeds of less than 50,000 rpm. Disposable diamond burs recently gained popularity from maintenance and OSHA viewpoints because of three factors: (1) optimal instrument efficiency, (2) concerns over the reuse of disinfected abrasive devices, and (3) minimal heat build-up.

Diamond instruments are preshaped and trued; they are not treated as other bonded abrasives. *Diamond cleaning stones* are used on the super-coarse through

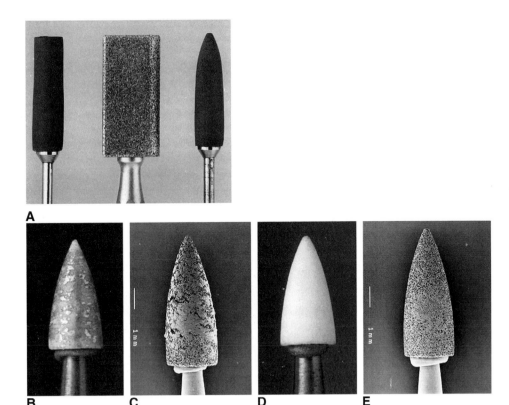

Fig. 13-7 A dressing tool is used to true, shape, and clean bonded abrasive instruments both before and during the finishing procedure. **A,** A rubber-bonded abrasive cylinder *(left)* shows irregular external contours that will cause it to run eccentrically. The cylinder is first trued against a diamond-coated abrasive dressing tool *(center)* to make it rotate around the central axis of the instrument. Once trued, the abrasive is further dressed to a desired working shape *(right).* **B,** Instruments that are blinded with debris lose cutting efficiency and generate more heat during operation. Note the coating of debris on the abrasive surface. **C,** A scanning electron micrograph of the same instrument reveals the significant amount of debris that is clogging the instrument surface. **D,** Frequent dressing of the abrasive on the dressing tool shown in the first photograph removes accumulated debris and restores cutting efficiency. **E,** A scanning electron micrograph of the blinded abrasive after dressing reveals that the debris has been removed and the abrasive surface has been restored.

fine grades to remove debris build-up and to maintain grinding efficiency. An example of a diamond cleaning stone is shown in Figure 13-8. Cleaning stones should not be used on finishing diamonds because their bonded particles are quickly removed. Manufacturers provide special operating and cleaning instructions for these instruments.

Coated Abrasive Disks and Strips

Coated abrasives are fabricated by securing abrasive particles to a flexible backing material (heavyweight paper, metal, or Mylar) with a suitable adhesive material. These abrasives typically are supplied as disks and finishing strips. Disks are available in different diameters and with thin and very thin backing thicknesses. A further designation is made in regard to whether or not the disk or strip is moisture-resistant. It is advantageous to use abrasive disks or strips with moisture-resistant backings because their stiffness is not reduced by water degradation.

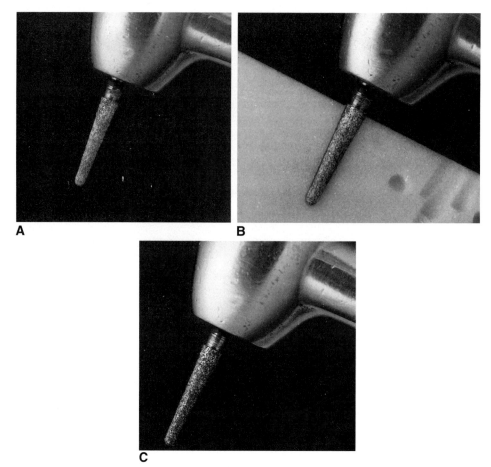

Fig. 13-8   A diamond cleaning stone is used to remove debris from diamond instruments. **A,** Diamond bur in high-speed rotary handpiece before cleaning. Note the accumulated debris. **B,** The bur is cleaned by running it against the moistened diamond cleaning stone for 2 to 4 sec. **C,** The cleaned diamond bur has no debris remaining between the diamond abrasive particles.

Furthermore, moisture acts as a lubricant to improve cutting efficiency. Examples of coated abrasives are shown in Figure 13-9.

Nonbonded Abrasives

Polishing pastes are considered as nonbonded abrasives and are primarily used for final polishing. They need to be applied to the substrate with a nonabrasive device such as synthetic foam, rubber, felt, or chamois cloth. The abrasive particles are dispersed in a water-soluble medium such as glycerin for dental applications. Aluminum oxide and diamond are the most popular nonbonded abrasives.

Abrasive Motion

The motion of abrasive instruments is classified as rotary, planar, or reciprocal. In general, burs are considered rotary, disks are planar, and reciprocating handpieces provide a cyclic motion and are reciprocal in relationship to their direction of motion. Different sizes of abrasives can be incorporated with each motion.

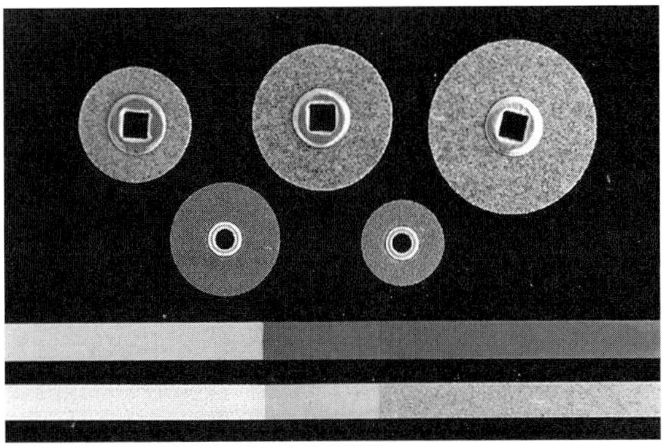

Fig. 13-9 Coated abrasive disks and strips. Disks are available in several sizes with both paper and moisture-resistant backings. Paper-backed disks are represented by the *top row of disks,* and moisture-resistant Mylar-backed disks are shown in the *second row.* Mylar-backed abrasive strips may be coated with two different grades of abrasive. The coatings are separated in the center of the strip by an uncoated area, which allows the strip to be passed between teeth.

Reciprocating handpieces especially provide the benefit of accessing interproximal and subgingival areas to remove overhangs, to finish subgingival margins without creating ditches, and to create embrasures.

TYPES OF ABRASIVES

Many types of abrasive materials are available, but only those commonly used in dentistry are discussed in this section. *Natural abrasives* include Arkansas stone, chalk, corundum, diamond, emery, garnet, pumice, quartz, sand, tripoli, and zirconium silicate. Cuttle and kieselguhr are derived from the remnants of living organisms. *Manufactured abrasives* are synthesized materials that are generally preferred because of their more predictable physical properties. Silicon carbide, aluminum oxide, synthetic diamond, rouge, and tin oxide are examples of manufactured abrasives.

Arkansas Stone

Arkansas stone is a semitranslucent, light gray, siliceous sedimentary rock mined in Arkansas. It contains microcrystalline quartz and is dense, hard, and uniformly textured. Small pieces of this mineral are attached to metal shanks and trued to various shapes for fine grinding of tooth enamel and metal alloys.

Chalk

One of the mineral forms of calcite is *chalk,* a white abrasive composed of calcium carbonate. Chalk is used as a mild abrasive paste to polish tooth enamel, gold foil, amalgam, and plastic materials.

Corundum

This mineral form of aluminum oxide is usually white. Its physical properties are inferior to those of manufactured alpha (α) aluminum oxide, which has largely replaced corundum in dental applications. Corundum is used primarily for grinding metal alloys and is available as a bonded abrasive in several shapes. It is most commonly used in an instrument known as a *white stone.*

CRITICAL QUESTION

What are the advantages and disadvantages of natural diamond abrasives versus synthetic diamond abrasives?

Natural Diamond

Diamond is a transparent, colorless mineral composed of carbon. It is the hardest known substance. Diamond is called a *superabrasive* because of its ability to abrade any other known substance. Diamond abrasives are supplied in several forms, including bonded abrasive rotary instruments, flexible metal-backed abrasive strips, and diamond polishing pastes. They are mostly used on ceramic and resin-based composite materials.

Synthetic Diamond Abrasives

The advantages of synthetic diamonds over natural diamonds include their controllable, consistent size and shape, as well as their lower cost compared with natural diamonds. The shape of the diamonds determines the binder needed for its use. The binders can be either resin or metal. Resin-bonded diamonds have sharp edges. During use, the sharp edges break down and expose new sharp edges and corners. On the other hand, metal-bonded diamonds are regular and more consistent in size. They function as cutting points or edges primarily through the benefit of their hardness rather than their shape. Larger synthetic diamond particles appear greenish because of the chemical reaction with nickel during the manufacturing process. Manufactured diamond is used almost exclusively as an abrasive and is produced at five times the quantity of natural diamond abrasive. This abrasive is used in the manufacture of diamond saws, wheels, and burs. Blocks with embedded diamond particles are used to true other types of bonded abrasives. Diamond polishing pastes are also produced from particles smaller than 5 μm in diameter. Synthetic diamond abrasives are used primarily on tooth structure, ceramic materials, and resin-based composite materials.

Emery

This abrasive is a grayish-black corundum that is prepared in a fine-grain form. Emery is used predominantly in the form of coated abrasive disks and is available in a variety of grit sizes. It may be used for finishing metal alloys or acrylic resin materials.

Garnet

The term *garnet* includes a number of different minerals that possess similar physical properties and crystalline forms. These minerals are the silicates of aluminum, cobalt, iron, magnesium, and manganese. The garnet abrasive used in dentistry is usually dark red. Garnet is extremely hard and, when fractured during the grinding operation, forms sharp, chisel-shaped plates, making it a highly effective abrasive. Garnet is available on coated disks and arbor bands. It is used in grinding metal alloys and acrylic resin materials.

Pumice

Volcanic activity produces this light-gray, highly siliceous material. It is used mainly in grit form but can be found in some rubber-bonded abrasives. Both pumice forms are used on acrylic resin materials. Flour of pumice is an extremely fine-grained volcanic rock derivative from Italy that is used in polishing tooth enamel, gold foil, dental amalgam, and acrylic resins.

Quartz

The most commonly used form of quartz is very hard, colorless, and transparent. It is the most abundant and widespread of minerals. Quartz crystalline particles are pulverized to form sharp, angular particles that are useful in making coated abrasive disks. Quartz abrasives are used primarily to finish metal alloys, and they may also be used to grind dental enamel.

Sand

Sand is a mixture of small mineral particles predominantly composed of silica. The particles represent a mixture of colors, making sand abrasives distinct in appearance. Sand particles have a rounded to angular shape. They are applied under air pressure to remove refractory investment materials from base metal alloy castings. They are also coated onto paper disks for grinding of metal alloys and acrylic resin materials.

Tripoli

This abrasive is derived from a lightweight, friable siliceous sedimentary rock. Tripoli can be white, gray, pink, red, or yellow. The gray and red types are most frequently used in dentistry. The rock is ground into very fine particles and formed with soft binders into bars of polishing compound. Tripoli is used for polishing metal alloys and some acrylic resin materials.

Zirconium Silicate

Zircon or zirconium silicate is supplied as an off-white mineral. This material is ground to various particle sizes and is used to make coated abrasive disks and strips. It is frequently used as a component of dental prophylaxis pastes.

Cuttle

Commonly referred to as *cuttlefish, cuttle bone,* or *cuttle,* this abrasive is a white calcareous powder made from the pulverized internal shell of a Mediterranean marine mollusk of the genus *Sepia.* Cuttle is available as a coated abrasive and is useful for delicate abrasion operations such as polishing of metal margins and dental amalgam restorations.

Kieselguhr

This material is composed of the siliceous remains of minute aquatic plants known as *diatoms.* The coarser form of kieselguhr is called *diatomaceous earth* and is used as a filler in many dental materials, such as the hydrocolloid impression materials.

Kieselguhr is an excellent mild abrasive; however, the risk for respiratory silicosis caused by chronic exposure to airborne particles of this material is significant, so appropriate precautions should always be taken.

Silicon Carbide

This extremely hard abrasive was the first of the *synthetic abrasives* to be produced. Green and blue-black types of silicon carbide are produced; both types have equivalent physical properties. The green form is often preferred because substrates are more visible against the green color. Silicon carbide is extremely hard and brittle. Particles are sharp, and they break to form new sharp particles. This results in highly efficient cutting of a wide variety of materials, including metal alloys, ceramics, and acrylic resin materials. Silicon carbide is available as an abrasive in coated disks and as vitreous-bonded and rubber-bonded instruments.

Aluminum Oxide

Fused aluminum oxide was the second synthetic abrasive to be developed. Synthetic aluminum oxide (alumina) is made as a white powder and can be much harder than corundum (natural alumina) because of its purity. Alumina can be processed with different properties by slight alteration of the reactants in the manufacturing process. Several grain sizes of alumina are available, and it has largely replaced emery for several abrasive uses. Aluminum oxide is widely used in dentistry to make bonded abrasives, coated abrasives, and air-propelled grit abrasives. Sintered aluminum oxide is used to make white stones, which are popular for adjusting dental enamel and for finishing metal alloys, resin-based composites, and ceramic materials.

Pink and ruby variations of aluminum oxide abrasives are made by adding chromium compounds to the original melt. These variations are sold in a vitreous-bonded form as noncontaminating mounted stones for the preparation of metal-ceramic alloys to receive porcelain. Remnants of these abrasives and other debris should be removed from the surface of metals used for metal-ceramic bonding so as not to prevent optimal bonding of porcelain to the metal alloy. A review by Yamamoto (1985) suggests that carbide burs are the most effective instruments for finishing this type of alloy because they do not contaminate the metal surface with entrapped abrasive particles.

Rouge

Iron oxide is the fine, red abrasive component of rouge. Like tripoli, rouge is blended with various soft binders into a cake form. It is used to polish high noble metal alloys.

Tin Oxide

Tin oxide is an extremely fine abrasive used extensively as a polishing agent for polishing teeth and metallic restorations in the mouth. It is mixed with water, alcohol, or glycerin to form a mildly abrasive paste.

Abrasive Pastes

The most commonly used abrasive pastes contain either aluminum oxide (alumina) or diamond particles. Alumina pastes should be used with a rotary instrument and increasing amounts of water as polishing proceeds from coarser to finer abrasives. Diamond abrasive pastes are used in a dry condition. The instruments that apply the paste to the material surface are equally important. These include ribbed prophy cups (the ribbed type or the more flexible, nonribbed type), brushes, and felt wheels. Abrasive pastes have several disadvantages. First, they are relatively thick and cannot gain access into embrasures. Second, the pastes tend to splatter off of the instruments. Third, heat is generated when insufficient coolant is used or when an intermittent polishing technique is not used.

FINISHING AND POLISHING PROCEDURES
Resin-Based Composite Restorations

Resin-based composites represent some of the most difficult materials to finish and polish to a high luster because they contain a relatively soft resin matrix with hard filler particles in its structure. This results in selective grinding associated with the soft material and the harder particles, a problem that is especially apparent with hybrid composites. In addition, the final finish of a composite restoration depends on the fillers and matrix, the preparation design, curing effectiveness, and the post-curing time required for the material to achieve its final properties. For some composite materials, a delay of 10 min or more is recommended after curing to allow complete polymerization to occur. Curing lights for polymerization, such as halogen lamps, must produce a minimal light output of 475 nm/mm^2 for most photo-initiated composites. Chemically cured composites must be properly placed within the working time of the materials.

Exposed filler particles create peaks and valleys that do not appear lustrous. During each stage of finishing and polishing, the operator should proceed in one direction only. Then, after the use of the next abrasive in the sequence, polishing should continue in a direction perpendicular to the previous one. This process ensures that scratches become more visible and that the effectiveness of scratch removal can be assessed more rapidly. The recommended abrasives and polishing instruments should be used in the proper sequence, and the clinician should never skip intermediate abrasive steps, for example, following a coarse abrasive disk with a fine abrasive rather than a medium grit abrasive. The operator can choose to use one system from start to finish (such as abrasive-coated or flexible abrasive-impregnated rubber disks) or combine different systems based on preference and the location of the restoration (such as sandpaper for anterior, brush for posterior).

The finishing and polishing technique consists of three essential steps: First, contour the restoration either with 12-flute carbide burs, 30 to 100 μm diamond burs, or coarse abrasive-coated disks, depending on the preference of the dentist. Next, finish with 16- to 30-flute carbide burs, fine and extra fine diamond burs, white stones (aluminum oxide), white Arkansas stones, or medium and fine abrasive-coated disks. Finally, polish with fine and extra-fine polishing paste (aluminum oxide or diamond); extra-fine abrasive-coated disks; silicon carbide–impregnated brushes; or diamond-impregnated rubber polishing disks, cups, or points.

Dental Amalgam

Burnishing alone will not provide a completely scratch-free and retention-free surface for the amalgam restorations. Slow-speed handpieces should be used in finishing and polishing amalgam restorations. In the past, a recommendation was made to wait 24 hr before polishing the amalgam restorations to allow the amalgam to set completely. However, if the restoration surface is finished initially with a very fine prophylaxis paste applied with a cotton pellet or a nonribbed rubber prophy cup rotated at slow speed and light pressure, a smooth, velvet-like finish is achieved that will acquire a luster as it is abraded normally in the mouth. Spherical amalgams set faster and can be finished and polished sooner.

If the amalgam has hardened to an advanced stage, at which the abrasion by a fine prophylaxis paste is no longer effective, the following procedure may be used at the next dental appointment: (1) contour with slow-speed green stones or diamond burs, brown and green rubber points, and (2) apply a mixture of fine pumice and water or alcohol with a rotary brush or felt wheel to polish the surface.

Gold Alloy

Gold is a relatively soft material. Therefore it requires a different approach than that used for other metals used in dentistry. Slow-speed handpieces should be used in finishing and polishing gold alloys. The technique consists of the following steps: (1) contour with carbide burs, green stones (silicone carbide), or heatless stones; (2) finish with pink stones (aluminum oxide), or medium-grade abrasive impregnated rubber wheels and points (brown and green); (3) apply fine abrasive-impregnated rubber wheels, cups, and points; and, if necessary, (4) apply tripoli or rouge with rag or leather wheels.

CRITICAL QUESTION

What are the differences between finishing and polishing a ceramic extraorally and intraorally?

Ceramic Restorations

The ideal surface for ceramic restorations is a polished and glazed surface. The production of a **glaze** layer through a **natural glaze** or **overglaze** process will not necessarily yield a smooth surface if the initial ceramic surface has significant roughness. The smoothest surfaces can be achieved extraorally before a prosthesis is cemented. In the mouth, however, minor roughness can be successfully polished without compromising the surface quality. In addition, polishing can improve the strength within the surface region of a ceramic prosthesis because it removes pores and microcracks. Adequate cooling is important in vivo when finishing and polishing ceramic restorations. Using an air-water spray and maintaining intermittent contact between the restoration and the rotary instrument are critical during the operation. Continuous contact between the restoration and the rotary instrument should be avoided. Heatless stones (silicone carbide) provide heat reduction and can be used as an alternative. Several kits are available for finishing and polishing ceramic restorations. Manufacturer's instructions should be followed when using different systems. Depending on the preference of the dentist, a general technique is as follows: (1) Contour with flexible diamond disks, diamond burs, heatless or polymer stones, or green stones (silicone carbide). (2) Finish with white stones or abrasive-impregnated rubber disks, cups, and points. This process may require two or three steps, depending on the system used. (3) Polish with fine abrasive-impregnated rubber disks, cups, and points, or, if necessary, use a diamond paste applied with a brush or felt wheel. (4) Apply an overglaze layer, or natural glaze the ceramic if necessary. For intraoral polishing, use intermittent application of rotating instruments with a copious amount of water as a coolant.

Acrylic Resins for Denture Bases and Veneers

Acrylic resins are relatively soft materials. To avoid overheating, apply a large amount of pumice slurry to the surface. Intermittent contact with the substrate also helps to avoid overheating. The following technique steps are recommended: (1) Contour with tungsten carbide burs and sandpaper. (2) Use a rubber point to remove the scratches. (3) Apply pumice with a rag wheel, felt wheel, bristle brush, or prophy cup, depending on the size of the area that needs to be polished. (4) Apply tripoli or a mixture of chalk and alcohol with a rag wheel.

Air-Abrasive Technology

As an alternative to the use of rotary instrument cutting, air-abrasive systems can deliver a fine, precisely controlled high-pressure stream of 25- to 30-μm aluminum oxide particles to remove enamel, dentin, and restorative materials. Because air abrasion generates minimal heat or vibration, the potential for tooth chipping or microfracturing is minimized. These systems have been used for the following applications: cavity preparation, removal of defective composite fillings, endodontic access through porcelain crowns, minimal preparation to repair crown margins, tunnel preparations, superficial removal of stains, cleaning of tooth surfaces before adhesive bonding, and roughening of internal surfaces of indirect porcelains or composite restorations before adhesive bonding.

Air-Abrasive Polishing for Dental Hygiene Procedures. Often referred to as air polishing, air-abrasive polishing is based on the controlled delivery of an air, water, and sodium bicarbonate slurry to remove plaque and stains from tooth surfaces. Compared with rubber cup and prophylaxis paste techniques, it is more time-effective, and it is possible to access many tooth surfaces with this technology. However, it is reported that surfaces of softer restorations, such as glass ionomers, can be damaged. Therefore it should be used with caution around cosmetic restorations.

DENTIFRICES

Dentifrices, available as toothpastes, gels, and powders, provide three important functions. First, their abrasive and detergent actions provide more efficient removal of debris, plaque, and stained pellicle compared with use of a toothbrush alone. Second, they polish teeth to provide increased light reflectance and superior aesthetic appearance. The high polish, as an added benefit, enables teeth to resist the accumulation of microorganisms and stains better than rougher surfaces. Finally, dentifrices act as vehicles for the delivery of therapeutic agents with known benefits; for example, fluorides, tartar control agents, desensitizing agents, and remineralizing agents. Fluorides improve resistance to caries and may, under a proper oral hygiene regimen, enhance the remineralization of incipient noncavitated enamel lesions. Tartar control agents, such as potassium and sodium pyrophosphates, can reduce the rate at which new calculus deposits form supragingivally. Desensitizing agents with proven clinical efficacy are strontium chloride and potassium nitrate. The therapeutic benefits of other additives such as peroxides and bicarbonates are under investigation. The products advertised as "whitening toothpastes" may contain an abrasive agent alone or a chemical agent and an abrasive agent. The former type of additive acts through a surface stain removal mechanism whereas the latter additives act through a combined mechanism of abrasion and bleaching.

Composition

Typical dentifrice components are listed in Table 13-3. The abrasive concentrations in paste and gel dentifrices are 50% to 75% lower than those of powder dentifrices. Therefore powders should be used more sparingly and with greater caution by patients (especially where cementum and dentin are exposed) to avoid excessive dentinal abrasion and pulpal sensitivity.

Table 13-3	Typical Dentifrice Components*			
	Composition (wt%)			
Component	**Pastes and gels**	**Powders**	**Materials**	**Purpose**
Abrasive	20–55	90–98	Calcium carbonate	Removal of plaque/stain Polish tooth surface
			Dibasic calcium phosphate dihydrate	
			Hydrated alumina	
			Hydrated silica	
			Sodium bicarbonate	
			Mixtures of listed abrasives	
Detergent	1–2	1–6	Sodium lauryl sulfate	Aids debris removal
Colorants	1–2	1–2	Food colorants	Appearance
Flavoring	1–2	1–2	Oils of spearmint, peppermint, wintergreen, or cinnamon	Flavor
Humectant	20–35	0	Sorbitol, glycerine	Maintains moisture content
Water	15–25	0	Deionized water	Suspension agent
Binder	3	0	Carrageenan	Thickener, prevents liquid-solid separation
Fluoride	0–1	0	Sodium monofluorophosphate	Prevents dental caries
			Sodium fluoride	
			Stannous fluoride	
Tartar control agents	0–1	0	Disodium pyrophosphate Tetrasodium pyrophosphate Tetrapotassium pyrophosphate	Inhibits formation of calculus above the gingival margin
Desensitization agents	0–5	0	Potassium nitrate Strontium chloride	Promotes occlusion of dentinal tubules

*Some compositional information provided by Dr. George Stookey.

Abrasiveness

The ideal dentifrice should provide the greatest possible cleaning action on tooth surfaces with the lowest possible abrasion rates. Dentifrices do not need to be highly abrasive to clean teeth effectively. This is fortunate because exposed root surface cementum and dentin are abraded at rates of 35 and 25 times that of enamel, respectively. Standardized laboratory tests have been developed to measure the cleaning ability and the abrasivity of a dentifrice. Only the abrasivity test is discussed in this section. Currently, the preferred means of evaluating dentifrice abrasivity is to employ irradiated dentin specimens and brush them for several minutes with test and reference dentifrices. An abrasivity ratio is then calculated by comparing the amounts of radioactive phosphorus (^{32}P) released by each dentifrice, and this value is multiplied by 1000. A dentifrice must obtain an abrasivity score of 200 to 250 or less to satisfy the abrasivity test requirements proposed by the American Dental Association (ADA) and the International Organization for Standardization (ISO). This means that a test dentifrice must abrade dentin at 20% to 25% of the rate of the reference standard to be considered safe for normal usage. A problem with this laboratory test is that it does not account for all variables that would affect abrasivity under in vivo conditions. Some of the factors affecting dentifrice abrasivity are listed in Box 13-1.

Another problem is that not all dentifrices respond in a similar manner under this test. For example, dentifrices that contain sodium bicarbonate yield poor test results because the particles completely dissolve approximately 1 min into the 8-min test. This illustrates that it is very difficult, if not impossible, to use a laboratory test to predict the actual abrasivity of various dentifrices in vivo. Patients should experience similar amounts of relative wear from the various dentifrices as those found in the laboratory tests. The majority of modern dentifrices are not exceedingly abrasive. In fact, one published document has rated four dozen dentifrices in regard to cleaning ability and abrasiveness. The products are ranked as high, moderate, or low in

BOX 13–1
Factors Affecting Dentifrice Abrasiveness

EXTRAORAL FACTORS

Abrasive particle type, size, and quantity in dentifrice

Amount of dentifrice used

Toothbrush type

Toothbrushing method and force applied during brushing

Toothbrushing frequency and duration

Patient's coordination and mental status

INTRAORAL FACTORS

Saliva consistency and quantity (normal variations)

Xerostomia induced by drugs, salivary gland pathology, and radiation therapy

Presence, quantity, and quality of existing dental deposits (pellicle, plaque, calculus)

Exposure of dental root surfaces

Presence of restorative materials, dental prostheses, and orthodontic appliances abrasiveness. It is highly probable that most of the evaluated products meet the American National Standards Institute/American Dental Association (ANSI/ADA) and ISO test requirements. Thus these rankings should be considered as a guide to products that do not exceed a maximum acceptable (safe) abrasivity value.

ADA Acceptance Program

A discussion of dentifrices would not be complete without mention of the ADA acceptance program for these materials. The ADA designates a dentifrice as "Accepted" only if the dentifrice meets specific requirements. First, the abrasivity of the dentifrice must not exceed the maximum acceptable abrasivity value of 250 (also a limit for the ISO standard). Second, the manufacturer must produce scientific data, usually from clinical trials, that verify any claims the manufacturer wishes to make on the product package or in commercial advertisements. The manufacturer's advertisements are also periodically reviewed by the appropriate ADA Council.

In advertising the product, a manufacturer may not claim or imply that the dentifrice confers benefits that have not been specifically proven. Some manufacturers produce excellent dentifrice products but do not seek ADA acceptance simply because they do not want such restrictions placed on their advertisements. For products that receive the ADA seal, a unique and individual statement for each product is provided that states what the dentifrice is intended to achieve.

Toothbrushes

Toothbrush bristle stiffness alone has been shown to have no effect on abrasion of hard dental tissues. However, when a dentifrice is used, there is evidence that more flexible toothbrush bristles bend more readily and bring more abrasive particles into contact with tooth structure, albeit with relatively light forces. This interaction should produce more effective abrasion and cleaning action on areas that the bristles can reach. Battery-powered toothbrushing devices provide a variety of cleansing actions that are claimed to improve tooth-cleaning actions even further than those achieved by manual toothbrushes.

Acknowledgment

The contributions of Charles DeFreest to the development of this chapter in the 10th edition is appreciated.

SELECTED READINGS

Carr MP, Mitchell JC, Seghi RR, and Vermilyea SG: The effect of air polishing on contemporary esthetic restorative materials. Gen Dent 50(3):238–241, 2002.
This article describes the effects of air polishing on different dental materials.

Consumer Reports, Toothpastes. September 1992, pp 602–606.
This reporting agency sent 48 toothpastes to independent laboratories for analysis of abrasivity and cleaning effectiveness. All toothpastes were subsequently ranked for these criteria. The American Dental Association no longer provides a ranking according to laboratory tests. Thus this report may serve as a screening guide in light of the fact that the tests were performed in vitro instead of in a clinical environment.

Cooley RL: Aerosol hazards. In: Goldman HS, Hartman KS, and Messite J (eds): Occupational Hazards in Dentistry. Chicago, Yearbook Medical, 1984, pp 21–33.
Sources of dental aerosols, their hazards, and preventive measures are presented.

Fairhust CW, Lockwood PE, Ringle RD, et al: The effect of glaze on porcelain strength. Dent Mater 8:203-207, 1992.

Fruits TJ, Miranda FJ, and Coury TL: Effects of equivalent grit sizes utilizing different polishing motions on selected restorative materials. Quintessence Int 27(4):279-285, 1996.

Hefferren JJ: Laboratory method for assessment of dentifrice abrasivity. J Dent Res 55:563, 1976.
This reference describes the dentifrice abrasivity test.

Hutchings IM: Tribology: Friction and Wear of Engineering Materials. Boca Raton, FL, CRC Press, 1992.

This publication thoroughly describes the scientific basis of friction, wear, and lubrication.

Kroschwitz JI, and Howe-Grant M (eds): Kirk-Othmer Encyclopedia of Chemical Technology, 4th ed, Vol 1. New York, John Wiley and Sons, 1991, pp 17–37.

This encyclopedia presents a thorough review of specific abrasives, their physical properties, and their methods of manufacture.

Mackert JR: Side effects of dental ceramics. Adv Dent Res 6:90–93, 1992.

Presents information on silicosis and the potential hazards of porcelain dust generation during grinding procedures.

Nakazato T, Takahashi H, Yamamoto M, Nishimura F, and Kurosaki N: Effects of polishing on cyclic fatigue strength of CAD/CAM ceramics. Dent Mater J 18(4):395-402, 1999.

Powers JM, and Bayne SC: Friction and wear of dental materials: In: Henry SD (ed): Friction Lubrication and Wear Technology, ASM Handbook, Vol 18. Materials Park, OH, American Society of Metals International, 1992, pp 665-681.

This article, a compilation of information from more than 200 sources, presents a review of friction and wear as they relate to human dental tissues and restorative materials.

Ratterman E, and Cassidy R: Abrasives: In: Lampman SR, Woods M, and Zorc TP (eds): Engineered Materials Handbook, Vol 4, Ceramics and Glasses. Materials Park, OH, ASM International, 1991, pp 329-335.

Presents a system for selecting abrasives for glasses and ceramics based on a comparison of physical properties. Mechanical property tables are presented for several materials.

Stookey GK, Burkhard TA, and Schemehorn BR: In vitro removal of stain with dentifrices. J Dent Res 61:1236, 1982.

The method used to measure the cleaning effectiveness of a dentifrice is presented.

Williamson RT, Kovarik RE, Mitchell RJ: Effects of grinding, polishing, and over glazing on the flexure strength of a high-leucite feldspathic porcelain. Int J Prosthodont 9(1):30-37, 1996.

Yamamoto M: Metal-Ceramics. Chicago, Quintessence, 1985, pp 124-130.

Discusses the preparation of metal-ceramic alloys for porcelain application, using several excellent photographs.

III

DIRECT RESTORATIVE MATERIALS

14

Bonding

Barry K. Norling

OUTLINE

Mechanisms of Adhesion

Acid-Etch Technique

Dentin Bonding Agents

Measurement of Bond Strength and Microleakage

Glass Ionomer Restoratives

Amalgam Bonding

Pit and Fissure Sealants

KEY TERMS

Adhesive—Substance that promotes adhesion of one substance or material to another.

Adhesive bonding—Process of joining two materials by means of an adhesive agent that solidifies during the bonding process.

Dentin bonding—The process of bonding a resin to conditioned dentin.

Dentin bonding agent—A thin layer of resin between conditioned dentin and the resin matrix of a composite.

Dentin conditioner—An acidic agent that dissolves the inorganic structure in dentin, resulting in a collagen mesh that allows infiltration of an adhesive resin.

Hybrid layer—An intermediate layer of resin, collagen, and dentin produced by acid etching of dentin and resin infiltration into the conditioned dentin.

Microleakage—Flow of oral fluid and bacteria into the microscopic gap between a prepared tooth surface and a restorative material.

Preventive-resin restoration (PRR)—A conservative, sealed, resin-based composite restoration, usually placed in a minimally prepared occlusal fissure area, with the sealant extending into contiguous uncut fissures.

Primer—A hydrophilic, low-viscosity resin that promotes bonding to a substrate, such as dentin.

Resin tag—Extension of resin that has penetrated into etched enamel or dentin.

Sandwich technique—The process of restoring a prepared tooth by initially placing a layer of Type II glass ionomer cement for fluoride release followed by an overlayer of resin-based composite for strength and durability.

Smear layer—Poorly adherent layer of ground dentin produced by cutting a dentin surface.

CRITICAL QUESTION

Why is good wetting of tooth structure by a dental adhesive not adequate for long-term adhesive bonding of a restorative material?

True adhesion has been the "holy grail" of dental restorative materials for many decades. If true adhesion of restorative materials to tooth structure is to be achieved, three conditions must be satisfied:

1. Sound tooth structure must be conserved.
2. Optimal retention must be achieved.
3. **Microleakage** must be prevented.

As we have progressed into the twenty-first century, we have seen an exponential growth in the development of adhesive materials and techniques. Although adhesion alone cannot be relied on for retention except in very select circumstances, we are now well into the era of *adhesive dentistry* and its associated field of *aesthetic dentistry*.

MECHANISMS OF ADHESION

The science of adhesion has been covered in Chapter 2. For our purposes, we will briefly summarize only the essential principles of adhesion that are needed for an understanding of dental bonding.

The oral hard tissues and their environment are complex. Not surprisingly, the mechanisms of adhesion that have been successfully employed are also complex. In general, the following factors can play major or minor roles in achieving adhesive bonds:

1. Wetting
2. Interpenetration (formation of a hybrid zone)
3. Micromechanical interlocking
4. Chemical bonding

Wetting is essential for the success of all other adhesion mechanisms. An adhesive cannot form micromechanical interlocks, chemical bonds, or interpenetrating networks with a surface unless it can intimately contact the surface, spread onto the surface, and fill microscopic and submicroscopic irregularities. These conditions are achieved if the adhesive wets the surface. Although wetting is an essential requirement for intraoral adhesion, it is not sufficient to ensure durable bonding. This insufficiency is very unusual in the field of adhesives. For example, one can readily form strong, durable bonds between sheets of plate glass by using an epoxy resin. This combination involves no primary chemical bonding between adhesive and adherend, no micromechanical interlocking, and no interpenetration. However, one cannot expect the same result when tooth structure is the substrate.

Wetting of tooth structure alone does not achieve lasting intraoral bonds because the principal substrates (adherends), enamel and dentin, are hydrated, hydrophilic, and permeable to water. Such adherends require a hydrophilic, hydrolytically stable adhesive for wetting to occur. However, even if the surface is initially dried before adhesive application, diffusion results in one or more monolayers of water that strongly bond to both the tissue and the adhesive. Unfortunately, water has a very low shear strength, so the net shear bond strength between two perfectly flat surfaces is insignificant.

ACID-ETCH TECHNIQUE

Before the introduction of acid etching of enamel and the use of enamel bonding agents, leakage of oral fluids within the microscopic space between prepared teeth and restorative materials was a greater concern for resin-based composites than for any other restorative material. Other types of dental restorative products involve some type of mechanism to counteract the effects of marginal leakage. For example, the corrosion of amalgam over time produces a deposit such as tin oxide and/or tin oxychloride along the tooth-restoration interface to form a relatively leakproof seal. Although they are not capable of reducing microleakage, fluoride-releasing restoratives inhibit secondary caries at the tooth margin, within the interface, and to a limited extent, the released fluorine ions may protect the surfaces of adjacent teeth.

The first meaningful proof of intraoral adhesion was reported in 1955 by Michael Buonocore. He etched the enamel surface with acids and then placed an acrylic restorative material on the micromechanically roughened surface. The monomers of the acrylic resin wet the etched surface, flowed into the etch pits, and generated retentive **resin tags**. One of the surface conditioning agents he used, phosphoric acid, is still the most widely used etchant today for bonding to enamel and dentin.

Acid etching of enamel is one of the most effective ways to improve mechanical bonding and to ensure sealed interfacial gaps. This procedure has markedly expanded the use of resin-based restorative materials because it provides a strong bond between resin and enamel, forming the basis for many innovative dental procedures, such as resin-bonded metal retainers, porcelain laminate veneers, and bonded orthodontic brackets. It has also solved, to a great extent, all of the previous problems that plagued resin-based restorations, namely, marginal staining caused by interfacial leakage (Fig. 14-1). Without micromechanical bonding, current composite materials would be unable to resist the effects of marginal penetration, and the leakage of oral fluids would occur adjacent to these restorations. However, because of advances in adhesive technology, bonding of resin-based composites to tooth structure yields durable restorations.

To produce a bond between enamel and resin-based restorative materials, sufficient etching of enamel is required to provide selective dissolution and associated microporosity such as that shown in Figure 14-2. Unlike the normal, untreated enamel surface, etched enamel has a higher total surface energy, which ensures that a resin will readily wet the surface and penetrate into the resulting microporosity. Once the resin penetrates into the microporosity, it can be polymerized to form resin tags that produce a mechanical bond to the enamel. These resin tags may penetrate 10 to 20 μm into the enamel porosity, as shown in Figure 14-3, but their

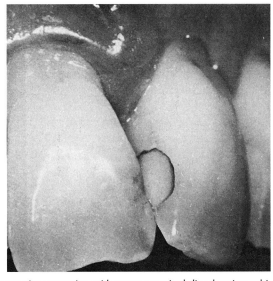

Fig. 14-1 Clinical composite restoration with severe marginal discoloration, which resulted from poor adaptation and subsequent leakage. (Courtesy of J. Osborne.)

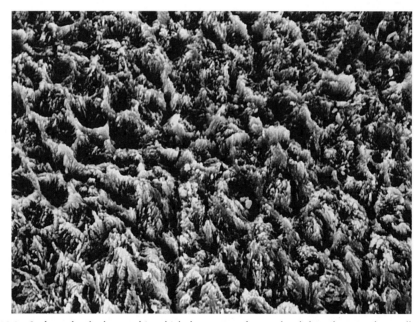

Fig. 14-2   Surface of etched enamel in which the centers of enamel rods have been preferentially dissolved by the phosphoric acid. (Courtesy of K-J. Söderholm.)

lengths are dependent on whether the enamel etching time and the rinsing time are sufficient to produce an adequate etching pattern and to eliminate etching debris that has deposited on the conditioned surface.

A number of acidic agents have been used to produce the required microporosity. However, phosphoric acid at a concentration between 30% and 50%, typically 37%, is the preferred etching agent. Concentrations greater than 50% result in the deposition of an adherent layer of monocalcium phosphate monohydrate on the etched surface, which inhibits further dissolution. Although aqueous fluids are available,

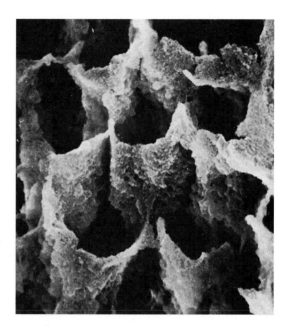

Fig. 14-3   Scanning electron microscopy image of tags formed by the penetration of resin into etched areas of enamel. The resin was applied to the etched enamel, and the enamel was then dissolved by acid to reveal the tags. (×5000.) (Courtesy of K-J. Söderholm.)

generally the etchant is supplied as an aqueous gel to allow precise placement over a specific area. These gels are often made by adding colloidal silica (the same fine particles used in microfilled composites) or polymer beads to the acid. Brushes are used to place the acidic gel material, or the acid may be supplied in a disposable syringe from which it can be expressed onto the enamel and dentin. During placement, it is important to be aware of the risk for air bubbles that may be introduced at the interface. If these voids remain, these regions will not be etched.

The application time of the etchant may vary somewhat, depending on previous exposure of the tooth surface to fluoride. For example, a permanent tooth with a high fluoride content derived from a fluoride water supply may require a somewhat longer etching time, as does a primary tooth. In the latter instance, increased surface conditioning time is needed to enhance the etching pattern on primary tooth enamel that is more aprismatic than permanent tooth enamel. Currently, the etching time for most etching gels is approximately 15 sec. The advantage of such short etching times is that they yield acceptable bond strength in most instances, while conserving enamel and reducing treatment time.

Once the tooth is etched, the acid should be rinsed away thoroughly with a stream of water for about 20 sec, and the enamel must be dried completely. When the enamel is dry, it should have a white, frosted appearance, indicative of the proper etching treatment. This surface must be kept clean and dry until the resin is placed to form a sound mechanical bond. Although enamel etching raises the surface energy of the enamel, contamination can readily reduce the energy level of the etched surface. Reducing the surface energy, in turn, makes it more difficult to wet the surface with a bonding resin that may have a higher surface energy than that of the contaminated surface. Thus even momentary contact with saliva or blood can prevent effective resin tag formation and severely reduce the bond strength. Another potential contaminant is oil that is released from the air compressor and transported along the airlines to the air-water syringe. If contamination occurs, the contaminant should be removed, and the enamel should be etched again for 10 sec.

Bond strengths to etched enamel range from 15 to 25 MPa, depending on the resin and testing method used. A bis-GMA/triethylene glycol dimethacrylate (TEGDMA) resin tends to yield lower bond strength values, whereas some of the newer enamel and **dentin bonding agents** can increase bond strength. These differences in bond strength are small, and because of large variations during testing, they are unlikely to be clinically significant. However, these in vitro differences may be associated with the better wetting capability of the etched enamel by the newer materials. Drying of the enamel with warm air or using an ethanol rinse can increase the bond strength, suggesting that moisture may still be trapped in the micropores even when the surface appears dry. In summary, the acid-etch technique has resulted in a simple, conservative, and effective use of resin in many dental procedures.

The etch pits result from selective dissolution of either the enamel rod cores (Type I etching) as shown in Figure 14-2, or the peripheral areas (Type II etching) as indicated by the resin tags in Figure 14-3. In either case, the resin tags are approximately 6 μm in equivalent diameter and 10 to 20 μm in length. (In aged extracted teeth, the tags may be 100 to 200 μm in length.)

The acid-etch technique was not widely used in the years following its introduction. The principal reason was the inferior properties of acrylic filling materials. Curing and thermal dimensional changes can generate interfacial stresses sufficient to rupture the bond with etched enamel, because of large polymerization shrinkages (>6 vol%) and coefficients of thermal expansion in excess of 100 ppm/° C. The acid-etch technique was rediscovered after highly filled resin-based composites were marketed beginning in the mid-1960s. Today, enamel etching is used to achieve stable bonds in procedures as diverse as orthodontic bracket bonding and porcelain laminate veneer bonding.

Even with the lower shrinkage and low coefficient of thermal expansion of today's resin-based composites, etched enamel cannot be relied on as the sole source of retention for any but the smallest restoration with enamel surrounding the entire periphery. However, conditioned enamel is essential to ensure a marginal seal even though retention relies on retentive cavity features and/or **dentin bonding**.

CRITICAL QUESTION

Why doesn't chemical bonding occur when using dentin bonding agents?

DENTIN BONDING AGENTS

Before the total-etch technique was adopted for enamel and dentin, enamel bonding agents were used. Because resin-based composites are more viscous than are unfilled acrylic resins, enamel bonding agents were developed to enhance the wetting and adaptation of resin to the conditioned enamel surface. Generally, the compositions of these materials were derived from those of the resin matrix, which was diluted by other monomers to lower the viscosity and to enhance wetting. These agents had no potential for adhesion, but they improved mechanical bonding by optimum formation of resin tags within the enamel. These materials have now been largely replaced by agents designed to provide adhesion to enamel and dentin, as discussed in the following sections.

Traditionally, enamel bonding agents were made by combining different dimethacrylates such as bis-GMA and TEGDMA to control viscosity. Because enamel can be kept fairly dry, these rather hydrophobic resins worked well as long as they were restricted to enamel. During the last few years, these bonding agents have been replaced by the same systems that are used on dentin. This transition occurred because of the benefit of simultaneously bonding resin to both enamel and dentin, not because of any substantial improvement in bond strength.

Dentin poses greater obstacles to adhesive bonding than does enamel, because dentin is a living tissue. It is heterogeneous and consists of 50 vol% of inorganic material (hydroxyapatite), 30 vol% of organic material (mainly Type I collagen), and 20 vol% of fluid. Its high fluid content places stringent requirements on materials that can be effective adhesive agents between dentin and a restorative material. The tubular nature of dentin provides a variable area through which dentinal fluid may flow to the surface and adversely affect adhesion. The tubules with their branching channels may also be used to enhance mechanical retention. Further challenges to adhesion involve the presence of the **smear layer** on the cut dentin surface and the potential biological side effects that different chemicals can cause within the pulp. It is for these reasons that the development of dentin bonding agents has been delayed compared with the development of enamel bonding agents.

An important breakthrough in dentin bonding occurred when Fusayama et al (1979) used 37% phosphoric acid to etch both enamel and dentin. This study demonstrated that the procedure did not increase pulp damage and that it did improve the restoration retention substantially. A subsequent study by Nakabayashi et al (1982) revealed that hydrophilic resins infiltrated a surface layer of collagen fibers in demineralized dentin to form a **hybrid layer** consisting of resin-infiltrated dentin. However, the dentin-etching procedure was not generally accepted initially. It was not until the early 1990s that dentin etching gained world-wide acceptance.

Ideally, dentin adhesives should be hydrophilic to wet the surface of slightly moist, conditioned dentin. Because most matrix resins of composites are hydrophobic, the bonding agent should contain hydrophilic groups to interact with the moist dentin surface and hydrophobic groups to ensure bonding to the restorative resin. The key to adhesion is to develop hydrophilic monomers that can easily infiltrate the collagen mesh produced by etching dentin with an acid often called a **conditioner**.

Several years ago, the general belief was that dentin bonding could be achieved by forming chemical bonds between a resin system and either the inorganic or the organic component of dentin. The most commonly targeted components were either collagen or the calcium ions within hydroxyapatite. The molecules that were designed for these purposes can be represented by an M–R–X molecule, where M is a methacrylate group, R is a spacer such as a hydrocarbon chain, and X is a functional group that is targeted for adhesion to tooth tissue. Typical phosphate X groups were believed to bond to calcium during dentin priming. Then, during polymerization, the methacrylate group of the M–R–X molecule would react with the resin matrix of the composite material and form a chemical bond between composite and dentin. Compounds that were believed to possess these properties were NPG-GMA (a condensation product of *N*-phenyl glycine and glycidyl methacrylate), polymerizable phosphates, and poly(alkenoic) acids (Fig. 14-4). In spite of theoretical evidence that chemical bonding to tooth structure is possible, there is no substantial scientific proof that demonstrates the development of significant chemical bonding between dentin adhesives and tooth surfaces under intraoral conditions.

A direct restoration could be reliably bonded without using retentive features if a method were available to bond to dentin as strongly as to acid-etched enamel. The intermediate link between dentin and/or enamel and unfilled resin is known as *dentinal bonding* or *dentin bonding*. The relatively thin resin layer is referred to as a *dentin bonding agent*. A wide variety of chemistries has been explored and marketed in the search for species that can produce strong, permanent bonds to dentin.

When discussing dentin bonding agents, it has become customary to describe the generations of bonding agents that have led sequentially from the earliest, relatively ineffective materials to the current materials, which provide reliable functional bonds. This organization into generations of bonding agents is a somewhat artificial device to mark key advances in materials and techniques along a more-or-less continuous developmental pathway.

First-Generation Dental Adhesives

Early dentin bonding agents were based on the successful model of silane coupling agents. Silane coupling agents are used to bond the inorganic filler to the matrix resin in composites, to bond porcelain laminate veneers through resin cements to acid-etched enamel, and to repair fractured porcelain with composites. Generically, a silane coupling agent may be represented as M–R–X, where M is an unsaturated methacrylate group capable of copolymerizing with the unfilled resin or the matrix/resin of a composite, X is a group capable of chemically reacting with the siliceous substrate, and R is a spacer group that ensures mobility of the M group after the X group has been immobilized by reaction with the surface. For all dental applications, the silane coupling agent used is γ-methacryloxypropyl trimethoxysilane (Fig. 14-5).

In use, the methoxy groups are hydrolyzed and yield silanol groups, which can condense with silanol groups that cover the surface of any siliceous substrate exposed to (moist) air. (A schematic representation of the silanation process on a silica structure is shown in Fig. 14-6.) The pendant methacrylate group may then copolymerize with unfilled resin or the resin matrix of a composite to form an interface in which resin is linked to siliceous filler through primary chemical bonds.

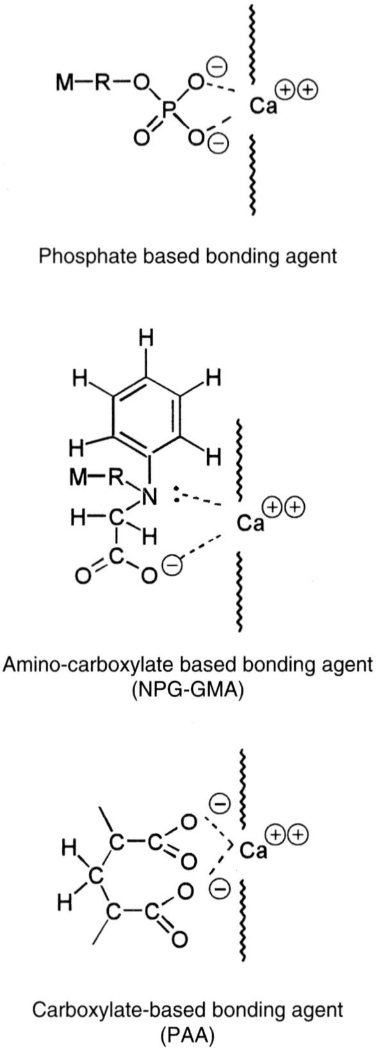
M—R—O
Ca
Phosphate based bonding agent
M—R
Ca
Amino-carboxylate based bonding agent
(NPG-GMA)
Ca
Carboxylate-based bonding agent
(PAA)

Fig. 14-4 Chemical bonding mechanisms to hard tooth tissues. (Courtesy of K-J. Söderholm.)

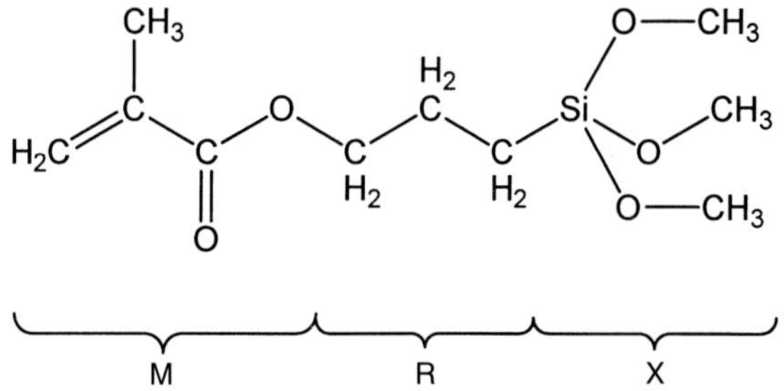
M
R
X

Fig. 14-5 M-R-X structure of γ-methacryloxypropyl trimethoxysilane.

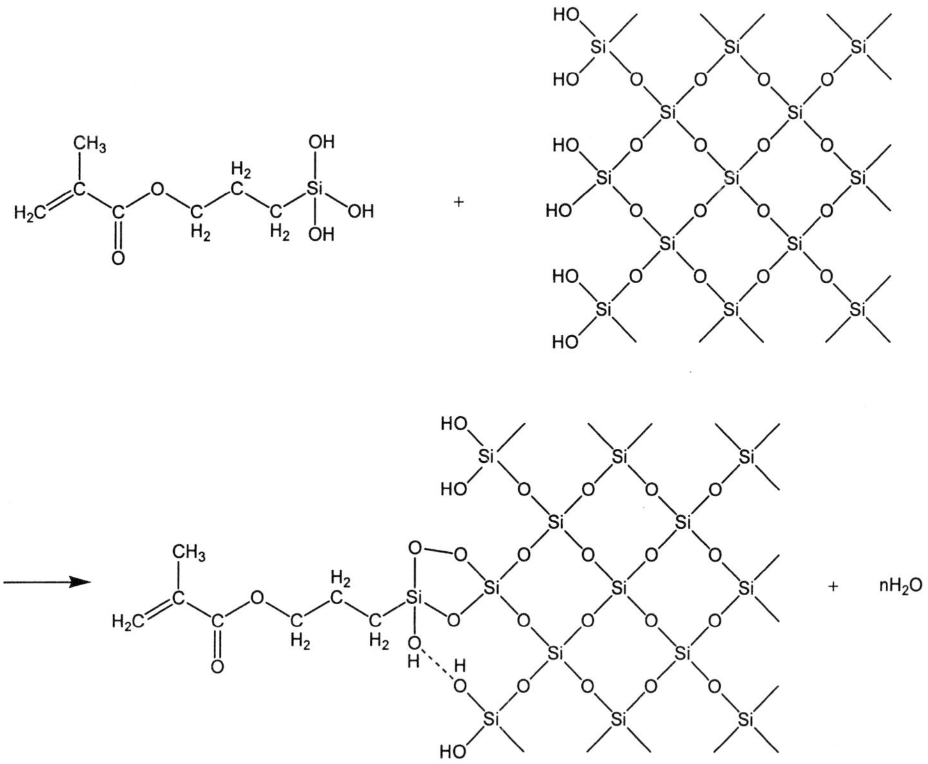

Fig. 14-6 Silanation of a siliceous substrate.

In the silane structure above, the M-R-X components are:
M: methacrylate group
R: $(CH_2)_3$
X: $OSi(OH)_3$
In the dentin bonding agent analogues, M is also a methacrylate group. The variations occur in the spacer R group and, particularly, in the dentin reactive (X) group. Initially, the search for a suitable X group involved simple recognition of the composition of dentin (Table 14-1). Note the relatively high organic component of dentin and its higher water content compared with enamel.

Not surprisingly, the early dentin bonding agents contained acidic X groups designed to react with the mineral portion, specifically the calcium in the hydroxyapatite. The first product, marketed in the early 1950s, contained the active agent glycerolphosphoric acid dimethacrylate, which is shown in Figure 14-7. This material achieved little clinical success for the same reasons that plagued the enamel

Table 14-1 Composition of Enamel and Dentin

	Enamel		Dentin	
	wt%	vol%	wt%	vol%
Mineral	97	92	70	45
Organic	1	2	20	33
Water	1	6	10	22

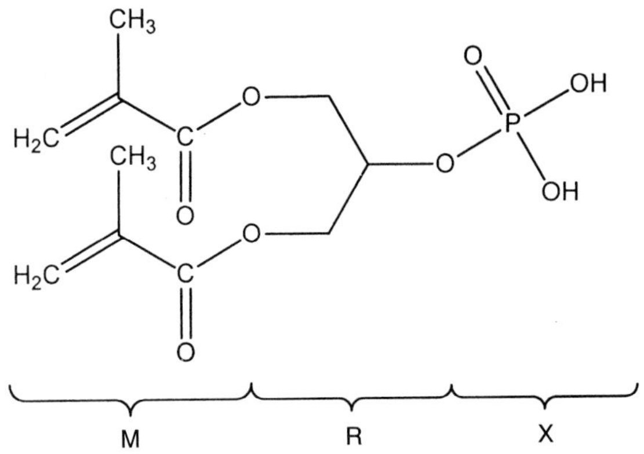

Fig. 14-7 Glycerophosphoric acid dimethacrylate.

etching applications, that is, the high polymerization shrinkage and high coefficient of thermal expansion of the unfilled acrylic restorative resins that were commonly used in this period.

Second-Generation Dental Adhesives

The clinical success of composite materials led to the rapid introduction of dentin bonding agents in the late 1960s and early 1970s. A general belief developed that dentin bonding could revolutionize the practice of restorative dentistry by minimizing the enlargement of cavity preparations required for retention of direct-filling restorations. Specifically, it was recognized that, if adequate dentin bonding could be achieved, composites might be used to restore cervical abrasion areas without supplementary tooth-retention features (such as shown in Fig. 14-8). Representative second-generation bonding agents include NPG-GMA (the adduct of *N*-phenyl glycine and glycidyl methacrylate), shown in Figure 14-8, and phenyl-P, 2-methacryloxy phenyl phosphoric acid, shown in Figure 14-9.

Evidence is lacking to demonstrate that significant chemical bonding occurs between these adhesives and tooth structure under in vivo conditions.

Third-Generation Dental Adhesives

The third generation of dentin adhesives was also based on the continued use of an acid group to react with Ca^{2+} ions and a methacrylate group to copolymerize with unfilled resin that was applied before placement of the composite restorative material. However, the second generation of adhesives also included an attempt to deal with the smear layer. Whenever dentin is cut or ground, an unstructured or amorphous smear layer is formed that consists of dentin particles, bacteria, and occasionally salivary constituents. This layer is weakly bonded to the underlying dentin. The first and second generations of adhesives achieved low bond strengths partly because of failures within the smear layer or between the smear layer and underlying dentin.

The third generation of adhesive procedures for conditioning dentin involved two approaches: (1) modification of the smear layer to improve its properties or (2) removal of the smear layer without disturbing the plugs that occluded the dentinal tubules.

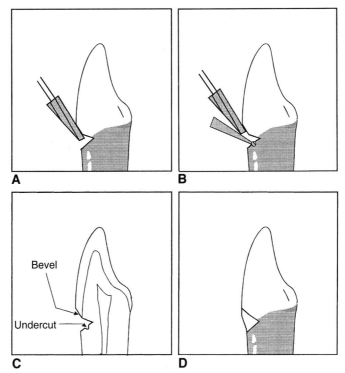

Fig. 14-8 **A,** Placement of incisal bevel in the enamel of Class V preparation. **B** and **C,** Placement of small retention groove in dentin using a small round bur. **D,** Finished composite restoration. (Courtesy of K-J. Söderholm.)

Although variations were common, the third-generation bonding procedures generally involved four steps:

1. Application of a **dentin conditioner**, which is a type of acid used to alter or remove the smear layer
2. Application of the **primer** (the dentin bonding agent)
3. Application of the adhesive, typically an unfilled resin
4. Placement of resin-based composite

Representative conditioning agents include a hydroxyethylmethacrylate (HEMA) solution of maleic acid such as that used in Scotchbond II (3M Dental Products, Minneapolis, MN) and 2% aqueous nitric acid, such as that used in Tenure (Den-Mat, Santa Maria, CA). The dentin bonding agents continued to involve M-R-X chemistries for the most part. For example, the Scotchbond bonding agent was a chlorophosphoric ester of bis-GMA (Fig. 14-10).

During this period another adhesive system was designed to react with the collagen rather than the hydroxyapatite. In this system, aqueous EDTA was used as the

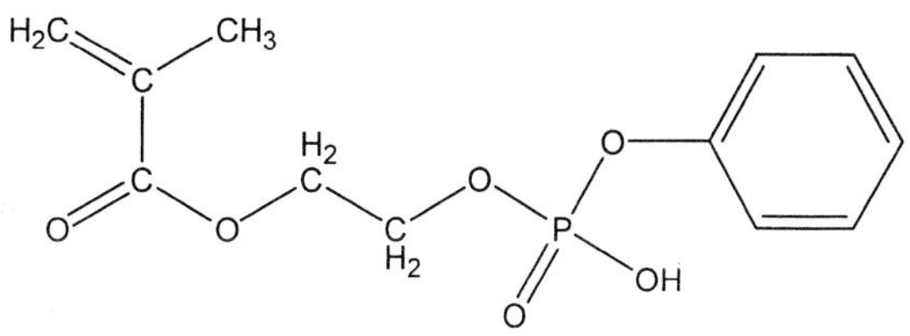

Fig. 14-9 Phenyl-P.

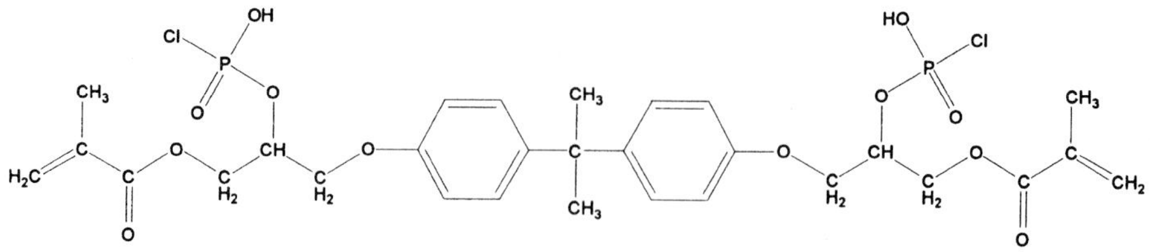

Fig. 14-10 Chlorophosphoric acid ester of bis-GMA.

conditioner while the bonding agent consisted of 35% glutaraldehyde in HEMA. No evidence is available on this system to demonstrate that any chemical bonding to collagen actually occurs.

Fourth-Generation Dental Adhesives

The fourth generation of adhesives was as much a result of a major change in thinking as an advance in materials development. In most of the world, it had been assumed that aggressively etching dentin, (for example, with the phosphoric acid used previously to etch enamel), was contraindicated because of the belief that opening the dentinal tubules by etching would result in pulpal irritation, inflammation, and, potentially, the death of pulpal tissue through exposure to the components of the etchant, bonding agents, and filling materials.

Previous research suggested that this belief might be mistaken. A variety of materials previously believed to be highly irritating to the pulp are now known to be well tolerated when they are placed in direct contact with the pulp tissue, provided that bacteria are excluded and microleakage is prevented. Similar work on gnotobiotic animals supported the conclusion that pulpal irritation was minimal in the absence of bacteria regardless of the presence of chemical irritants.

Subsequently, research conducted in Japan led to the development of dentin bonding systems that relied on total removal of the smear layer and smear plugs. Resin tags were produced in the dentinal tubules, and these extensions into dentin contributed to the retention of the restorative resin. Although these systems were contemporaneous with the third generation of adhesive systems described above, it was several years before the aggressive dentin etching approach was adopted for the dentin bonding systems in the rest of the world, leading to a new fourth generation of products.

It is important to recognize the simplification in the clinical technique afforded by the recognition that phosphoric acid could be used to etch both dentin and enamel. Previous generations relied on separate etching regimens for enamel and dentin. It can be easily appreciated that isolating the etchants to the two adjacent tissues was demanding at best. The so-called *total-etch technique*, in which the same conditioning agent was applied to both enamel and dentin, represented a major reduction in clinical complexity. Overall, however, the technique is still quite complex because of the large number of steps involved. The general procedures required for a fourth-generation system of dentin bonding are as follows:

1. Etch dentin and enamel simultaneously with conditioner (usually phosphoric acid). Most dentin bonding systems are provided with a conditioner, often an acid that can remove the smear layer and expose a collagen network. The dentin is conditioned most commonly for 15 sec and the conditioner and precipitate are subsequently rinsed away. Excess water is then removed from the etched and rinsed dentin surface, without desiccating the collagen

mesh. If the mesh is desiccated, the collagen network will collapse and form a dense film that is difficult to infiltrate with the primer.

2. Rinse to remove etchant and dissolved tooth minerals.
3. Dry with air to determine that enamel is adequately etched.
4. Slightly moisten the surface.
5. Absorb excess water with a cotton pellet.
6. Apply primer according to the recommended number of coats—from 1 to 6, depending on the product. The hydrophilic primer, in contrast with a hydrophobic resin, infiltrates the collagen network when placed on the slightly moist dentin surface. To optimize bonding, the clinician should cure the primer as efficiently as possible. This curing process, though not easy to achieve because both dentinal fluid and oxygen, which are present either in the dentin or in the air jet used for drying, inhibit polymerization. To avoid this situation, the primer should contain a solvent that evaporates easily and removes water without the need for excessive air drying. In addition, the primer should also contain a resin that produces a cross-linked polymer network that is well retained within the collagen mesh.
7. Dry thoroughly to remove primer solvent.
8. Apply adhesive to enamel and dentin. A bonding resin is placed on the primed surface region of conditioned tooth surface. The resin should be thinned with a brush rather than with an air jet to avoid oxygen inhibition. The thickness of the bonding resin should be at least 50 μm to prevent diffusion of oxygen from the atmosphere through the coating and thereby prevent oxygen inhibition of the primer and the adjacent bonding resin during polymerization. Because the light-activating compounds are contained commonly in the bonding resin, the primer and the bonding resin are cured simultaneously for the minimum time recommended by the manufacturer. Subsequently, layers of composites are placed and cured on the bonding agent layer.
9. Light-cure the adhesive.
10. Apply composite resin over adhesive.
11. Cure the matrix resin of the composite.

Obviously, there are ample opportunities for human error in this system; improper manipulation in any of the steps can lead to clinical failure.

The gentle drying procedure in Step 5 is critical. The demineralized collagen layer produced by etching is extremely fragile. Thorough drying of the dentin surface leads to its collapse and the consequent inability of the hydrophilic bonding agent solvents and monomers to penetrate and reinforce the conditioned dentin structure. Gentle air drying of dentin for as little as 3 sec can reduce bond strength to less than half the bond strength to moist dentin. The initial drying procedure in Step 3 is necessary to ensure that the enamel is adequately etched as revealed by its frosted or chalky appearance. Following the drying process, the dentin must be rehydrated in Step 4 to ensure that the collagen fiber network swells to its original permeable condition.

In summary, the unique features of the fourth-generation dentin bonding agents include the total etch technique and the wet bonding process. These concepts marked a clear break from traditional beliefs that one should never consider extensive etching of dentin and that good technique involved extensive drying of both dentin and enamel before the application of bonding agents.

Fifth-Generation Dental Adhesives

The fifth generation of dentin bonding agents was developed as the result of the recognition that clinical success should be more consistent if fewer steps were involved. Current dentin bonding agents rely on a complex combination of micro-mechanical retention by (1) penetration into partially opened dentinal tubules, (2) formation of a hybrid layer in which hydrophilic monomers penetrate and polymerize to form an interpenetrating network with a demineralized collagen fibril network, and (3) chemical interactions involving first-and second-order bonds.

Much emphasis has been placed on the importance of the interpenetrating network formed by polymerization of the dentin bonding agent monomers within the demineralized collagen layer. In fact, a comparable bond strength can be achieved in the laboratory by treating the conditioned surface also with sodium hypochlorite, which removes the demineralized collagen. These results suggest that formation of the hybrid layer is critical to avoid the weakening of a noninfiltrated demineralized zone.

The number of procedural steps was reduced by combining the conditioner and primer (self-etching primer) or the primer and adhesive (self-priming adhesive or one bottle system). These simplifications have increased the consistency of results. Although laboratory results suggest a similar effectiveness for either approach, initial clinical results suggest that self-etching primers generally produce superior results. One product has been designed to combine all three components, but early clinical findings suggest that this level of simplification may not produce optimal results. This single-step bonding is sometimes referred to as a *sixth-generation system*.

CRITICAL QUESTION

Why are dentin bond strength values so variable?

MEASUREMENT OF BOND STRENGTH AND MICROLEAKAGE

Evaluation of the efficacy of dentin adhesives is generally based on measurement of bond strength determined by loading bond test specimens in shear or in tension until fracture occurs. Such tests are indicative of how the adhesive is likely to perform in vivo. Data published on bond strengths for a given material often vary widely, and the standard deviation of the mean value for a given bond test is usually high. This wide variance in data may be attributed to the variables inherent at the dentin surface, such as water content, the presence or absence of the smear layer, dentin permeability, orientation of the tubules relative to the surface, and differences in the in vitro test design and stress distribution adjacent to the interface. Furthermore, although no universal agreement on the minimal bond strength necessary to provide successful bonding has been established, a value of 20 MPa or higher has been proposed as a reasonable goal.

Recently, a number of studies have adopted the microtensile test methodology. By using very small specimens (approximately 1 mm² in cross-section), one can prepare multiple specimens from a single tooth. Even with very high indicated strengths, for example, 30 MPa or higher, failure occurs at the adhesive interface rather than within dentin. This interfacial failure has led some proponents of the method to suggest that it is the only valid measure of bond strength because significant fractions of specimens rarely fail along the tooth/resin interface using traditional test specimen geometries.

Regardless of the numerical differences generated by different laboratory test methods, it is clear that current dentin bonding agents are capable of yielding higher bond strength values that can shift the site of clinical failure from the interface to within dentin adjacent to the restoration or, in some cases, within the restoration adjacent to the interface. Regardless of the bond test selected, it is clear that the inherent bond strength is no longer the limitation in the effectiveness of bonded restorations. The limiting factor now appears to be, at least for large restorations, induced stresses generated during curing shrinkage within the resin-based composite itself.

The degree of microleakage at the restoration/tooth interface can be monitored by the penetration of tracers and staining agents. As is true for bond testing, there is also a large variation in leakage data from one laboratory to another, depending on the technique used and the manipulative variables adopted during placement of the bonding agents. Often, there is not a good correlation between bond strength and microleakage. Nonetheless, the newer systems appear to be superior in inhibiting interfacial leakage between the conditioned tooth structure and adhesive resin.

CRITICAL QUESTION

Why are glass ionomer restoratives not used routinely as a pit and fissure sealant?

GLASS IONOMER RESTORATIVES

Although these materials are not considered dental adhesives, glass ionomers are of interest to this discussion because they represent a class of materials that exhibit chemical bonding to tooth structure. Glass ionomer cements are covered in some detail in the discussion of dental cements (Chapter 16). They consist of a powder, an acid-soluble aluminosilicate glass, and an aqueous solution of polyacrylic acid or an analogous polyacid. Ca^{2+} and Al^{3+} ions from the powder react with the carboxylate groups to cross-link the polymeric acid. The same carboxylate groups interact strongly with surface Ca^{2+} ions in enamel or dentin to yield chemical adhesion to tooth structure. Because of their fluorine-releasing capability, they are especially useful for patients who are at a high risk for carious lesions. For teeth requiring Class II restorations, a **sandwich technique** is sometimes used. This technique consists of placing a Type II glass ionomer cement in the cervical area of a proximal box or the floor of other tooth preparations and building the remainder of the restoration with a resin-based composite because of its greater strength and durability in occlusal sites.

Glass ionomer cements are translucent and are used as aesthetic filling materials, particularly in Class V erosion lesions. Although shear bond strengths measured in the laboratory are only approximately 3 MPa, clinical retention is excellent. Until recently, glass ionomers were the only materials that yielded 100% retention rates in Class V lesions without mechanical retention or enamel etching, based on certain clinical studies of 3 years or more in duration.

Clinical longevity depends not just on bond strengths, but also on dislodging forces. Composite restoratives undergo significant polymerization shrinkage, which creates stresses at the resin-dentin interface that can rupture dentinal bonds on the order of 20 MPa in all but the smallest restorations. Because glass ionomers generate low stresses on setting, they are well retained even with bond strengths as low as 3 MPa in areas such as Class V lesions, where occlusal forces and other external forces induce small stresses. However, they have also been used with limited success as pit and fissure sealants. Because of the higher stresses induced by intraoral forces in occlusal areas, a greater degree of dislodgement and fracture occurs in these sites.

CRITICAL QUESTION

How does amalgam bonding to dentin differ from composite bonding to dentin?

AMALGAM BONDING

Although retention and resistance forms were the hallmark of traditional amalgam preparation design, modern conservative philosophy and the desire to extend the use of amalgams to more extensive restorations (e.g., the amalgam crown) have stimulated a search for improved methods for retaining amalgam restorations. Mechanical adjuncts, including threaded pins or retentive grooves placed in dentin, have served well for years toward these ends. More recently, bonding agents employing M–R–X type coupling agents have achieved some clinical success. One system uses 4-methacryloxyethyl trimellitate anhydride (4-META; Fig. 14-11). However, the mechanism responsible for bonding amalgam to resin is predominantly mechanical in nature. It is produced by condensing the plastic amalgam mass into a plastic resin layer, thereby producing macroretentive areas within the resin after the resin has polymerized. The results of controlled clinical trials have been mixed, but it is safe to say that amalgam bonding agents have a place as an adjunct to conventional retentive means if properly employed.

CRITICAL QUESTION

Can sealant prevent secondary caries progression when it is placed over underlying carious enamel or dentin?

PIT AND FISSURE SEALANTS

Various materials and techniques have been advocated for preventing caries in the susceptible pit and fissure areas of posterior teeth, particularly in the child patient or for the high-caries-risk patient in general. The most popular sealant techniques make use of resin systems that can be applied to the occlusal surfaces of the teeth. The objective of sealant use is for the resin to penetrate into the pits and fissures and to seal these areas against the oral bacteria and debris. A cross-section of a tooth to which a pit and fissure sealant has been applied is shown in Figure 14-12.

Several types of resin, both filled and unfilled, have been employed as pit and fissure sealants. These resin systems include cyanoacrylates, polyurethanes, and bis-GMA. The commercially available products have been based on either the polyurethane resin or the bis-GMA resin. The bis-GMA material may be polymerized in a conventional manner by means of the amine-peroxide chemical activation-

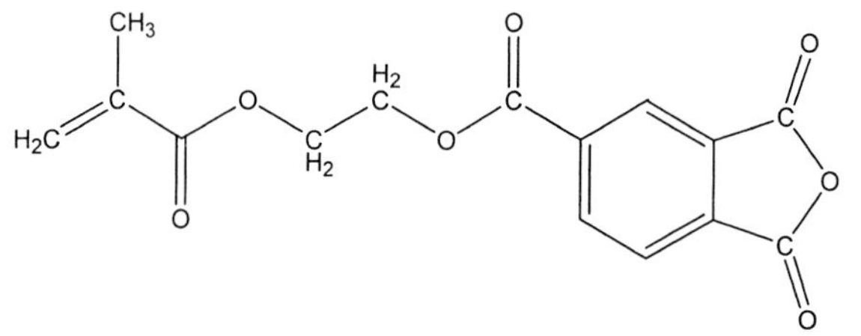

Fig. 14-11   4-methacryloxyethyl trimellitate anhydride.

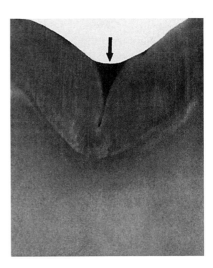

Fig. 14-12 Cross-section of a tooth, showing penetration of a sealant into an occlusal fissure **(arrow).** (Courtesy of K-J. Söderholm.)

initiation system or by light activation. The unfilled resins are available as colorless or tinted transparent materials. The filled resins are opaque and available either as tooth-colored or white materials.

The success of the sealant technique is highly dependent on obtaining and maintaining an intimate adaptation of the sealant to the tooth surface. Therefore the sealants must be of relatively low viscosity so that they will wet the tooth and flow readily into the depths of the pits and fissures. To enhance wetting and mechanical retention of the sealant, the tooth surface is first conditioned by etching with acid, as described earlier. The physical properties of the sealants are closer to those of unfilled direct resins than to those of resin-based composites.

The reduction in occlusal caries resulting from the careful use of pit and fissure sealants has been impressive. Consequently, the use of sealants has been endorsed as an effective therapy by the American Dental Association, the American Academy of Pediatric Dentistry, the American Society of Dentistry for Children, and the American Association of Public Health Dentistry.

Clinical studies have shown that the failure frequency of sealants is approximately 5% per year after one single application of the sealant. In one report, at the end of 10 years 78% of first permanent molars were free of caries when a single application of sealant had been placed, as compared with only 31% of caries-free teeth in the unsealed matched pairs. Mertz-Fairhurst et al (1998) reported even more dramatic results in a study of sealed Class I composite restorations where carious dentin was not removed. They showed that the lesions did not progress over a period of 10 years as long as the sealants remained intact.

If doubt exists about whether the pit or fissure is free from caries or not, it is still justified to place a sealant. Clinical trials in which sealants were intentionally placed in pits and fissures that were diagnosed as having caries have shown that as long as a sealant is well retained, no caries progression will occur.

If a dentist feels uncomfortable about sealing in a potential carious lesion and believes that a visual inspection of the potential lesion is required, another conservative approach can be taken. This option consists of a minimal cavity preparation and the placement of an enamel-dentin bonded composite restoration combined with a sealant application. With such an approach, most of the occlusal surface is sealed. This restoration is called a **preventive-resin restoration (PRR).** The PRR treatment has exhibited a success rate of 75% after 9 years, a remarkably high success rate even when compared with traditional amalgam treatment.

SELECTED READINGS

Asmussen E, and Munksgaard EC: Bonding of restorative resins to dentine: Status of dentine adhesives and impact on cavity design and filling techniques. Int Dent J 38:97, 1988.

The chemistry of dentin bonding agents is described, and bond strength data are presented. Also, factors involved in clinical usage that influence retention are cited.

Bowen RL, Eichmiller FC, Marjenhoff WA, and Rupp NW: Adhesive bonding of composites. J Am Coll Dent 56:10, 1989.

This article discusses the merits of several of the popular dentin and enamel bonding systems, noting differences in chemical components and instructions for use.

Buonocore MG: A simple method of increasing the adhesion of acrylic filling materials to enamel surfaces. J Dent Res 34:849, 1955.

In this paper, published approximately 50 years ago, Buonocore suggested that etching enamel would improve mechanical bonding of an unfilled resin (composites were nonexistent at that time). The technique is now an essential step in the use of all modern composites.

Buonocore MG: The Use of Adhesives in Dentistry. Springfield, IL, Charles C Thomas, 1975.

In this book, Buonocore, the developer of the acid-etch technique, identifies potential problems associated with the use of adhesives in dentistry that are still germane to current systems, for example, dentin bonding agents.

Douglas WH: Clinical status of dentine bonding agents. J Dent 17:209, 1989.

An excellent review and update of the evolution of earlier dentin bonding agents, the problems associated with adhesion, and the clinical criteria involved in phenomena such as microleakage and tooth strengthening. This reference is essential for individuals interested in this highly controversial area.

Fusayama T, Nakamura M, Kurosaki M, and Iwaku M: Nonpressure adhesion of a new adhesive restorative resin, J Dent Res 58:1364, 1979.

A breakthrough in dentin bonding was demonstrated when acid etching of dentin was reported to increase retention of restorations, but with no increase in pulpal trauma.

Houpt M, Fuks A, and Eidelman E: The preventive resin (composite resin/sealant) restoration: nine-year results. Quintessence Int 25:155, 1994.

Nine-year data presented to show the efficiency of using PRRs to treat cavities with carious lesions.

Mertz-Fairhurst EJ: Current status of sealant retention and caries prevention. National Institutes of Health Consensus Development Conference. Dental sealants in the prevention of tooth decay. J Dent Res 48:18, 1984.

Ten-year data presented to show a substantial reduction in caries following the placement of sealant as compared with untreated control surfaces.

Mertz-Fairhurst EJ, Curtis JW, Ergle JW, Rueggeberg FA, and Adair SM: Ultraconservative and cariostatic sealed restorations: Results at year 10, J Am Dent Assoc 129:55, 1998.

A classic 10-year study that demonstrates the efficacy of sealed composites in preventing caries progression even when the carious dentin was not removed.

Nakabayashi N, Kojima K, and Masuhara E: Sealants consensus development conference statement on dental sealants and the prevention of tooth decay. J Am Dent Assoc 108:233, 1984.

Recommendations are made from a consensus conference on the state of the art of sealant therapy. The data presented were strongly supportive of sealant use.

Pashley DH, Carvalho RM, Sano H, Nakajima M, Yoshiyama M, Shono Y, Fernandes CA, and Tay F: The microtensile bond test: A review, J Adhes Dent 1(4):299, 1999.

A review of the microtensile bond test, which permits true interfacial bond strength measurement in modern bonded systems for which conventional shear bond tests yield cohesive dentin failure.

Perdigao J, Lopes M: Dentin bonding—Questions for the new millennium. J Adhes Dent 1(3):19, 1999.

An update on the state of dentin bonding with a discussion of unanswered questions.

Simonsen RJ: Retention and effectiveness of dental sealant after 15 years. J Am Dent Assoc 122:34-42, 1991.

This paper represents a long-term evaluation of sealants based on a single application.

15

Restorative Resins

H. Ralph Rawls and J. Esquivel-Upshaw

OUTLINE

Aesthetic Restorative Materials

Composite Restorative Materials

Curing of Resin-Based Composites

Classification of Resin-Based Composites

Composites for Posterior Restorations

Use of Composites for Resin Veneers

Finishing of Composites

Biocompatibility of Composites

Repair of Composites

Survival Probability of Composites

KEY TERMS

Activation—The process through which sufficient energy is provided to induce an initiator to generate free radicals and cause polymerization to begin. The three sources of energy commonly used with dental resins include heat, chemicals, and light.

Activator—A source of energy used to activate an initiator and produce free radicals. Three possible energy sources can be used to dissociate an initiator into free radicals: (1) heat that supplies thermal energy; (2) an electron-donating chemical such as a tertiary amine that forms a complex and reduces the necessary thermal energy to that available at ambient temperature; or (3) visible light that supplies energy for photoinitiation in the presence of a photosensitizer such as camphorquinone (CQ).

C-factor—The configuration factor or ratio between the bonded surface area of a resin-based composite restoration to the unbonded or free surface area.

Chemically activated resin—A resin system consisting of two pastes (one containing a benzoyl peroxide [BP] initiator and the other an aromatic tertiary amine activator) which, when mixed together, release free radicals that initiate polymerization.

Chemically cured composite—A particle-filled resin that is polymerized through a chemically activated process.

Composite—In materials and science, a solid formed from two or more distinct phases (e.g., particles in a metal matrix) that have been combined to produce properties superior to or intermediate to those of the individual constituents; also a term used in dentistry to describe a dental composite.

Coupling agent—A bonding agent applied to filler particles to ensure chemical bonding to the resin matrix.

Degree of conversion (DC)—The percentage of carbon-carbon bonds converted to single bonds to form a polymeric resin; also, the percentage of polymerized methacrylate groups.

KEY TERMS—cont'd

Dental composite—A highly cross-linked polymeric material reinforced by a dispersion of amorphous silica, glass, crystalline, or organic resin filler particles and/or short fibers bonded to the matrix by a coupling agent.

Depth of cure—The thickness of a resin that can be converted from a monomer to a polymer under a specific light-curing condition.

Dual-cure resin—A dental composite that contains both chemically activated and light-activated components to initiate polymerization and potentially overcome the limitations of the chemical cure or light-cure systems, which include porosity incorporated during mixing and limits on depth of cure, respectively.

Estrogenicity—The potential of synthetic chemicals with a binding affinity for estrogen receptors to cause reproductive alterations.

Filler—The inorganic and/or organic resin particles that are designed to strengthen a composite, decrease thermal expansion, minimize polymerization shrinkage, and reduce the amount of swelling caused by water sorption.

Flowable composite—A hybrid composite with reduced filler level and a more narrow particle size distribution that increases flow and promotes intimate adaptation to prepared tooth surfaces.

Hybrid composite—A particle-filled resin that contains a graded blend of small and colloidal silica filler particles to achieve an optimal balance among the properties of strength, polymerization shrinkage, wear resistance, and polishability.

Inhibitor—A chemical added to resin systems to provide increased working time and extended storage life by minimizing spontaneous polymerization.

Initiator—A free radical–forming chemical used to start the polymerization reaction. It enters into the chemical reaction and becomes part of the final polymer compound; thus it is not a catalyst.

Light-cured composite—A particle-filled resin consisting of a single paste that becomes polymerized through the use of a photosensitive initiator system (CQ and an amine initiator) and a light source activator (visible blue light).

Microfiller—Colloidal silica filler particles, approximately 0.04 μm in size, which reinforce resin materials and form a composite that can be polished to a highly smooth surface.

Oxygen-inhibited layer—The thin surface region of a polymerized resin that contains unreacted methacrylate groups associated with exposure to oxygen.

Packable composite—A hybrid resin composite designed for use in posterior areas, where a stiffer consistency facilitates condensation in posterior teeth.

AESTHETIC RESTORATIVE MATERIALS

During the first half of the 20th century, silicates were the only tooth-colored aesthetic materials available for cavity restoration. Although silicates release fluoride, they are no longer used for permanent teeth (see Chapter 16) because they become severely eroded within a few years. Acrylic resins similar to those used for custom impression trays and dentures (polymethylmethacrylate [PMMA]) replaced the silicates during the late 1940s and the early 1950s because of their toothlike appearance, insolubility in oral fluids, ease of manipulation, and low cost. Unfortunately, these acrylic resins also have relatively poor wear resistance and they shrink severely during curing, which causes them to pull away from the cavity walls and produce leakage along margins. Their excessive thermal expansion and contraction cause further stresses to develop at the cavity margins when hot or cold beverages and foods are consumed. These problems were reduced somewhat by the addition of quartz powder to form a **composite** structure. Incorporation of inert **filler** particles became a practical means of reducing curing contraction as well as thermal expansion. The filler occupies space, but it does not take part in the setting reaction. In addition, commonly used fillers have extremely low coefficients of thermal expansion, approaching that of tooth structure. Thus the stresses resulting from thermal expansion and contraction were greatly reduced as well.

The early composites based on PMMA were not very successful, in part because the filler particles simply reduced the volume of polymer resin but were not bonded (coupled) to the resin. Thus defects developed between the mechanically retained particles and the surrounding resin, producing leakage, staining, and poor wear resistance. A major advance was made when Dr. Ray L. Bowen (1962) of the American Dental Association research unit at the National Bureau of Standards (now the National Institute of Standards and Technology) developed a new type of composite material. Bowen's main innovations were bisphenol A glycidyl methacrylate (bis-GMA), a dimethacrylate resin (see Chapter 7), and an organic silane **coupling agent** to form a bond between the filler particles and the resin matrix.

CRITICAL QUESTIONS

What are the essential components of resin composite materials? What are the potential uses of composites in dentistry? What roles do coupling agents, fillers, bis-GMA, and other high-molecular–weight dimethacrylates play in the function and performance of dental resins?

Uses and Applications

Improved matrix properties and filler-matrix coupling have largely overcome the problems of the earlier restorative materials. Consequently, since the early 1970s, resin-based composite systems and their dimethacrylate resins have become the material of choice for direct aesthetic anterior restorations. These materials are also gaining acceptance for restoration of posterior occlusal areas and other high-stress–bearing sites and are used in a variety of other dental applications, such as pit and fissure sealants, bonding of ceramic veneers, and cementation of other fixed prostheses. Furthermore, the mean longevity of posterior composites (7 yr) is approaching that of amalgam (10 yr).

COMPOSITE RESTORATIVE MATERIALS

There are three structural components in dental resin-based composites:
1. Matrix—A plastic resin material that forms a continuous phase and binds the filler particles
2. Filler—Reinforcing particles and/or fibers that are dispersed in the matrix
3. Coupling agent—Bonding agent that promotes adhesion between filler and resin matrix

Dental Composites

Dental composites are highly cross-linked polymeric materials reinforced by a dispersion of glass, crystalline, or resin filler particles and/or short fibers bound to the matrix by silane coupling agents.

CRITICAL QUESTION

Dentin and enamel are natural composites. Which components of enamel and dentin represent the filler and matrix structures in teeth analogous to those of resin-based composites?

Composition and Function of Components

Tooth enamel and dentin are two examples of the many composite materials found in nature. Enamel contains approximately 95 wt% inorganic structure, 90% to 92% of which is hydroxyapatite. The other components of enamel are 1 wt% of an organic enamelin structure and 4 wt% water. Dentin contains approximately 75 wt% of inorganic structure, primarily small hydroxyapatite crystals, 20 wt% organic matter (90% of which is collagen), and 5 wt% water. In both of these "natural tooth composites" the reinforcing filler particles are hydroxyapatite crystals. The difference in the properties of these two tissues is associated in part with differences in the matrix-to-filler ratios. This is analogous to the situation of synthetic restorative materials, in which the amount of filler in the composite has a major influence on the material's properties.

Composite restorative materials contain a number of components in addition to the resin matrix, inorganic filler particles, and a coupling agent. An **activator-initiator** system is required to convert the resin paste from a soft, moldable filling material to a hard, durable restoration. Other components are included to enhance the performance, appearance, and durability of the material. Pigments help to match the color of tooth structure. Ultraviolet (UV) absorbers and other additives improve color stability, and polymerization **inhibitors** extend storage life and provide increased working time for **chemically activated resins**. These components are discussed below.

Resin Matrix

Most dental composites use a blend of aromatic and/or aliphatic dimethacrylate monomers such as bis-GMA, one of the most widely used ingredients (see Fig. 7-16), triethylene glycol dimethacrylate (TEGDMA; see Fig. 7-17), and urethane dimethacrylate (UDMA; see Fig. 7-18). UDMA, bis-GMA, and TEGDMA are widely used resin matrix ingredients that form highly cross-linked polymer structures (see Fig. 7-3) in composites and sealant materials.

CRITICAL QUESTION

What problems result from shrinkage and contraction during polymerization of dental restorative resins?

As discussed previously, shrinkage occurs during curing as monomers are converted from an aggregate of freely flowing molecules to a rigid assembly of cross-linked polymer chains. Before polymerization, the monomers are held loosely together by van der Waal forces at a spacing that produces minimum potential energy (Chapter 2). As a polymer, the mer units are connected by covalent bonds with a minimum potential energy spacing approximately 20% less than that in the unreacted monomer. The result is a substantial volume contraction during curing. In turn, this curing shrinkage produces unrelieved stresses in the resin when the point is reached after which the resin has "gelled" and begins to harden. These stresses tend to develop at the tissue/composite interfaces, thereby weakening the bond and eventually producing a gap at the restoration margins. This can lead to staining, secondary caries, and other clinical problems. Because bis-GMA and UDMA have almost five times the molecular weight of methyl methacrylate, the density of methacrylate double-bond groups is approximately one-fifth as high in these monomers, which reduces polymerization shrinkage proportionately. The use of a dimethacrylate also results in extensive cross-linking, which increases the strength and rigidity of the polymer.

Although the high molecular weight of a monomer reduces curing shrinkage and improves mechanical properties, it also increases viscosity, as explained in Chapter 7. Bis-GMA has a particularly high viscosity (similar to honey), which makes it very difficult to blend and manipulate. Thus it is necessary to use lower-molecular–weight, highly fluid monomers to dilute bis-GMA and similar resins to attain sufficiently high filler levels (discussed in the following section), while also producing resin pastes with consistencies suitable for clinical manipulation. These diluent monomers can be any fluid methacrylate but are usually dimethacrylates such as TEGDMA. The reduction in viscosity is significant when TEGDMA is added to bis-GMA. A blend of 75 wt% bis-GMA and 25 wt% TEGDMA has a viscosity of 4300 centipoise, whereas the viscosity of a 50 wt% bis-GMA/50 wt% TEGDMA blend is 200 centipoise (like thin syrup).

The dimethacrylate monomers also have the advantage of producing extensive cross-linking among polymer chains. This results in a rigid resin matrix that is highly resistant to softening and/or degradation by heat and solvents such as water and alcohol. Unfortunately, the tradeoffs in polymerization shrinkage, wear resistance, and manipulation properties place severe limits on the ability to optimize the performance of composite materials. The need for a better balance of properties among these conflicting requirements has made the development of a "universal" composite difficult and has resulted in a proliferation of restorative resin products, each designed for a specialized application.

CRITICAL QUESTIONS

How is curing shrinkage affected by the presence of reinforcing fillers in dental composites? What are the relationships and tradeoffs among particle size, composition, and filler loading relative to their effect on the consistency, polishability, radiopacity, durability, and appearance of resin-based composite materials?

Filler Particles and Proportion of Filler

Incorporation of filler particles into a resin matrix greatly improves material properties, provided that the filler particles are well bonded to the matrix. If not, the filler particles do not provide reinforcement and can actually weaken the material. Because of the importance of well-bonded filler particles, the use of an effective coupling agent is extremely important to the success of a composite material.

Benefits of Fillers

The primary purposes of filler particles are to strengthen a composite and to reduce the amount of matrix material. Several important properties of dental composites are improved by increased filler "loading" (volume fraction): (1) reinforcement of the matrix resin, resulting in increased hardness, strength, and decreased wear; (2) reduction in polymerization shrinkage; (3) reduction in thermal expansion and contraction; (4) improved workability by increasing viscosity (liquid monomer plus filler yields a paste consistency); (5) reduction in water sorption, softening, and staining; and (6) increased radiopacity and diagnostic sensitivity through the incorporation of strontium (Sr) and barium (Ba) glass and other heavy metal compounds that absorb x-rays. Several of these improvements can only be realized if the filler particles are strongly coupled to the matrix.

Another benefit of filler particles is that curing shrinkage is offset in proportion to the volume fraction (loading) of filler. Although shrinkage varies from one composite product to another, it ranges from 1.5 to 4 vol% within 24 hr after curing. Another advantage is that there is less water sorption and less softening of composites compared with unfilled resins. Composites also have a lower coefficient of thermal expansion that is closer to that of tooth tissue. Hence less interfacial stress is produced. Mechanical properties such as compressive strength, tensile strength, and modulus of elasticity (stiffness) are increased, as is abrasion resistance. An increase in the volume fraction of well-bonded filler particles enhances physical and mechanical properties to levels comparable with those of tooth tissue, thereby increasing clinical performance and durability.

Filler particles are most commonly produced by grinding or milling quartz or glasses to produce particles ranging in size from 0.1 to 100 μm (Fig. 15-1). Submicron silica particles of colloidal size (~0.04 μm), referred to collectively as **microfiller** or individually as *microfillers*, are obtained by a pyrolytic or precipitation process. In these processes, a silicon compound (e.g., $SiCl_4$) is burned in an O_2 and H_2 atmosphere to form macromolecule chains of SiO_2 (Fig. 15-2). These macromolecules are of a colloidal size and constitute the inorganic filler particles (Fig. 15-3).

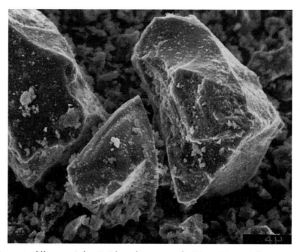

Fig. 15-1 Ground quartz filler particles (with a diameter of ~20 to 30 μm) that were used in early formulations of traditional composites. The smaller particles seen in the background contribute to a broad particle-size distribution. (Courtesy of K-J.M. Söderholm.)

$$4 \left\{ \begin{array}{c} Cl \\ | \\ Cl-Si-Cl \\ | \\ Cl \end{array} \right\} + 12\,H_2 + 6\,O_2 \xrightarrow{\text{Heat}} \begin{array}{c} OH \qquad\quad OH \\ | \qquad\qquad | \\ HO-Si-O-Si-OH \\ | \qquad\qquad | \\ O \qquad\qquad O \\ | \qquad\qquad | \\ HO-Si-O-Si-OH \\ | \qquad\qquad | \\ OH \qquad\quad OH \end{array} + 16\,HCl$$

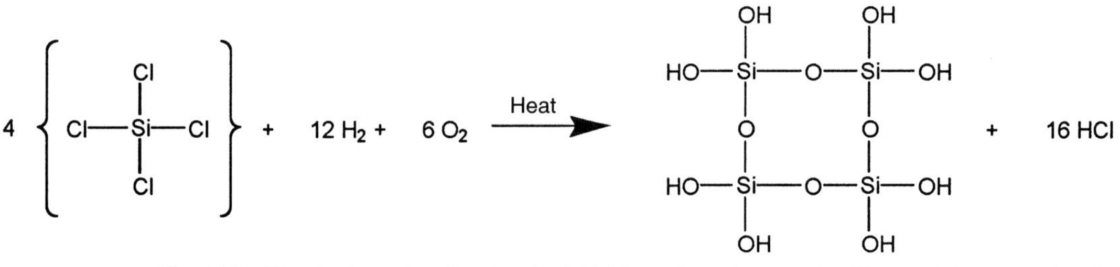

Fig. 15-2 Chemical reaction showing the initial formation of pyrogenic silica particles, as used in the microfill resins. (Courtesy of K-J.M. Söderholm.)

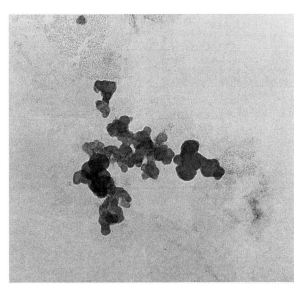

Fig. 15-3 Transmission electron microscopy image of pyrogenic silica particles. The diameter of the particles is approximately 0.04 μm. (Courtesy of K-J.M. Söderholm.)

Composites are classified on the basis of the average size of the major filler component. In addition to filler volume level, other important factors that determine the properties and the clinical application of the resultant composites include the filler size, size distribution, index of refraction, radiopacity, and hardness of the filler.

A distribution of particle sizes is necessary to incorporate a maximum amount of filler into a resin matrix. Obviously, if a uniform particle size is used, even with close packing, a space will exist between particles. This concept can be visualized as the presence of larger voids in a box filled with spheres of the same size compared with the voids present in a mixture of larger and smaller spheres or a combination of spheres and irregular-shaped particles. These spaces can be filled by smaller particles, such as small beads among the spheres. By extending this process, a continuous distribution of particles can yield a maximum filler loading. Most composites also contain some colloidal silica. In total, inorganic filler particles account for between 30 and 70 vol%, or 50 to 85 wt% of a composite. The maximum theoretical packing fraction for close-packed structures is 74 vol%.

The practical amount of filler that can be incorporated into a resin is greatly influenced by the total filler surface area, which is a function of particle size, with surface area increasing as size decreases for a constant volume of filler. Colloidal silica particles, because of their extremely small size, have extremely large surface areas ranging from 50 to as much as 400 m^2 per gram. The silica surfaces form polar bonds with the monomer molecules; this inhibits their flow, increases the viscosity, and "thickens" the resin paste, even with very small amounts. Because of this effect, the microfilled composites contain only 20 to 59 vol% colloidal silica as the only inorganic component. The remainder is pulverized, precured resin, the so-called "organic" filler with a particle size between 5 and 30 μm. In many composite formulations colloidal fillers are added in amounts of less than 5 wt% solely to increase paste viscosity and to enhance cavity packing consistency. Hybrids, with 10 to 15 wt% colloidal silica, can be filled to only approximately 5% less inorganic filler content than the small-particle composites.

For acceptable aesthetics, the translucency of a composite restoration must be similar to that of tooth structure. Thus the index of refraction of the filler must closely match that of the resin. For bis-GMA and TEGDMA, the refractive indices are approximately 1.55 and 1.46, respectively, and a mixture of the two components in equal proportions by weight yields a refractive index of approximately 1.50. Most of the glasses and quartz that are used for fillers have refractive indices of approximately 1.50, which is adequate to achieve sufficient translucency.

Quartz has been used extensively as a reinforcing filler, particularly in the early versions of dental composites. It has the advantage of being chemically inert and yet also very hard, making it abrasive as well as difficult to grind into very fine particles. However, this hardness also makes quartz composites difficult to polish and potentially abrasive to opposing teeth or restorations. So-called amorphous silica has the same composition and refractive index as quartz, but it is not crystalline and not as hard, thus greatly reducing the abrasiveness of the composite surface structure.

The radiopacity of filler materials is provided by a number of glasses and ceramics that contain heavy metals such as barium (Ba), strontium (Sr), and zirconium (Zr). These glasses also have indices of refraction of approximately 1.50 to match that of the resin. The most commonly used glass filler is Ba glass. Although glass fillers containing metals of a high atomic number provide radiopacity, they are not as inert as quartz and amorphous silica and are slowly leached and weakened in acidic juices and other oral fluids. The glass filler is also attacked over time by acidulated phosphate fluoride solutions or gels. Because of differences in the composition of saliva among patients, it is difficult to predict the clinical effects of exposure to saliva, but the implication is that glass-filled composites would gradually become more susceptible to abrasive wear and hence have a shorter functional lifetime compared with silica-reinforced resins.

Coupling Agents

As stated previously, it is essential that filler particles be bonded to the resin matrix. This allows the more flexible polymer matrix to transfer stresses to the higher modulus (more rigid and stiffer) filler particles. The bond between the two phases of the composite is provided by a coupling agent. A properly applied coupling agent can impart improved physical and mechanical properties and inhibit leaching by preventing water from penetrating along the filler-resin interface.

Although titanates and zirconates can be used as coupling agents, organosilanes such as γ-methacryloxypropyl trimethoxysilane are used most commonly (Fig. 15-4). In the presence of water, the methoxy groups ($-OCH_3$) are hydrolyzed to silanol ($-Si-OH$) groups that can bond with other silanols on the filler surfaces by formation of a siloxane bond ($-Si-O-Si-$; see Fig. 15-4). The organosilane methacrylate groups form covalent bonds with the resin when it is polymerized, thereby completing the coupling process. Proper coupling by means of organosilanes is extremely important to the clinical performance of resin-based composite restorative materials.

CRITICAL QUESTION

What are the similarities and differences in the mechanisms involved in chemically activated and light-activated dental resins?

Activator-Initiator System

Both monomethacrylate and dimethacrylate monomers polymerize by the addition polymerization mechanism initiated by free radicals, as described in Chapter 7. Free radicals can be generated by chemical **activation** or by external energy

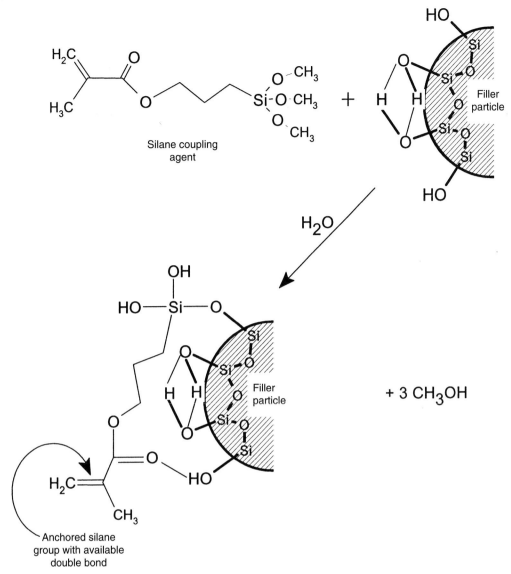

Fig. 15-4 The chemical structure of γ-methacryloxypropyltrimethoxy silane and an idealized diagram of how a silane is hydrolyzed and becomes attached to silica and glass filler particle surfaces. Such silanized particles are then reactive and can "couple" the particles to the resin matrix by copolymerization with the double bond in the silane propylmethacrylate group $(CH_2=C(CH_3)COO–C_3H_6–Si–)$. (Adapted from Söderholm K-JM, and Shang S-W: Molecular orientation of silane at the surface of colloidal silica. J Dent Res 72:1050, 1993.)

activation (heat, light, or microwave). Because dental composites for direct placement use chemical activation or light activation, or a combination of the two, only these systems are discussed.

Chemically Activated Resins

Chemically activated products are supplied as two pastes, one of which contains the benzoyl peroxide (BP) initiator and the other an aromatic tertiary amine activator (e.g., N, N-dimethyl-*p*-toluidine), as previously described in Chapter 7 for the acrylic resins. When the two pastes are mixed together, the amine reacts with the BP to form free radicals, and additional polymerization is initiated. Today, these materials are mainly used for restorations and large foundation structures (buildups) that are not readily cured with a light source.

Light-Activated Resins. The first light-activated systems were formulated for UV light to initiate free radicals. Today, the UV light–cured composites have been replaced by visible blue-light–activated systems with greatly improved **depth of cure,** a controllable working time, and other advantages. Because of these advantages, visible light-activated composites are more widely used than are chemically activated materials.

Light-curable dental composites are supplied as a single paste contained in a light-proof syringe. The free radical initiating system, consisting of a photosensitizer and an amine initiator, is contained in this paste. As long as these two components are not exposed to light, they do not interact. However, exposure to light in the blue region (wavelength of ~468 nm) produces an excited state of the photosensitizer, which then interacts with the amine to form free radicals that initiate addition polymerization (Fig. 15-5).

Camphorquinone (CQ) is a commonly used photosensitizer that absorbs blue light with wavelengths between 400 and 500 nm. Only small quantities of CQ are required (0.2 wt% or less in the paste). A number of amine initiators are suitable for interaction with CQ, such as dimethylaminoethyl methacrylate (DMAEMA), which is also present at low levels, that is, approximately 0.15 wt%.

CRITICAL QUESTION

What roles do inhibitors play in dental resin materials?

Inhibitors

Inhibitors are added to the resin systems to minimize or prevent spontaneous or accidental polymerization of monomers. Inhibitors have a strong reactivity potential with free radicals. If a free radical is formed, for example, by brief exposure to room lighting when the material is dispensed, the inhibitor reacts with the free radical faster than the free radical can react with the monomer. This prevents chain propagation by terminating the reaction before the free radical is able to initiate polymerization. After all of the inhibitor is consumed, chain propagation begins. A typical inhibitor is butylated hydroxytoluene (BHT), which is used in concentrations on the order of 0.01 wt%. BHT and similar free radical scavengers are also used as food preservatives to prevent oxidation and rancidity. Thus inhibitors have two functions: they extend the storage lifetime for all resins and they ensure sufficient working time.

Optical Modifiers

For a natural appearance, dental composites must have visual shading and translucency that are similar to the corressponding properties of tooth structure. Shading is achieved by adding various pigments. These pigments usually consist of minute amounts of metal oxide particles. Translucency and opacity are adjusted as necessary to simulate enamel and dentin. For example, if a Class IV incisal area is reconstructed, the translucency of an unmodified composite might allow too much light

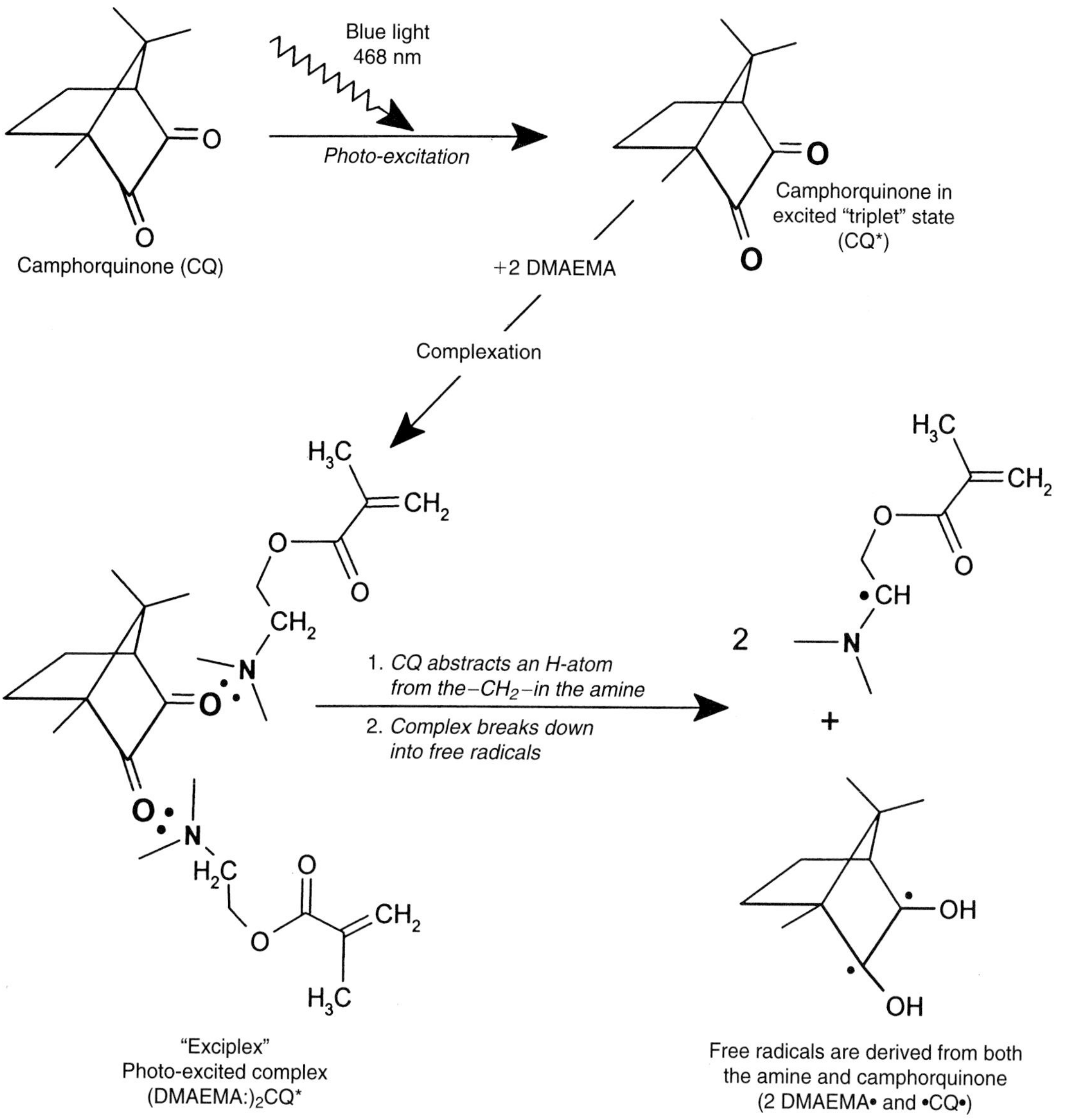

Fig. 15-5 The light-cure process is activated when a diketone photosensitizer such as camphorquinone (CQ) absorbs a quantum of blue light and forms an excited-state complex (exciplex) with an electron donor such as an amine (e.g., dimethylaminoethyl methacrylate [DMAEMA]). In the figure ":"denotes the unshared pair of electrons "donated" by the amines to the >C=O (ketone) groups in CQ. While in this activated complex, CQ extracts a hydrogen atom from the α-carbon adjacent to the amine group, and the complex decomposes into amine and CQ free radicals. The CQ free radical is readily inactivated. Thus in photoinitiation only the amine free radicals act to initiate the addition polymerization reaction (see Fig. 7-8).

to pass through the restoration. As a result, less light is reflected or scattered back to the observer, who perceives the incisal edge as too dark. This deficiency can be corrected by adding an opacifier. However, if an excessive amount of opacifier is added, too much light may be reflected and the observer then perceives that the restoration is "too white," or more correctly, "too high in value" (see Chapter 3). To increase the opacity, the manufacturer adds titanium dioxide and aluminum oxide to composites in only minute amounts (0.001 to 0.007 wt%) because these oxides are highly effective opacifiers.

It is important to realize that all optical modifiers affect light transmission through a composite. Thus darker shades and greater opacities have a decreased depth of light-curing ability and require either an increased exposure time or a thinner layer when cured. Studies have shown that for optimum polymerization, darker shades and opacifier resins should be placed in thinner layers. This consideration has added importance when a bonding agent covered with a composite layer is being cured. These concepts are discussed below in greater detail.

CRITICAL QUESTION

What are the relative advantages and drawbacks of chemically-activated and light-activated restorative resins?

CURING OF RESIN-BASED COMPOSITES
Chemical Activation

As discussed previously, the first composites were cured by a chemically activated polymerization process. This is also referred to as *cold curing* or *self-curing*. Chemically activated polymerization is initiated by mixing two pastes just before use (see Chapter 7). During mixing it is almost impossible to avoid incorporating air into the mix, thereby forming pores that weaken the structure and trap oxygen, which inhibits polymerization during curing. Another problem with chemical activation is that the operator has no control over the working time after the two components have been mixed. Therefore both insertion and contouring must be completed quickly once the resin components are mixed.

Light Activation

To overcome the problems of chemical activation, manufacturers developed resins that do not require mixing. This was achieved by use of a photosensitive initiator system and a light source for activation.

In addition to avoiding the porosity of chemically activated resins, light-cured materials also allow the operator to complete insertion and contouring before curing is initiated. Furthermore, once curing is initiated, an exposure time of 40 sec or less is required to light-cure a 2-mm–thick layer, as compared with several minutes for chemically cured materials. Another advantage of light-cured systems is that they are not as sensitive to oxygen inhibition as are the chemically cured systems. However, there are substantial limitations with light-cured composites. First, they must be placed incrementally when the bulk exceeds approximately 2 to 3 mm because of the limited depth of light penetration. Thus light-cured composites can actually require more time when producing large restorations (e.g., in Class II cavity preparations). Other drawbacks include the cost of the light-curing unit and several complicating factors associated with light sources and photocuring, as discussed in the following.

CRITICAL QUESTION

What are the tradeoffs among the several types of light sources used to photoactivate dental restorative resins?

Photocuring with Visible (Blue) Light

Dentists produce cross-linked resin when a diacrylate monomer containing a photoinitiator system is irradiated with a blue light. The advantages of using **light-cured composites** instead of chemically cured products include the following: (1) mixing is not required, which results in less porosity, less staining, and increased strength; (2) an aliphatic amine can be used instead of the aromatic amines required with chemical curing, thereby enhancing color stability; and (3) command polymerization on exposure to blue light, providing control of working time. There are also several drawbacks to light-cured composites: (1) limited curing depth, requiring buildup layers of 2 mm or less; (2) relatively poor accessibility in certain posterior and interproximal locations; (3) variable exposure times because of shade (hue, value, and chroma) differences, resulting in longer exposure times for darker shades and/or increased opacity; and (4) sensitivity to room illumination, which may lead to formation of a skin or crust when an opened tube is exposed too long to room light.

Curing Lamps

Most curing lamps are hand-held devices that contain the light source and are equipped with a relatively short, rigid light guide made up of fused optical fibers. A few have the power unit connected to the handpiece by a long, flexible, liquid-filled light guide. At present the most widely used light source is a quartz bulb with a tungsten filament in a halogen environment, similar to those used in automobile headlights and slide projectors. More recently, other types have been introduced with advantages that should make them increasingly popular (see text in sections below that describe types of lamps). Light-emitting diodes (LEDs), plasma arc curing (PAC), and laser lamps offer several advantages over quartz-tungsten-halogen (QTH) lamps but at generally higher costs and with other offsetting drawbacks. LED lamps require much less power than other light sources, and they do not produce heat or require filters. They are lightweight and can be operated by battery. PAC and argon laser lamps are higher-powered, more intense light sources that allow shorter exposure times for curing a given thickness of composite.

Types of Lamps Used for Photoinitiator Curing

Four types of lamps may be used for photoinitiation of the polymerization process. The following lists these lamps in order of lowest intensity to highest intensity.

1. **LED lamps.** Using a solid-state, electronic process, these light sources emit radiation only in the *blue* part of the visible spectrum between 440 and 480 nm, and they do not require filters. LEDs require low wattage, can be battery-powered, generate no heat, and are quiet because a cooling fan is not needed. Although they produce the lowest intensity radiation, new technology is rapidly overcoming this limitation.
2. **QTH lamps.** QTH lamps have a quartz bulb with a tungsten filament that irradiates both UV and white light that must be filtered to remove heat and all wavelengths except those in the *violet-blue* range (~400 to 500 nm). The intensity of the bulb diminishes with use, so a calibration meter is required to measure the output intensity.
3. **PAC lamps.** PAC lamps use a xenon gas that is ionized to produce a plasma. The high-intensity white light is filtered to remove heat and to allow blue light (~400 to 500 nm) to be emitted.

4. **Argon laser lamps.** Argon laser lamps have the highest intensity and emit at a single wavelength. Lamps currently available emit ~490 nm.

The tungsten and plasma arc lamps are filtered to transmit light only in the part of the *violet-blue* region of the spectrum that matches the photoabsorption range of CQ. CQ, as explained earlier, is a photosensitizer that is widely used for dental resins. Currently available LED and laser dental curing lamps are designed to emit light only in the *blue* spectral range that falls within the 400 to 500 nm photoabsorption range of CQ. Thus they do not require filters. A few photosensitizers and light sources have been introduced that absorb or emit, respectively, at wavelengths outside the 400 to 500 nm range, which will provide inadequate curing unless the lamp and resin/photosensitizer are matched to each other.

Polymerization is initiated when a critical concentration of free radicals is formed. This requires that a particular number of photons be absorbed by the initiator system, which is directly related to the wavelength, intensity, and time of exposure. There can be substantial differences in the wavelength range and intensity among various brands and types of manufactured lamps. Commonly available QTH lamps emit a radiant power density that ranges from approximately 300 to 1200 milliwatts/cm^2 (mW/cm^2) in the violet-blue region, and it is not unusual for two brands to vary in intensity by a factor of 2 or more.

For maximum curing, which is about 50% to 60% monomer conversion (see the following), a radiant energy influx of approximately 16,000 millijoules/cm^2 (16 joules/cm^2) is required for a 2-mm–thick layer of resin. This can be delivered by a 40-sec exposure to a lamp emitting 400 mW/cm^2 (40 sec × 400 mW/cm^2 = 16,000 mJ/cm^2 or 16 J/cm^2). The same result can be produced by a 20-sec exposure at 800 mW/cm^2, or an exposure of ~13 sec with a 1200-mW/cm^2 lamp. Thus increasing the power density of the lamp increases the rate and degree of cure. However, faster curing with higher-intensity light sources is not without its tradeoffs, as discussed in the following (see Reduction of Residual Stresses).

CRITICAL QUESTIONS

Can increasing the intensity of curing lamps shorten the time needed to adequately cure composite resins? How does lamp intensity affect the depth of cure?

Depth of Cure and Exposure Time

Recently QTH, PAC, and laser lamps have been introduced with substantially increased intensities (>1,000 mW/cm^2), thus opening the possibility of reduced exposure times and/or greater depth of cure. These are highly desirable benefits that can greatly reduce restoration treatment time and therefore cost to the patient.

However, light absorption and scattering in resin composites reduces the power density and **degree of conversion (DC)** exponentially with depth of penetration. Intensity can be reduced by a factor of 10 to 100 in a 2-mm–thick layer of composite. This reduces monomer conversion to an unacceptable level at depths greater than 2 to 3 mm. Thus the surface must be irradiated for a longer time to deliver sufficient power density well below the surface. Given the limits imposed by the light scattering and absorption inherent in current restorative resins, the tradeoffs are such that increased intensity will allow either shorter curing times for a given depth of cure, or increased depth of cure for a given exposure time, but there is little advantage in attempting to achieve both simultaneously. The practical consequence is that curing depth is limited to 2 to 3 mm unless excessively long exposure times are used, regardless of lamp intensity. Thus solutions to this problem are more likely to come through advances in the chemistry and technology of composite structures rather than through advances in clinical technique or the technology of curing lamps.

CRITICAL QUESTION

What are the most important factors that affect depth of cure for a lamp with a given intensity?

Light attenuation can also vary considerably from one type of composite to another, depending on the opacity, filler size, filler concentration, and pigment shade. As described earlier, darker shades and/or more opaque resins require longer curing times. For these reasons, manufacturers usually recommend curing times based on a particular curing device for each shade and type of resin. These recommended times are usually the absolute minimum. To maximize both degree of polymerization and long-term clinical durability, the clinician should adjust the exposure time and curing technique to the intensity of the light source used, and the lamp intensity should be evaluated frequently.

Light is also absorbed and scattered as it passes through tooth structure, especially dentin, thereby causing incomplete curing in such critical areas as proximal boxes. When attempting to polymerize the resin through tooth structure, the exposure time should be increased by a factor of 2 to 3 to compensate for the reduction in light intensity.

For the halogen lamps, light intensity can decrease depending on the quality and age of the light source, orientation of the light tip, distance between light tip and restoration, and presence of contamination, such as composite material residue on the light tip. Consequently, the lamp output intensity should be checked regularly, and the operator should always place the light tip as close as possible to the restorative material.

Despite the many advantages of light-cured resins, there is still a need for **chemically cured composites** and resins in certain situations. For example, only chemically cured materials can be used with reliable results as a luting agent under metallic restorations.

Dual-Cure Resins and Extraoral Curing

One way to overcome limits on curing depth and some of the other problems associated with light curing is to combine chemical curing and visible-light curing components in the same resin. So-called **dual-cure resins** are commercially available and consist of two light-curable pastes, one containing benzoyl peroxide (BP) and the other containing an aromatic tertiary amine. When these two pastes are mixed and then exposed to light, light curing is promoted by the amine/CQ combination and chemical curing is promoted by the amine/BP interaction. Dual-cure materials are intended for any situation that does not allow sufficient light penetration to produce adequate monomer conversion, for example, cementation of bulky ceramic inlays. Like the chemically cured resins, air inhibition and porosity are problems with dual-cure resins.

As an alternative to intraoral chemical curing and/or light curing, extraoral heat or light can be used to promote a higher level of cure. For example, a chemical- or light-cured composite can be used to produce an inlay on a tooth or a die. This inlay can be cured directly within the tooth or on the die and then transferred to an oven, where it receives additional heat or light curing. After completion, the inlay is cemented to the tooth with a resin-based composite.

CRITICAL QUESTIONS

How does the extent to which monomer is converted to polymer affect the longevity of composite restorations? What factors related to the curing process affect the integrity of the seal between a photocured composite resin and the margins of a cavity preparation?

Degree of Conversion

The DC is a measure of the percentage of carbon-carbon double bonds that have been converted to single bonds to form a polymeric resin (Fig. 15-6). The higher the DC, the better the strength, wear resistance, and many other properties essential to resin performance. A conversion of 50% to 60%, typical of highly cross-linked

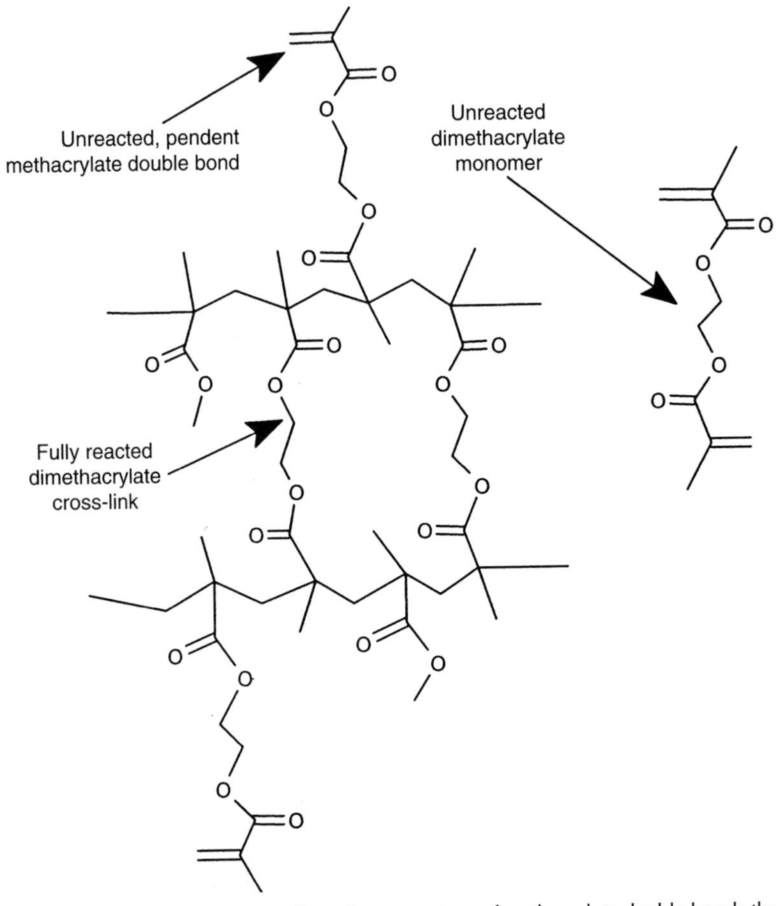

Unreacted, pendent
methacrylate double bond

Unreacted
dimethacrylate
monomer

Fully reacted
dimethacrylate
cross-link

Fig. 15-6   Degree of conversion (DC) reflects the percentage of methacrylate double bonds that are converted to single bonds during the curing reaction. This figure shows that a cured resin can contain dimethacrylates (DM) with zero, one, or two unreacted double bonds. If at least one double bond has reacted, the DM is bound to the polymer network as a "pendant" group with one double bond available for further reaction. Any completely unreacted monomers can migrate out of the cured resin. Cross-linked groups strengthen and make the resin rigid while pendant groups plasticize the resin (see Fig. 7-14), and unreacted monomer softens and swells the resin structure, as explained in Chapter 7.

bis-GMA–based composites, implies that 50% to 60% of the methacrylate groups have polymerized. However, this does not imply that 40% to 50% of the monomer molecules are left in the resin because one of the two methacrylate groups per dimethacrylate molecule could still have reacted and could be covalently bonded to the polymer structure, forming a pendant group (see Fig. 15-6). Conversion of the monomer to polymer depends on several factors, such as resin composition, the transmission of light through the material, and the concentration of sensitizer, initiator, and inhibitor. As discussed earlier, transmission of light through the material is controlled by lamp intensity, absorption, and scattering of light by filler particles and opacifiers, as well as by any tooth structure interposed between the light source and composite.

The total DC within resins does not differ between chemically activated and light-activated composites containing the same monomer formulations, as long as adequate light curing is employed. Conversion values of 50% to 70% are achieved at room temperature for both types of curing system. Likewise, polymerization shrinkage of comparable light-activated and chemically activated resins is not significantly different. However, in light-cured materials, curing shrinkage leads to substantially greater stress buildup and leakage at the resin margins, in turn leading to staining, sensitivity and secondary caries.

Reduction of Residual Stresses

The light-activated resins have overcome many of the deficiencies of chemically activated resins, including lack of control over working time, yellowing, and porosity. However, the internal pores in chemically cured resins act to relax residual stresses that build up during curing (the pores enlarge during hardening and reduce the concentration of stresses at the margins). Also, the slower curing rate of chemical activation allows a larger portion of the shrinkage to be compensated by internal flow among the developing polymer chains, before formation of extensive cross-linking (i.e., before gelation). After the gel point, stresses cannot be relieved but instead continue to increase and concentrate within the resin and the tooth structure adjacent to the bonded interfaces.

CRITICAL QUESTION

How can the composite clinical manipulation technique be used to improve the integrity of the marginal seal in a composite restoration?

Two general approaches have been followed in seeking to overcome the problem of stress concentration and marginal failure experienced with light-activated resins: (1) reduction in volume contraction by altering the chemistry and/or composition of the resin system and (2) clinical techniques designed to offset the effects of polymerization shrinkage. The former is the more desirable solution, and intensive research and development efforts are currently in progress to develop resins with low shrinkage and low thermal expansion. In the meantime, a variety of techniques have been investigated that can immediately be put into practice by the clinician. These techniques are associated with incremental buildup and curing rate control.

Incremental Buildup and Cavity Configuration

One technique attempts to reduce the so-called **C-factor (configuration factor).** The C-factor is related to the cavity preparation geometry and is represented by the ratio of bonded to nonbonded surface areas. Residual polymerization stress increases directly with this ratio. During curing, shrinkage leaves the bonded cavity surfaces in a state of stress and the nonbonded, free surfaces (i.e., those that reproduce the original external tooth anatomy) relax some of the stress by contracting inward toward the bulk of the material. A layering technique (Fig. 15-7) in which the restoration is built up in increments, curing one layer at a time, effectively reduces polymerization stress by minimizing the C-factor. That is, thinner layers reduce bonded surface area and maximize nonbonded surface area, thus minimizing the associated C-factor. In any case, as discussed previously, limitations on the depth of cure of photoinitiated resins dictate the use of incremental buildup of the composite. Thus an incremental technique overcomes both limited depth of cure and residual stress concentration, but adds to the time and difficulty of placing a restoration. Several variations on this idea are described in numerous texts and articles on operative dentistry.

Soft-Start, Ramped Curing and Delayed Curing

Another approach to offsetting photopolymerization stress buildup is to follow the example of chemical initiation by providing an initial low rate of polymerization, thereby extending the time available for stress relaxation before reaching the gel point. This can be accomplished by using a soft-start technique. In this technique, curing begins with a low intensity and finishes with a high intensity. The approach allows for a slow initial rate of polymerization and a high initial level of stress relaxation during the early stages, and it ends at the maximum intensity once the gel point has been reached. This drives the curing reaction to the highest possible conversion only after much of the stress has been relieved. A number of studies have shown that varying levels of stress reduction in tooth-cavity walls can be achieved in this way, while not increasing total exposure time or sacrificing either DC or depth of cure. Consequently, a variety of protocols have been developed and the necessary lamps made available that automatically provide one or more soft-start exposure sequences.

Variations on this technique include ramping and delayed cure. In ramping, the intensity is gradually increased, or "ramped up," during the exposure. This ramping consists of either stepwise, linear, or exponential modes. In delayed curing, the

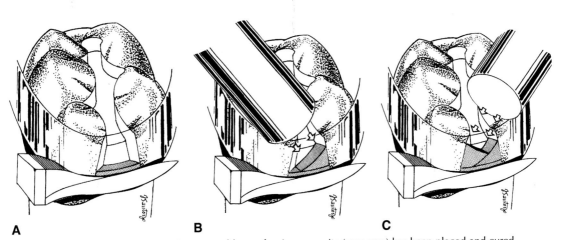

A   **B**   **C**

Fig. 15-7 **A,** First incremental layer of resin composite (gray area) has been placed and cured. **B,** Second increment being cured with a light source. **C,** Third composite increment during curing.

restoration is initially incompletely cured at low intensity. The clinician then sculpts and contours the resin to the correct occlusion and later applies a second exposure for the final cure. This delay allows substantial stress relaxation to take place. The longer the time period available for relaxation, the lower the residual stress. Delayed curing and exponential ramp curing appear to provide the greater reductions in curing stress.

High-Intensity Curing

As discussed earlier, increased lamp intensity allows for shorter exposure times for a given depth of cure in a particular shade and type of resin. Curing depths equivalent to that of a 500 mW/cm^2 QTH lamp (2 mm at 40 sec) have been demonstrated using an exposure time of 10 sec with certain PAC lights, and 5 sec with an argon laser. Thus these high-intensity lamps could provide substantial savings in chair time. However, high-intensity, short exposure times cause accelerated rates of curing, and there may be substantial residual stress buildup because insufficient time is allowed for stress relaxation, even when used in combination with incremental buildup and soft-start curing. At present, this aspect has not been well investigated. In the meantime, the clinician should carefully consider the tradeoffs before investing in these more expensive types of curing lamps.

The technology of photoinitiated curing is advancing rapidly on a number of fronts, some of which may well result in substantially greater latitude for the practice of restorative dentistry. A grasp of the fundamental principles will aid the clinician in keeping pace with these changes and avoiding the pitfalls, which inevitably accompany any potential advances in composite technology.

Precautions for Using Curing Lamps

The light emitted by curing units can cause retinal damage if a person looks directly at the beam for an extended period or even for short periods in the case of lasers. To avoid such damage, never look directly into the light tip and minimize observation of the reflected light for longer periods. Protective eyeglasses and various types of shields that filter the light are available for increased protection for both clinical personnel and patients.

CRITICAL QUESTION

How can particle size and size distribution of resin-based composites be used to select clinical materials to match the needs of various restorative situations?

CLASSIFICATION OF RESIN-BASED COMPOSITES

A useful classification system for resin composites is one based on filler particle size and size distribution, as shown in Table 15-1. Subgroups and overlapping may exist, particularly for the hybrid category. A **hybrid composite** combines filler from either the small or the traditional category, with microfillers (submicron, colloidal filler particles). Any resin with fillers from two or more size ranges can, in principle, be considered a hybrid. Future composites that contain fiber and and/or nanoparticle fillers can be classified in a similar way.

A single classification of hybrid composite is not very meaningful because most modern dental composites that use fillers in the micrometer (μm) size range also

Table 15-1	Classification of Resin-Based Composites and Indications for Use	
Class of composite	**Particle size**	**Clinical use**
Traditional (large particle)	1–50 μm glass	High-stress areas
Hybrid (large particle)	(1) 1–20 μm glass (2) 0.04 μm silica	High-stress areas requiring improved polishability (Classes I, II, III, IV)
Hybrid (midifiller)	(1) 0.1–10 μm glass (2) 0.04 μm silica	High stress areas requiring improved polishability (Classes III, IV)
Hybrid (minifiller/SPF)	(1) 0.1–2 μm glass (2) 0.04 μm silica	Moderate stress areas requiring optimal polishability (Classes III, IV)
Packable hybrid	Midifiller/minifiller hybrid, but with lower filler fraction	Situations in which improved condensability is needed (Classes I, II)
Flowable hybrid	Midifiller hybrid, but with finer particle size distribution	Situations in which improved flow is needed and/or where access is difficult (Class II)
Homogeneous microfill	0.04 μm silica	Low-stress and subgingival areas that require a high luster and polish
Heterogeneous microfill	(1) 0.04 μm silica (2) Prepolymerized resin particles containing 0.04 μm silica	Low-stress and subgingival areas where reduced shrinkage is essential

SPF, Small-particle filled.

contain small amounts (<5 wt%) of microfillers to adjust the paste to the desired viscosity. The most commonly used hybrid composites in the early 2000s usually refer to resins that contain fillers having an average particle size of ~0.5 to 1.0 μm in combination with 10 to 15 wt% microfiller. Hybrid composites that fall within these guidelines are discussed subsequently. Two special categories of hybrids that vary somewhat from this definition are also described: flowable and **packable composites**. The properties of the major composite classifications are summarized in Table 15-2.

Traditional Composites

As can be seen in Tables 15-1 and 15-2, the traditional composites have comparatively large filler particles. This category was developed during the 1970s and modified slightly over the years. These composites are also referred to as *conventional* or *macrofilled composites*. Because these materials are no longer widely used, the term *traditional* is more meaningful than is *conventional*. The most commonly used filler for these materials is finely ground amorphous silica and quartz. As can be seen in the photomicrograph of the ground quartz filler in Figure 15-1, there is a wide distribution in particle size. Although the average size is 8 to 12 μm, particles as large as 50 μm may also be present. Filler loading generally is 70 to 80 wt% or 60 to 70 vol%. Exposed filler particles, some quite large, are surrounded by appreciable amounts of the resin matrix (Fig. 15-8).

Table 15-2 Properties of Composite Restorative Materials

Characteristic/property	Unfilled acrylic	Traditional	Hybrid (small-particle)	Hybrid (all-purpose)	Microfilled	Flowable hybrid	Packable hybrid	Enamel	Dentin
Size (μm)	—	8-12	0.5-3	0.4-1.0	0.04-0.4	0.6-1.0	Fibrous	—	—
Inorganic filler (vol%)	0	60-70	65-77	60-65	20-59	30-55	48-67	—	—
Inorganic filler (wt%)	0	70-80	80-90	75-80	35-67	40-60	65-81	—	—
Compressive strength (MPa)	70	250-300	350-400	300-350	250-350	—	—	384	297
Tensile strength (MPa)	24	50-65	75-90	40-50	30-50	—	40-45	10	52
Elastic modulus (GPa)	2.4	8-15	15-20	11-15	3-6	4-8	3-13	84	18
Thermal expansion coefficient (ppm/° C)	92.8	25-35	19-26	30-40	50-60	—	—	—	—
Water sorption (mg/cm^2)	1.7	0.5-0.7	0.5-0.6	0.5-0.7	1.4-1.7	—	—	—	—
Knoop hardness (KHN)	15	55	50-60	50-60	25-35	—	—	350-430	68
Curing shrinkage (vol%)	8-10	—	2-3	2-3	2-3	3-5	2-3	—	—
Radiopacity (mm Al)	0.1	2-3	2-3	2-4	0.5-2	1-4	2-3	2	1

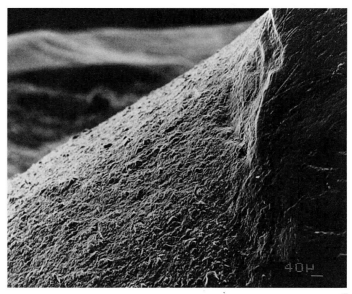

Fig. 15-8 A scanning electron micrograph of the posterior, occlusal surface of a traditional composite restoration that had been in clinical service for 5 yr. The composite has been worn away from the occlusal margins on the right, and coarse filler particles have been exposed, making the surface very rough. (Courtesy of K-J.M. Söderholm.)

Properties of Traditional Composites

Physical and mechanical properties of traditional composite resins are listed in Table 15-2. Individual products may exhibit properties that deviate from these values, but those shown are representative of the property values for the composite categories.

In comparing the properties of traditional composites with those for unfilled acrylic materials, it is obvious that significant improvements have been obtained through use of composite structures. Compared with the unfilled acrylics, the compressive strength of the six composite groups in Table 15-2 is improved by 300% to 500% because of the transfer of stress from the matrix to the filler particles. Similarly, the elastic modulus (i.e., stiffness) is four to six times greater, and the tensile strength is more than doubled. Likewise, water sorption, polymerization shrinkage, and thermal expansion are substantially reduced compared with unfilled acrylic; nevertheless, these values still exceed those of tooth structure. This difference contributes to expansion- and contraction-induced stresses at the resin-tooth interface, and these stresses must be reduced further to promote longer-term durability.

Hardness is considerably greater for composites than for unfilled acrylic resins (Knoop hardness number [KHN] of approximately 55 compared with 15 KHN, respectively). The increase is associated with both the filler reinforcement and the cross-linked resin structure. In general, these composites are more resistant to abrasion than are unfilled acrylics. However, except for the microfilled category, they suffer from roughening of the surface as a result of the selective abrasion of the softer resin matrix surrounding the harder filler particles. Composites that contain quartz or amorphous silica as fillers are radiolucent. A radiopacity approximately equal to or greater than that of enamel is needed to provide sufficient contrast to detect marginal gap formation and/or secondary caries on diagnostic radiographic film.

Clinical Considerations of Traditional Composites

A major clinical disadvantage of traditional composites is the rough surface that develops during abrasive wear of the soft resin matrix, thus exposing the more wear-resistant filler particles, which protrude from the surface, as illustrated in Figure 15-8. Finishing of the restoration produces a roughened surface, as does toothbrushing and masticatory wear over time. These restorations also tend toward discoloration, undoubtedly caused in part by the susceptibility of the rough textured surface to retain stain.

Fracture of the traditional composites is not a common problem even when they are used for stress-bearing restorations such as those in Class IV and Class II sites. However, the poor resistance of traditional composites to occlusal wear has been a clinical problem. From this standpoint, they are inferior to materials specifically designated as "posterior composites," as is discussed in a subsequent section.

Small-Particle–Filled Composites

To improve surface smoothness and retain or improve the physical and mechanical properties of traditional composites, inorganic fillers are ground to a size range of ~0.5 to 3 μm, but with a fairly broad size range distribution, as shown in Figure 15-9. This broad particle-size distribution facilitates a high filler loading, and small-particle–filled (SPF) composites generally contain more inorganic filler (80 to 90 wt% and 65 to 77 vol%) than traditional composites. This is particularly true for those composites designed for posterior restorations. The high density of filler

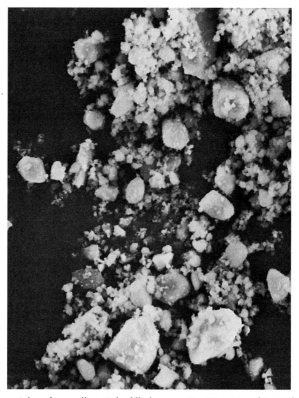

Fig. 15-9 Typical particles of a small-particle–filled composite. (Courtesy of E.A. Glasspoole and R. Erickson.)

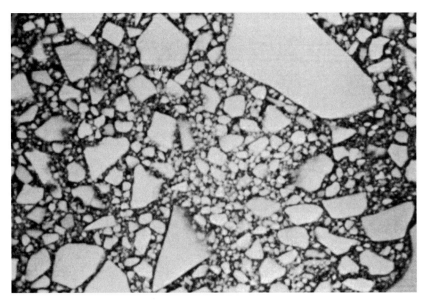

Fig. 15-10   Polished surface of a small-particle–filled composite. (Courtesy of W.H. Douglas.)

particles, compared with that of the matrix resin, is evident in the polished specimen of the small-particle–filled hybrid composite shown in Figure 15-10.

Some SPF composites use amorphous silica as filler, but most incorporate glasses that contain heavy metals for radiopacity. The matrix resin of these materials is similar to that of traditional and microfilled composite materials. The primary filler consists of silane-coated ground particles. Colloidal silica is usually added in amounts of approximately 5 wt% to adjust the viscosity of the paste for packing into a cavity.

This category of composite generally exhibits superior physical and mechanical properties. With the increased filler content, there is an improvement in virtually all of the relevant properties (see Table 15-2). Compressive strength and elastic modulus of SPF composites exceed those of both traditional and microfilled composites. The tensile strength of SPF composites is double that of the microfilled materials and 1.5 times greater than that of the traditional composites. The coefficient of thermal expansion is less than that of other composites, although it is still approximately twice that of tooth structure. The use of small and highly packed filler imparts a surface smoothness approaching that of the microfilled resins. These superior properties result in greater wear resistance and some decrease in polymerization shrinkage.

Those materials filled with heavy metal–containing glass are radiopaque. Radiopacity is an important property for materials used for restoration of posterior teeth to facilitate the diagnosis of secondary caries and other features. Unfortunately, the heavy metal glass fillers are softer and more prone to hydrolyze and leach in water than are amorphous silica and quartz. Over time they soften and become more prone to wear and deterioration, which reduces the long-term durability of the restoration.

Clinical Considerations of SPF Composites

Because of their higher filler loading and, consequently, greater strength and other physical properties, SPF composites are indicated for high-stress and abrasion-prone applications, such as in Class IV sites. The particle sizes of some SPF composites make it possible to attain reasonably smooth surfaces for anterior applications, but they cannot form as smooth a polished surface as microfilled composites.

Microfilled Composites

The problems of surface roughening and low translucency associated with traditional and small-particle composites can be overcome through the use of colloidal silica particles as the inorganic filler. The individual particles are approximately 0.04 μm (40 nm) in size. This value is one-tenth of the wavelength of visible light and 200 to 300 times smaller than the average particle in traditional composites. The concept of the microfilled composite entails the reinforcement of the resin by means of the filler; yet these composites exhibit a smooth surface, similar to that obtained with the unfilled direct-filling acrylic resins.

CRITICAL QUESTION

Why is it that although the inorganic filler loading in microfilled composites is substantially lower than in other composites, polymerization shrinkage is not higher?

These tiny colloidal silica particles tend to agglomerate. Agglomerates of colloidal silica filler can be seen in Figure 15-11. During mixing, some, but not all, of the agglomerates are broken up. Consequently, agglomerates account for the 0.04 to 0.4 μm size range in Table 15-2.

Ideally, this colloidal silica filler would be added in large amounts directly to the resin matrix. However, this is not easily done because of the large surface area that must be wetted by the monomer and especially because of the formation of polymer-like chains among the colloidal particles. These phenomena significantly increase the viscosity and produce undue thickening, even with very small additions of microfillers. Although several approaches may be used to increase the filler loading, each compromises the idealized concept of a homogeneous resin filled with dispersed colloidal silica. One approach is to sinter the colloidal silica so that particles

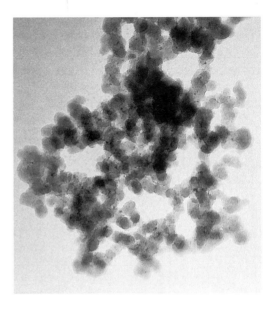

Fig. 15-11 The pyrogenic silica used in microfilled composites has a very large total surface area because of its extremely small average particle size of ~0.04 μm. These particles agglomerate and form long chains, as seen in this transmission electron micrograph. The chains of silica particles act similarly to resin polymer chains and dramatically increase the viscosity of the monomer, as described in Chapter 7. (Courtesy of K-J.M. Söderholm.)

several tenths of a micrometer in size are obtained. This larger agglomerate results in a reduced surface area, allowing more filler to be incorporated before compromising the rheology of the material. However, the most common method for increasing filler loading is to make new filler particles by grinding a prepolymerized composite that is highly loaded with colloidal silica particles. Particles of this highly microfilled material are then incorporated into the resin paste to produce a filling material with acceptable handling characteristics.

The preparation of the prepolymerized filler involves adding 60 to 70 wt% (about 50 vol%) of silane-treated colloidal silica to the monomer at a slightly elevated temperature to lower its viscosity. When the filler is thoroughly mixed into the resin, the composite paste is heat-cured using BP initiator. The DC of the resin is very high, approximately 80%. The cured composite is then ground into particles of sizes that may be larger than the quartz particles used in traditional composites. The prepolymerized particles are often called *organic fillers*, a term that is somewhat misleading because they contain a high percentage of inorganic filler. These "composite particles," along with additional silane-treated colloidal silica, are then blended with monomer to form the composite paste. A diagram representing the preparation of the filler in microfilled resins of this type is shown in Figure 15-12.

The final inorganic filler content may be only approximately 50 wt%, but if the composite particles are counted as filler particles, the filler content is closer to 80 wt% (approximately 60 vol%). This is an important consideration in understanding certain properties of these materials, such as the volumetric shrinkage during polymerization. The composite particles do not shrink when the composite is cured. Thus a microfilled composite, despite having a much lower volume fraction of inorganic filler than a traditional or small particle composite, will not shrink as much as expected based on the total resin volume. A major shortcoming of these materials is that the bond between the composite particles and the clinically cured matrix is relatively weak, facilitating wear by a chipping mechanism (Fig. 15-13). Because of this deficiency, most microfilled composites are not suitable for use as stress-bearing surfaces, with some notable exceptions.

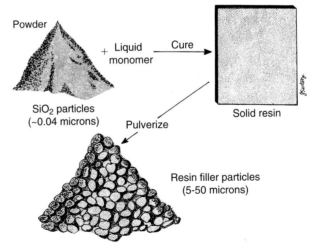

Fig. 15-12 Preparation of resin filler particles for use in microfilled composites. The filler particles in a microfilled composite consist of pulverized "composite filler particles" dispersed in a cured resin matrix. Pyrogenic colloidal silica particles (~0.04 μm) are incorporated into both the precured resin filler particles and the curable monomer, but the precured resin contains a substantially higher concentration. (Modified from P. Lambrechts: Basic Properties of Dental Composites and Their Impact on Clinical Performance. Thesis, Katholieke University, Leuven, Belgium, 1983.)

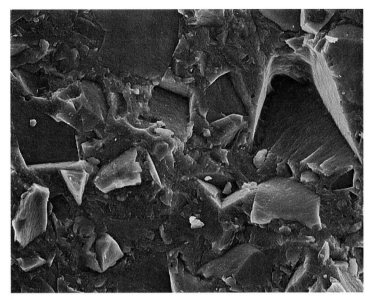

Fig. 15-13 Fractured microfilled composite. The fracture surface shows that the "organic filler" or "composite filler" particles have been pulled out, suggesting a weak bond between these particles and the surrounding matrix. (Courtesy of K-J.M. Söderholm.)

CRITICAL QUESTIONS

Which properties of microfilled resins are generally inferior to those of other composite resin materials, and what are the clinical implications of these deficiencies? What features of microfilled resins make them the material of choice for certain types of restorations? Which restorations are produced ideally from microfilled composites?

Properties of Microfilled Composites

Microfilled composites have physical and mechanical properties that are generally inferior to those of traditional composites (see Table 15-2). This is to be expected, because 40 to 80 vol% of the restorative material is made up of resin. The larger amount of resin compared with inorganic filler results in greater water sorption, a higher coefficient of thermal expansion, and decreased elastic modulus. In addition, the weak bond of the prepolymerized particles to the clinically cured resin matrix results in decreased tensile strength similar to that of composites with nonsilanized filler particles. Nevertheless, microfilled composites remain remarkably wear-resistant for several years, with rates of wear comparable with those of the highly filler-loaded composites designed for the occlusal surfaces of posterior restorations. However, in the longer term, if microfilled composites are placed in wear-prone areas, they eventually begin to break down and wear at a rate too fast for acceptable clinical performance. If placed in areas of proximal contact, anterior tooth "drifting" may occur. The wear process has been related to fracture propagation around the poorly bonded "organic" filler particles (Fig. 15-13).

Compared with unfilled acrylic resins, microfilled composites have significantly improved properties, and they provide the smoothest surface finish available among aesthetic composite restorations. Thus they are often preferred for restoring teeth with carious lesions in smooth surfaces (Classes III and V). The inorganic filler particles are smaller than the abrasive particles used for finishing the restoration. Thus the silica filler is removed along with the resin in which it is embedded, leaving a very smooth, polished surface that is retained for the life of the restoration.

Clinical Considerations of Microfilled Composites

For most applications, the decreased physical properties do not create problems. However, in stress-bearing situations, such as Class II and Class IV sites, the potential for fracture is greater. The occasional chipping that has been observed at the margins of restorations has been attributed to debonding of the prepolymerized composite filler. Diamond burs, rather than fluted tungsten-carbide burs, are recommended for trimming microfilled composites to minimize the risk for chipping. Nonetheless, microfilled composites are widely used today. Because of their smooth surface, they have become the resin of choice for aesthetic restoration of anterior teeth, particularly in non-stress–bearing situations and for restoring subgingival areas.

CRITICAL QUESTIONS

What advantages are conferred by combining filler particles of two or more size ranges? What are the clinical consequences of this filler combination?

Hybrid Composites

This category of composite materials was developed in an effort to obtain even better surface smoothness than that provided by the small-particle composites, while still maintaining the desirable properties of the latter. The hybrid composites are viewed by some as having surface smoothness and aesthetic characteristics that are competitive with these properties for microfilled composites used in anterior restorative applications.

As the name implies, hybrid composites contain two kinds of filler particles. Most modern hybrid fillers consist of colloidal silica and ground particles of glasses containing heavy metals, constituting a filler content of approximately 75 to 80 wt% (see Table 15-1). The glasses have an average particle size of about 0.4 to 1.0 μm, with a trend to steadily reduce this size range as improvements are made. In a typical size distribution, 75% of the ground particles are smaller than 1.0 μm. Colloidal silica represents 10 to 20 wt% of the total filler content. In this case, the microfillers also contribute significantly to the properties. The smaller filler particle size, as well as the greater amount of microfillers, increase the surface area. Thus the overall filler loading is not as high as it is for some of the SPF composites. A polished surface is shown in Figure 15-14. The smaller filler particle size is evident compared with that for the traditional and SPF composites.

Physical and mechanical properties for these systems generally range between those of the traditional and SPF composites. However, as can be seen in Table 15-2, these properties are generally superior to those of the microfilled composites. Because the filler particles contain heavy metal atoms, they have a radiopacity sufficient for radiographic detection of secondary caries and various other diagnostic tasks.

Clinical Considerations of Hybrid Composites

Because of their surface smoothness and reasonably good strength, these composites are widely used for anterior restorations, including Class IV sites (Figures 15-15 and 15-16). Although the mechanical properties of hybrid composites generally are somewhat inferior to those of SPF composites, the hybrid composites are widely employed for stress-bearing, posterior restorations. Because there are few practical differences between hybrid and SPF composites, these two terms are often used interchangeably to describe the two materials. From a clinical standpoint, this confusion in terminology is not significant.

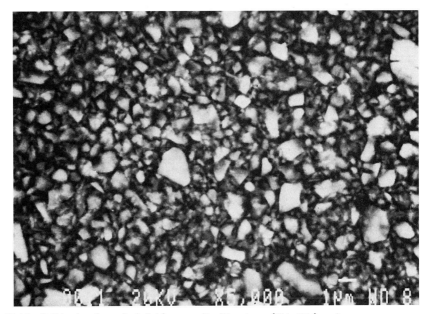

Fig. 15-14 Polished surface of a hybrid composite. (Courtesy of R.L. Erickson.)

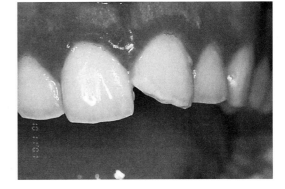

Fig. 15-15 Hybrid composites have sufficient strength to restore fractured incisal edges. See also color plate. (Courtesy of Dr. William Rose.)

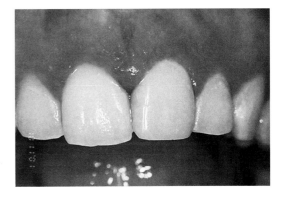

Fig. 15-16 Class IV restoration made with a hybrid composite. See also color plate. (Courtesy of Dr. William Rose.)

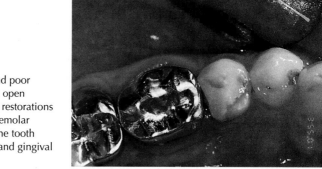

Fig. 15-17 Difficult access and poor manipulation usually results in open contacts for Class II composite restorations (proximal surface of second premolar tooth). This deficiency makes the tooth susceptible to food impaction and gingival trauma. See also color plate.

Flowable Composites

A modification of the SPF and hybrid composites results in the so-called **flowable composites.** These resins have a reduced filler level so as to provide a consistency that enables the material to flow readily, spread uniformly, and intimately adapt to a cavity form to produce a desired dental anatomy. The reduced filler makes them more susceptible to wear, but improves the clinician's ability to form a well-adapted cavity base or liner, especially in Class II posterior preparations and other situations in which access is difficult. Because of their greater ease of adaptation and greater flexibility as a cured material, flowable composites are useful in Class I restorations in gingival areas. Shown in Figure 15-17 is a poorly made Class II composite indicated by poor anatomical form in the proximal area of the second premolar tooth. Note also the missing restoration in the first premolar tooth.

Another application is in minimal Class I restorations to prevent caries, when used in a manner similar to the use of fissure sealants. Flowable composites are also indicated for applications in which there is poor accessibility and little or no exposure to wear and for applications in which excellent adaptation is needed. The properties and clinical uses of flowable composite materials are similar to those of the so-called compomers, which are hybrids between resin composites and glass ionomer materials (see Chapter 16).

CRITICAL QUESTION

Compared with amalgam, what disadvantages are associated with the use of resin composites as aesthetic posterior resins?

COMPOSITES FOR POSTERIOR RESTORATIONS
Direct Posterior Composites

Amalgam has long been the direct filling material of choice for restoration of posterior teeth. Its attributes are ease of placement, good mechanical properties, excellent wear resistance, and the unique characteristic of being "self-sealing" (i.e., reducing leakage within marginal gaps as the restoration ages). However, the increasing demand for aesthetic dentistry and the concern of some individuals regarding the potential toxicity of mercury has resulted in an increased interest and frequency in use of composites for Class I and Class II (Figs. 15-18, 15-19, 15-20) restorations.

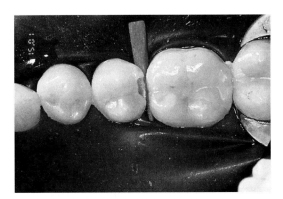

Fig. 15-18 Composite allows conservative tooth preparation in the posterior area of a second premolar tooth. See also color plate.

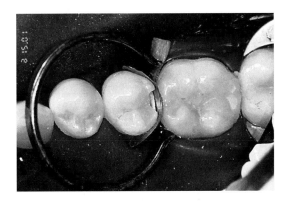

Fig. 15-19 Use of a segmental matrix band is best for restoring proximal contacts with composite. See also color plate.

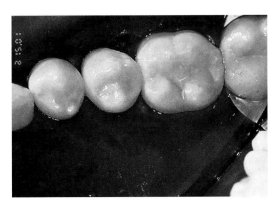

Fig. 15-20 Class II composite restoration (DO in second premolar tooth). See also color plate.

CRITICAL QUESTION

What are the main advantages and drawbacks of fibrous and/or textured filler particles that tend to interlock and resist flow?

Packable Composites

Except for the flowable composites, materials in each of the composite categories in Tables 15-1 and 15-2 have been used for posterior restorations. Compared with amalgam, the technique of composite placement is far more time-consuming and demanding. Because of the highly plastic, pastelike consistency in the precured state, composites cannot be packed vertically into a cavity in such a way that the material flows laterally as well as vertically to ensure intimate contact with the cavity walls. In particular, in the restoration of a tooth in which a proximal contact with the adjacent tooth is required, the paste consistency of most composites dictates that a matrix band be carefully contoured and wedged to obtain an acceptable proximal contact. These are tedious, time-consuming procedures and can produce variable results without a high level of skill. (A textbook on operative dentistry should be consulted for detailed information on this subject.) Such composites are somewhat analogous in their handling characteristics to amalgams made from spherical particles. A solution to this problem is offered by resin composites with filler characteristics that increase the strength and stiffness of the uncured material and that provide a consistency similar to that of lathe-cut amalgams.

The so-called packable and **condensable composites** form two special categories of hybrid composites. These materials were introduced in the late 1990s to provide resin composites that enable clinicians to apply techniques similar to those used for amalgam restorations. The packable/condensable characteristics derive from inclusion of elongated, fibrous, filler particles of about 100 μm in length, and/or textured surfaces that tend to interlock and resist flow. This causes the uncured resin to be stiff and resistant to slumping, yet moldable under the force of amalgam-condensing instruments ("pluggers"). Rough surfaces and blends of fibrous and particulate fillers produce a packable consistency and enable other properties to be optimized for clinical performance. Although this is a useful approach, many of the limitations of resin composites prevail, and approximately twice the time required for amalgam placement is still required. At the present time these materials have not demonstrated any advantageous properties or characteristics over the hybrid resins, other than being somewhat similar to amalgam in their placement technique. Despite manufacturers' claims to the contrary, packable composites have not yet proven to be an answer to the general need for highly wear-resistant, easily placeable posterior resins with low curing shrinkage and a depth of cure greater than 2 mm. A classification of composites by use is given in Table 15-1.

Marginal Leakage

When the gingival margins of the cavity preparation are located in dentin, cementum, or both, and the resin is firmly anchored to the etched enamel at the other margins, the material tends to pull away from the gingival margins during curing because of polymerization shrinkage. This leads to formation of a gap at that interface. Subsequently, the risk for marginal leakage and its ensuing problems of marginal staining and secondary caries, is enhanced. Undoubtedly, this is one of the greatest problems of composites used for Class II and Class V restorations. Every measure must be taken to maintain the integrity of the dentin-resin or cementum-resin interfaces. The role of dentin-bonding agents in this regard is discussed in Chapter 14.

Radiopacity

Resins are inherently radiolucent. However, leaking margins, secondary caries, poor proximal contacts, wear of proximal surfaces, and other problems cannot be detected unless adequate radiographic contrast can be achieved. Thus radiopacity is an especially important property for any posterior restorative material. Radiopacity is imparted by certain glass filler particles containing heavy metal atoms. Although not all composite resins are radiopaque, most demonstrate sufficient radiopacity so this seldom poses a problem. It is interesting to note that some of the flowable composites are still radiolucent and the common practice of using them for access to proximal boxes necessitates caution. For optimum diagnostic contrast, the restoration should have a radiopacity approximately equal to that of enamel, which is about twice that of dentin. A wide range of radiopacity values have been considered to be adequate, but exceeding the radiopacity of enamel by a large degree will have the effect of obscuring radiolucent areas caused by gap formation or secondary caries.

Wear

In addition to polymerization shrinkage, another frequent clinical problem has been occlusal wear (see Fig. 15-21). The mechanism of occlusal wear is a complex problem that has been the subject of much research. Unfortunately, before clinical usage, abrasion and wear resistance can be measured only by a laboratory test that simulates simplified environmental conditions. As yet, no test method has been agreed upon as a valid predictor of clinical performance. Although several laboratory test methods are useful to guide research and development efforts, controlled clinical evaluations are the only reliable means of evaluating the durability and useful lifetime of restorative materials. However, based on such studies, the best composites designed for posterior restorations still wear more than natural enamel under identical conditions. Although wear rate differences of 10 to 20 μm/yr may seem small, posterior composites still wear 0.1 to 0.2 mm more than the enamel over 10 yr. Because of these wear rates and the potential implications of wear on occlusion, it is still important to select with caution the clinical cases to be treated with posterior composites.

Germane to this critical property of posterior composites is the nature of wear mechanics. Two principal mechanisms of composite wear have been proposed. One mode, two-body wear, is based on direct contact of the restoration with an opposing cusp or with adjacent proximal surfaces so that high stresses develop in the small

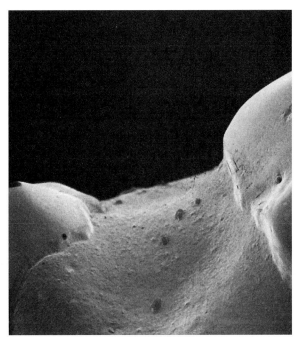

Fig. 15-21 Scanning electron micrograph of a 9-yr-old small-particle–filled composite, illustrating generalized, three-body wear. (Courtesy of R.L. Erickson.)

area of contact. The wear process in this region are related to the higher force levels exerted by the opposing cusp or forces transferred to proximal surfaces.

Loss of material in noncontacting areas is most probably caused by contact with a food bolus as it is forced across the occlusal surface. This type of three-body wear is probably controlled in a complex way by a number of composite properties, such as toughness, porosity, stability of the silane coupling agent, degree of monomer conversion, filler loading, and the size and type of filler particles. Variations among patients, such as differences in chewing habits, force levels, and variations in oral environments also play a significant role in the wear process. A typical wear pattern for a composite is shown in Figure 15-15 for a 9-yr-old, chemically activated, SPF composite restoration. Although the loss of material shown in this figure is more severe than for current restorative materials, it illustrates the wear phenomenon. Notice the smoother anatomical contours and the exposed cavity walls where the composite has been worn away by abrasion.

Clinically, the loss of material caused by direct wear in areas of tooth-to-tooth contact appears to be greater than that associated with abrasion by food in non-contacting areas. Composites in which the filler particles are small, high in concentration, and well bonded to the matrix are the most resistant to wear. Large restorations tend to wear more than do smaller ones, as do restorations in molars compared with those in premolars. The major indications for composites for Class II restorations place emphasis on the demand for aesthetics. A conservative preparation is preferred so that the tooth, rather than the composite, absorbs more of the stress. The dentist must also be familiar with the rigorous placement procedures that are essential to success, as described in textbooks on operative dentistry.

However, there are obvious contraindications. A composite Class II restoration is doomed to failure in the mouth of a patient who bruxes because of the greater potential for wear. Use of posterior composites in a caries-active mouth is questionable, because the current materials have no capability to provide an anticariogenic effect or to resist leakage. If composites are used for such situations, the application of a hydrophilic sealing resin along the margins may be beneficial. Nonetheless, with the greater demands on aesthetics and the improved composite formulations, the use of these materials in stress-bearing situations will continue to increase. In response, academic and industry research can be expected to continue to improve the clinical durability of composite materials.

Selection Criteria

Not all patients should be considered as candidates for these posterior restorations. The primary indication for using direct posterior composites in place of amalgam is aesthetics. Unless the patient's aesthetic demands are high, there are minimal advantages to using resin restorations in posterior regions. Often, the disadvantages coupled with the difficulty in manipulation far outweigh the benefits. Other indications might include the need for conservative preparations along with conservation of tooth structure. Because composite restorations do not depend on mechanical undercuts for retention, the concepts of resistance form and retention form do not really apply to resin preparations. However, because of their inferior physical properties, composites should not be used for cuspal coverage or for large restorations exceeding one-third the buccolingual width of the tooth. If possible, occlusal load should always be borne by sound tooth structure and never by resin. Because wear is also an issue, posterior composites should not be placed in patients experiencing parafunctional habits. Another lesser indication is the use of composites to minimize thermal conduction. Because amalgam is metallic, it tends to conduct heat more rapidly, leading to tooth sensitivity and pain. Placement of composites, which are good thermal insulators, often reduces this occurrence.

Indirect Posterior Composites

The problem of wear in posterior resin applications has been considerably reduced by ongoing advances in composite technology, but difficulties still exist in high-stress situations, which are related to inherent problems with both mechanical and chemical degradation of composites. However, polymerization shrinkage, technique sensitivity, and difficulty in obtaining a predictable, reliable bond to dentin or cementum margins are probably more important. These deficiencies raise a major concern regarding the potential leakage associated with Class II restorations.

Indirect composites for fabrication of onlays are polymerized outside the oral environment and luted to the tooth with a compatible resin cement. Indirect composite inlays or onlays reduce wear and leakage and overcome some of the limitations of resin composites. Several different approaches to resin inlay construction have been proposed. These include (1) the use of both direct and indirect fabrication methods; (2) the application of light, heat, pressure, or a combination of these curing systems; and (3) the combined use of hybrid and microfilled composites.

The fabrication process for direct composite inlays first requires the application of a separating medium (agar solution or glycerin) to the prepared tooth. The restorative resin pattern is then formed, light-cured, and removed from the preparation. The rough inlay is then exposed to additional light for approximately 4 to 6 min or heat-activated at approximately 100° C for 7 min, after which the preparation is etched, the inlay is cemented into place with a dual-cure resin, and it is then polished.

Composite systems are also available as indirect products. Indirect inlay resins require an impression and a dental laboratory technician to fabricate the inlay. In addition to conventional light and heat curing, laboratory processing may employ heat (140° C) and pressure (0.6 MPa for 10 min). The potential advantage of these materials is that a somewhat higher degree of polymerization is attained, which improves physical properties and resistance to wear. The polymerization shrinkage does not occur in the prepared teeth, so induced stresses and bond failures are reduced, which reduces the potential for leakage. Furthermore, these resins are repairable in the mouth and they are not as abrasive to opposing tooth structure as ceramic inlays.

Although laboratory studies support some of these expectations, long-term clinical studies are needed to verify the longevity of these restorations in the oral environment. In addition, the technique sensitivity of these systems remains high, and their appropriateness as a substitute for amalgam or cast restorations in all posterior applications needs additional investigation, even though the aesthetics are appealing.

USE OF COMPOSITES FOR RESIN VENEERS

Originally, resin-veneering materials were heat-polymerized poly(methyl methacrylate), which were improved subsequently by the addition of fillers and cross-linking agents. Microfilled materials, which use bis-GMA, UDMA, or 4,8-di(methacryloxy methylene)-tricyclodecane as resin matrices, have created renewed interest in resin-veneered metal restorations. These resins are polymerized by using visible light in the violet-blue range or by a combination of heat and pressure. In general, the new microfilled resins have physical properties superior to those of the original unfilled resin.

The first resin veneers were mechanically bonded to metal substrates using wire loops or retention beads. Recent improvements in bonding mechanisms have included micromechanical retention created by acid etching the base metal alloy and the use of chemical bonding systems such as 4-META, phosphorylated methacrylate, epoxy resin, or silicon dioxide that is flame-sprayed to the metal surface followed by the application of a silane coupling agent (Silicoating™).

Prosthetic resin-veneering materials have several advantages and disadvantages compared with ceramics. The advantages include ease of fabrication, predictable intraoral repairability, and less wear of opposing teeth or restorations. The drawbacks include low proportional limit and pronounced plastic deformation that contributes to distortion on occlusal loading. Therefore the resin should be protected with metal occlusal surfaces whenever feasible. Leakage of oral fluids and staining below the veneers, particularly those attached mechanically, are caused by dimensional changes from water sorption, heating, and cooling. Surface staining and intrinsic discoloration tend to occur with these resins.

Resins are also susceptible to wear during tooth brushing. Thus it is necessary to instruct the patient on proper cleaning procedures using a soft toothbrush and mild abrasive toothpastes. Resin-veneered metal restorations are not suitable for use as removable partial denture abutment retainers where the clasp arm engages an undercut on the veneered surface because the resin is not as wear-resistant as porcelain.

Resin composites can also be used as a conservative alternative to conventional prosthodontic restorations, such as veneers for masking tooth discoloration or malformation. The resins are used as preformed laminate veneers, in which resin shells are adjusted by grinding and the contoured facing is bonded to tooth structure using the acid-etching technique with either chemically activated, visible light-activated, or dual-cure luting resin cements. Resins used to cement indirect restorations, veneers, and prosthetic devices are similar to flowable restorative resins, but are adjusted to match the needs of luting applications. This type of resin material is discussed further in Chapter 16.

FINISHING OF COMPOSITES

Optimum finishing and polishing of composite resins is a very important step in the completion of the restoration. Residual surface roughness can encourage bacterial growth, which can lead to a myriad of problems including secondary caries, gingival inflammation, and surface staining. Several methods for the finishing and polishing of composite resins have been advocated. The best possible finish is produced by not polishing the surface at all, at least for surfaces that have polymerized next to a matrix strip. The smoothest surface on a restoration can be obtained by curing the composite against a smooth matrix strip. This minimizes porosities as well as the **oxygen-inhibited layer.** However, it is often difficult to achieve proper contours and margin adaptation without some amount of finishing because the plastic strip is often difficult to adapt to the different convex and concave surfaces of the tooth. As such, different finishing and polishing systems are being marketed to achieve the best possible surface.

Research has been conducted to examine the effect of three significant factors on the finish and polish of a composite restoration: (1) environment, (2) delayed versus immediate finish, and (3) the type of material. The term *finishing* usually refers to the process of adapting the restorative material to the tooth (e.g., removing overhangs and shaping occlusal surfaces), whereas *polishing* refers to removing surface irregularities to achieve the smoothest possible surface.

The first factor, environment, refers to whether the process of finishing and polishing should be performed in a wet or dry field in the mouth. Some advocates say that finishing in a dry field with the finishing equipment mounted on a slow-speed handpiece allows for better visualization of the restoration margins. However, studies have shown that a dry polishing technique results in an increase in marginal leakage, possibly because of heat production that disturbs the marginal sealing ability of the adhesive resins. Other studies have shown that structural and chemical changes occur on the surface of restorations as a result of a dry environment. However, other research has confirmed that the dry polish technique has no effect on the hardness or surface structure. As with many dental procedures, grinding and finishing procedures are best accomplished in moderation. The clinician should finish the restoration in an environment in which the margins are clearly discernible and where minimal heat is generated. Excessive heat results in smearing of the surface and depolymerization. Water cooling during grinding and finishing should ensure standard surface quality.

The elapsed time between curing of the composite and finishing and polishing may also have an effect on the type of surface characteristics and resistance to leakage. Some advocate delaying the finishing of composite restorations for up to 24 hr because polymerization is incomplete at placement, although composite manufacturers recommend that finishing be accomplished shortly after placement. Studies have shown that delayed finishing can actually increase marginal leakage and has no effect on surface characteristics compared with immediate finishing. Also, delayed finishing has a minimal effect on hardness. Thus for all practical purposes, almost all composite restorations should be finished and polished shortly after placement, during the same appointment, although the finishing should be delayed for approximately 15 min after curing.

Several systems can be used to finish and polish composite restorations. Use of a scalpel blade or any thin, sharp-edged instrument to remove flash on the proximal areas is recommended. However, this is a very risky procedure, especially if the trimming procedure involves shearing in a direction away from the gingival margin. This can lead to localized debonding and leakage. Trimming forces should be applied either parallel to the margin or toward the gingival tissue. Coarse to ultrafine aluminum oxide discs can be applied to areas with difficult access around the proximal surfaces or in embrasures (see Chapter 13). Tungsten carbide burs or fine diamond tips can be used to adjust occlusal surfaces and blend the composite to the surfaces of the teeth. Several studies in the literature have rated many of these systems as to their effect on surface smoothness and microleakage. Currently, aluminum oxide discs produce the best surface and induce minimal trauma. Other systems include resin-finishing devices with use of fine and extra fine polishing pastes, silicone-based systems, and silicon carbide–impregnated polishing brushes and points. Although high stresses may be associated with surface grinding and polishing, a recent study has shown that microleakage is not significantly affected by the type of polishing system used. Perhaps the most important step in finishing and polishing is the application of a bonding agent or a surface sealer. It has been widely documented that the finishing (and possibly polishing) process is detrimental to composite surfaces, in that it introduces microcracks and removes the most highly polymerized area of the restoration. Application of a surface sealer or a low-viscosity resin with little or no filler ensures that surface porosities are filled and microcracks are sealed. Studies have shown that this "rebonding" technique significantly decreases microleakage by improving the marginal seal of restorations.

Additional information on the finishing and polishing of restorative materials is presented in Chapter 13.

BIOCOMPATIBILITY OF COMPOSITES

Concerns about the biocompatibility of restorative materials usually relate to the effects on the pulp from two aspects: (1) the inherent chemical toxicity of the material and (2) the marginal leakage of oral fluids.

The chemical insult to the pulp from composites is possible if components leach out or diffuse from the material and subsequently reach the pulp. Adequately polymerized composites are relatively biocompatible because they exhibit minimal solubility, and unreacted species are leached in very small quantities. From a toxicological point of view, these amounts should be too small to cause toxic reactions. However, from an immunological point of view, under extremely rare conditions, some patients and dental personnel can develop an allergic response to these materials.

Inadequately cured composite materials at the floor of a cavity can serve as a reservoir of diffusible components that can induce long-term pulp inflammation. This situation is of particular concern for light-activated materials. If a clinician attempts to polymerize too thick a layer of resin or if the exposure time to the light is inadequate (as discussed previously), the uncured or poorly cured material can release leachable constituents adjacent to the pulp.

The second biological concern is associated with shrinkage of the composite during polymerization and the subsequent marginal leakage. The marginal leakage might allow bacterial ingrowth, and these microorganisms may cause secondary caries or pulp reactions. Therefore the restorative procedure must be designed to minimize polymerization shrinkage and marginal leakage, as described earlier in this chapter. A comprehensive review of biocompatibility is presented in Chapter 8.

Bisphenol A (BPA), a precursor of bis-GMA has been shown to be a xenoestrogen, or a synthetic compound found in the environment that mimics the effects of estrogen by having an affinity for estrogen receptors. BPA and other endocrine-disrupting chemicals (EDCs) have been shown to cause reproductive anomalies, especially in the developmental stages of fetal wildlife. Although the effects on humans are still unclear, testicular cancer, decreased sperm count, and hypospadias (displacement of the urethral meatus) have been seen as the result of exposure to EDCs.

BPA has recently also been shown to exhibit antiandrogenic activities, which may prove to be detrimental in organ development. Studies have shown that the **estrogenicity** of resin compounds are mainly associated with BPA and BPA dimethacrylate (BPA-DM), which are monomers found in the base paste of some dental sealants. In vitro reports have confirmed that BPA and BPA-DM applied to cancer cells significantly increase cell proliferation and DNA synthesis, similar to the effect of estrogen. In vivo studies with mammals have revealed numerous effects such as delayed and sustained hyperprolactinemia changes in estrogen receptors in the hypothalamus and pituitary glands.

Controversy surrounds this issue because it is unclear how much BPA or BPA-DM is released to the oral cavity and what dosage is enough to affect human health. A clinical study (Olea et al, 1996) revealed that BPA was collected in saliva after 1 hr of sealant placement, leading the authors to conclude that sealant application led to xenoestrogen exposure in children. This led to a deluge of follow-up examinations to determine the validity of the results. More recent studies have shown that BPA-DM should be restricted for use in resin-based composites because of its very potent estrogenic effect and because of high levels found in the body; however, the effect of BPA is negligible. Further research should be conducted in vivo to show the chemical activity of these compounds and their effects on human development.

Additional information on the biocompatibility of restorative materials is presented in Chapter 8.

REPAIR OF COMPOSITES

Composites may be repaired by placing new material over the old composite. This is a useful procedure for correcting defects or altering contours on existing restorations. The procedures for adding new material differ, depending on whether the restoration is freshly polymerized or whether it is an older restoration.

When a restoration has just been placed and polymerized, it may still have an oxygen-inhibited layer of resin on the surface. Additions of new composite can be made directly to this layer because this represents, in essence, an excellent bonding substrate. Even after the restoration has been polished, a defect can still be repaired by adding more material. A restoration that has just been cured and polished may still have more than 50% of unreacted methacrylate groups to copolymerize with the newly added material.

As the restoration ages, fewer and fewer unreacted methacrylate groups remain, and greater cross-linking reduces the ability of fresh monomer to penetrate into the matrix. The strength of the bond between the original material and the new resin decreases in direct proportion to the time that has elapsed between polymerization and addition of the new resin. In addition, polished surfaces expose filler surfaces that are free from silane. Thus the filler surface area does not chemically bond to the new composite layer. Under the most ideal condition, that is, the addition of a silanate bonding agent to the surface before the addition of new composite, the strength of repaired composite is less than half the strength of the original material (Fig. 15-22).

SURVIVAL PROBABILITY OF COMPOSITES

The clinical performance of dental restorations is best judged on the basis of long-term clinical trials, preferably those based on randomized, controlled experimental designs. Very few studies of this type exist in the dental literature. However, a recent evidence-based review of the longevity of amalgam and composite restorations was based on a critical review of clinical data over 10 yr (Chadwick et al, 2001). The survival probability for restorations in permanent teeth is shown in Figure 15-23. Note that the most consistent survival levels are exhibited by amalgam restorations. The variability among studies is much larger for the composite restorations compared with amalgam restorations. The comparative survival probabilities for amalgam versus composite restorations in permanent teeth at 3, 4, 5, and 7 yr are summarized in Table 15-3. Similar comparative data for restorations in primary teeth after 3 yr and 4 yr are also listed in this table. The survival rate overall for composites in permanent teeth after 7 yr was 67.4% compared with 94.5% for amalgam

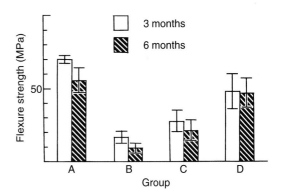

Fig. 15-22 The influence of the method of composite repair on strength. Flexural strength after storage in distilled water at 37° C for 3 and 6 months. **A,** Original, unbroken samples serving as a control. **B,** Repair without first acid-etching. **C,** Repair after acid-etching and the application of an unfilled resin. **D,** Repair after toluene/silane treatment to soften the broken surfaces and make them more receptive to new monomer. (From K-JM Söderholm: Scand J Dent Res 94:364-369, 1986.)

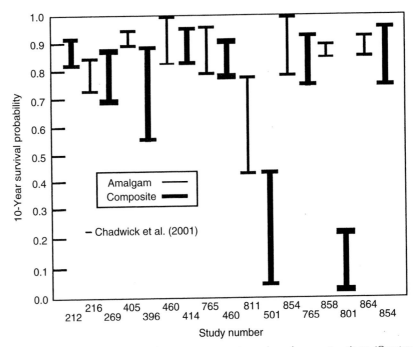

Fig. 15-23   10-yr survival probability of posterior composite and amalgam restorations. (Courtesy of K.J. Anusavice.)

restorations. More than 90% of amalgam restorations in permanent teeth survived longer than 9 yr. In comparison, only 64% of glass ionomer restorations survived after 5 yr. Only 41% of Class V composites placed with dentin bonding agents survived longer than 5 yr. Chadwick et al (2001) concluded that the Class II glass ionomer/composite restorations should be avoided because of a high percentage of failures at the gingival margin of the proximal box.

Table 15-3   **Comparison of Survival Probabilities (%) for Various Types of Restorations After 3, 4, 5, and 7 Yr**

Restoration type	3 Yr		4 Yr		5 Yr		7 Yr	
	Primary teeth	Permanent teeth	Primary teeth	Permanent teeth	Primary teeth	Permanent teeth	Primary teeth	Permanent teeth
Amalgam	95.3	97.2	95.1	96.6	90.8	95.4	—	94.5
Composite	82.4	90.0	67.2	85.6	—	78.2	—	67.4
Glass Ionomer	51.5	73.8	51.5	73.8	31.2	64.9	—	—
DBA and Composite	—	83.7	—	47.7	—	41.5	—	—
Ceramic or Composite Inlay	—	93.3	—	90.1	—	85.3	—	—

(Modified from Chadwick et al, 2001.)
DBA, Dentin bonding agent.

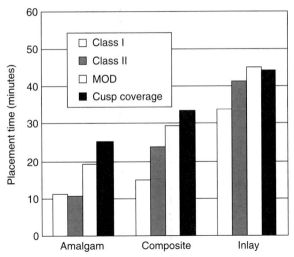

Fig. 15-24 Placement time for posterior amalgam, composite, and ceramic and composite inlay restorations. (Courtesy of K.J. Anusavice.)

Table 15-4 Comparison of Average Time (Min) Required for Initial (I) and Replacement (R) Restorations

Restoration type	Amalgam		Composite		Composite and ceramic inlay	
	I	R	I	R	I	R
Class I	11	11	15	16	34	34
Class II	15	13	24	24	41	40
MOD	19	19	29	31	45	45
CRWP	25	26	33	34	44	44

(Adapted from Chadwick et al, 2001.)
I, Initial restoration; *R*, replacement restoration; *MOD*, mesio-occluso-distal restoration; *CRWP*, cusp replacement with pin(s).

Although the performance of posterior composites has greatly improved during the past decade relative to amalgams, the placement time is significantly higher for composites, as shown in Figure 15-24. The placement time of ceramic and composite inlays is significantly higher than for either amalgam or composite restorations. Obviously, the cost of the restorations for the patient is also proportionately higher for the inlay prostheses. In fact the relative cost per tooth per yr over a 5-yr period for amalgam, composite, and ceramic or composite inlay restorations is 1×, 1.62×, and 6.35×, respectively. The relative cost per tooth per yr of amalgam restorations is significantly less than that of composite after 10 yr (1× versus 3.36×, respectively). A comparative analysis of the placement times is summarized in Table 15-4 for Class I, Class II (2-surface), Class II (3-surface, mesial-occlusal-distal), and pin-retained cusp replacement restorations.

In summary, it is clear that the clinical use of amalgam has continued in many countries because of its ease of use, relatively low cost, wear resistance, freedom from excessive shrinkage during setting, and its high survival probabilities. In spite of the controversies surrounding its use, amalgam continues to exhibit superior clinical characteristics compared with several of the currently available tooth-colored restorative materials.

SELECTED READINGS

Academy of Dental Materials: International Congress on Dental Materials, Transactions. Houston, TX, Academy of Dental Materials, Baylor College of Dentistry, 1990.

A host of review papers are presented on many aspects of dental composite chemistry, systems usage, dentin bonding agents, and microleakage.

Albers H: Tooth-Colored Restoratives: Principles and Techniques, 9th ed. Hamilton, Ontario, Canada, BC Decker Inc, 2002.

The author discusses a complete array of composite systems, with emphasis on clinical applications. The book combines the science of dental polymers with discussions of clinical applications.

Baum L, Phillips RW, and Lund MR: Textbook of Operative Dentistry, 3rd ed. Philadelphia, WB Saunders Co, 1995.

The technical procedures in the placement of composite resins in various types of restorations are discussed and illustrated.

Bowen RL: Dental filling material comprising vinyl-silane treated fused silica and a binder consisting of the reaction product of bisphenol A and glycidyl methacrylate. US Patent 3,006,112, 1962, Washington, DC, US Patent and Trademark Office.

This patent is a milestone in dentistry. It resulted in superior resin-based materials and was issued a few years after Buonocore's discovery that resins could be bonded to acid etched enamel. With Bowen's and Buonocore's inventions, it became possible to restore Class IV restorations in a conservative and predictable way, something that had been impossible previously.

Burgess JO, Walker RS, Porche CJ, and Rappold AJ: Light curing—An update. Compendium 23(10):889-908, 2002.

This article provides an excellent overview of the performance and limitations of four types of curing lights for resin-based composites: LED, QTH, PAC, and laser curing.

Chadwick BL, Dummer PMH, Dunstan F, Gilmour ASM, Jones RJ, Phillips CJ, Rees J, Richmond S, Stevens J, and Treasure ET: The Longevity of Dental Restorations: A Systematic Review. National Health Service Centre for Reviews and Dissemination, University of York, 2001.

A comprehensive evidence-based review of dental restorations.

Gallegos Ll, and Nicholls JI: In vitro two-body wear of three veneering resins. J Prosthet Dent 60:172, 1988.

Three veneering resins were tested for wear. A significant difference in wear against porcelain was found among the three resins, but no difference in wear was found against enamel.

Joniot SB, Gregoire GL, Auther AM, and Roques YM: Three dimensional optical profilometry analysis of surface states obtained after finishing sequences for three composite resins. Oper Dent 2000; 25:311-315.

Khurana S, Rammal S, and Ben-Jonathan N: Exposure of newborn male and female rats to environmental estrogens: Delayed and sustained hyperprolactinemia and alterations in estrogen receptor expression. Endocrinology 141:4512-4517, 2000.

Lambrechts P, Braem M, and Vanherle G: Evaluation of clinical performance for posterior composite resins and dentin adhesives. J Oper Dent 12:53, 1987.

These authors have been leaders in the clinical evaluation of resin systems. This paper is a superb treatment of the subject and emphasizes the limitations of current adhesives and composites.

Lopes GC, Franke M, and Maia HP: Effect of finishing time and techniques on marginal sealing ability of two composite restorative materials. J Prosthet Dent 88:32-36, 2000.

Lutz F, and Phillips RW: A classification and evaluation of composite resin systems. J Prosthet Dent 50:480, 1983.

This article presents a structure-based classification scheme for composites, one that has been almost universally accepted since its publication. A knowledge of the structure makes it possible to make decisions as to the inherent properties and selection for specific situations. (See also Willems et al [1992], below).

Manhart, J, Chen, HV, and Hickel, R: The suitability of packable resin-based composites for posterior restorations. J Am Dent Assoc 132(5):639-645, 2001.

Manhart J, Kunzelmann K-H, Chen HY, and Hickel R: Mechanical properties of new composite restorative materials. J Biomed Mater Res (A) 53: 353-361, 2000.

An evaluation of the new class of hybrid composites known as "packable" or "condensable." These authors demonstrate that although the handling character of these materials is analogous to that of lathe-cut amalgams, they do not offer any other advantage compared with other hybrid composites as restorative resins.

Naciff JM, Jump ML, Torontalli SM, Carr GJ, Tiesman JP, Overmann GJ, and Daston GP: Gene expression profile induced by 17 alpha-ethynyl estradiol, bisphenol A and genistein in the developing female reproductive system of the rat. Toxicol Sci 68: 184-199, 2002.

Olea N, Pulgar R, Perez P, Olea-Serrano F, Rivas A, Novillo-Fertrell A, Pedraza V, Soto AM, and Sonnenschein C: Estrogenicity of resin-based composites and sealants used in dentistry. Environ Health Perspect 104: 298-305, 1996.

Paris F, Balaguer P, Terouanne B, Servant N, Lacoste C, Cravedi JP, Nicolas JC, and Sultan C: Phenylphenols, biphenols, bisphenol-A and 4-tert-octylphenol exhibit α and β estrogen activities and antiandrogen activity in reporter cell lines. Mol Cell Endocrinol 193: 43-49, 2002.

Ramos RP, Chinelatti MA, Chimello DT, and Dibb RG: Assessing microleakage in resin composite restorations rebounded with a surface sealant and three low-viscosity resin systems. Quintessence Int 33: 450-456, 2002.

Roeder LB, Tate WH, and Powers JM: Effect of finishing and polishing procedures on the surface roughness of packable composites. Oper Dent 25: 534-543, 2000.

Roulet JF: Degradation of Dental Polymers, Basel and New York, Karger AG, 1987.

A thorough discussion is presented of the chemistry and composition of modern dental restorative resins. Emphasis is placed on how composition and clinical usage influences the longevity of a restorative material in vivo.

Roulet JF: The problems associated with substituting composite resins for amalgam: A status report on posterior composites. J Dent 16:101, 1988.

A comprehensive review is presented of the factors to be considered in the use of posterior composites as an alternative to dental amalgam. Author concludes that the indications for posterior composites are very limited.

Schafer TE, Lapp CA, Hanes CM, Lewis JB, Wataha JC, and Schuster GS: Estrogenicity of bisphenol A and bisphenol

A dimethacrylate in vitro. J Biomed Mater Res 45: 192-197, 1999.

Setcos JC, Tarim B, and Suzuki S: Surface finish produced on resin composites by new polishing systems. Quintessence Int 30:169-173, 1999.

Swartz ML, Phillips RW, and Rhodes B: Visible light-activated resins: Depth of cure. J Am Dent Assoc 106:634, 1983.

Depth of cure, as determined by hardness measurements, is influenced by a number of parameters, such as color of the resin, type of system, and time of exposure to the light source.

Vanherle G, and Smith DS: Posterior Composite Resin Dental Restorative Materials. St Paul, MN, Dental Products Division, 3M Co, 1985.

Proceedings from an international symposium provide a basis for clinical decisions and for further research and development of resin-based composites.

Wendt SL, Jr, and Leinfelder KF: The clinical evaluation of heat-treated composite resin inlays. J Am Dent Assoc 120:177, 1990.

One of a few papers available at this time that report the clinical performance of heat-polymerized composite inlays. Although marginal integrity was superior, no difference was detected in wear resistance as compared with light-cured inlays.

Willems G, Lambrechts P, Braem M, and Celis JP: A classification of dental composites according to morphological and mechanical characteristics. Dent Mater 8l:310-319, 1992.

A classification scheme for composites, based on structure, that revises and updates the earlier one of Lutz and Phillips (1983; see above).

Yap AUJ, Sau CW, and Lye KW: Effects of finishing/polishing time on surface characteristics of tooth-colored restoratives. J Oral Rehab 25:456-461, 1998.

Yap AU, Wong ML, and Lim AC: The effect of polishing systems on microleakage of tooth-coloured restoratives. Part 2: Composite and polyacid-modified composite resins. J Oral Rehabil 27:205-210, 2000.

16

Dental Cements

Chiayi Shen

KEY TERMS

Acid-base reaction—Chemical reaction between a compound with replaceable hydrogen ions (acid) and a substance with replaceable hydroxide ions (base) that yields water and a salt; for aqueous cements, the liquid is the acid and the powder is the base.

Acidogenic—Capable of producing an acid.

Anticariogenic—Capable of inhibiting or preventing dental caries.

Atraumatic restorative treatment (ART)—Clinical procedure performed without dental burs, air/water spray, or anesthesia that consists of manual excavation of carious tissue and restoration of the tooth cavity with a Type II fluoride-releasing cement.

Base—Layer of insulating, sometimes medicated, cement, placed in the deep portion of the preparation to protect pulpal tissue from thermal and chemical injury.

Cavity liner—Thin layer of cement, such as a calcium hydroxide suspension in an aqueous or resin carrier (after evaporation), used for protection of the pulp; certain glass ionomer cements that are used as an intermediate layer between tooth structure and composite restorative material are also considered liners.

Cement—Substance that hardens to act as a base, liner, filling material, or adhesive to bind devices and prostheses to tooth structure or to each other.

KEY TERMS—cont'd

Cermet—A glass ionomer cement that has been reinforced with filler particles prepared by fusing silver particles to glass.

Compomer—Resin-based composite material containing silicate glass filler particles and methacrylate and acidic monomers as matrices; also known as *polyacid-modified resin-based composite;* the term *compomer* is derived from the words *composite* and *ionomer.*

Craze—Network of fine, interconnected cracks formed within the surface of aqueous-based cement as a result of rapid dehydration.

Demineralization—Loss of mineral, typically calcium and phosphate ions, from tooth structure caused by exposure to organic acids produced by oral microorganisms.

Dew point—Temperature at which moisture in air begins to condense (e.g., the temperature at which dew deposits on a cooled glass mixing slab).

Dual-cure—Pertaining to setting of a material via two mechanisms; for glass ionomer cements, an acid-base reaction and a chemical- or light-activated polymerization process; for resin cement, a chemical- and a light-activated polymerization process.

Film thickness—Height of the space between two surfaces that are separated by a cement (e.g., the distance between the tooth surface and a cemented prosthesis); a property of luting cements, this dimension is measured after pressure is applied between two flat surfaces that are separated by the cement layer.

Fluorapatite—Compound formed in the tooth enamel when a fluorine ion replaces a hydroxyl (OH) ion in hydroxyapatite.

Fluoride recharging—Phenomenon in which glass ionomer cement absorbs fluoride from a solution with a high fluoride concentration.

Flux—Substance that reduces the fusing temperature of minerals during the melting of glass.

Glass—Hard, brittle, amorphous noncrystalline material typically made by fusing silicates with various types of mineral oxides.

Glass ionomer cement (GIC)—An aqueous-based material that hardens following an acid-base reaction between fluoroaluminosilicate glass powder and a polyacrylic acid solution; also referred to as *conventional GIC.*

Intermediate restoration—Tooth filling or prosthesis that is placed for a limited period, from several days to months, and is designed to seal teeth and maintain their position until a long-term restoration is placed; also called a *temporary restoration.*

Luting agent—A viscous material placed between tooth structure and a prosthesis that hardens through chemical reactions to firmly attach the prosthesis to the tooth structure.

Maturation—Process of hardening a cement matrix through hydration to achieve greater mechanical strength.

Metal-reinforced glass ionomer cement—A modified glass ionomer cement that incorporates metal particles to improve mechanical properties.

"Permanent" restoration—A long-lasting replacement or restoration for missing, damaged, or discolored teeth. Because of the tendency of any material to degrade or fracture over time, the term *permanent* does not signify an unlimited life expectancy.

Remineralization—Process of restoring mineral content in demineralized tooth structure.

Resin cement—Flowable resin-based composite material used for attaching orthodontic brackets and fixed prostheses to tooth structure following the application of either an enamel or dentin-bonding agent to achieve bonding.

Resin-modified glass ionomer cement—Modified glass ionomer cement that incorporates polymerizable monomer and a cross-linking agent; this type of cement has a longer working time and is less sensitive to water contamination than conventional glass ionomer cement; also called *hybrid ionomer cement.*

Restoration—Filling material or prosthesis used to restore or replace a tooth, a portion of a tooth, multiple teeth, or other oral tissues.

Sandwich technique—Process of placing glass ionomer cement as an intermediate layer between the tooth structure and a resin-based composite; this restoration design benefits from the adhesive quality and fluoride-releasing ability of glass ionomer cement and the aesthetic quality and durability of resin-based composite.

Self-adhesive—Ability of a material to adhere to tooth structure without the aid of a dentin-bonding agent or enamel-bonding agent.

Setting time—The elapsed time from the start of mixing to the point at which the mixture reaches a desired hardness or consistency.

Silicate cement—Restorative material, made from a matrix-forming mixture of a liquid (phosphoric acid) and a fluoride-containing silicate glass powder.

Silver alloy admix—A type of metal-reinforced glass ionomer cement.

Temporary restoration—See **intermediate restoration.**

Tri-cure—Pertaining to the setting reaction of a glass ionomer cement via three mechanisms: (1) an acid-base reaction between the powder particles and acid, (2) a chemically activated polymerization reaction, and (3) a light-activated polymerization process.

Varnish—A solution of natural gum, synthetic resins, or resins dissolved in a volatile solvent, such as acetone, ether, or chloroform.

Working time—Elapsed time from the start of mixing to the point at which the consistency of a material is no longer suitable for its intended use.

Zinc oxide–eugenol (ZOE) cement—One of several types of products formulated for use as a base, luting agent, restorative, and impression material that is based on the reaction between zinc oxide (powder) and eugenol (liquid).

Zinc phosphate cement—Substance formed by the reaction between zinc oxide powder and phosphoric acid liquid that can be used either as a base or as a luting agent.

DENTAL CEMENTS

Most dental cements are supplied as two components, a powder and a liquid. An increasing number of these are packaged in capsule form to be triturated by an amalgamator. Some have been reformulated in two pastes. With the exception of resin cements, the liquids are usually acidic solutions or proton donors, and the powders are basic in nature, consisting typically of either **glass** or metallic oxide particles. Depending on the particle size and powder/liquid (P/L) ratio, these components, when mixed, yield a pastelike or a flowable material, which hardens (or sets) to a rigid solid within a reasonable time. The reaction between the powder and liquid is essentially an **acid-base reaction.** Upon setting, these cements gain sufficient strength for use as a **base,** as a restorative material for temporary or **permanent restorations,** or as a **luting agent.**

Cements must exhibit a sufficiently low viscosity to flow along the interfaces between hard tissue and a fixed prosthesis, and they must be capable of wetting both surfaces to hold the prosthesis in place. This type of material is called a *luting agent.* Before placement of a **restoration** or seating of a prosthesis, the pulp may have been irritated or damaged from a variety of sources, such as the caries process or cavity preparation. As a means of protecting the pulp against further thermal and chemical trauma, some dental cements can be used to prepare bases that are placed under restorations and as pulp-capping agents and **cavity liners** that are placed on prepared tooth surface areas close to the pulp chamber.

Advances in resin chemistry for dental applications have led to the development of resin-based composite cements in consistencies suitable for luting of various prostheses. These materials are called *resin cements.* Other materials associated with the protection of the pulp, such as cavity **varnish** and cavity liners also fall into the category of dental cements by virtue of their application. Thus dental cements are classified according to their chief chemical ingredients and their applications. Examples of the various types of cement are shown in Figure 16-1.

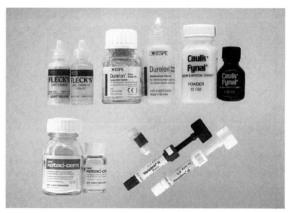

Fig. 16-1   Commercial products representative of zinc phosphate, zinc polycarboxylate, glass ionomer, reinforced zinc oxide–eugenol, and resin luting cements.

CRITICAL QUESTION

Dental cements are not as strong as composites or amalgams. Why do we use some cements for restorations in certain situations?

FLUORIDE-RELEASING CEMENTS FOR DIRECT-FILLING RESTORATIONS

Fluoride-releasing dental cements used as restorative materials have low strengths compared with those of resin-based composites and amalgams, so they must be used in low-stress areas. This relatively low strength is beneficial when used for temporary and **intermediate restorations** because the materials are easier to remove when they need to be replaced with more durable restorations. The use of **glass ionomer cement (GIC)** for long-term restoration is contraindicated. Nevertheless, fluoride-releasing cements must often be used for restorations in patients at a high risk for caries.

The use of dental cement as a restorative material began with **silicate cement,** which is based on silicate glass and phosphoric acid. Silicate cement, like most brittle material is relatively strong in compression but weak in tension after it sets. Despite its high rate of disintegration over time, silicate cement is more aesthetic than amalgam. Observation of 20,000 existing amalgam and silicate cement restorations revealed that a 12% incidence of secondary caries occurred adjacent to amalgam restorations, whereas the incidence of secondary caries was only 3% adjacent to silicate restorations. Also, the incidence of proximal surface caries adjacent to silicate cement restorations was less than that associated with proximal surfaces adjacent to amalgam restorations.

The glass for silicate cement was made by fusing compounds of silica (SiO_2), alumina (Al_2O_3), fluoride compounds, and calcium salts at approximately 1400° C. Type II GIC has evolved from silicate cement, and several other cements have subsequently been derived from GIC. Laboratory studies show that fluoride is released into an aqueous medium from silicate cement and other fluoride-containing cements. The impressive **anticariogenic** potential of silicate cement confirms the ability of F⁻ ions to inhibit **demineralization** and the role of fluoride-releasing cements to serve as direct restorative materials. However, there is no consensus on the precise mechanism of its anticariogenic action. It is known that a fluoride concentration of 5 parts per million (ppm) or more is maintained in the immediate region of a glass ionomer restoration. Because secondary caries is inhibited adjacent to restorations that release fluoride, this effect is especially important in areas where plaque is likely to accumulate.

Currently, there are three major theories to explain the anticariogenic mechanism of fluoride: increased acid resistance of enamel, enhancement of **remineralization,** and inhibition of carbohydrate metabolism by the acidogenic plaque microflora.

Acid Resistance of Enamel

The acid resistance of enamel theory suggests that fluoride, when taken up in the apatite in the form of **fluorapatite,** reduces the solubility of apatite. Although the posteruptive fluoride uptake by enamel is minimal, the continuous release of fluorine ions from silicate cement provides a localized, but high concentration, of a fluoridated environment at the enamel/restorative material interface. Thus this mechanism is analogous to that of topically applied fluoride solutions, except that it is concentrated at the margin of the cavity preparation. The increase in fluoride content of the surface layer of enamel adjacent to a fluoride-releasing silicate restoration and the reduction in the enamel acid solubility are shown in Table 16-1. When similar experiments were performed with a silicate cement prepared with a nonfluoride **flux,** no appreciable change occurred in the fluoride content of the enamel. In fact, the enamel solubility actually increased.

This theory implies that caries resistance, once obtained, will last the lifetime of the tooth. However, it has also been observed that caries protection by fluoride ceases when the fluoride intake or its administration is terminated. For example, individuals who are born and raised in an area with fluoridated water and then move to an area with nonfluoridated water quickly experience a caries incidence characteristic of the new community. A similar prevention effect can be achieved through the application of fluoride varnishes or through the application of a fluoride gel in a dental office. Individuals at a high risk for caries who have acquired a high concentration of fluorapatite in their enamel through previous applications of fluoride varnish and other fluoride supplements may ultimately develop new caries lesions when they stop receiving the fluoride varnish or supplements.

Remineralization-Demineralization Balance

The ionic fluorides are present in aqueous solution, in plaque, and within enamel and dentin. The remineralization-demineralization balance theory indicates that the presence of 0.2 to 1.0 ppm of fluoride lowers the solubility of enamel, and increased uptake in enamel results from an enhanced balance between remineralization and

Table 16-1	Changes in Fluoride Content and Acid Solubility of Enamel Induced by Cements	
Cement type	**Change in fluoride content**	**Change in acid solubility**
Silicate (without fluoride)	0%	20%
Silicate (with fluoride)	3500%	−40%
Zinc silicophosphate	5000%	−50%
Glass ionomer	3000%	−30%

Mean values connected by a straight line are not significantly different from one another.

demineralization. Because fluoride in oral fluids is rinsed and swallowed, a continuous supply of fluoride is needed to maintain fluoride protection. It appears that the two mechanisms are mutually inclusive. However, chemical, clinical, and epidemiological evidence indicates that the remineralization-demineralization mechanism is by far the most important factor in caries prevention.

Two types of fluorides deposit on enamel after topical fluoride treatment or fluoride varnish application: bound fluoride in the form fluorapatite and unbound fluoride as crystal deposits of calcium fluoride. The bound enamel fluoride is unrelated to caries inhibition, whereas the unbound calcium fluoride dissolves in response to decreased pH in the oral cavity, releasing fluorine ions that shift the equilibrium balance toward remineralization rather than toward demineralization.

Fluoride and Plaque Metabolism

Fluoride accumulates in dental plaque. The sources of plaque fluoride include saliva, gingival fluid, diet, topically applied fluoride gel or fluoride varnish, and demineralizing enamel. It is well established that fluoride inhibits carbohydrate metabolism by **acidogenic** plaque microflora. Fluoride enters microorganisms against a concentration gradient and accumulates intracellularly as the pH of extracellular fluid decreases. The transport of hydrogen fluoride (HF) into the extracellular fluid of cells leads to dissociation into H^+ and F^- ions within the more alkaline intracellular fluid. Ionic fluoride then induces enzyme inhibition, leading to a slower rate of acid production. Meanwhile the fluoride increases cell permeability and it can rapidly diffuse out of the cariogenic bacterium, contributing again to the fluoride content within the plaque matrix.

In vitro experiments have shown that high concentrations of fluoride in the range of 100 ppm reduce sensitive bacterial populations. Sublethal concentrations alter carbohydrate metabolism by reducing acidogenicity, altering the production of extracellular, insoluble polysaccharides, and possibly by reducing adhesion. The fluoride concentration in saliva rarely exceeds a few ppm. The effect of additional fluoride on plaque metabolism is insignificant, except for individuals with a severely reduced saliva flow rate (<0.5 mL/min) and except for periods of up to 2 hr after a topical fluoride treatment.

The presence of fluoride-containing cements should have little impact on the fluoride concentration in saliva. The effectiveness is limited only to areas adjacent to fluoride-releasing restorations. Chemical analyses of plaque collected at the margins of resin, amalgam, and cast gold restorations reveal a difference in composition when compared with plaque that accumulates at the margins of silicate cement restorations.

Sources of Fluoride Release

Our understanding of the caries prevention mechanism for silicate cement has led to numerous investigations designed to capture the anticariogenic characteristic by the addition of fluoride compounds to resins, amalgam, **zinc phosphate cement, zinc oxide–eugenol (ZOE) cement,** pit and fissure sealants, cavity varnishes, and even chewing gums. Addition of fluoride can be achieved by physically incorporating a soluble fluoride salt within the bulk material or by using nearly insoluble fluoride minerals as filler. Another alternative for fluoride release is chemical in nature and uses monomers with fluorine in pendant groups as the matrix former. These monomers release fluorine ions by means of ion exchange with hydroxyl groups.

GICs remain the most significant fluoride-releasing material compared with fluoridated composites and amalgams, which release fluoride at a much lower level and for a shorter duration. The effect of fluoride loss on the pertinent properties of a material is a significant long-term concern.

Fluoride Recharging

Although in vitro data have shown that fluoride release from glass ionomer remains detectable for years, the rate of release is reduced by as much as a factor of 10 within the first few months. It has also been shown that silicate cements are capable of absorbing fluoride from their environment. To investigate the phenomenon of **fluoride recharging** in GICs, researchers stored aged specimens in fluoridated toothpaste (250 ppm) or sodium fluoride solutions as high as 2500 ppm for up to 15 min. The rerelease data show that recharged specimens exhibit a significantly increased release initially and a rapid decrease to its preexposure level within weeks. The level of rerelease depends on the concentration of the storage medium and the duration of storage. The efficiency of recharging seems to decrease with the frequency of recharging. The clinical efficacy of recharging glass ionomer to improve caries inhibition is yet to be proved.

CEMENTS AS LUTING AGENTS

Numerous dental treatments necessitate attachment of prostheses and appliances to the teeth by means of a luting agent. These include metal, metal-ceramic, composite, and ceramic restorations; provisional or interim acrylic restorations; laminate veneers for anterior teeth; orthodontic appliances; and pins and posts used for retention of restorations. The word *luting* implies the use of a moldable substance to seal a space or to cement two components together; hence the term is descriptive of dental cementing agents.

Table 16-2 shows the chief components of zinc phosphate, ZOE, zinc polycarboxylate, glass ionomer, resin-modified glass ionomer (hybrid ionomer), **compomer,** and **resin cements.**

Listed in Table 16-3 are the mechanical and physical properties of the different types of luting agents, in addition to the requirements set forth in American National Standards Institute/American Dental Association (ANSI/ADA) Specification No. 96 for water-based dental cements. The values listed in this table are taken from a variety of sources; therefore they are representative of typical cements. Although variation occurs from one brand to another, the differences induced by manipulative variables are usually considerably greater than those inherent between brands.

As shown in Table 16-3, the properties of various cements differ from one another. Hence the choice of cement is mandated to a large degree by the functional and biological demands of the specific clinical situation. If optimal performance is to be attained, the physical and biological properties and the handling characteristics (such as **working time, setting time,** consistency, and ease of removal of excess material) must be considered when selecting a cement for a specific task.

CRITICAL QUESTION

During the initial seating of a three-unit fixed partial denture (bridge), the prosthesis fits the prepared tooth perfectly and appears to be retained on the tooth so tenaciously that removal requires a great deal of force. Why is a cement required for retention under this condition?

Table 16-2	Reacting Components and Reaction of Dental Cements	
Materials	**Formulation and reacting components**	**Reaction type**
Zinc phosphate	Powder: Zinc oxide and magnesium oxide Liquid: Phosphoric acid	Acid-base reaction
Zinc oxide–eugenol	Powder: Zinc oxide Liquid: Eugenol	Acid-base reaction
Zinc oxide–eugenol (EBA modified)	Powder: Zinc oxide Liquid: Eugenol and ethoxybenzoic acid	Acid-base reaction
Zinc polycarboxylate	Powder: Zinc oxide and magnesium oxide Liquid: Polyacrylic acid	Acid-base reaction
Glass ionomer	Powder: Fluoroaluminosilicate glass Liquid: Polyacrylic acid, polybasic carboxylic acid, water	Acid-base reaction
Resin modified glass ionomer	Powder: Fluoroaluminosilicate glass, chemical- and/or light-activated initiator(s) Liquid: Polyacrylic acid, water-soluble methacrylate monomer, water, activator	Light- or chemical-activated polymerization and acid-base reaction
	Paste A: Fluoroaluminosilicate glass, chemical-activated initiator Paste B: Polyacrylic acid, water-soluble methacrylate monomer, water, activator	Chemical-activated polymerization and acid-base reaction
Compomer	One paste: Methacrylate monomer, acidic monomer, initiator	Light-activated polymerization
	Powder: Fluoroaluminosilicate glass, metallic oxides, sodium fluoride, chemical- and/or light-activated initiator(s) Liquid: Dimethacrylate/carboxylic monomers, multiple functional acrylate monomers, water, activator (for chemical-cure)	Light- or chemical-activated polymerization and acid-base reaction
Resin cement	One Paste: Methacrylate monomers, initiator	Light-activated polymerization
	Base paste: Methacrylate monomers, fillers, chemical- and/or light-activated initiator(s) Catalyst paste: Methacrylate monomers, fillers, activator (for chemical-cure)	Light- and chemical-activated polymerization or chemical-activated polymerization only
	Powder: Polymethyl methacrylate beads (for thickening) Liquid 1: Methacrylate monomers Liquid 2: Catalyst	Chemical-activated polymerization

Characteristics of the Abutment-Prosthesis Interface

When two relatively flat surfaces are brought into contact, analogous to a fixed prosthesis being placed on a prepared tooth, a space exists between the substrates on a microscopic scale. As shown in Figure 16-2, *A*, prepared surfaces on a microscopic scale are rough; that is, the surface exhibits peaks and valleys. When two surfaces are placed against each other, there are only point contacts along the peaks (Fig. 16-2, *B*). The areas that are not in contact then become open spaces. The space created can be substantial in terms of oral fluid flow and bacterial invasion. One of the main

Table 16-3 Properties of Dental Cements Used for Bonding Applications

Cement type	Setting time (min)	Film thickness (μm)	24-hr Compressive strength (MPa)	24-hr Diametral tensile strength (MPa)	Elastic modulus (GPa)	Solubility in water (wt%)	Pulp response
ANSI/ADA Specification 8 (Type I)	5.0 (minimum)	25 (maximum)	69	N/A	N/A	0.20 (maximum)	See note*
Zinc phosphate	5.5	20	104	5.5	13.5	0.06	Moderate
ZOE (Type I)	4.0-10	25	6-28	—	—	0.04	Mild
ZOE-EBA (Type II)	9.5	25	55	4.1	5.0	0.05	Mild
ZOE plus polymer (Type II)	6.0-10	32	48	4.1	2.5	0.08	Mild
Silicophosphate	3.5-4.0	25	145	7.6	—	0.40	Moderate
Resin	2.0-4.0	<25	70-172	—	2.1-3.1	0-0.01	Moderate
Polycarboxylate	6.0	21	55	6.2	5.1	0.06	Mild
Glass Ionomer	7.0	24	86	6.2	7.3	1.25	Mild to moderate

*Note: Based on comparison with silicate cement, a severe irritant.
ANSI, American National Standards Institute, *ADA*, American Dental Association; *ZOE*, zinc oxide–eugenol; *EBA*, orthoethoxy-benzoic acid

purposes of luting is to fill and seal this space completely. The clinician can seal the space by placing between the two surfaces a soft substance such as an adhesive, which can conform under pressure to the surface undercuts.

The current approach for cementing prostheses or appliances is to use adhesive technology. Adhesive bonding involves the placement of a third material, often called a *luting agent* that flows within the rough surfaces and sets to a solid form within a few minutes (Fig. 16-2, *C*). The solid matter not only seals the space, but also improves the retention of the prosthesis. Materials used for this application are classified as luting agents. If the cement is not fluid enough or incompatible with the surfaces, voids can develop around deep and narrow valleys (Fig. 16-2, *D*) and undermine the effectiveness of the luting agent. For example, large voids in cement adjacent to a ceramic crown in the occlusal region of the prepared tooth can substantially increase the tensile stress within the crown when a biting force is exerted on the occlusal surface near this area.

Procedure for Luting Prostheses

To be effective, a luting agent must be sufficiently fluid to flow into a continuous film of 25 μm thickness or less without fragmentation. The procedure consists of placing the cement on the inner surface of a prosthesis, seating the prosthesis on the preparation, and removing the excess cement at an appropriate time. Luting of a single crown described in the following as an example (Fig. 16-3, *A*).

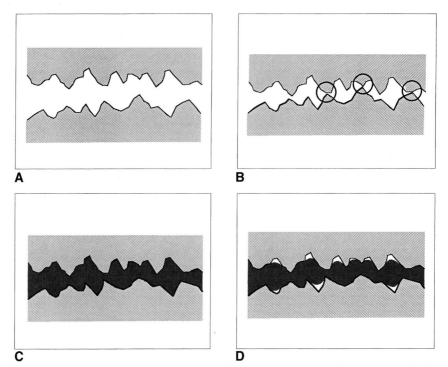

Fig. 16-2 Microscopic image of the abutment-prosthesis interfaces. **A,** Irregular surface morphology of the two surfaces to be bonded. **B,** Two surfaces pressed against each other without an intermediate cement layer. Note the small number of points of contact illustrated by the circles. **C,** Continuous interface when a third material, either cement or adhesive, is used as the intermediate layer. **D,** Voids generated as a result of the inability of the intermediate layer to wet the surfaces.

Placement of Cement

The cement paste should coat the entire inner surface of the crown and extend slightly over the margin to ensure that the space between the crown and tooth is completely sealed. It should fill approximately half of the interior crown volume (Fig. 16-3, *B*). The occlusal aspect of the tooth preparation must be free of voids. This is to ensure that there is no air entrapment in this critical area during the early stage of the seating. If voids remain in the occlusal region, any occlusal force applied above the voids to a resin or ceramic inlay, onlay, or crown will result in excessive tensile stress in the ceramic and a greater risk for fracture. Completely filling the crown with cement is not advisable for at least four reasons: (1) The risk for bubble entrapment increases, (2) the time for seating increases, (3) increased pressure may be required, and (4) the time for removal of excess cement increases.

Seating

Use moderate finger pressure to displace excess cement and to seat the crown on the prepared tooth. After the marginal gap area is evaluated for closure at three or more points with an explorer, the patient may be asked to bite on a soft piece of wood or a cotton roll to ensure complete seating. During this stage, the last increment of excess cement is expelled through the space between the prosthesis and the tooth. As the prosthesis reaches its final position on the prepared tooth, the space for expelling the excess cement becomes smaller, making seating more difficult (Fig. 16-3, *C*).

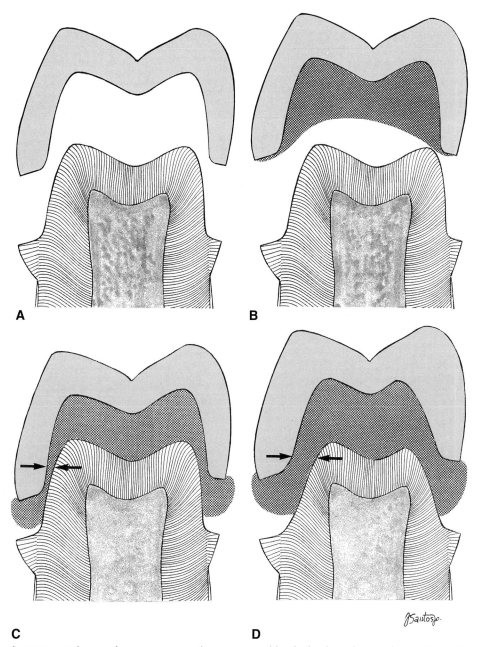

Fig. 16-3 Mechanics of cementing a prosthesis. **A,** Assembly of a fixed prosthesis and respective tooth preparation. **B,** Luting agent placed in the prosthesis should cover the entire surface. **C,** Space for expelling excess cement decreases as the prosthesis reaches its final position. **Arrows** show the thickness of space for displacement of excess cement. **D,** A higher degree of the abutment taper will provide a greater space for displacing excess cement.

Variables that facilitate seating include using a cement of lower viscosity, increasing the taper, and decreasing the height of the crown preparation (Fig. 16-3, *D*) and creating vibration by tapping on the prosthesis as the pressure is applied. Hand-held vibrators that use ultrasound to increase cement flow characteristic and eliminate air voids in cement are commercially available to assist complete seating of the crown. Note that increasing the degree of taper can compromise retention.

It is important to ensure that a prosthesis is completely seated during cementation. This concern can be alleviated in at least two ways, including evaluation of occlusion and evaluation of the margin at a minimum of three points before the cement has set. The latter step ensures that if the margin is closed completely at these three points, it will be closed at all other points along the margin.

The effect of increased viscosity of the luting cement on the ability to seat a cast restoration is illustrated in Figure 16-4. A crown cemented with a mixture of zinc phosphate cement that was prepared on a cool slab and seated properly on the prepared tooth is shown in Figure 16-4, A. However, because of the high viscosity of the mix prepared on a warm slab, the crown in Figure 16-4, B, failed to seat completely, and a thick layer of cement is exposed at the cervical margin. An ultrasonic vibrator could have been used to seat the crown more completely. The thick layer poses two potential problems: (1) The prosthesis may be in hyperocclusion, and (2) the thicker cement gap may increase the risk for marginal "ditching," which may occur when using a hard scaling and root-planing instrument.

Removal of Excess Material

Excess cement accumulates around the marginal area at the completion of seating. Its removal depends on the properties of the cement used. If the cement sets to a brittle state and does not adhere to the surrounding surfaces, the tooth and the prosthesis, it is best to remove it after it sets. Zinc phosphate and ZOE cements should set completely before the excess cement is removed. The procedures for removal of excess glass ionomer, zinc polycarboxylate, and resin cements, which are potentially capable of adhering both chemically and/or physically to the surrounding surfaces, vary among the products. The surrounding surfaces can be coated with a separating medium, such as petroleum jelly, thereby inhibiting cement adherence to the surfaces and facilitating removal of excess after the cement sets. However, care should

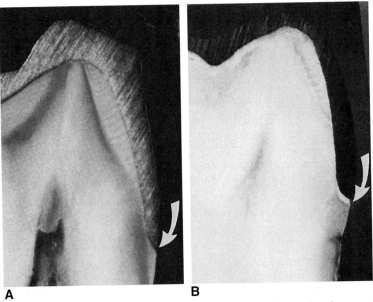

A   **B**

Fig. 16-4   Section through gold crowns cemented with the same mix of zinc phosphate cement. The crown shown in **A** was cemented 2.5 min after the start of the mix, whereas that shown in **B** was cemented at 5 min. Because of the increase in viscosity of the cement over time, the casting in **B** failed to seat completely, leaving a thick layer of cement exposed at the margin (**arrow**).

be taken to avoid contact of the medium with the marginal area of the tooth or prosthesis. Another technique requires the removal of excess cement as soon as the seating is completed, thus preventing the materials from adhering to the adjacent surfaces.

Some instructions from the manufacturer for Type I GIC and **dual-cure** resin cements indicate that once the prosthesis is seated, the cement should be allowed to set for 1.5 to 3 min after the completion of cement mixing, but before the excess cement is removed. The rationale is that the cement becomes more viscous, but not rigid during this period. In this consistency, removal of the excess cement is facilitated. For light-curable cements, including dual-cure cements, a short duration of light irradiation (e.g., 10 sec) has also been recommended to achieve the same goal.

The viscosity of the cement increases as it sets, and eventually it becomes a solid. If the clinician attempts to remove the excess cement immediately before it turns into a solid, the integrity of the marginal seal may be breached. At this stage the cement is so thick that any attempt to remove the excess may inadvertently pull the cement from the marginal area. The most relevant material in this regard is polycarboxylate cement, which transforms to a rubbery stage before setting.

Postcementation

Aqueous-based cements continue to mature over time well after they have passed the defined setting time. If they are allowed to mature in an isolated environment, that is, free of contamination from surrounding moisture and loss of water through evaporation, the cements will acquire additional strength and become more resistant to dissolution. As a precaution, the clinician should apply a varnish coat or a bonding agent along the accessible marginal area of cemented restorations before discharging the patient. Further details are discussed later in this chapter.

Mechanism of Retention

Prostheses can be retained by mechanical or chemical means or by a combination of the two. On a microscopic level, the interface region is similar to that in Figure 16-5. Both surfaces are rough, and the cement fills the irregular crevices along both

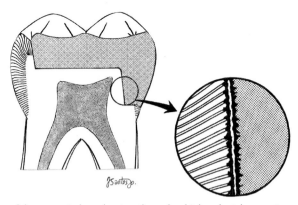

Fig. 16-5 Diagram of the suggested mechanism through which a dental cement provides mechanical retention of a gold inlay. The cement penetrates into irregularities in the tooth structure and the casting. Upon hardening, these retentive sites aid in retaining the restoration in place. The enlargement shows fracture of these tiny cement projections and loss of retention, possibly resulting in dislodgement of the inlay. See also color plate. (From Phillips RW, Swartz ML, and Norman RD: Materials for the Practicing Dentist. St Louis, Mosby, 1969.)

surfaces. The cement/prosthesis and cement/tooth interfacial regions then exhibit a void-free sealed continuum, and the cement layer can resist shear stress acting along the interface. This represents the principle of mechanical retention. The strength of retention depends on the strength of the luting agent to resist applied forces, which may act to dislodge the prosthesis. For certain situations, mechanical retention alone is insufficient to ensure retention and incomplete wetting of the prosthesis margin can also leave voids in the surface that may allow an influx of oral fluid.

Because clinicians cannot always rely on mechanical bonding effectiveness for retention, chemical bonding as a means of retention is the ideal goal. In theory, chemical bonds can resist interfacial separation and thereby improve retention. Aqueous cements based on polyacrylic acids provide some chemical bonding through chelation of acrylic acids to both organic and inorganic components of teeth. Resin cements based on N-phenylglycine and glycidyl methacrylate (NPG-GMA), polymerizable phosphates, and 4-methacrylethyl-trimellitic anhydride (4-META) are believed to bond to calcium within dentin. Contemporary dentin-bonding agents, which are hydrophilic and can penetrate porosities in dentin resulted from acid etching, exhibit high bond strength through micromechanical retention.

CRITICAL QUESTION

The "film thickness" of a dental cement has two meanings. What is the clinical significance of each meaning?

Dislodgment of Prostheses

Fixed prostheses can debond because of biological factors, physical reasons, or a combination of the two. Secondary caries results from a biological origin. Disintegration of the luting agents can result from fracture or erosion of the cement. For a brittle prosthesis, such as a glass-ceramic crown, fracture of the prosthesis may also occur because of physical factors, including intraoral forces and flaws within the crown surfaces and porosity within the cement.

In the oral environment luting agents are immersed in aqueous solutions. In this environment the cement layer near the margin can dissolve and erode, leaving a space (Fig. 16-6). This space can be susceptible to plaque accumulation and secondary caries. Because of these risks, the margin should be protected with a coating to allow continuous long-term setting of the cement. Two modes of failure are associated with cements: fracture of the cement (Fig. 16-7, *A*) and leakage along the interface (Fig. 16-7, *B*). Because the cement layer is the weakest link of the entire assembly, higher-strength luting agents should be chosen to enhance retention and prevent prosthesis dislodgment by providing a firm support base against applied forces.

Several factors can influence the retention of these fixed prostheses. First, the **film thickness** of cement beneath the prosthesis should be thin. A thinner film has fewer internal flaws compared with a thicker one. Second, the cement should have high strength values. It has been shown that generally greater forces are required to dislodge appliances cemented with luting agents that have a high compressive, shear, or tensile strength than with cements of lower strength. It is also well established that the stresses in cement, which develop during mastication, are exceedingly complex. Although compressive strength is a good indicator of fracture resistance, other factors such as tensile strength, shear strength, fracture toughness, and film

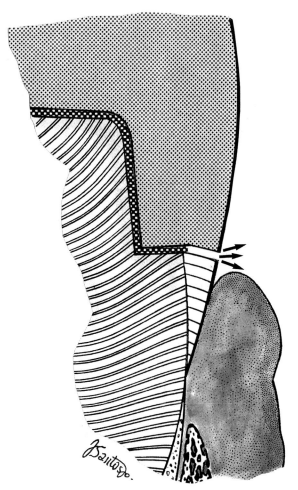

Fig. 16-6 Loss of cement at the marginal area resulting from exposure to oral fluid. See also color plate.

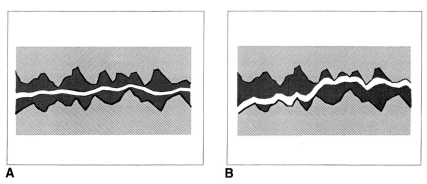

A   **B**

Fig. 16-7 Failure modes of the interface. **A,** Cleavage through the cement layer. This is probably not associated with the dimension of the cement involved. **B,** The most likely failure occurs at the luting agent/prosthesis interface. Remnants of the luting agent often remain on the opposing surface.

thickness are also important. Third, the dimensional changes occurring in the cement during setting should be minimized. Sources include gain or loss of water and differences in the coefficients of thermal expansion among the tooth, the prosthesis, and the cement. Therefore it is important to isolate the cement immediately after removal of the excess cement. Fourth, a cement with the potential to chemically bond to teeth and prosthesis surfaces or to enhance bonding of restorative material to tooth structure should be used. Such a cement layer can reduce the potential of separation at the interface and maximize the effect of the inherent strength of the cement on retention.

When mechanical undercuts are the principal mechanism of retention, failure tends to occur along the interfaces. When chemical bonding is involved, the failure often occurs cohesively through the cement itself. The prosthesis becomes dislodged only when the luting cement fractures or dissolves.

Film Thickness

With regard to cementation, the film thickness of cements can be described in one of two ways. The first is that described in ANSI/ADA Specification No. 96 (ISO 9917-1) for the consistency of the cement. Freshly mixed cement is placed between two optically flat surfaces and a 150 Newton (N) vertical load is applied 10 sec before the end of the measured working time. When at least 10 min have elapsed after application of the load, the thickness of the film between the two flat surfaces is measured. The film should be continuous, and no voids should exist through the entire body of the film. For luting applications the maximum allowable film thickness is 25 μm; a low value of film thickness is preferred because excess cement can be expressed more easily. The size of particles and the P/L ratio significantly affect the film thickness. For restorative applications, including temporary and final cementations, the maximum thickness is typically about 40 μm. For comparison, the diameter of human hair ranges between 40 and 80 μm.

Film thickness also refers to the thickness of the cement between a cast crown, inlay, onlay, or veneer and the tooth structure. As discussed in the previous section, the thickness of this film plays a significant role in the retention of the prosthesis. This film thickness varies with (1) the amount of force applied during seating of a prosthesis, (2) the manner in which the force is applied to the prosthesis during seating, (3) the configuration of the prosthesis relative to its hindering or facilitating the flow of cement, and (4) the fit of the prosthesis on the prepared tooth. The film thickness values reported in the literature typically range between 25 and 150 μm.

AGENTS FOR PULP PROTECTION

Metallic restorations, which are excellent thermal conductors, can cause thermal sensitivity during drinking of hot and cold foods or beverages. Other restorative materials, such as the phosphoric acid-containing cements, direct filling resins, and, in some instances, GICs can produce chemical irritation. Also, the interfacial leakage that occurs as a result of the setting contraction of amalgam and composite restorations may also cause pulpal irritation.

Cavity varnishes, liners, and bases are used as adjuncts to the use of restorative materials to protect the pulp against these types of injury. In addition to serving as insulation against temperature change, as a barrier against irritants released from restorative materials, and as sealing agents against interfacial leakage with associated bacterial invasion, some of these agents may also provide caries prevention benefits.

CRITICAL QUESTION

Why are copal-based varnishes no longer used as often as they were in the 1960s through 1990s?

Cavity Varnishes

Typical cavity varnishes are principally natural gums, such as copals or rosins, or synthetic resins dissolved in an organic solvent, such as acetone, chloroform, or ether. They form a coating on the tooth by evaporation of the solvent and are not generally applied in a sufficient thickness to provide the required thermal insulation. The literature generally suggests that varnish reduces pulpal irritation. This conclusion is likely drawn from in vitro studies showing a reduction in the infiltration of irritating fluids through marginal areas. Clinical observations based on the tooth sensitivity reported by patients have yet to confirm the applicability of in vitro data to clinical performance. Varnish is also claimed to prevent penetration of corrosion products of amalgams into the dentinal tubules, thereby reducing the unsightly tooth discoloration often associated with amalgam restorations. To attain a uniform and continuous coating on all surfaces of the prepared cavity, the clinician should apply at least two thin layers of varnish. When the first layer dries, small pinholes usually develop. A second or third application fills in most of these voids, thereby producing a more continuous coating. The varnish must be applied in a thin consistency, using a brush or a small pledget of cotton. It is advisable that a disposable applicator be used and discarded after each use to prevent introduction of microorganisms into the varnish bottle.

A varnish is not indicated when adhesive materials, such as GIC and resin-based composite, are used. Research on dentin-bonding agents has shown that they can be used in areas that traditionally require varnish and that they potentially can serve the same role as varnish.

Cavity Liners

The original purpose of cavity liners was to utilize the beneficial effects of calcium hydroxide in accelerating the formation of reparative dentin. Thus these liners were formulated by dispersing calcium hydroxide in aqueous or resin carrier solutions to facilitate their application to the walls of a cavity preparation. The carrier evaporates and leaves a thin layer of calcium hydroxide residue on the cavity walls. In addition, a film of calcium hydroxide with a pH of 11 can neutralize or react with acid released from adjacent phosphoric acid-containing cements. Because calcium hydroxide is soluble in oral fluids regardless of the type of carrier used, it is mandatory that this type of liner not be left on the margins of the cavity preparation.

Several chemical setting materials have been introduced as liners and liner/base materials; these include calcium hydroxide materials, low viscosity ZOE, and glass ionomer. These materials are placed in a thin layer on the pulpal floor. As such, the function of a cavity liner has expanded to include maintaining adhesion at the tooth-restoration interface and sealing the dentin from an influx of microorganisms and irritants resulting from restorative procedures.

Cement Bases

In contrast to liners, bases are applied in much thicker layers (>0.75 mm) under restorations to protect the pulp against thermal injury, galvanic shock, and chemical

Table 16-4	Thermal Conductivity of Cement Base Materials Compared with Two Insulation Materials
Material	**Thermal conductivity (mcal • cm/cm² • sec •°K)**
Zinc phosphate cement (dry)	3.11
Zinc phosphate cement (wet)	3.88
Zinc oxide–eugenol	3.98
Asbestos	1.90
Cork	7.00

irritation, depending on the particular restorative materials used. In addition, the material should also be strong enough to withstand condensation forces during placement of restorations and to resist fracture under any masticatory stress induced on the restoration. Zinc phosphate cement has been used for this purpose for many years, as have numerous ZOE formulations. In addition, both zinc polycarboxylate and GICs have properties that make them suitable for use as bases. Several fast-setting ionomer cements are available for this purpose.

Table 16-4 shows that the thermal conductivity of zinc phosphate and ZOE cements is in the same range as that of recognized insulators, such as cork and asbestos. The insulation abilities of other cements (e.g., polycarboxylate, glass ionomer, and calcium hydroxide) also fall within this range. Clinical experience has shown that temperature changes in the mouth have a more acute effect on the pulp when teeth containing large amalgam restorations are not insulated by a base. Heat transfer through a material depends not only on the coefficients of thermal conductivity and thermal diffusivity of the substance, but also on its thickness.

Calcium hydroxide and ZOE provide effective barriers against the penetration of irritating constituents from restorative materials. Bases of zinc polycarboxylate and GICs can also be used as chemical barriers. There is some concern that if zinc phosphate is employed as a base for thermal insulation, the low pH may require pulp protection. However, if zinc phosphate cement is mixed as a thick, non-tacky, puttylike mass, this risk is negligible because minimal free acid remains. In the case of using glass ionomer as a base, any deep areas should be protected by a thin layer of a calcium hydroxide paste.

Studies have shown that dental cements develop sufficient strength to resist condensation stress after they attain an initial set. Placement of restorative material should begin only after the initial set of the base material has occurred. Table 16-5 shows the compressive strength of representative dental cements. The minimal

Table 16-5	Compressive Strength of Cement Base Materials					
	7 min		**30 min**		**24 hr**	
Material	**MPa**	**psi**	**MPa**	**psi**	**MPa**	**psi**
Zinc oxide–eugenol	2.8	400	3.5	500	5.2	750
	15.9	2300	20.7	3000	24.1	3500
	6.2	900	6.9	1000	12.4	1800
Calcium hydroxide	7.6	1100	6.2	900	8.3	1200
	3.8	550	4.8	700	10.3	1500
Zinc phosphate	6.9	1000	86.9	12,600	119.3	17,300

strength required to resist masticatory forces has not been determined. Unquestionably, the design of the prepared tooth cavity is an important factor. For a Class I tooth preparation in which the base is supported on all lateral sides by tooth structure, less strength is necessary than is required for Class II preparations. A study involving more than 350 amalgam restorations placed over bases of a hard-setting calcium hydroxide revealed no unusual evidence of failure. Insufficient clinical data are available on this subject to make specific conclusions on the minimal strength necessary to resist clinical fracture.

Clinical Considerations

The selection of a base is governed to an extent by the design of the cavity, the type of direct restorative material used, and the proximity of the pulp relative to the cavity wall. For amalgam restorations, calcium hydroxide or ZOE base materials serve effectively as the sole base. For direct filling gold, it may be necessary to use a stronger material for the base, for example, zinc phosphate, zinc polycarboxylate, or a GIC. Thus in those cases in which it is desirable to place a calcium hydroxide or ZOE cement liner on the floor of the cavity, the liner should be overlaid with a stronger cement. For resin-based composites, calcium hydroxide and GICs applied as a thin base are also satisfactory for this purpose.

Note that use of a base in conjunction with amalgam or gold foil does not prevent microleakage and acid penetration. If a cavity varnish or dentin-bonding agent is selected to ensure sealing of the restoration, the type of base often governs the respective order of applying the materials. If a zinc phosphate cement base is to be used, then the sealing material should be applied to the cavity walls before placement of the base. On the other hand, if the base cement is biocompatible (e.g., calcium hydroxide, ZOE, zinc polycarboxylate or GIC), the cement should be placed first, followed by the sealing agent after the base material has hardened.

ZINC PHOSPHATE CEMENT

Zinc phosphate is the oldest of the luting cements. Thus it has the longest clinical "track record" and serves as a standard with which newer systems can be compared. It consists of powder and liquid in two separate bottles.

Composition and Setting

The main ingredients of the powder are zinc oxide (90%) and magnesium oxide (10%). The ingredients of the powder are sintered at temperatures between 1000° C and 1400° C into a cake that is subsequently ground into a fine powder. The powder particle size influences the setting rate of the cement mixture. Generally, the smaller the particle size, the faster the set of the cement.

The liquids contain phosphoric acid, water, aluminum phosphate, and, in some cases, zinc phosphate. The acid content of most liquids is 33 ± 5 wt%. The water controls the ionization of the acid, which in turn influences the rate of the liquid-powder (acid-base) reaction.

When the powder is mixed with the liquid, the phosphoric acid attacks the surface of the particles and releases zinc ions into the liquid. Aluminum, which already forms a complex with the phosphoric acid, reacts with zinc and yields a zinc aluminophosphate gel on the surface of the remaining portion of the particles. Thus the set cement is a cored structure consisting primarily of unreacted zinc oxide particles embedded in a cohesive amorphous matrix of zinc aluminophosphate.

Because water is critical to the reaction, the composition of the liquid should be preserved to ensure consistent reactions from one mix to the next. Changes in composition and reaction rates may occur either because of degradation of the liquid or by water evaporation from the liquid. This means that changes in the composition can affect the reaction. Liquid degradation effects are exhibited as a clouding of the liquid over time. Loss of water from the acid can lengthen the setting reaction, whereas incorporation of some additional water during mixing accelerates the reaction.

CRITICAL QUESTION

Why is it that prolonged spatulation of zinc phosphate cement can increase the setting time of the cement, but the same prolonged spatulation shortens the setting time of gypsum products?

Working and Setting Times

Working time is measured as the time from the start of mixing to the maximum time at which the viscosity (consistency) of the mix is still low enough to flow readily under pressure to form a thin film. It is obvious that the rate of matrix formation dictates the length of working time. On the other hand, setting time refers to the period during which the matrix formation has reached a point at which an external physical disturbance will not cause permanent dimensional changes. Setting time can be measured with a 1-mm–diameter needle indenter at a load of 400 g, a temperature of 37° C, and relative humidity greater than 90%. Setting time is defined as the elapsed time from the start of mixing to the point at which the needle no longer makes a complete circular indentation in the cement. Clinically, this represents the time at which the excess zinc phosphate cement should be removed from the margins of the restoration. A reasonable setting time for zinc phosphate cement is between 2.5 and 8 min, as specified in ANSI/ADA Specification No. 96 (ISO9917).

Working and setting times of a commercial product are inherent properties determined by the manufacturing process. Generally, it is desirable to extend the setting time of the cement to provide sufficient working time for manipulation. The following four procedures can extend the setting time of zinc phosphate cement at chair side:

1. Reducing the P/L ratio produces a thinner mixture, which increases the working and setting times of zinc phosphate cement. However, this change will adversely affect the physical properties and result in a lower initial pH of the cement. Thus it is not an acceptable means of extending the setting time. The compressive strength as a function of decreasing P/L ratio is clearly demonstrated in Figure 16-8.
2. Mixing cements in increments and introducing smaller quantities of powder into the liquid for the first few increments increases the working and setting times and permits more powder to be incorporated into the mix. These steps are consistent with the recommended procedure for mixing zinc phosphate cement.
3. If an operator prolongs the spatulation of the last increment, the matrix will be effectively destroyed as it is forming. Fragmentation of the matrix means that extra time is needed to rebuild the bulk of the matrix. This is different from the phenomenon observed for dental stones, in which a fragmented matrix represents new nuclei for crystallization that control the setting time and microstructure of the gypsum product.

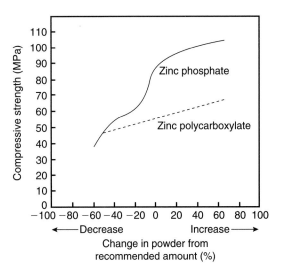

Fig. 16-8 Effect of powder/liquid (P/L) ratio on the strength of two cements. Cement specimens were prepared with greater and lesser amounts of powder (higher and lower P/L ratios) than those recommended by the manufacturers (represented by a 0% change).

4. Because the reaction between powder and liquid is exothermic, the most effective method of controlling the working and setting times is to regulate the temperature of the mixing slab. Cooling the slab markedly retards the chemical reaction between the powder and the liquid, thereby retarding formation of the matrix. This permits incorporation of the optimum amount of powder into the liquid without the mix developing an unduly high viscosity. For the same P/L ratio and mixing technique, the cement prepared on a cool slab (Fig. 16-9, *A*) is still fluid and suitable for cementation of cast restorations, whereas the mix made on a slab at room temperature (Fig. 16-9, *B*) may be too viscous for use in cementing precision castings.

Physical Properties of Zinc Phosphate Cement

Two physical properties of the cement that are relevant to the retention of fixed prostheses are the mechanical properties and solubilities. The prosthesis can become dislodged if the underlying cement is stressed beyond its strength. High solubility can induce loss of the cement needed for retention and may create plaque retention sites.

Zinc phosphate luting cements, when properly manipulated, exhibit a compressive strength of up to 104 megapascals (MPa) and a diametral tensile strength of approximately 5.5 MPa (Table 16-3). Zinc phosphate cement has a modulus of elasticity of approximately 13.7 gigapascals (GPa). Thus it is quite stiff and should be resistant to elastic deformation even when it is employed as the luting agent for restorations that are subjected to high masticatory stress.

As illustrated in Figure 16-8, the compressive strength, and perhaps the tensile strength, vary with the P/L ratio. The recommended P/L ratio for zinc phosphate cement is about 1.4 g powder to 0.5 mL liquid. The increase in strength attained by addition of powder in excess of the recommended amount is modest compared with the reduction incurred by decreasing the amount of powder in the mix. A reduction in the P/L ratio of the mix produces a markedly weaker cement. A loss or gain in the water content of the liquid reduces both the compressive strength and the tensile strength of the cement.

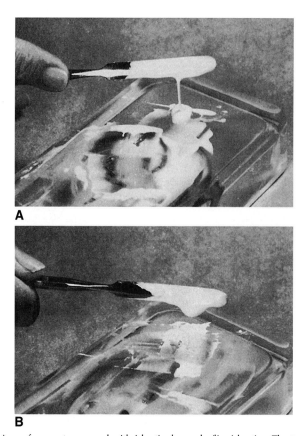

Fig. 16-9 Two mixes of cement prepared with identical powder/liquid ratios. The temperature of the mixing slab in **A** was 18° C; the temperature of the slab in **B** was 29.5° C. (From Phillips RW, Swartz ML, and Norman RD: Materials for the Practicing Dentist. St Louis, Mosby, 1969.)

Zinc phosphate cements have a relatively low solubility in water when they are tested in accordance with the ANSI/ADA Specification. However, this test is performed for quality control and does not reflect the relative rates of disintegration of various types of cement in the oral cavity. In vivo disintegration will be discussed later. Also, the solubility rate of zinc phosphate cement is appreciably greater in dilute organic acids, such as lactic, acetic, and citric acids.

Retention

Setting of zinc phosphate cement does not involve any reaction with surrounding hard tissue or other restorative materials. Therefore bonding occurs by mechanical interlocking at interfaces, not by chemical interactions, and any coating applied on the tooth surface for pulp protection reduces retention.

Biological Properties

As might be expected from the presence of the phosphoric acid, the acidity of zinc phosphate cement is quite high at the time when a prosthesis is placed on a prepared tooth. Two min after the start of the mixing, the pH of the cement is approximately 2 (Table 16-6). The pH then increases rapidly, but still is only about 5.5 at 24 hr. From these data it is evident that any damage to the pulp from acid attack by zinc phosphate cement probably occurs during the first few hours after insertion.

Table 16-6	pH of Cements for Luting Applications				
Time (min)	Zinc phosphate	Zinc silicophosphate	Zinc polycarboxylate	Glass ionomer	
2	2.14	1.43	3.42	2.33	1.76
5	2.55	1.74	3.94	3.26	1.98
10	3.14	2.15	4.42	3.78	3.36
15	3.30	2.46	4.76	3.91	3.88
20	3.62	2.56	4.87	3.98	4.19
30	3.71	2.79	5.03	4.18	4.46
60	4.34	3.60	5.08	4.55	4.84
1440	5.50	5.55	5.94	5.67	5.98

Manipulation

The following five points should be observed in the manipulation of zinc phosphate cements:

1. It is probably not necessary to use a measuring device for proportioning the powder and liquid because the desired consistency may vary to some degree with the clinical situation. For example, because more working time may be needed for cementation of a fixed partial denture with multiple crowns, a slightly thinner mix is often accepted. However, the maximum amount of powder possible for the particular application should be used to ensure minimum solubility and maximum strength.

2. A cool mixing slab should be employed. The cool slab prolongs the working and setting times and permits the operator to incorporate the maximum amount of powder before matrix formation proceeds to the point at which the mixture stiffens. The liquid should not be dispensed onto the slab until mixing is to be initiated because water will be lost to the air by evaporation, as shown in Figure 16-10.

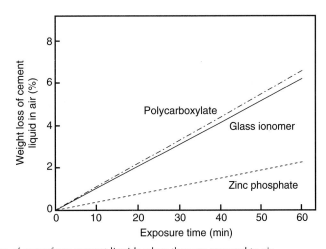

Fig. 16-10 Loss of water from cement liquids when they are exposed to air.

3. The powder should be divided into several portions indicated by the instructions. Mixing is initiated by the addition of a small amount of powder. Small quantities are incorporated initially, with brisk spatulation. A considerable area of the mixing slab should be used. A good rule to follow is to spatulate each increment for 15 to 20 sec before adding another increment. The mixing time is not unduly critical. Completion of the mix usually requires approximately 1.5 to 2 min. It is important to follow the instructions provided with the material. As stated previously, the appropriate consistency varies according to the purpose for which the cement is to be used. However, the desired consistency is always attained by the addition of more powder and never by allowing a very thin mix to stiffen. For a fixed partial denture, additional time is required to apply the cement. In this case, a slightly decreased viscosity may be acceptable.

4. The prosthesis should be seated immediately, before matrix formation occurs. After the prosthesis has been seated, it should be held under pressure until the cement sets. The field of operation should be kept dry during the entire procedure.

5. Excessive cement can be removed after it has set. It is advisable to apply a layer of varnish or other nonpermeable coating to the margin. The purpose of the varnish coating is to allow the cement more time to mature and to develop an increased resistance to dissolution in oral fluid.

ZINC POLYCARBOXYLATE CEMENT

In the quest for an adhesive luting agent that can bond strongly to tooth structure, zinc polycarboxylate evolved as the first cement system that developed an adhesive bond to tooth structure.

Composition and Chemistry

The polycarboxylate cements are powder-liquid systems. The liquid is an aqueous solution of polyacrylic acid or a copolymer of acrylic acid with other carboxylic acids, such as itaconic acid. The molecular weight of the polyacids is in the 30,000 to 50,000 range. The acid concentration varies from 32% to 42% by weight.

The composition and manufacturing procedures for the powder are similar to those of zinc phosphate cement. The powder contains mainly zinc oxide with some magnesium oxide. Stannic oxide may be substituted for magnesium oxide. Other oxides, such as bismuth and aluminum, can be added. The powder may also contain small quantities of stannous fluoride, which modifies the setting time and enhances the manipulative properties. Stannous fluoride is an important additive because it increases strength. However, the fluoride released from this cement is only a small fraction (15% to 20%) of that released from GICs.

The setting reaction of this cement involves particle surface dissolution by the acid that releases zinc, magnesium, and tin ions, which bind to the polymer chain via the carboxyl groups, as illustrated in Figure 16-11, A. These ions react with carboxyl groups of adjacent polyacid chains so that a cross-linked salt is formed as the cement sets. The hardened cement consists of an amorphous gel matrix in which unreacted particles are dispersed. The microstructure resembles that of zinc phosphate cement in appearance.

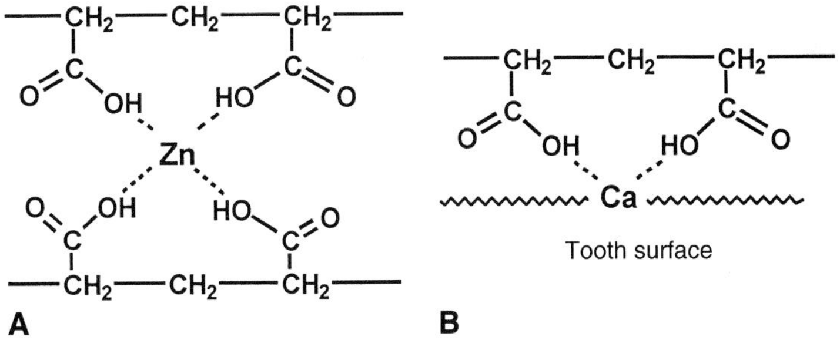

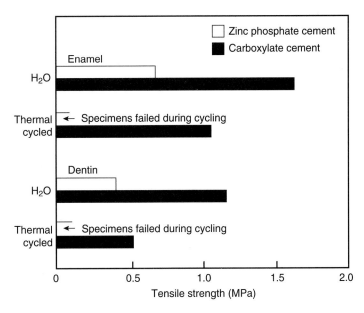

Fig. 16-11 The role of carboxylate functional groups. **A,** Matrix formation. **B,** Binding to tooth sturcture.

Bonding to Tooth Structure

As noted previously, an outstanding characteristic of zinc polycarboxylate cement is that the cement bonds chemically to the tooth structure. The mechanism is not entirely understood but is probably analogous to that of the setting reaction. As shown in Figure 16-11, *B,* the polyacrylic acid is believed to react with calcium ions via carboxyl groups on the surface of enamel or dentin. Thus the bond strength to enamel is greater than that to dentin. This is illustrated in Figure 16-12, which compares the bond strengths of a zinc polycarboxylate cement to enamel and to dentin.

Film Thickness

When zinc polycarboxylate cements are mixed at the recommended P/L ratio, they appear to be much more viscous than a comparable mix of zinc phosphate cement. However, the zinc polycarboxylate mix is classified as pseudoplastic and it

Fig. 16-12 The tensile strength required to separate enamel and dentin surfaces luted with a polycarboxylate cement after storage in water for 1 wk. Thermally stressed specimens were subjected to 2500 cycles between water baths maintained at 10° C and 50° C.

undergoes thinning at an increased shear rate. This means that the actions of spatulation and seating reduce the viscosity of the cement and the procedures can yield a film thickness of 25 μm or less.

Working and Setting Times

The working time for this cement is much shorter than that for zinc phosphate cement (i.e., approximately 2.5 min compared with approximately 5 min for zinc phosphate). This is illustrated in Figure 16-13, in which the viscosities of zinc phosphate, zinc polycarboxylate, and GICs are plotted as a function of time. The flat plateaus of the curves represent the working times. Lowering the temperature of the reaction can increase the working time. Unfortunately, the temperature of the cool slab can cause the polyacrylic acid to thicken. This increased viscosity makes the mixing procedure more difficult. It is suggested that only the powder should be refrigerated before mixing. The rationale for this procedure is that the reaction occurs on the surface and the cool temperature retards the reaction without thickening the liquid. The setting time ranges from 6 to 9 min, which is in the acceptable range for a luting cement.

Mechanical Properties

The compressive strengths of zinc polycarboxylate cements range from approximately 55 to 67 MPa; hence the compressive strength is inferior to that of zinc phosphate cement in this respect. However, the diametral tensile strength is slightly higher. It is not as stiff (2.4 to 4.4 GPa) as zinc phosphate cement (13.7 GPa) as indicated by its modulus of elasticity, which is less than half that of zinc phosphate cement. Also it is not as brittle as zinc phosphate cement. Because of its plastic deformation potential, it is more difficult to remove the excess cement after setting.

Solubility

The solubility of zinc polycarboxylate cement in water is low, but when it is exposed to organic acids of less than pH 4.5, the solubility markedly increases.

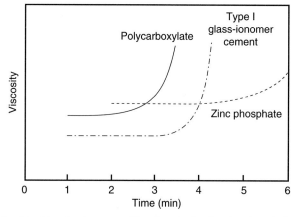

Fig. 16-13 Viscosity of freshly mixed cements. The viscosity is related to the relative ability to allow complete seating of a prosthesis. Zinc phosphate cement is more viscous initially, but it provides a longer working time for seating compared with either zinc polycarboxylate or glass ionomer cements. (From Mount GJ: An Atlas of Glass-Ionomer Cements, London, Martin Dunitz, 1990.)

Also, a reduction in the P/L ratio results in a significantly higher solubility and disintegration rate in the oral cavity.

Biological Considerations

The pH of the cement liquid is approximately 1.7. However, the liquid is rapidly neutralized by the powder. Thus the pH of the mix rises rapidly as the setting reaction proceeds, as can be seen in Table 16-6. The pH of a zinc polycarboxylate cement is higher than that of a zinc phosphate cement at various time intervals. Despite the initial acidic nature of the zinc polycarboxylate cements, they produce minimal irritation to the pulp.

Several theories have been advanced to explain the difference in the reaction of the pulp to zinc polycarboxylate and zinc phosphate cements. The pH of zinc polycarboxylate cement rises more rapidly than that of zinc phosphate cement. Also it is possible that the larger size of the polyacrylic acid molecule compared with phosphoric acid molecule may limit its diffusion through the dentinal tubules. Its excellent biocompatibility with the pulp is a major factor in the popularity of this cement system. In this regard, zinc polycarboxylate cement is equivalent to ZOE cement. Postoperative sensitivity effects are negligible for both cements.

CRITICAL QUESTION

Why should zinc polycarboxylate cement be applied on the tooth preparation before the cement loses its glossy appearance?

Manipulation

The cement liquids for zinc polycarboxylate cement are quite viscous. The viscosity is a function of the molecular weight and concentration of the polyacrylic acid and varies from one brand of cement to another. Thus the P/L ratios required to produce a cement of suitable cementing consistency may vary from product to product. Generally, these ratios are in the range of 1.5 parts of powder to 1 part of liquid by weight.

This cement should be mixed on a surface that will not absorb liquid. A glass slab affords an additional advantage over paper pads supplied by manufacturers because, once the glass slab is cooled, it maintains that temperature for a longer time. As stated previously, cooling the slab and the powder provides a somewhat longer working time, but under no circumstances should the liquid be stored in a refrigerator.

The liquid should not be dispensed before the time when the mix is to be made. It loses water to the atmosphere very rapidly, as shown in Figure 16-10. The loss of water from the liquid results in a very marked increase in its viscosity.

The powder is rapidly incorporated into the liquid in large quantities. Shown in Figure 16-14 is the consistency of the cement immediately after completion of the 30-sec mix as compared with the consistency after a longer mixing time or an additional time on the mixing slab. If good bonding to tooth structure is to be achieved, the cement must be adapted against the tooth surface before it loses its glossy appearance. The glossy appearance indicates a sufficient number of free carboxylic acid groups on the surface of the mixture that are vital for bonding to tooth structure. A dull-looking mixture, on the other hand, means that an insufficient number of unreacted carboxyl groups are available to bond to the calcium in the tooth surface.

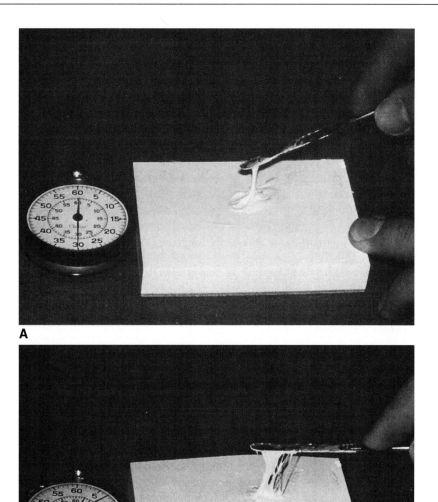

Fig. 16-14 **A,** Consistency of zinc polycarboxylate cement upon completion of 30 sec of mixing. **B,** If the mixing time is prolonged or the mix is allowed to remain on the slab, the cement becomes dull in appearance and the material becomes tacky to the touch. (Courtesy of M. Jendresen.)

Surface Preparation and Retention

Despite the adhesion of the cement to tooth structure, zinc polycarboxylate cements are not superior to zinc phosphate cement in the retention of cast noble metal restorations. A comparable force is required to remove gold inlays cemented either with zinc phosphate cement or with zinc polycarboxylate cement. Examination of the fractured surface shows that failure usually occurs at the cement-tooth interface with zinc phosphate cement. In the case of the zinc polycarboxylate cements, the failure occurs usually at the cement-metal interface, rather than at the cement-tooth interface.

The cement does not bond to the noble metal in the chemically contaminated as-cast or pickled condition. Thus it is essential that this contaminated surface on the cavity side of the casting be removed to improve wettability and the mechanical bond at the cement-metal interface. The surface can be carefully abraded with a small stone, or it can be sandblasted with high-pressure air and alumina abrasive, for example. However, long sandblasting times should be avoided to minimize the risk for margin deformation on cast metals. After exposure of the fresh metal, the casting should be thoroughly rinsed to remove debris and the surface should be dried.

Because this type of cement affords an opportunity to obtain adhesion to tooth structure, a meticulously clean cavity surface is necessary to ensure intimate contact and interaction between the cement and the tooth. A recommended procedure is to apply a 10% polyacrylic or maleic acid solution for 10 to 15 sec, followed by rinsing with water.

After cleansing, the cavity should be isolated to prevent further contamination by oral fluids. Blotting the surface before cementation is considered sufficient as a drying procedure. Drying with an air syringe is acceptable, although some discomfort may be experienced by the patient if the tooth is not anesthetized.

Removal of Excess Cement

During setting, the zinc polycarboxylate cement passes through a rubbery stage that makes removal of the excess cement quite demanding. The excess cement that has extruded beyond the margins of the casting should not be removed while the cement is in this stage because there is danger that some of the cement may be pulled out from beneath the margins, leaving a void. Excess cement can be removed when the cement becomes hard. It is important that the outer surface of the prosthesis be coated carefully with a thin layer of a separating medium, such as petroleum jelly, to prevent excess cement from adhering to its surface. Care should be taken not to allow the medium to touch the margin of the prosthesis. Another approach is to start removing excess cement as soon as seating is completed. The goal of these two methods is to avoid removing the excess during the rubbery stage.

GLASS IONOMER CEMENT

Glass ionomer is the generic name of a group of materials based on the reaction of silicate glass powder and polyacrylic acid. This material acquires its name from its formulation of a glass powder and an ionomer that contains carboxylic acids. Originally, the cement was intended for the aesthetic restoration of anterior teeth, and it was recommended for use in restoring teeth with Class III and Class V cavity preparations. Because of its adhesive bond to tooth structure and its caries prevention potential, the types of glass ionomers have expanded to include their use as luting agents, orthodontic bracket adhesives, pit and fissure sealants, liners and bases, core buildups, and intermediate restorations. The type of application depends on the consistency of the cement, which ranges from a low viscosity to very high viscosity by adjusting the particle size distribution and P/L ratio. The maximum particle sizes are 50 µm for restorative cement and 15 µm for luting agents.

The chemistry of GIC has also evolved over time. The need of improving its mechanical properties has led to the incorporation of metal particles that result in a **metal-reinforced glass ionomer cement.** Replacing part of the polyacrylic acid with hydrophilic monomers results in a light-curable or chemical-curable material called **resin-modified glass ionomer cement** or hybrid ionomer cement. The acid-base reaction is a part of the curing process. Therefore these materials are considered dual-cured glass ionomers. Use of both methods of initiating polymerization results in a **tri-cure** glass ionomer. This material has a longer working time and is less sensitive to moisture during setting. Using liquid water-free polyacid monomer in place of polyacrylic acid has yielded polyacid-modified composite resin, commonly called *compomer* (derived from *composite* and *ionomer*). The chemical makeup of the glass particles also varies with each modification, but it is essentially a fluoroaluminosilicate cement. The original material is now called *conventional GIC*. In this section, we will focus on the characteristics and manipulation of conventional GIC.

Composition

The glass ionomer powder is an acid-soluble calcium fluoroaluminosilicate glass. The composition of two commercial glass ionomer powders is given in Table 16-7. The raw materials are fused to a uniform glass by heating them to a temperature of 1100° C to 1500° C. Lanthanum, strontium, barium, or zinc oxide additions provide radiopacity. The glass is ground into a powder having particles in the range of 15 to 50 μm. Originally, the liquids for GIC were aqueous solutions of polyacrylic acid in a concentration of about 40% to 50%. The liquid was quite viscous and tended to gel over time. In most of the current cements, the acid is in the form of a copolymer with itaconic, maleic, or tricarboxylic acids (Fig. 16-15). These acids tend to increase the reactivity of the liquid, decrease the viscosity, and reduce the tendency for gelation. Tartaric acid is also present in the liquid. It improves the handling characteristics and increases working time, but it shortens the setting time (Fig. 16-16). The viscosity of the tartaric acid-containing cement does not generally change over the shelf life of the cement. However, a viscosity change can occur if the cement is out of date.

As a means of extending the working time of GIC, freeze-dried polyacid powder and glass powder are placed in the same bottle as the powder. The liquid consists of water or water with tartaric acid. When the powders are mixed with water, the acid powder dissolves to reconstitute the liquid acid and this process is followed by the acid-base reaction. This type of cement is referred to occasionally as *water-settable glass ionomer* or erroneously as *anhydrous glass ionomer*.

CRITICAL QUESTION

Water plays two critical roles in the setting of conventional GIC. What are they, and how do they work?

Table 16-7	Composition of Two Glass Ionomer Cement Powders	
Compound	Composition A (wt%)	Composition B (wt%)
SiO_2	41.9	35.2
Al_2O_3	28.6	20.1
AlF_3	1.6	2.4
CaF_2	15.7	20.1
NaF	9.3	3.6
$AlPO_4$	3.8	12.0

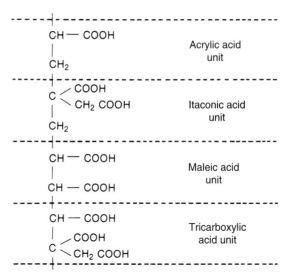

Fig. 16-15 Structure of various types of alkenoic acids that make up polyacids of glass ionomer cements.

Chemistry of Setting

When the powder and liquid are mixed to form a paste, the acid etches the surface of the glass particles and calcium, aluminum, sodium, and fluorine ions are leached into the aqueous medium. The polyacrylic acid chains are cross-linked by the calcium ions that are replaced by aluminum ions within the next 24 hr. Sodium and fluorine ions do not participate in the cross-linking of the cement. Some of the sodium ions may replace the hydrogen ions of carboxylic groups, whereas the remaining ions are dispersed uniformly within the set cement along with fluorine ions. The cross-linked phase becomes hydrated over time with the same water used for mixing. This process is called **maturation.** The unreacted portion of glass particles are sheathed by a silica gel that develops during removal of cations from the surface of the particles. Thus the set cement consists of an agglomeration of unreacted

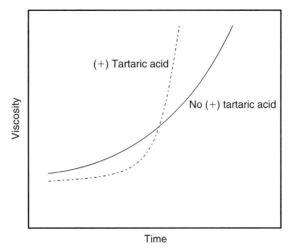

Fig. 16-16 Effect of tartaric acid on the viscosity-time relationship for a glass ionomer cement during setting. (From Wilson AD, and McLean JW: Glass Ionomer Cement. Chicago, Quintessence, 1988, p 37.)

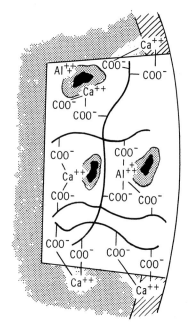

Fig. 16-17 Diagram depicting the structure of the glass ionomer cement. The **solid black particles** represent unreacted glass particles surrounded by the gel (**shaded structure**) that form when Al^{+++} and Ca^{++} ions are leached from the glass as a result of attack by the polyacrylic acid. The Ca^{++} and Al^{+++} ions form polysalts with the COO^- groups of the polyacrylic acid to form a cross-linked structure. The carboxyl groups react with the calcium in enamel and dentin.

powder particles surrounded by a silica gel in an amorphous matrix of hydrated calcium and aluminum polysalts. This mechanism is illustrated in the diagram in Figure 16-17, and the micrograph of the set cement is shown in Figure 16-18.

Water plays a critical role in the setting of GIC. It serves as the reaction medium initially and then slowly hydrates the cross-linked matrix, thereby yielding a stable gel structure that is stronger and less susceptible to moisture. If freshly mixed cements are exposed to ambient air without any protective covering, the surface will **craze** and crack as a result of desiccation. Any contamination by water that occurs at this stage can cause dissolution of the matrix-forming cations and anions to the surrounding areas. Both desiccation and contamination compromise the integrity of the material. Therefore conventional GIC must be protected against desiccation and water changes in the structure during placement and for a few weeks after placement if possible.

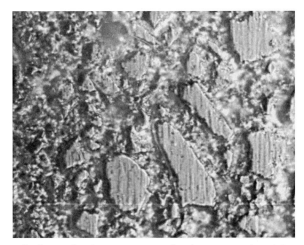

Fig. 16-18 Micrograph of a set glass ionomer cement showing unreacted particles surrounded by the continuous matrix.

Mechanism of Adhesion

The mechanism by which the glass ionomer bonds to tooth structure has not been clearly identified. However, there seems little doubt that it primarily involves chelation of carboxyl groups of the polyacids with the calcium in the apatite of the enamel and dentin (see Fig. 16-17). The adhesive mechanism of glass ionomer is comparable to that of zinc polycarboxylate cement (see Fig. 16-11). The bond strength to enamel is always higher than that to dentin because of the greater inorganic content of enamel and its greater homogeneity from a morphological standpoint.

Biological Properties

Glass ionomers release fluoride in amounts comparable to those released initially from silicate cement and continue to do so over an extended period. The minimal amounts of fluoride release and subsequent uptake by the enamel necessary to inhibit caries have not been defined. Several controlled clinical studies of glass ionomer used for restorations or fissure sealants show that the number of secondary carious lesions that developed ranged from zero to a number as high as that associated with composite restorations that were placed in the same study. Surveys of dentists show that the frequency of secondary caries in teeth with glass ionomer restorations compared with that of teeth with posterior composites was lower for one group of dentists but higher for another group of dentists. However, many studies have shown that fluoride ions released from GIC inhibit the progression of secondary caries.

Most histological studies indicate that glass ionomers are relatively biocompatible. They elicit a greater pulp reaction than ZOE but generally less than that from zinc phosphate cement. Glass ionomer used as a luting agent has a lower P/L ratio and can pose a greater hazard than that from glass ionomer restorations because a cement made of a lower P/L ratio remains at a lower pH for longer periods. With any GIC, it is wise to place a thin layer of a protective liner, such as $Ca(OH)_2$, within 0.5 mm of the pulp chamber in a deep preparation.

CRITICAL QUESTION

Under what condition might zinc phosphate cement be preferred over GIC for luting of an all-ceramic crown?

Physical Properties of Glass Ionomer Cement

Table 16-3 shows the properties of a typical glass ionomer luting cement. The compressive strength is comparable to that of zinc phosphate, and its diametral strength is slightly higher. The modulus of elasticity is only about one-half that of zinc phosphate cement. Thus the GIC is less stiff and more susceptible to elastic deformation. In this regard, it is not as desirable as zinc phosphate cement to support an all-ceramic crown, because greater tensile stress would develop in the crown under occlusal loading. For example, in one study the mean failure load for a feldspathic porcelain crown increased from 963 N to 2800 N as the elastic modulus of the supporting substrate increased from 3 to 14 GPa.

Table 16-8 shows the relative properties of the restorative glass ionomers. Another property that is particularly pertinent to its use as a restorative material is

Table 16-8	Properties of Restorative Cements				
	Compressive strength (MPa)	Diametral tensile strength (MPa)	Knoop hardness (KHN)	Solubility (ANSI/ADA Test)	Anticariogenic/ pulp response
Silicate cement	180	3.5	70	0.7	Yes/Severe
Glass ionomer (Type II)	150	6.6	48	0.4	Yes/Mild
Cermet	150	6.7	39	—	Yes/Mild
Hybrid ionomer	105	20	40	—	Yes/Mild

ANSI, American National Standards Institute, *ADA*, American Dental Association.

its fracture toughness (Table 16-9), a measure of the energy required to cause crack propagation that leads to fracture. Restorative GICs are much inferior to composites in this respect. They also are more vulnerable to wear than are composites when subjected to in vitro toothbrush abrasion tests and simulated occlusal wear tests. However, the following positive aspects of GICs make them attractive: (1) they are reasonably biocompatible, (2) they bond to enamel and dentin, and (3) they provide an anticariogenic benefit.

Manipulation Considerations for GIC

To achieve long-lasting restorations and retentive fixed prostheses, the following conditions for GIC must be satisfied: (1) the surface of the prepared tooth must be clean and dry, (2) the consistency of the mixed cement must allow complete coating of the surface irregularities and complete seating of prostheses, (3) excess cement must be removed at the appropriate time, (4) the surface must be finished without excessive drying, and (5) protection of the restoration surface must be ensured to prevent cracking or dissolution. These conditions are similar for luting applications, except that no surface finishing is needed.

Surface Preparation

Clean surfaces are essential for promoting adhesion. A pumice slurry can be used to remove the smear layer that is produced during cavity preparation. The commonly used method is etching with phosphoric acid (~34%-37%) or an organic acid like polyacrylic acid (~10%-20%) for 10 to 20 sec, followed by a 20 to 30 sec of water

Table 16-9	Fracture Toughness of Cements and Other Restorative Materials
Type of material	Fracture toughness (MPa•m$^{1/2}$)
Admixed amalgam	1.29
Light-cured glass ionomer	1.37
Hybrid composite	1.17
Glass ionomer lining cement	0.88
Cermet	0.51
Metal-reinforced glass ionomer	0.30

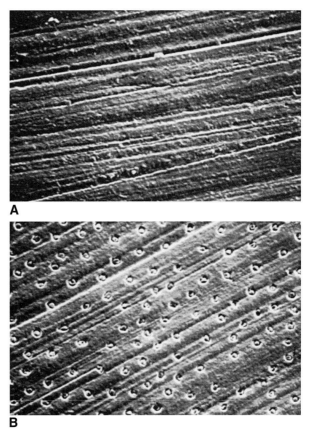

Fig. 16-19 **A,** Prepared dentin surface showing the presence of the smear layer. **B,** After cleansing with polyacrylic acid, the smear layer is removed, yet the tubules remain plugged.

rinsing time. Figure 16-19 shows the result of 10 sec of swabbing action on a cut dentin surface with a 10% solution. After conditioning and rinsing of the preparation, the surface should be dried, but it should not be unduly desiccated. It must remain clean because any further contamination by saliva or blood impairs bonding of the cement.

Preparation of the Material

The P/L ratio recommended by the manufacturer for GIC should be followed. A paper pad is sufficient for mixing. A cool and dry glass slab may be used to retard the reaction and extend the working time. It is important that the slab not be used if its temperature is below the **dew point.** The powder and liquid should not be dispensed onto the slab until just before the mixing procedure is begun. Prolonged exposure to the atmosphere can alter the precise acid/water ratio of the liquid. The powder should be incorporated rapidly into the liquid using a stiff spatula for restorative applications and a metal or plastic spatula for luting applications. The mixing time should not exceed 45 to 60 sec, depending on the individual products. At this time, the mix should have a glossy appearance, which indicates unreacted polyacid on the surface. This residual acid on the surface is critical for bonding to the tooth. A dull appearance indicates that there is inadequate free acid for bonding.

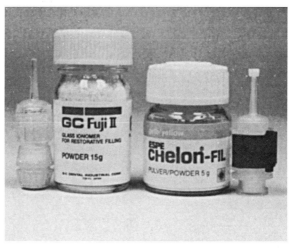

Fig. 16-20   Representative Type II restorative glass ionomer cements. Only the powder is shown for the cement. The respective capsules contain both powder and liquid.

Glass ionomers are also supplied in capsules containing preproportioned powder and liquid (Fig. 16-20). The mixing is accomplished in an amalgamator (triturator) after the seal that separates the powder and liquid has been broken. Note that the capsule contains a nozzle, so the mix can be injected directly on the prepared tooth and/or on a fixed prosthesis for bonding. The precise protocol for the mixing time and speed should be followed. The main advantages of capsules are convenience, consistent control of the P/L ratio, and elimination of the variations associated with hand spatulation.

CRITICAL QUESTION

Why are faster-setting GICs more durable as dental fillings than slower-setting products?

Placement of GIC as a Restorative Material and Removal of Excess

The restorative cement mixture is applied by a plastic instrument or injected on the prepared tooth surface. Tooth cavities should be slightly overfilled with cement. After placement, the surface should be covered with a plastic matrix to protect the setting cement from losing or gaining water during the initial set. The matrix is left in place for at least 5 min, although this time varies according to the product, based on the setting rate. Upon removal of the matrix, the surface must immediately be protected while the excess material is trimmed from the margins. Further finishing procedures, if needed, should be delayed for at least 24 hr. However, because this is clinically unrealistic, finishing of the restoration should be completed in the same appointment. Thus faster-setting cements are desirable. Even so, the longer the dentist waits to properly protect the surface, the more mature the cement becomes, the lower the risk for surface cracks, and the lower the tendency for the restoration to become slightly more opaque.

In the case of luting applications, no matrix protection is needed. The excess cement can be removed immediately upon seating or after a length of time as prescribed in the manufacturer's instructions.

Postoperative Procedures

Before the patient leaves, the Type II GIC restoration should be coated again with a protective agent, because the exposed cement around trimmed areas and margins is still vulnerable to the environment until it reaches full maturity. If these recommended procedures for providing protection to the setting cement are not followed, a chalky or a crazed surface will inevitably result (Fig. 16-21).

In summary, protection of glass ionomer restorations depends on meticulous attention to recommended procedures related to: (1) conditioning of the tooth surface, (2) proper manipulation, and (3) protection of the cement during setting and during potential situations when desiccation might occur. When these parameters are controlled, high-quality restorations should be produced (Fig. 16-22).

METAL-REINFORCED GLASS IONOMER CEMENTS

GICs lack toughness. Hence they cannot withstand high-stress concentrations that promote crack propagation. GICs can be reinforced by physically incorporating silver alloy powder with glass powder, usually referred to as a **silver alloy admix,** or by fusing glass powder to silver particles through sintering. The latter formula is often referred to as a **cermet.** Metal-reinforced GICs based on each of these two systems are commercially available (Fig. 16-23).

General Properties

Table 16-8 and Table 16-9 indicate that metallic fillers have little or no influence on the mechanical properties of restorative glass ionomers. In vitro wear tests show that these materials, which are indicated for use on occlusal surfaces in primary molars, perform well initially but do not perform any better than conventional glass ionomers when placed in long-term contact-free surfaces. Under in vitro acidic conditions, both conventional and metal-reinforced glass ionomers exhibit similar degrees of wear at contact-free areas at a solution pH between 6 and 7, but considerably greater wear is evident at pH 5.

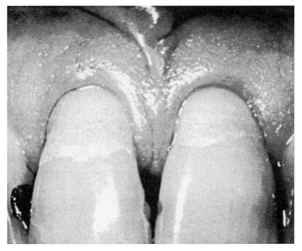

Fig. 16-21 Crazed, chalky surface on glass ionomer restorations resulting from inadequate protection of the cement during its maturation. (Courtesy of G. Mount.)

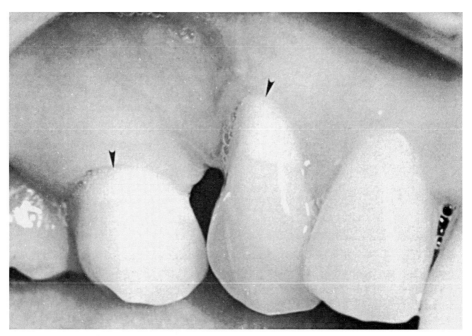

Fig. 16-22   Six-yr-old glass ionomer restorations, shown by **arrows.** A conservative and aesthetic treatment for the eroded area. (Courtesy of G. Mount.)

Both metal-reinforced systems release appreciable amounts of fluoride initially, but the magnitude decreases substantially over time (Table 16-10). Less fluoride is released from the cermet cement, because a portion of the glass particle is metal-coated. For the admix cement, the metal filler particles may not bond well to the cement matrix; thus the filler-cement interfaces become additional surface areas for fluoride leaching.

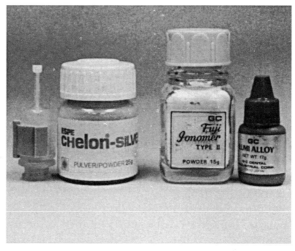

Fig. 16-23   Representative metal-reinforced glass ionomer cements. Cermet products are at **left.** At **right** is an admix of amalgam alloy added to Type II ionomer cement (Miracle Mix).

Table 16-10	Cumulative Fluoride Release from Various Glass Ionomer Products	
	Fluoride Released (μg)	
Cement Type	**14 Days**	**30 Days**
Type II glass ionomer	440	650
Cermet	200	300
Alloy admix glass ionomer (silver alloy admix)	3350	4040
Type I glass ionomer	470	700
Glass ionomer liner (conventional)	1000	1300
Glass ionomer liner (light-cured)	1200	1600

Clinical Considerations

The presence of metal fillers has made the material radiopaque and grayish in color. They have been suggested for limited use as an alternative to amalgam or composite for posterior restorations. However, clinical data indicate that these cements fall short of expectations. They exhibit frequent fracture when used for Class II restorations, as do the conventional glass ionomers. On the other hand, these cements harden rapidly, so they can be finished in a relatively short time. Along with their potential for adhesion and caries resistance, these characteristics have prompted the use of metal fillers for core buildup of teeth to be restored with cast crowns. However, a conservative approach should be taken because of their low fracture toughness and brittle nature. It is recommended that metal-reinforced GICs not be used wherever the cement will constitute greater than 40% of the total core buildup. Likewise, the auxiliary use of pins or other retention forms may be desirable.

CRITICAL QUESTION

For the atraumatic restorative treatment technique, why is a highly viscous GIC the most appropriate material?

HIGHLY VISCOUS CONVENTIONAL GLASS IONOMER CEMENT

Modern restorative dentistry requires an assortment of auxiliary equipment, such as water, electricity, and power-driven tools, to support various procedures. Unfortunately, basic restorative procedures that are common in industrialized countries are not possible in disadvantaged countries that lack the infrastructure to provide water, electricity, and equipment to remote areas. In such areas, practitioners often rely on the **atraumatic restorative treatment (ART)** technique, which was designed to retain as many teeth as possible under these adverse circumstances. Only hand instruments are used to remove carious tissue. Caries removal with hand instruments is often incomplete, increasing the risk for secondary caries. Materials that bond chemically to tooth structure are needed as cavity restoratives or as pit and fissure sealants. Glass ionomer, because of its adhesiveness and release of fluoride, is the natural choice to fill that gap. In addition, placing ART as a filling and as a sealing material using a GIC relies on a technique of pressing the material into the excavated tooth cavities and to pits and fissures, in contrast to the flow technique used with resin-based sealant. To simplify insertion of the material in a manner similar to that used for amalgam, a highly viscous version of glass ionomer is available.

The clinical procedures in the ART technique include the following: (1) isolating the tooth with cotton rolls, (2) obtaining access to the carious lesion with hand instruments, (3) removing the carious tissue with an excavator, (4) placing the highly viscous GIC restorative materials, and (5) removing excess cement. Ideally, the tooth surface should be prepared with a weak acid to enhance chemical bonding to the GIC. However, air-water spray and suction equipment are not available in remote areas where this technique has often been used.

Results of a recent study indicated that the survival rate of partially and fully retained single-surface restorations on permanent teeth was 99% after 1 yr and 88% after 3 yr. The same study showed that the partial and full retention of sealants in the permanent dentition were 90% after 1 yr and 71% after 3 yr.

Because the ART approach is based on the sound concept of maximum prevention, minimal surgical intervention, and minimal tooth preparation, these materials should be considered as fillings in deciduous teeth and as intermediate restorations of permanent posterior teeth. This material should provide better protection of the restored tooth than nonfluoridated materials. Recent introduction of encapsulated versions of these materials will facilitate the use of these materials and should increase their acceptance (Fig. 16-24).

RESIN-MODIFIED GLASS IONOMER CEMENT (HYBRID IONOMER)

Moisture sensitivity and low early strength of GICs are the result of slow acid-base setting reactions. Polymerizable functional groups can be added to impart more rapid curing when activated by light or chemicals to overcome these two inherent drawbacks and still allow the acid-base reaction to take its course long after polymerization. These products are considered to be dual-cure cements if only one polymerization mechanism is used; if both mechanisms are used, they are considered tri-cure cements. These materials are classified as resin-modified glass ionomers or hybrid ionomers (Fig. 16-25).

Depending on the manufacturer's formulation and P/L ratios, clinical applications of resin-modified glass ionomers include their use as liners, fissure sealants, bases, core buildups, restoratives, adhesives for orthodontic brackets, repair materials for damaged amalgam cores or cusps, and retrograde root-filling materials.

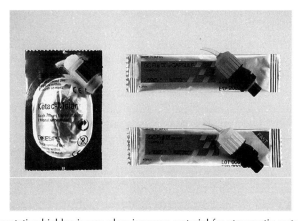

Fig. 16-24 Representative highly viscous glass ionomer material for atraumatic restorative treatment applications.

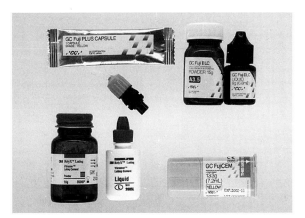

Fig. 16-25   Representative commercial resin-modified glass ionomer cements.

For these applications, surface conditioning of the tooth structure with a mild acid is still essential for bond formation.

Composition and Setting Reactions

The powder component consists of ion-leachable fluoroaluminosilicate glass particles and initiators for light curing and/or chemical curing. The liquid component usually contains water and polyacrylic acid or polyacrylic acid modified with methacrylate and hydroxyethyl methacrylate (HEMA) monomers. The last two components are responsible for polymerization. The initial setting reaction of the material occurs by the polymerization of methacrylate groups. The slow acid-base reaction will ultimately be responsible for the unique maturing process and the final strength. The overall water content is less for this type of material to accommodate the polymerizable ingredients.

Characteristics of Hybrid Ionomer Cements

One noted change from conventional glass ionomer is the improvement of translucency because the inclusion of monomer brings the refractive index of the liquid close to that of the particle. In vitro testing of resin-modified GIC (hybrid GIC) indicates a fluoride release at the same level as conventional GICs. The diametral tensile strengths of hybrid glass ionomers are higher than those of conventional GICs (see Table 16-8). This increase in strength is mainly attributable to their lower elastic modulus and the greater amount of plastic deformation that can be sustained before fracture occurs. Other properties are difficult to compare because of differences in material formulations and in testing protocols.

The mechanism for bonding to tooth structure is the same as that for conventional GICs. Less ionic activity is expected because of the reduction in carboxylic acid in the liquid of resin-modified glass ionomers; however, their bond strength to tooth structure can be higher than that of conventional GICs. Compared with conventional glass ionomers, resin-modified glass ionomers exhibit a higher bond strength to resin-based composites. It is likely controlled by the residual nonpolymerized functional groups within the former material.

Polymerization results in a greater degree of shrinkage upon setting. Lower water and carboxylic acid content also reduce the ability of the cement to wet the tooth substrates, which can greatly increase microleakage compared with conventional glass ionomers.

The biocompatibility of hybrid glass ionomers is comparable to that of conventional glass ionomers. Similar precautions should be followed, such as the use of calcium hydroxide for deep preparations. The transient temperature increase associated with the polymerization process may also be a concern.

Fissure Sealant Application

The traditional GIC is somewhat viscous, which prevents penetration to the depth of the fissures. The use of glass ionomers in sealant therapy may increase as less viscous formulations become available. One clinical study shows that the retention rate of glass ionomer sealant is poor after 1 yr, but no signs of carious lesions were observed. Close examination of the occlusal surface revealed that patches of GIC were retained within the fissures.

Liner/Base Applications

The handling characteristics of hybrid glass ionomers have been adjusted so that they can be used either as a liner or a base. The compressive and tensile strengths of liners are lower than those of the restorative cements. The primary purpose of a glass ionomer liner is to serve as an intermediate bonding material between the tooth and composite restoration. As a result of the adhesion to dentin, it tends to reduce the probability of gap formation at gingival margins located in dentin, cementum, or both caused by polymerization shrinkage of the resin.

The advantage of glass ionomer over resin bonding agents lies in the proven adhesive bond, reduced technique sensitivity, and an established anticariogenic mechanism by fluoride release (see Table 16-10). When it is used in this context, this procedure is often referred to as the **sandwich technique.** This technique takes advantage of the desirable qualities of the glass ionomer yet provides the aesthetics of the composite restoration. The sandwich technique is recommended for Class II and V composite restorations when individual patients are at a moderate to high risk for caries. They are available both as conventional GIC and light-curable hybrid GIC formulations (Fig. 16-26).

COMPOMER

The search for a material that has the fluoride-releasing capability of conventional glass ionomer and the durability of composites has led to the introduction of

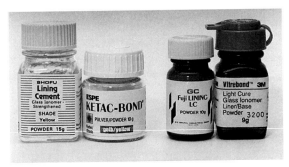

Fig. 16-26　Commercial glass ionomer liners. The two at left are based on the conventional powder/liquid system, whereas the two at right are light-cured.

polyacid-modified composite, or compomer. This material has a structure and physical properties similar to those of composites. It also has the ability to release fluoride, and it undergoes an acid-base reaction in the presence of saliva.

CRITICAL QUESTION

Resin-modified glass ionomers and one-paste compomers exhibit both polymerization and acid-base reactions. What is the difference in the role of the acid-base reaction for each material?

Composition and Chemistry

Compomer is usually provided as a one-paste, light-curable material for restorative applications (Fig. 16-27). It consists of silicate glass particles, sodium fluoride, and polyacid-modified monomer without any water. It is sensitive to moisture, so it is often packaged in a moisture-proof pouch. Setting is initiated by photopolymerization of the acidic monomer that yields a rigid material. During the service life of the restoration, the set material begins to absorb water in the saliva that contributes the acid-base reaction between the acidic functional groups within the matrix and silicate glass particles. It is this acid-base reaction induced by water absorption that eventually sustains fluoride release. Because of the absence of water in the formulation, the cement mixture is not **self-adhesive** like conventional GIC and hybrid GIC. Thus a separate dentin-bonding agent is needed for compomers used as restoratives.

Recently, some two-component materials, consisting of powder and liquid or of two pastes, have been marketed as compomers for luting applications (see Fig. 16-27). The powder is composed of strontium aluminum fluorosilicate, metallic oxides, and chemically activated and/or light-activated initiators. The liquid contains polymerizable methacrylate/carboxylic acid monomers, multifunctional acrylate monomers, and water. The pastes have the same ingredients corresponding to those in the powder and liquid. Because of the presence of water in the liquid, these materials are self-adhesive and an acid-base reaction starts at the time of mixing.

Characteristics of Compomers

One-paste compomers used as a restorative material release less fluoride than do conventional and hybrid GICs. The bond strength of compomer to tooth structure

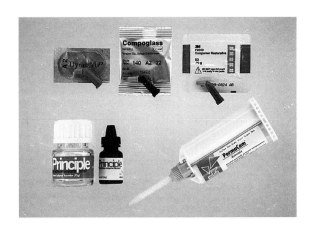

Fig. 16-27 Commercial compomer cement.

is in the same range as that of GIC to tooth structure because of the use of a dentin-bonding agent. Although the main application of a one-paste compomer is as a restorative for low-stress bearing areas, current clinical data are limited regarding the use of compomer to restore Class III and V cavities as an alternative to glass ionomer or resin-based composite. The two-component luting systems are indicated primarily for cementing of prostheses fabricated with a metallic substrate.

Manipulation of Compomers

For the one-paste system, the tooth structure should be etched before application of dentin-bonding agent and the cement. Finishing of the restoration requires the same process as that used for resin composites.

For the two-component luting system, the cement mixture is placed only on the prosthesis, and the prosthesis is seated with finger pressure. After 90 sec have elapsed from the end of mixing, the material should reach a gel state, at which time the excess cement is removed. The margin should be light-cured immediately to stabilize the prosthesis. The chemical cure should complete the setting reaction in approximately 3 min in the oral environment. It may take 10 min or more to set in ambient air.

RESIN CEMENTS

Resin cement has become attractive as a luting agent because of the development of direct-filling resins with improved properties, the benefit of the acid-etch technique for attaching resins to enamel, and the potential to bond to dentin conditioned with organic or inorganic acid. Some cements are designed for general use and others for specific uses, such as the cementation of ceramic crowns and fixed partial dentures (FPDs) and attachment of orthodontic brackets or resin-bonded crowns and FPDs. Resin cements are essentially flowable composites of low viscosity.

Composition and Chemistry

The composition of most current resin cements is similar to that of resin-based composite filling materials: a resin matrix with silane-treated inorganic fillers. The fillers are those used in composites, that is, silica or glass particles and/or colloidal silica used in microfilled resins. Except for anterior veneer tooth preparations that are made in enamel, the majority of a tooth surface prepared for a full crown is dentin. In the latter case, most resin cements require a dentin-bonding agent to promote adhesion to tooth structure. The adhesive monomer incorporated in the bonding agent and the resin cement includes HEMA, 4-META, and an organophosphate, such as 10-methacryloyloxydecamethylene phosphoric acid (MDP). This 4-META system is a liquid adhesive that acquires a cement consistency by incorporating polymer beads. No separate bonding agent is needed.

Polymerization can be achieved by a conventional chemical-cure system or by light activation. Several systems use both mechanisms and are referred to as *dual-cure systems* (Fig. 16-28).

Characteristics of Resin Cements

Resin cements as a group are virtually insoluble in oral fluids, but, as indicated in Table 16-3, there is a wide variation in the range of other properties from one

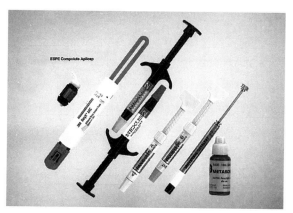

Fig. 16-28   Commercial resin cement.

product to another. These variations undoubtedly are associated with compositional differences, the diluent concentration, and filler contents.

With respect to bonding to dentin, resin cement should perform as well as resin-base composites. The monomeric component of the resin cements, which is the same as that used in restorative composites, is irritating to the pulp. Thus pulp protection with a calcium hydroxide or glass ionomer liner is important when the remaining dentin thickness is not sufficient (e.g., <0.5 mm) to prevent the infiltration of irritants.

Chemically activated resin cements are supplied as two-component systems, consisting of either a powder and a liquid or two pastes. The two components are combined by mixing on a paper pad for 20 to 30 sec. Removal of the excess cement is difficult if it is delayed until the cement has polymerized. It is best to remove the excess cement immediately after the prosthesis is seated. This cement is suitable for all types of prostheses.

Light-curable cements are single-component systems just as are the light-curable resin-based composites. They are indicated for cementation of thin ceramic prostheses, resin-based prostheses, and direct bonding of ceramic and plastic orthodontic brackets when the thickness of the appliance in the bonded area is less than 1.5 mm, thereby allowing adequate transmission of light. The required time of exposure to the light for polymerization of the resin cement depends on the intensity of the light transmitted through the ceramic restoration or bracket and the layer of polymeric cement. However, the time of exposure to the light should never be less than 40 sec. Excess cement should be removed as soon as seating is completed, unless the instructions for the specific resin cement indicate otherwise. For example, a 10-sec light exposure has been indicated in some instructions.

The dual-cure cements are two-component systems and require mixing in a manner similar to that used for chemically activated systems. Chemical activation is very slow and provides extended working time until the cement is exposed to the curing light, at which point the cement hardens rapidly. It then continues to gain strength over an extended period because of the chemically activated polymerization process. These dual-cure cements should not be used with light-transmitting prostheses thicker than 2.5 mm; anything thicker than 2.5 mm should be bonded with chemically curable cement. Removal of excess cement may proceed upon completion of seating or after waiting for a specific period as indicated in the instructions.

Manipulation

Resin cements are often designed for specific applications rather than general uses. They are formulated to provide the handling characteristics required for particular applications. The procedure for the tooth surface remains the same for each system, but the treatment of the prostheses differs depending on their composition.

Metallic Prostheses

The bondable surface of base metal can be roughened by grit blasting with 30- to 50-μm alumina particles at an air pressure of 0.4 to 0.7 MPa or by electrochemical etching. Some systems use a metal primer that contains an adhesive promoter. Naturally formed oxide on the base metal surface also contributes to the bonding when MDP- or 4-META–based resin is used. Noble metals used for metal-ceramic prosthesis do not form a stable oxide at room temperature. However, to enhance bonding, the clinician can electrochemically deposit a thin layer of tin, ($\sim$ 0.5 μm) on noble metal and heat it to an appropriate temperature to form a metal oxide. A silica coating can also be used to improve bonding to noble and base alloys. The bond strength values are in the same range as those resulting from grit blasting and electrochemical etching.

Orthodontic Brackets

The success of bonding orthodontic brackets depends on proper isolation and etching of the enamel surface and the bond between the tooth and the bracket. The tissue side of the bracket requires some means of mechanical retention, such as that available in the metal mesh of a metallic bracket. Bonding of resin to ceramic brackets is achieved either by etching the bracket and/or coating it with an organosilane analogous to the coupling agents employed to bond inorganic fillers to the resin matrix of resin-based composite. A plastic bracket, on the other hand, is primed with a solvent containing methylmethacrylate monomer.

The bond strength of the resin cement to tooth structure appears to be adequate if proper procedures are followed. Debonding of metal brackets often occurs at the cement/bracket interface. For plastic and ceramic brackets, failure often occurs at the wing of the brackets. A bonding agent is also needed for the etched enamel. Bracket removal is sometimes troublesome when the bond of the cement to the bracket and etched enamel is strong. When an attempt is made to pry the bracket from the tooth, the brittle ceramic bracket sometimes fractures and it may become necessary to remove remnants by grinding. Occasionally, fragments of enamel may fracture during removal of ceramic brackets.

Bonding of Resin-Based Veneers, Inlays, Onlays, Crowns, and Fixed Partial Dentures

Composites have been used to fabricate veneers and crowns; they are not strong enough for posterior full crown coverage, so their use is limited to long-term provisional crowns. During the 1980s and 1990s the wear resistance of composites significantly improved and their fracture toughness increased. Currently, several material systems are available to fabricate composite-based inlays, onlays, crowns, and bridges as final restorations. Special equipment and procedures are often required for processing these components. Depending on the cement of choice, the surface for bonding can be grit-blasted to increase roughness for bonding and/or it can be treated with a designated adhesive. This adhesive is often based on the same monomer that is used to fabricate the prosthesis. Sufficient time must be allowed for adequate penetration and diffusion to occur (e.g., 30 min) into the cross-linked network of the prosthesis.

Bonding of Ceramic Prostheses

Ceramic restorations can be quite translucent, and they require specific shades of luting cements to maximize their aesthetic appearance. Resin cements are the luting agent of choice for all-ceramic inlays, crowns, and bridges because of their ability to reduce fracture of the ceramic structures and because of the range of shades available to produce an optimal aesthetic appearance. The inner surfaces of ceramic prostheses with a glassy phase usually are etched and a silane coating may be applied before cementation to achieve optimal retention.

To assist the clinician in selecting the proper shade of cement, some systems provide water-soluble try-in materials with the same shades as the cements (Fig. 16-29). The material is applied like a cement, and the prosthesis is seated and examined in situ for its aesthetic appearance; after the proper shade has been selected, the residual try-in paste can be rinsed away with a water spray. This process can be repeated until the clinician is satisfied with the aesthetic appearance. The cementation process is then completed using a cement with the same shade after cleaning the try-in material from the preparation and the prosthesis.

ZINC OXIDE–EUGENOL CEMENT

These cements are usually dispensed in the form of zinc oxide powder and eugenol liquid or sometimes as two pastes. Their pH is approximately 7 at the time of placement, which potentially makes them the least irritating of all dental materials.

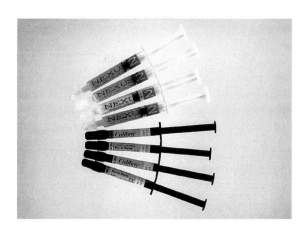

Fig. 16-29 Try-in gels.

Composition and Setting Chemistry

The chief ingredients of the cements are zinc oxide and eugenol. It is fairly well established that the setting mechanism for ZOE materials consists of zinc oxide hydrolysis and a subsequent reaction between zinc hydroxide and eugenol to form a chelate. Water is needed to initiate the reaction, and it is also a by-product of the reaction. This is why the reaction proceeds more rapidly in a humid environment. The setting reaction is also accelerated by the presence of zinc acetate dihydrate, which is more soluble than $Zn(OH)_2$ and which can supply zinc ions more rapidly. Acetic acid is a more active catalyst for the setting reaction than is water because it increases the formation rate of zinc hydroxide. High atmospheric temperature also accelerates the setting reaction.

There are numerous means by which the handling characteristics and physical properties of ZOE preparations can be altered. As a result, cements suitable for a wide range of uses are produced. The versatile uses of this material are reflected in ANSI/ADA Specification No. 30 (ISO 3107), which lists four types of cement. Type I ZOE cement is used for temporary cementation, and Type II cement is intended for long-term cementation of fixed prostheses. Type III cement is used for temporary fillings and thermal insulating bases, whereas Type IV cement is indicated for intermediate restorations. Varieties of ZOE cements also serve as root canal sealers and periodontal dressings.

CRITICAL QUESTION

Why does ZOE exhibit a faster setting rate when mixed on a chilled glass slab that has condensed water on its surface?

Characteristics of ZOE Cements

The higher the P/L ratio, the faster the material sets. Cooling a glass mixing slab slows the setting reaction unless the temperature is below the dew point. Below the dew point, water condensate is incorporated into the mix and the setting reaction is accelerated.

Particle size affects strength. In general, smaller particle sizes correspond to a stronger-set cement. The compressive strength of ZOE cement ranges from 3 to 55 MPa, depending on the intended use and individual formulation designed for each specific purpose.

Temporary ZOE Restorations (Type III)

Materials used for **temporary restorations** are expected to last for a few days to a few weeks at most. They can provide a temporary restorative treatment while the pulp heals or until a more long-lasting restoration can be fabricated and cemented.

Intermediate ZOE Restorations (Type IV)

Clinical experience with this type of material indicates that it can serve effectively as a restorative material for at least 1 yr. To achieve the properties necessary for this use, sufficient powder must be added to achieve a stiff, puttylike restorative consistency.

Temporary ZOE Luting Cement (Type I)

The strength of temporary cement must be sufficiently low to permit removal of the restoration without trauma to the teeth and damage to the restoration. It seals the cavity surprisingly well against the ingress of oral fluids, at least for a short time; hence irritation caused by microleakage is minimized. The presence of residual free eugenol from temporary luting cement is thought to interfere with the proper setting of resin-bonded composites; various types of carboxylic acids can be used to replace eugenol and produce a ZOE-like material. These products are called zinc oxide–noneugenol cements.

Long-Term ZOE Luting Cement (Type II)

Commercial cements largely have been based on two systems with improved strength and abrasion resistance. One system substitutes a part of the eugenol liquid with orthoethoxybenzoic acid (EBA) liquid, and alumina is added to the powder. The other system consists of a powder made up of 20 wt% to 40 wt% of fine polymer particles and zinc oxide particles that have been surface treated with carboxylic acid. The liquid used in this system is eugenol.

The compressive strength of these improved ZOE cements (see Table 16-3) is acceptable, but overall their strength values are inferior to those of other cements. The cements are also somewhat difficult to manipulate in the oral cavity. The film thickness of some products tends to be high, and the cement excess after setting may be quite difficult to remove. For these reasons, the use of ZOE cements for long-term applications has been confined primarily to those situations in which tooth sensitivity might be a problem. An excellent application for these cements is for short-term or intermediate-term luting of provisional acrylic crowns and fixed partial dentures. However, these cements should never be used for temporary cementation of final fixed prostheses because they would be difficult to remove without risking the integrity of the prepared teeth or the prosthesis.

CALCIUM HYDROXIDE

Calcium hydroxide is the chief ingredient in cavity liners. Reformulation of the materials has expanded its application as a cement base.

Cavity Liners

Calcium hydroxide, used as a cavity liner, is suspended in a solvent carrier with a thickening agent. When it is placed on the pulpal floor, the solvent evaporates and leaves a thin film of calcium hydroxide. The liner does not possess significant mechanical strength or thermal insulation capability, but it can neutralize acids that migrate toward the pulp and, in the process, it can induce the generation of reparative dentin.

Bases

The cements are usually produced as a two-paste system with radiopaque fillers; the setting reaction occurs between calcium hydroxide and salicylate, yielding calcium disalicylate. A one-component light-curable base is also available. It can be used to line the cavity, or it can be applied as a direct pulp-capping material.

CRITICAL QUESTION

Why is the standard laboratory solubility test of dental cements not capable of predicting their solubility resistance in the mouth?

SOLUBILITY AND DISINTEGRATION OF CEMENTS

With the exception of resin cements, an important requirement of dental cements is that they be resistant to solubility and disintegration in the oral cavity. If the luting cement dissolves or deteriorates so that fragments are lost from beneath a restoration, leakage ensues with subsequent adverse effects including sensitivity, caries, or both. Dissolution or disintegration of restorative cement results in the loss of surface material, which leads to eventual replacement of restorations.

Cements in the oral environment are continually exposed to a variety of acids produced by microorganisms during the breakdown of fermentable carbohydrates. Some of the acids are components of foods and drinks. Both the pH and temperature of the oral cavity fluctuate. This complexity of the oral environment, coupled with the fact that different cements behave in different ways, has hindered the development of a standard laboratory test to accurately predict the relative resistance to degradation of various cements in the mouth. ANSI/ADA Specification No. 96 describes the use of 0.1 M lactic acid/sodium lactate (pH = 2.74) to test the erosion rate of glass ionomer, zinc polycarboxylate, and zinc phosphate cements. The maximum allowable loss in 24 hr is 0.1 mm for GICs, 0.2 mm for zinc phosphate cement, and 0.3 mm for zinc polycarboxylate cement. The solubility of GIC by weight in distilled water is higher than that of any other cement, except for calcium hydroxide; the solubility decreases as the resin content increases. ANSI/ADA Specification 30 describes the maximum allowable disintegration of ZOE and zinc oxide–noneugenol cements in distilled water to be 2.5 wt% for Type I materials and 1.5 wt% for the other cements. Laboratory data show that their solubility is much lower than the limit allowed by the specification. Calcium hydroxide has the highest solubility; it ranges from 0.4 wt% to 7.8 wt% in distilled water in 24 hr. Properly cured resin cement is not soluble in oral fluid. Weight changes after immersion in water is caused by the leaching of the unreacted monomer or solubility of the filler particles.

Because of problems with in vitro tests, the most reliable data on the durability of cementing agents have been obtained in vivo by placing small specimens of the cements in intraoral appliances that can be removed from the mouth to measure the loss of material. In one study cements were inserted in tiny wells placed in the proximal surfaces of cast crown restorations. These crowns were cemented with temporary ZOE cement. After 1 yr, they were removed and the cement loss was measured. GIC exhibited the least degradation, followed in increasing order of degradation by zinc polycarboxylate cement, zinc phosphate cement, and zinc polycarboxylate cement mixed in a low P/L ratio. The relative disintegration rates of the cements apparently bear no relationship to the solubility data presented in Table 16-3. The solubility of zinc polycarboxylate cement, when it is mixed at the recommended P/L ratio, and zinc phosphate cement were not significantly different. However, a reduction in the amount of powder in the zinc polycarboxylate mixture produced a cement that disintegrated rapidly.

Another study that employed this test procedure revealed that the "permanent" ZOE cements exhibit more rapid degradation than either zinc phosphate or polycarboxylate cement.

SUMMARY

Zinc phosphate cement has long served as the universal luting cement. Its advantages include good handling characteristics and a proven longevity in the oral cavity when it is used for cementation of well-designed and well-fitting restorations. Its disadvantages include pulp irritation, lack of adhesiveness to tooth structure, and lack of anticariogenic properties. Zinc phosphate cement is not suitable when the mechanical retention is poor or when the aesthetic demand is high.

The main advantage of improved ZOE cements is their biocompatibility. The physical and mechanical properties and the handling characteristics generally are inferior to those of other long-term luting cements.

The properties of zinc polycarboxylate cements are good compared with those of zinc phosphate cement. The outstanding characteristics are their blandness to the pulp and formation of an adhesive bond to tooth structure. Disadvantages include the short working time and limited capability for fluoride release. Their short working time limits their use to single units or three-unit fixed partial dentures (bridges). These cements have decreased in popularity, but they are still often used for patients who have reported a history of postoperative sensitivity.

Glass ionomer luting cements bond to tooth structure and release fluoride. Compared with zinc phosphate cements, GICs show a greater resistance to disintegration in the oral cavity and comparable mechanical properties, with the exception of a lower elastic modulus. A primary disadvantage of these cements is the slow maturing process that is required to develop their ultimate strength. The translucency of GICs makes them useful for cementing ceramic prostheses. However, their low stiffness may allow excessive elastic deformation of the ceramic prosthesis, which may result in fracture of the brittle prosthesis. Nevertheless, the fluoride-releasing capability makes GIC the material of choice for the replacement of restorations that have failed because of secondary caries, and for patients living in areas where fluoridated drinking water is not available.

The durability of compomers is inferior to that of resin-based composites. Thus they should only be used for low-stress areas.

Resin cements are virtually insoluble in oral fluids, and their fracture toughness is higher than that of other cements. Through the use of bonding agents, resin cements bond to dentin and form a strong attachment to enamel. A primary problem of modern resin cements centers on the poor handling characteristics of some specialty resins. It is critical to remove the cement flash before the initial set or immediately after seating of the prosthesis or orthodontic attachment device. To ensure optimal performance, follow the instructions for the product. Resin cement can be used for all types of cementation, most notably for prostheses with poor retention and for all-ceramic prostheses when the demand for aesthetic "perfection" is very high. Although the elastic modulus of resin cements is generally lower than that of zinc phosphate cement, this deficiency does not appear to affect the fracture resistance of ceramic prostheses luted with resin cements.

Thus it is readily apparent that no single type of cement satisfies all the ideal characteristics. One system may be better suited to one task than another, and it is prudent for the dentist to have several types available. Each situation should be evaluated on the basis of the pertinent environmental, biological, and mechanical factors. This chapter provides a framework for making appropriate clinical decisions for use of the cement system that is best suited for each specific case.

SELECTED READINGS

American Dental Association Council on Scientific Affairs: Products of excellence. J Am Dent Assoc 129(suppl):1, 1998.

Balderamos LP, O'Keefe KL, and Powers JM: Color accuracy of resin cements and try-in paste. Int J Prosthodont 10:111, 1997.

Berekally TL, Makinson OF, and Pietrobon RA: A microscopic examination of bond surfaces in failed electrolytically etched cast metal fixed prostheses. Aust Dent J 38:229, 1993.

Blalock KA, and Powers IM: Retention capacity of the bracket bases of new esthetic orthodontic brackets. Am J Orthod Dentofac Orthop 107:596, 1995.

Costa CAS, Mesas AN, and Hebling J: Pulp response to direct capping with an adhesive system. Am J Dent 13:81, 2000.

Crisp S, Kent BE, Lewis BG et al: Glass ionomer cement formulations. II. The synthesis of novel polycarboxylic acids. J Dent Res 59:1055, 1980.

Davidson CL, and Mjör IA (eds): Advances in Glass Ionomer Cements. Chicago, Quintessence, 1999.

Forsten L: Fluoride release from a glass ionomer cement. Scand J Dent Res 85:503, 1977.

Goldman M: Fracture properties of composite and glass ionomer dental restorative materials. J Biomed Mater Res 19:771, 1985.

Hilton TJ: Cavity sealers, liners, and bases: Current philosophies and indications for use. Oper Dent 21:134, 1996.

Hunt TR (ed): The Next Generation: Proceedings of the 2nd International Symposium on Glass Ionomers. Philadelphia, 1994.

Knibbs PJ, and Walls AWG: A laboratory and clinical evaluation of three dental luting cements. J Oral Rehabil 16:467, 1989.

McKinney JE, Antonucci JM, and Rupp NW: Wear and microhardness of a silver-sintered glass ionomer cement. J Dent Res 67:831, 1988.

McLean JW: Limitations of posterior composite resins and extending their use with glass ionomer cements. Quintessence Int 18:517, 1987.

Mennemeyer VA, Neuman P, and Powers JM: Bonding of hybrid ionomers and, resin cements to modified orthodontic band materials. Am J Orthod Dentofac Orthop 115:143, 1999.

Mount GJ: An Atlas of Glass Ionomer Cements. London, Martin Dumitz, 1990.

O'Keefe KL, Miller BH, and Powers JM: In vitro tensile bond strength of adhesive cements to new post materials. Int J Prosthodont 13:47, 2000.

Pameijer CH, and Nilner K: Long-term clinical evaluation of three luting materials. Swed Dent J 18:59, 1994.

Phillips RW, Crim G, Swartz ML, and Clark HE: Resistance of calcium hydroxide preparations to solubility in phosphoric acid. J Prosthet Dent 52:358, 1984.

Phillips RW, Swartz ML, Lund MS, et al: In vivo disintegration of luting agents. J Am Dent Assoc 114:489, 1987.

Powis DR, Folleras T, Merson SA, and Wilson AD: Improved adhesion of a glass ionomer cement to dentin and enamel. J Dent Res 61:1416, 1982.

Sasanaluckit P, Albustany KR, Doherty PJ, and Williams DF: Biocompatibility of glass ionomer cements. Biomaterials 14:906, 1993.

Sidhu SK, and Watson TF: Resin-modified Glass Ionomer materials—A status report for the American Journal of Dentistry. Am J Dent 8:59-67, 1994.

Sipahier M, and Ulusu T: Glass-ionomer-cermet cements applied as fissure sealants—II. Clinical evaluation. Quintessence Int 26(1):43-47, 1995.

Smith DC, and Ruse ND: Acidity of glass ionomer cements during setting and its relation to pulp sensitivity. J Am Dent Assoc 112:654, 1986.

Swartz ML, Phillips RW, and Clark HE: Long-term F release from glass ionomer cements. J Dent Res 63:158, 1984.

Ten Cate JW, and Featherstone JD: Mechanistic aspect of the interactions between fluoride and dental enamel. Crit Rev Oral Biol Med, 2:283-296, 1991.

Wefel, JS: Effects of fluoride on caries development and progression using intra-oral models. J Dent Res 69:626-636, 1990.

Welburg RR, McCabe JF, Murray JJ, and Rusby S: Factors affecting the bond strength of composite resin to etched glass ionomer cement. J Dent 16:188, 1988.

Wilson AD, and McLean JW: Glass Ionomer Cements. Chicago, Quintessence, 1988.

Wolff MS, Barretto MT, Gale EN, et al: The effect of the powder-liquid ratio on in vivo solubility of zinc phosphate and polycarboxylate cements. J Dent Res 64:316, 1985.

17

Dental Amalgams

Sally J. Marshall, Grayson W. Marshall Jr., and Kenneth J. Anusavice

OUTLINE

Alloy Composition

Manufacture of Alloy Powder

Amalgamation and Resulting Microstructures

Dimensional Stability

Strength

Creep

Clinical Performance of Amalgam Restorations

Factors Affecting the Success of Amalgam Restorations

Mercury/Alloy Ratio

Mechanical Trituration

Condensation

Carving and Finishing

Clinical Significance of Dimensional Change

Side Effects of Mercury

Marginal Deterioration

Repaired Amalgam Restorations

KEY TERMS

Alloy for dental amalgam—See *dental amalgam alloy.*

Amalgam—An alloy containing mercury.

Amalgamation—The process of mixing liquid mercury with one or more metals or alloys to form an amalgam.

Creep—The time-dependent strain or deformation that is produced by a stress. The creep process can cause an amalgam restoration to extend out of the cavity preparation, thereby increasing its susceptibility to marginal breakdown.

Delayed expansion—The gradual expansion of a zinc-containing amalgam over weeks to months, which is associated with hydrogen gas development caused by contamination of the plastic mass with moisture during its manipulation in a cavity preparation.

Dental amalgam—An alloy of mercury, silver, copper, and tin, which may also contain palladium, zinc, and other elements to improve handling characteristics and clinical performance. The general term *amalgam* is also used as a synonym by the dental profession.

Dental amalgam alloy—An alloy of silver, copper, tin, and other elements that is formulated and processed in the form of powder particles or as a compressed pellet. Also known as *alloy for dental amalgam.*

KEY TERMS—cont'd

Marginal breakdown—The gradual fracture of the perimeter or margin of a dental amalgam restoration that leads to the formation of gaps or ditching at the external interfacial region between the amalgam and the tooth.

Trituration—The process of grinding powder, especially within a liquid. In dentistry, the term is used to describe the process of mixing the amalgam alloy particles with mercury in an amalgamator.

CRITICAL QUESTION

After reacting with liquid mercury, how do some or all of the original powder particles become structural components of the set dental amalgams?

An **amalgam** is an alloy that contains mercury as one of its constituents. Because mercury is liquid at room temperature, it can be alloyed with solid metals. The process of **amalgamation** in a clinic consists of releasing mercury droplets from a sealed chamber within a capsule into another chamber within the capsule that contains an alloy powder and then mixing the components together in a device called an *amalgamator*. The amalgamation process continues while segments of the plastic mass are condensed under firm pressure against the walls of prepared teeth and, if present, a matrix band. The reaction continues during the manipulation period in the mouth and decreases within a few minutes as the **dental amalgam** increases in strength and hardness. Although the reaction can continue for several days, the dental amalgam becomes sufficiently strong to support moderate biting forces within the first hour.

The general descriptive reaction is as follows:

$$\text{Alloy Particles for Amalgam} + \text{Mercury} \rightarrow$$
$$\text{Dental Amalgam} + \text{Nonreacted Alloy Powder Particles} \qquad (1)$$

ALLOY COMPOSITION

American National Standards Institute (ANSI)/American Dental Association (ADA) Specification No. 1 requires that amalgam alloys contain predominantly silver and tin. Unspecified amounts of other elements, for example, copper, zinc, gold, and mercury, are allowed in concentrations less than the silver or tin content. Alloys that contain in excess of 0.01% zinc are required to be designated as *zinc-containing alloys* for dental amalgam. Alloys that contain 0.01% zinc or less are designated as *nonzinc alloys* for dental amalgam. There is no specification for a low- or high-copper alloy per se.

It is less common to use the silver-tin alloys (low-copper alloys) of G.V. Black in preparing amalgam restorations. Nevertheless, the silver-tin alloy is still important for amalgam because a silver-tin alloy powder makes up the largest part of many high-copper alloy powders. Therefore it is important to understand the characteristics of both low-copper and high-copper alloys.

Before these alloys combine with mercury, they are known as **dental amalgam alloys** or **alloys for dental amalgam.** Historically, amalgam alloys contained at least 65 wt% silver, 29 wt% tin, and less than 6 wt% copper, a composition close to that recommended by G.V. Black in 1896. During the 1970s, many amalgam alloys containing between 6 wt% and 30 wt% copper were developed. Many of these high-copper alloys produce amalgams (high-copper amalgams) that are superior in many respects to the traditional low-copper amalgams.

To produce dental amalgam, mercury is mixed with a powder of the amalgam alloy. The powder may be produced by milling or lathe cutting a cast ingot of the amalgam alloy. The particles of this lathe-cut powder are irregularly shaped, as seen in Figure 17-1. Alternatively, the powder may be produced by atomizing the liquid alloy, thereby producing essentially spherical particles. As can be seen in Figure 17-2, they may not be true spheres and can even have an oblong shape, depending on the atomizing and solidification technique that is employed. The alloy also may be supplied as a mixture of lathe-cut and spherical particles.

The powder may also be supplied in the form of pellets. In this case, the fine particles are subjected to pressure sufficient to cause them to form a "skin" over the outside of the pellet and to cohere slightly on the inside. Yet the cohesion is not so great that the particles cannot be readily separated when they are properly amalgamated.

Amalgam alloy is mixed with mercury by the dentist or the assistant. In dentistry, the mixing procedure is technically known as **trituration.** The product of trituration is a plastic mass similar to the one that occurs in the melt of alloys between the liquidus and solidus temperatures. Special instruments are used to force the plastic mass into the prepared cavity by a process known as *condensation.* The complete technique is discussed in detail later in this chapter.

During trituration of an alloy powder with mercury, the mercury dissolves the surface of alloy particles, and some new phases form. These new phases have melting points well above any temperature that might normally occur in the mouth. The transformation of the mercury-powder mixture to a composite plastic mass is followed by the setting and hardening of the amalgam as the liquid mercury is consumed in the formation of new solid phases.

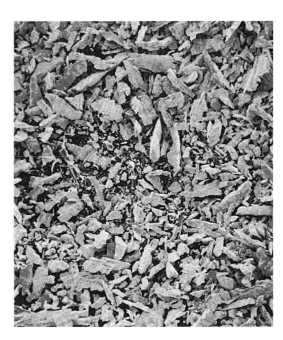

Fig. 17-1 Particles of a conventional lathe-cut amalgam alloy. (×100.)

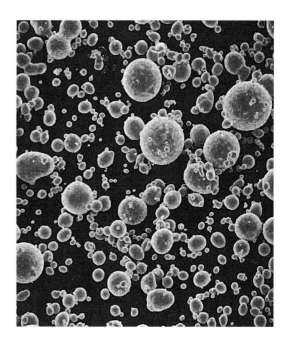

Fig. 17-2 Particles of a spherical amalgam alloy. (×500.)

The clinical success of the amalgam restoration is based on meticulous attention to detail. Each manipulative step from the time the cavity is prepared until the restoration has been polished can have an effect on the physical and chemical properties of the amalgam and the success or failure of the restoration. Violation of the fundamental principles of cavity preparation has contributed substantially to failure. These matters are treated in operative dentistry texts. The following discussions are concerned with failures associated with the alloy itself and its manipulation.

In a sense, the dentist and the dental assistant (or dental nurse) produce dental amalgam. The two components, the alloy and the mercury, are purchased. In the process of combining the alloy and mercury and producing the restoration, the dental amalgam is formed. The manner in which this is accomplished controls the properties and performance of the amalgam.

The factors governing the quality of a dental amalgam restoration can be divided into two groups: those that can be controlled by the dentist and those that are under the control of the manufacturer. The factors governed by the dentist are (1) selection of an alloy, (2) mercury/alloy ratio, (3) trituration procedures, (4) condensation technique, (5) marginal integrity, (6) anatomical characteristics, and (7) final finish. Because many modern amalgam alloys are furnished by manufacturers in a capsule containing both alloy and mercury, selection of a specific pre-encapsulated alloy results in selection of the mercury/alloy ratio as well.

The manufacturer controls (1) the composition of the alloy; (2) the heat treatment of the alloy; (3) the size, shape, and method of production of the alloy particles; (4) the surface treatment of the particles; and (5) the form in which the alloy is supplied.

CRITICAL QUESTION

Why is zinc a beneficial additive to alloy for dental amalgam, but also a component that can potentially cause significant postoperative discomfort to the patient?

Table 17-1	Symbols and Stoichiometry of Phases that Are Involved in the Setting of Dental Amalgams
Phases in amalgam alloys and set dental amalgams*	**Stoichiometric formula**
γ	Ag_3Sn
γ_1	Ag_2Hg_3
γ_2	$Sn_{7-8}Hg$
ε	Cu_3Sn
η	Cu_6Sn_5
Silver-copper eutectic	Ag-Cu

*The Greek letters are named as follows: γ (gamma); ε (epsilon); η (eta).

Metallurgical Phases in Dental Amalgams

The setting reactions of alloys for dental amalgam with mercury are usually described by the metallurgical phases that are involved. These phases are named with Greek letters that correspond to the symbols found in the phase (constitution) diagram for each alloy system. The Greek letters and stoichiometric information for these phases are provided in Table 17-1 to facilitate the reader's understanding of subsequent sections.

The Silver-Tin System

Figure 17-3 is an equilibrium phase diagram of the silver-tin alloy system. Because silver and tin make up the major portion of amalgam alloys, the phase relations shown in this diagram are found in many amalgam alloys.

The low-copper alloys have a narrow range of compositions that fall within the β (beta) + γ (gamma) and the γ areas of the diagram shown in Figure 17-3. These areas are enclosed by the lines ABCDE. At point C is the intermetallic compound Ag_3Sn, the γ phase, which forms by a peritectic reaction (see Chapter 6) from the liquid plus β area above it. The more silver-rich β phase is crystallographically similar to the γ phase.

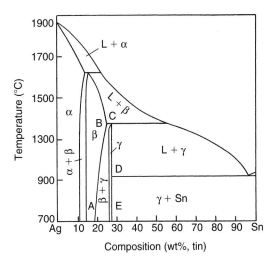

Fig. 17-3 Equilibrium phase diagram of the silver-tin system.

The Influence of Ag-Sn Phases on Amalgam Properties

In the range of compositions near the γ phase, increases or decreases of silver influence the amounts of β and γ phases formed and the properties of the amalgam. Most commercial alloys fall within the limited composition range of B to C and are not exactly at the peritectic composition (point C). Because the effect of these phases is relatively pronounced, their control is essential if an alloy of uniform quality is to be produced.

If the tin concentration exceeds 26.8 wt%, a mixture of γ and tin-rich phases is formed. Presence of the tin-rich phase increases the amount of the tin-mercury phase formed when the alloy is amalgamated. The tin-mercury phase lacks corrosion resistance and is the weakest component of the dental amalgam. However, amalgams of tin-rich alloys display less expansion than silver-rich alloys.

Silver-tin alloys are quite brittle and difficult to comminute uniformly unless a small amount of copper is substituted for silver. This atomic replacement is limited to about 4 wt% to 5 wt%, above which Cu_3Sn is formed. Within the limited range of copper solubility, an increased copper content hardens and strengthens the silver-tin alloy.

The use of zinc in an amalgam alloy is a subject of controversy. Zinc is seldom present in an alloy to an extent greater than 1 wt%. Alloys without zinc are more brittle, and their amalgams tend to be less plastic during condensation and carving. The chief function of zinc in amalgam alloys is that of a deoxidizer. It acts as a scavenger during melting, uniting with oxygen to minimize the formation of other oxides. Zinc may have some beneficial effects related to early corrosion and marginal integrity, as shown in clinical trials. It is unfortunate that zinc, even in small amounts, causes an abnormal expansion of the amalgam over time as a result of the incorporation of water into the amalgam during condensation. This phenomenon is discussed later in the chapter.

The ANSI/ADA specification for amalgam alloys allows mercury to be incorporated in the alloy powder. Some preamalgamated alloys are sold in Europe, but they have not been marketed extensively in the United States. Other elements may be included in the amalgam alloy if clinical and biological data show that the alloy is safe to use in the mouth. Small amounts of indium or palladium have been included in some commercial systems.

MANUFACTURE OF ALLOY POWDER
Lathe-Cut Powder

To produce lathe-cut powder, an annealed ingot of alloy is placed in a milling machine or in a lathe and is fed into a cutting tool or bit. The chips removed are often needlelike, and some manufacturers reduce the chip size by ball-milling.

Homogenizing Anneal

Because of the rapid cooling conditions from the as-cast state, an ingot of a silver-tin alloy has a cored structure and contains nonhomogeneous grains of varying composition. A homogenizing heat treatment is performed to reestablish the equilibrium phase relationship (see Chapter 6). The ingot is placed in an oven and heated at a temperature below the solidus for a sufficient time to allow diffusion of the atoms to occur and the phases to reach equilibrium. The time of heat treatment may vary depending on the temperature used and the size of the ingot, but 24 hr at the selected temperature is not unusual.

At the conclusion of the heating cycle, the ingot is brought to room temperature for the succeeding steps in manufacture. The manner in which the ingot is cooled influences the proportion of phases present in the ingot after cooling. If the ingot is withdrawn from the heat treatment oven rapidly and then quickly quenched, the phase distribution remains essentially unchanged. On the other hand, if the ingot is permitted to cool very slowly, the proportions of phases continue to adjust toward the room temperature equilibrium ratio. For example, in an Ag-Sn alloy, rapid quenching of the alloy ingot results in the maximum amount of β phase retained, whereas slow cooling results in the formation of the maximum amount of the γ phase.

Particle Treatments

Once the alloy ingot has been reduced to lathe-cut segments, many manufacturers perform some type of surface treatment of the particles. Although specific treatments are proprietary, treatment of the alloy particles with acid has been a manufacturing practice for many years. The exact function of this treatment is not entirely understood, but it is probably related to the preferential dissolution of specific components from the alloy. Amalgams made from acid-washed powders tend to be more reactive than those made from unwashed powders.

The stresses induced into the particle during cutting and ball-milling must be relieved or they will slowly decrease over time, causing a change in the alloy characteristics, particularly in the amalgamation rate and the dimensional change occurring during hardening. The stress-relief process involves an annealing cycle at a moderate temperature, usually for several hours at approximately 100° C. The alloy is generally then stable in its reactivity and properties when it is stored for an indefinite time.

Atomized Powder

Atomized powder is made by melting together the desired elements. The liquid metal is atomized into fine spherical droplets of metal. If the droplets solidify before hitting a surface, the spherical shape is preserved; these atomized powders are frequently called *spherical powders.* Like the lathe-cut powders, spherical powders are given a heat treatment that coarsens the grains and slows the reaction of the particles with mercury. As with the lathe-cut alloys, spherical powders are usually washed with acid.

Particle Size

Maximum particle size and the distribution of sizes within an alloy powder are controlled by the manufacturer. The average particle sizes of modern powders range between 15 and 35 μm. The most significant influence on amalgam properties is the distribution of sizes around the mean value. For example, very small particles (less than 3 μm) greatly increase the surface area per unit volume of the powder. A powder containing tiny particles requires a greater amount of mercury to form an acceptable amalgam.

In producing lathe-cut alloys, the cutting rate is precisely controlled to maintain the desired average particle size and size distribution. Similarly, parameters of the atomizing process are controlled to produce the desired particle sizes of spherical alloys. The particles may be graded according to size and the graded particles remixed to produce a powder with an optimum size distribution. The present trend in amalgam technique favors the use of a small average particle size, which tends to produce a more rapid hardening of the amalgam with greater early strength.

As is discussed in more detail later, the bulk of the finished restoration is composed of particles of the original alloy surrounded by reaction products. The particle size distribution can affect the character of the finished surface. When the amalgam has partially hardened, the tooth anatomy is carved in the amalgam with a sharp instrument. During this carving, the larger particles may be pulled out of the matrix, producing a rough surface. Such a surface is probably more susceptible to corrosion than a smooth surface.

Lathe-Cut Powder Compared with Atomized Spherical Powder

Amalgams made from lathe-cut powders, or admixed powders of a blend of lathe-cut and spherical powders, tend to resist condensation better than amalgams made entirely from spherical powders. Because amalgams of spherical powders are very plastic, the clinician cannot rely on the pressure of condensation to establish proximal contour. A contoured and wedged matrix band is essential to prevent flat proximal contours, improper contacts, and overhanging cervical margins. Good technique requires a matrix band, regardless of the amalgam's resistance to condensation.

Spherical alloys require less mercury than typical lathe-cut alloys because spherical alloy powder particles have a smaller surface area per volume than do the lathe-cut alloy particles. Amalgams with a low mercury content generally have better properties.

CRITICAL QUESTION

Through what mechanism does the addition of 6 wt% or more of copper prevent the formation of the undesirable γ_2 phase?

AMALGAMATION AND RESULTING MICROSTRUCTURES
Low-Copper Alloys

Amalgamation occurs when mercury contacts the surface of the silver-tin alloy particles. When a powder is triturated, the silver and tin in the outer portion of the particles dissolve into mercury. At the same time, mercury diffuses into the alloy particles. The mercury has a limited solubility for silver (0.035 wt%) and tin (0.6 wt%).

When the solubility in mercury is exceeded, crystals of two binary metallic compounds precipitate into the mercury. These are the body-centered cubic Ag_2Hg_3 (γ_1) phase and the hexagonal $Sn_{7-8}Hg$ (γ_2) phase. Because the solubility of silver in mercury is much lower than that of tin, the γ_1 phase precipitates first, and the γ_2 phase precipitates later.

Immediately after trituration, the alloy powder coexists with the liquid mercury, giving the mix a plastic consistency. γ_1 and γ_2 crystals grow as the remaining mercury dissolves the alloy particles. As the mercury disappears, the amalgam hardens. As the particles become covered with newly formed crystals, mostly the γ_1 phase (Ag_2Hg_3), the reaction rate decreases. The alloy is usually mixed with mercury in about a 1:1 ratio. This is insufficient mercury to completely consume original alloy particles; consequently, unconsumed particles are present in the set amalgam. Alloy particles (smaller now, because their surfaces have dissolved in mercury) are surrounded and bound together by solid γ_1 and γ_2 crystals.

Thus a typical low-copper amalgam is a composite in which the unconsumed particles are embedded in γ_1 and γ_2 phases. The sequence of amalgamation of the silver-tin alloy is shown schematically in Figure 17-4.

The micrograph shown in Figure 17-5 illustrates the features found in a typical amalgam made from a lathe-cut, low-copper alloy. The features include the remaining alloy particles of β and γ Ag-Sn phases (larger dark gray areas labeled P), ε (Cu$_3$Sn) particle (black area labeled E), γ_1 (Ag$_2$Hg$_3$) phase (labeled G1), γ_2 (Sn$_{7\text{-}8}$Hg) grains (labeled G2), and voids (left center and right center areas labeled V). These voids are always formed during γ_1 and γ_2 crystal growth when amalgam is condensed by the usual methods. The reaction can be conveniently expressed in terms of the phases that form during amalgamation:

$$\text{ALLOY PARTICLES } (\beta + \gamma) + \text{Hg} \rightarrow$$
$$\gamma_1 + \gamma_2 + \text{UNCONSUMED ALLOY PARTICLES } (\beta + \gamma) \qquad (2)$$

The physical properties of the hardened amalgam depend on the relative percentages of each of the microstructural phases. The more unconsumed Ag-Sn particles that are retained in the final structure, the stronger the amalgam. The weakest

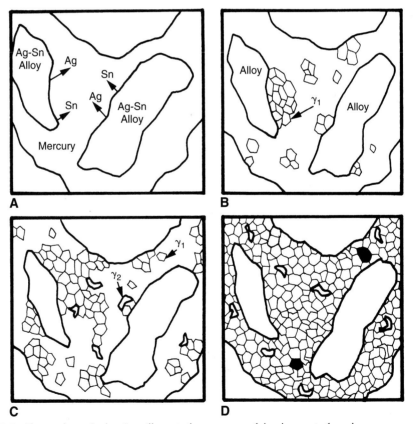

Fig. 17-4 These schematic drawings illustrate the sequence of development of amalgam microstructure when lathe-cut low-copper alloy particles are mixed with mercury. **A,** Dissolution of silver and tin into mercury. **B,** Precipitation of γ_1 crystals in the mercury. **C,** Consumption of the remaining mercury by growth of γ_1 and γ_2 grains. **D,** The final set amalgam. (Courtesy of T. Okabe, R. Mitchell, and C.W. Fairhurst.)

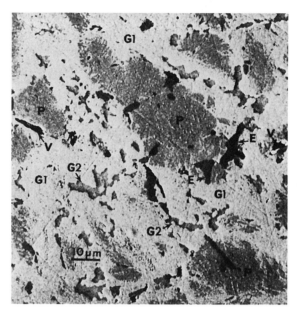

Fig. 17-5 A scanning electron micrograph of a low-copper silver-tin amalgam. (×1000.) (Courtesy of T. Okabe and M.B. Butts.)

component is the γ_2 phase. The hardness of γ_2 is approximately 10% of the hardness of γ_1, whereas the γ phase hardness is somewhat higher than that of γ_1.

The γ_2 phase is also the least stable in a corrosive environment and may suffer corrosion attack, especially in "crevices" of the restorations. In general, γ (Ag$_3$Sn) and pure γ_1 (Ag$_2$Hg$_3$) phases are stable in an oral environment. However, γ_1 in amalgam does contain small amounts of tin, which can be lost in a corrosive environment.

The interface between the γ phase and the γ_1 matrix is important. The high proportion of the unconsumed γ phase will not strengthen the amalgam unless the particles are bound to the matrix.

CRITICAL QUESTION

Compared with amalgams made from admixed high-copper alloys, what are the benefits and risks associated with amalgams made from high-copper, single composition, spherical particles?

High-Copper Alloys

Compared with traditional low-copper amalgams, high-copper amalgams have become the materials of choice because of their improved mechanical properties, corrosion characteristics, better marginal integrity, and improved performance in clinical trials. Two different types of high-copper alloy powders are available. The first is an admixed alloy powder, and the second is a single-composition alloy powder. Both types contain more than 6 wt% copper.

Admixed Alloys

In 1963, Innes and Youdelis added spherical silver-copper eutectic alloy (71.9 wt% Ag and 28.1 wt% Cu) particles to lathe-cut low-copper amalgam alloy particles. This was the first major change in the composition of alloys for dental amalgam since

Black's formulation was introduced in the late 1800s. These alloys are often called *admixed alloys* because the final powder is a mixture of at least two kinds of particles. An admixed powder, showing lathe-cut low-copper alloy particles and spherical silver-copper alloy particles, is illustrated in Figure 17-6. Amalgam made from these powders is stronger than amalgam made from lathe-cut, low-copper powder, because of the increase in residual alloy particles and resultant decrease in matrix rather than the *dispersion strengthening* mechanism originally suggested. It is known that composite materials (materials that consist of a matrix and a filler) can be strengthened by the addition of strong fillers (see Chapter 15). The silver-copper particles as well as the Ag-Sn particles probably act as strong fillers in amalgam, thereby strengthening the amalgam matrix.

Several classic studies have shown that restorations made with this prototype of admixed amalgam were clinically superior to those made from low-copper amalgam restorations when they were evaluated for resistance to **marginal breakdown.** The suggested characteristics of the alloy that bring about this improved clinical performance are discussed later.

Admixed alloy powders usually contain 30 wt% to 55 wt% spherical high-copper powder. The total copper content in admixed alloys ranges from approximately 9 wt% to 20 wt%. The phases present in the copper-containing particles depend on their composition. The silver-copper alloy consists of mixtures of two phases, a silver-rich phase and a copper-rich phase, with the crystal structures of pure silver and pure copper, respectively. Each phase contains a small amount of the other element. In the atomized powder (which is fast-cooled), the eutectic two-phase mixture forms very fine lamellae. Compositions on either side of the eutectic form relatively large grains of copper-rich phase or silver-rich phase amid the eutectic mixture (see Chapter 6).

When mercury reacts with an admixed powder, silver dissolves into the mercury from the silver-copper alloy particles and both silver and tin dissolve into the mercury from the silver-tin alloy particles. The tin in solution diffuses to the surfaces of the silver-copper alloy particles and reacts with the copper to form the η phase

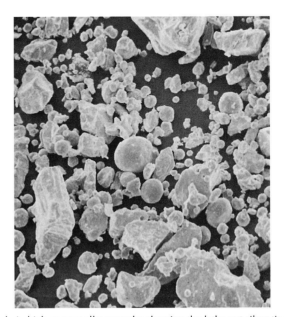

Fig. 17-6 Typical admix high-copper alloy powder showing the lathe-cut silver-tin particles and the silver-copper spheres. (×500.)

(Cu_6Sn_5). A layer of η crystals forms around unconsumed silver-copper alloy particles. The η layer on Ag-Cu alloy particles also contains some γ_1 crystals. The γ_1 phase forms simultaneously with the η phase and surrounds both the η-covered silver-copper spherical alloy particles and the silver-tin lathe-cut alloy particles. As in the low-copper amalgams, γ_1 is the matrix phase, that is, the phase that binds the unconsumed alloy particles together.

Figure 17-7 illustrates the microstructure of an admixed amalgam. Included in the structures are the γ phase, Ag-Cu particles, ε particles, γ_1 matrix areas, and η reaction layers. In some admixed amalgams, a small number of η crystals are also found amidst the γ_1 matrix.

Thus the reaction of the admixed alloy powder with mercury can be summarized as follows:

$$\text{ALLOY PARTICLES } (\beta + \gamma) + \text{Ag-Cu eutectic} + \text{Hg} \rightarrow$$
$$\gamma_1 + \eta + \text{UNCONSUMED ALLOY OF BOTH TYPES OF PARTICLES} \qquad (3)$$

Note that the γ_2 phase has been eliminated in this reaction. The γ_2 phase actually forms at the same time as η but is later replaced by it. There is not a precise definition for an amalgam alloy to qualify as a "high-copper" system, but it is generally accepted that it is a formulation whereby the γ_2 is virtually eliminated during the hardening reactions. To accomplish this, it is probably necessary to have a net copper concentration of at least 12% in the alloy powder.

Some set admixed amalgams do contain γ_2, although the percentage is less than that in low-copper amalgams. The effectiveness of the copper-containing particles in preventing γ_2 formation depends on their percentage in the mix.

Single-Composition Alloys

Success of the admixed amalgams has led to the development of another type of high-copper alloy. Unlike admixed alloy powders, each particle of these alloy

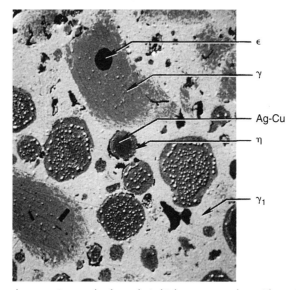

Fig. 17-7 Scanning electron micrograph of an admix high-copper amalgam. The various phases and reaction layer are labeled. The small, very light, drop-shaped areas are high in mercury owing to the freshly polished specimen. (×1000.)

powders has the same chemical composition. Therefore they are called *single-composition alloys*. The major components of the particles are usually silver, copper, and tin. The first alloy of this type contained 60 wt% silver, 27 wt% tin, and 13 wt% copper. The copper content in various single-composition alloys ranges from 13 wt% to 30 wt%. In addition, small amounts of indium or palladium are included in some of the currently marketed single-composition alloys, as noted earlier.

A number of phases are found in each single-composition alloy particle, including the β phase (Ag-Sn), γ phase (Ag_3Sn), and ε phase (Cu_3Sn). Some of the alloys may also contain some η phase (Cu_6Sn_5). Atomized particles have dendritic microstructures, consisting of fine lamellae.

When triturated with mercury, silver and tin from the Ag-Sn phases dissolve in mercury. Very little copper dissolves in mercury. The γ_1 crystals grow, forming a matrix that binds together the partially dissolved alloy particles. The η crystals are found as meshes of rodlike crystals at the surfaces of alloy particles, as well as dispersed in the matrix. These are much larger than the η crystals found in the reaction layers surrounding Ag-Cu particles in admixed amalgams.

Figure 17-8 shows the microstructure of a typical single-composition amalgam. The structure includes unconsumed alloy particles labeled P, γ_1 grains (G1), and η crystals (H).

Figure 17-9, *A*, shows a scanning electron micrograph of a high-copper single-composition amalgam fractured a few minutes after condensation, when the amalgamation reaction was still taking place. Two kinds of crystals are seen on the surface: polyhedral crystals *(arrow A)* between the unconsumed alloy particles, and meshes of η rod crystals *(arrow B)*, which cover the unconsumed alloy particles.

Figure 17-9, *B*, shows details of the marked areas in Figure 17-9, *A*. In addition to a mesh of η crystals *(arrow B)* that formed on an unconsumed particle, η rods *(arrow C)* are seen embedded in a γ_1 crystal *(arrow A)*. Meshed η crystals on unconsumed alloy particles may strengthen bonding between the alloy particles and

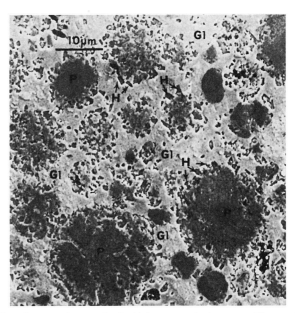

Fig. 17-8 A scanning electron micrograph of a high-copper single-composition amalgam. A relief polish technique was used to reveal the structure. (×560.) (Courtesy of M.B. Butts, T. Okabe, and C.W. Fairhurst.)

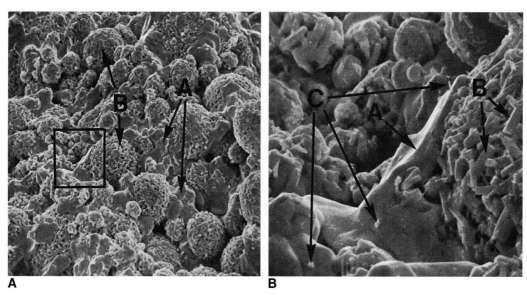

Fig. 17-9 **A,** Scanning electron micrograph of a high-copper single-composition amalgam fractured shortly after condensation, showing reaction products being formed: γ **(arrow A),** and η **(arrow B).** (×1000.) **B,** Higher magnification of marked area. η rods embedded in γ; crystals can be identified **(arrow C).** (×5000.) (Courtesy of T. Okabe, R. Mitchell, M.B. Butts, and C.W. Fairhurst.)

γ_1 grains, and η crystals dispersed between γ_1 grains may interlock γ_1 grains. This interlocking is believed to improve the amalgam's resistance to deformation.

To summarize, the reaction of the single-composition alloy powder with mercury is as follows:

$$\text{Ag-Sn-Cu ALLOY PARTICLES} + \text{Hg} \rightarrow$$
$$\gamma_1 + \eta + \text{UNCONSUMED ALLOY PARTICLES} \tag{4}$$

The undesirable γ_2 phase can also form in single-composition amalgams. This is particularly true if the atomized powder has not been heat treated or if the powder has been treated for too long at too high a temperature. Nevertheless, in most single-composition amalgams, little or no γ_2 forms.

CRITICAL QUESTION

How does the mercury content and condensation method affect the expansion or contraction that may occur during setting of an amalgam restoration?

DIMENSIONAL STABILITY

Ideally, an amalgam should set with no change in dimensions and then remain stable for the life of the restoration. However, a variety of factors influence both the initial dimensions on setting and the long-term dimensional stability.

Dimensional Change

Amalgam can expand or contract, depending on its manipulation. Ideally, the dimensional change should be small. Severe contraction can lead to microleakage, plaque accumulation, and secondary caries. Excessive expansion can produce pressure on the pulp and postoperative sensitivity. Protrusion of a restoration can also result from excessive expansion.

The dimensional change of amalgam depends on how much the amalgam is constrained during setting and on when the measurement is initiated. ANSI/ADA Specification No. 1 requires that amalgam neither contract nor expand more than 20 μm/cm, measured at 37° C, between 5 min and 24 hr after the beginning of trituration, with a device that is accurate to at least 0.5 μm. The specimen size is essentially equivalent to the bulk used in large amalgam restorations.

Theory of Dimensional Change

Most modern amalgams exhibit a net contraction when triturated with a mechanical amalgamator and evaluated by the ADA procedure. The classic picture of dimensional change is one in which the specimen undergoes an initial contraction for approximately 20 min after the beginning of trituration and then begins to expand. However, as Figure 17-10 illustrates, modern amalgams do not exhibit such simple behavior.

When the alloy and mercury are mixed, contraction results as the particles begin to dissolve (hence become smaller) and the γ_1 grows. Calculations show that the final volume of the γ_1 phase is less than the sum of the initial volumes of dissolved silver and liquid mercury that are used to produce the γ_1 phase. Therefore contraction continues as long as growth of the γ_1 phase continues. As γ_1 crystals grow, they impinge against one another. If conditions are appropriate, this impingement of γ_1 can produce an outward pressure, tending to oppose the contraction.

If there is sufficient liquid mercury present to provide a plastic matrix, expansion will occur when γ_1 crystals impinge upon one another. After a rigid γ_1 matrix has formed, growth of γ_1 crystals cannot force the matrix to expand. Instead γ_1 crystals grow into interstices containing mercury, consuming mercury, and producing a continued reaction.

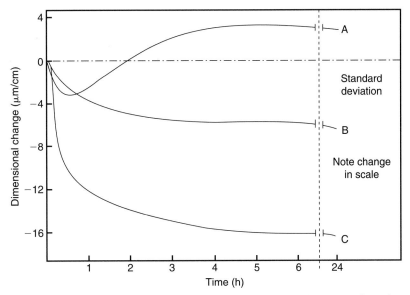

Fig. 17-10 Dimensional change curves for three amalgam alloys. **A,** A high-copper admixed amalgam. **B,** A high-copper single-composition amalgam. **C,** A lathe-cut low-copper amalgam.

According to this model, if sufficient mercury is present in the mix when the measurement of dimensional change begins, expansion will be observed. Otherwise, contraction will occur. Therefore manipulation that results in less mercury in the mix, such as lower mercury/alloy ratios and higher condensation pressures, favors contraction. Higher condensation pressures squeeze mercury out of the amalgam, producing a lower mercury/alloy ratio and favoring contraction. In addition, manipulative procedures that accelerate setting and consumption of mercury also favor contraction, including longer trituration times and use of smaller particle size alloys. Smaller particle size accelerates the consumption of mercury because small particles have a larger surface area per unit mass than larger particles. Because a larger surface area is dissolving, silver enters the solution faster, γ_1 grows from the solution faster, and the consumption of mercury is accelerated.

Measurements of the dimensional change of many modern amalgams reveal a net contraction, whereas in the past, measurements invariably indicated that an expansion occurred. Two reasons for the difference are that older amalgams contained larger alloy particles and they were mixed at higher mercury/alloy ratios than present-day amalgams. Likewise, hand trituration was used in preparing the specimens. Now high-speed mechanical amalgamators are employed. The change in the modern method is equivalent to a large increase in trituration time, resulting in contraction of the specimens prepared by these techniques.

Effect of Moisture Contamination

All the observations thus far presented have been concerned with the dimensional change during the first 24 hr only. Some admixed amalgams continue to expand for at least 2 yr. This expansion may be related to the disappearance of some or all of the γ_2 phase in these high-copper amalgams or other solid-state transformations that continue to occur for long periods. Nevertheless, if they are manipulated properly, most amalgams exhibit little further dimensional change after 24 hr.

However, if a zinc-containing low-copper or high-copper amalgam is contaminated by moisture during trituration or condensation, a large expansion, such as that shown in Figure 17-11, can take place. This expansion usually starts after 3 to 5 days and may continue for months, reaching values greater than 400 µm (4%). This type of expansion is known as **delayed expansion** or *secondary expansion*.

Delayed expansion is associated with the zinc in the amalgam. The effect is caused by the reaction of zinc with water and is absent in nonzinc amalgams. It has been clearly demonstrated that the contaminating substance is water. Hydrogen is produced by electrolytic action involving zinc and water. The hydrogen does not combine with the amalgam; rather, it collects within the restoration, increasing the internal pressure to levels high enough to cause the amalgam to **creep,** thus producing the observed expansion. The contamination of the amalgam can occur at almost any time during its manipulation and insertion into the cavity. If the operative area is not kept dry, the amalgam may become contaminated by moisture from an air-water syringe, from direct contact with the hands, or by saliva during condensation. In short, any contamination of zinc-containing amalgam with moisture, whatever the source, causes a delayed expansion. It should be noted that the contamination must occur during trituration or condensation. After the amalgam is condensed, the external surface may come in contact with saliva without the occurrence of delayed expansion.

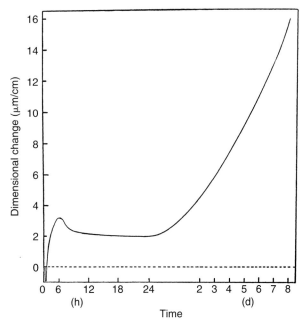

Fig. 17-11 Delayed expansion of an amalgam.

CRITICAL QUESTION

Describe the phenomenon of marginal breakdown and the steps that can be taken to reduce the risk for or extent of this process.

STRENGTH

A primary requisite for any restorative material is sufficiently high strength to resist fracture. Fracture of even a small area, especially at the margins, increases the risk for corrosion, secondary caries, and subsequent clinical failure. A lack of strength to resist masticatory forces and such fractures has been recognized as one of the inherent weaknesses of the amalgam restoration.

An example of bulk fracture of an amalgam restoration is shown in Figure 17-12. In properly designed restorations, such failures are relatively rare. More common are defects at the margins of amalgams. There is a difference of opinion as to whether the gaps produced at the interfacial region between the tooth and the amalgam are caused by fracture of the enamel or of the amalgam (marginal breakdown). Marginal defects are the most frequently occurring defects in amalgams. However, there are no general correlations of increased secondary caries incidence with increases in gap size. In fact, one study revealed that more lesions were found beneath amalgams with smaller marginal gaps and at locations far removed from the larger gaps. The incidence of secondary caries may be quite low in patients with severely deteriorated margins, if oral hygiene and dietary factors are well controlled. Özer (1998) reports that plaque accumulation is a major cause of secondary caries and that microleakage appears to be unrelated to the demineralization process. Thus a more conservative approach to replacement of amalgams with defective margins has gained acceptance in the absence of evidence of other pathological conditions.

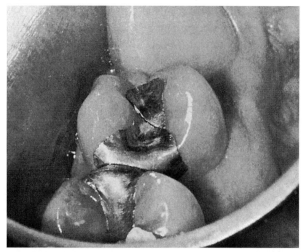

Fig. 17-12 A fractured amalgam restoration. Such failures may occur from improper manipulation of the material. (Courtesy of J.T. Andrews).

Measurement of Strength

It is difficult to identify the principal property, or properties, responsible for the fractured amalgam restoration shown in Figure 17-12. Traditionally, the strength of dental amalgam has been measured under compressive stress using specimens of dimensions comparable to the volume of typical amalgam restorations. When strength is measured in this manner, the compressive strength of a satisfactory amalgam probably should be at least 310 megapascals (MPa). When they are manipulated properly, most amalgams exhibit a compressive strength in excess of this value.

In Table 17-2, typical compressive strengths at 1 hr and 7 days after preparation are given for a low-copper amalgam and two high-copper amalgams. After 7 days, the compressive strengths of high-copper amalgams are generally higher than those of low-copper amalgams. In addition, note that the 1-hr compressive strength of the single-composition amalgam is almost double that of the other two amalgams. This trend is generally true for other single-composition amalgams.

The significance of the 7-day compressive strength relative to clinical performance has been questioned. The strength of amalgam is more than adequate to withstand potential compressive loads. It is unfortunate that amalgam is much weaker in tension than in compression. Both low- and high-copper amalgams have tensile strengths that range between 48 and 70 MPa (see Table 17-2).

Table 17-2	Comparison of Compressive Strength and Creep of a Low-Copper Silver-Tin Amalgam and High-Copper Amalgams			
	Compressive Strength (MPa)			
Amalgam	1 hr	7 Days	Creep (%)	Tensile strength—24 hr (MPa)
Low copper*	145	343	2.0	60
Admix[†]	137	431	0.4	48
Single composition[‡]	262	510	0.13	64

*Fine Cut, LD Caulk Company, Milford, DE.
[†]Dispersalloy, Johnson & Johnson Dental Products, East Windsor, NJ.
[‡]Tytin, SS White Dental Manufacturing Company, Philadelphia, PA.

Tensile stresses can easily be produced in amalgam restorations. For example, a compressive stress on the adjacent restored cusp introduces complex stresses that result in tensile stresses in the isthmus area. Because dentin has a relatively low elastic modulus, as much tooth structure as possible should be preserved to prevent the dentin from bending away from the restoration, or fracturing under masticatory forces. It is important to reemphasize that amalgam cannot withstand high tensile or bending stresses. The design of the restoration should include supporting structures whenever there is danger that it will be bent or pulled in tension. Use of a high-copper amalgam does not help. The tensile strengths of high-copper amalgams are not significantly different from those of the low-copper amalgams (see Table 17-2).

Effect of Trituration

The effect of trituration on strength depends on the type of amalgam alloy, the trituration time, and the speed of the amalgamator. Either undertrituration or overtrituration decreases the strength in both traditional and high-copper amalgams.

Effect of Mercury Content

A very important factor in the control of strength is the mercury content of the restoration. Sufficient mercury should be mixed with the alloy to coat the alloy particles and to allow a thorough amalgamation. Each particle of the alloy must be wet by the mercury; otherwise a dry, granular mix results. Such a mix results in a rough, pitted surface that may lead to corrosion. Any excess of mercury left in the restoration can produce a marked reduction in strength.

The effect of the mercury content on the compressive strength of amalgam is shown in Figure 17-13. For either low-copper or high-copper admixed amalgam, if the mercury content increases more than approximately 54%, the strength is markedly reduced. Similar decreases in strength with increased final mercury

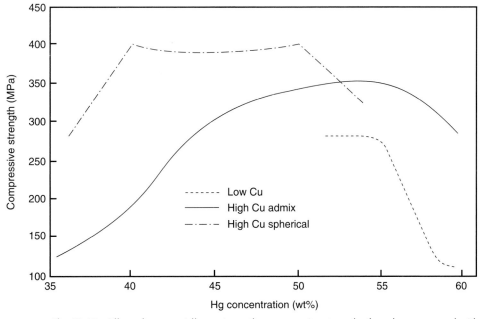

Fig. 17-13 Effect of mercury/alloy ratio on the compressive strength of amalgam prepared with representative low-copper, high-copper admix and high-copper single-composition spherical alloys.

content are observed for spherical high-copper amalgams, except that the critical mercury content at which the strength decrease occurs is less.

The strength of an amalgam is a function of the volume fractions of unconsumed alloy particles and mercury-containing phases. Low-mercury content amalgams contain more of the stronger alloy particles and less of the weaker matrix phases. Increasing the final mercury content increases the volume fraction of the matrix phases at the expense of the alloy particles. As a result, amalgams containing higher amounts of final mercury are weaker.

High-copper amalgams are particularly weakened by the presence of a small amount of γ_2 phase because it is the weakest phase within the dental amalgam. This problem can be minimized by using low mercury/alloy ratios because excess mercury promotes formation of the γ_2 phase in a high-copper amalgam.

Effect of Condensation

Condensation pressure, technique, and alloy particle shape affect amalgam properties. When typical condensation techniques and lathe-cut alloys are employed, the greater the condensation pressure, the higher the compressive strength, particularly the early strength (e.g., at 1 hr). Good condensation techniques express mercury and result in a smaller volume fraction of matrix phases. Higher condensation pressures are required to minimize porosity and to express mercury from lathe-cut amalgams. On the other hand, spherical amalgams condensed with lighter pressures produce adequate strength.

Effect of Porosity

Voids and porosity are possible factors influencing the compressive strength of set amalgam. Voids are seen in micrographs of a low-copper amalgam (see Fig. 17-5), an admixed amalgam (see Fig. 17-7), and a single-composition amalgam (see Fig. 17-8).

Porosity is related to a number of factors, including the plasticity of the mix. Plasticity of amalgam mixes decreases with increased time from the end of trituration and condensation (delayed condensation) and with undertrituration. It can be anticipated that, under such conditions, porosities are be greater and strength is lower. Increasing condensation pressure steadily improves adaptation at the margins and decreases the number of voids.

The previous comments are related to lathe-cut or admix amalgams, which offer resistance to condensation. For spherical alloys, the condenser simply punches through the amalgam if heavy pressures are employed. It is fortunate that voids are not such a problem with these amalgams. Thus lighter pressure can be used without danger of sacrificing properties.

Effect of Amalgam Hardening Rate

The amalgam hardening rate is of considerable interest to the dentist. Because a patient may be dismissed from the dental chair within 20 min after trituration of the amalgam, a vital question is whether the amalgam has gained sufficient strength for its function. It is probable that a high percentage of amalgam restorations that fracture (see Fig. 17-12) do so shortly after insertion. The clinical manifestation may not be evident for some months, but an initial crack within the restoration may occur within the first few hours.

Amalgams do not gain strength as rapidly as might be desired. For example, at the end of 20 min, compressive strength may be only 6% of the 1-wk strength. The

ANSI/ADA specification stipulates a minimum comprehensive strength of 80 MPa at 1 hr. The 1-hr compressive strength of high-copper single-composition amalgams is relatively high compared with admixed high-copper amalgams after 24 hr (see Table 17-2). This strength may have some advantages clinically. For example, fracture is less probable if the patient accidentally bites on the restoration soon after leaving the dental office. Also, these amalgams may be strong enough shortly after placement to permit amalgam build-ups to be prepared for crowns and to permit taking impressions for crowns.

Even if a fast-hardening amalgam is used, its strength is likely to be low initially. Patients should be cautioned not to subject the restoration to high biting stresses for at least 8 hr after placement. By that time, a typical amalgam has reached at least 70% of its strength.

It is of interest to note that even at the end of a 6-month period, some amalgams may still be increasing in strength. Such observations suggest that the reactions between the matrix phases and the alloy particles may continue indefinitely. It is doubtful whether equilibrium conditions between them are ever attained.

CREEP
Significance of Creep on Amalgam Performance

During the 1970s, it was shown that the resistance to fracture of hardened dental amalgams at slow strain rates seemed to correlate with long-term clinical performance. One such test measures the static creep of amalgam. Creep rate has been found to correlate with marginal breakdown of traditional low-copper amalgams; that is, the higher the creep magnitude, the greater the degree of marginal deterioration. This is illustrated in Figure 17-14, which shows marginal breakdown of amalgam restorations placed with low and high creep rate amalgams. The margins of the high creep amalgam are severely ditched.

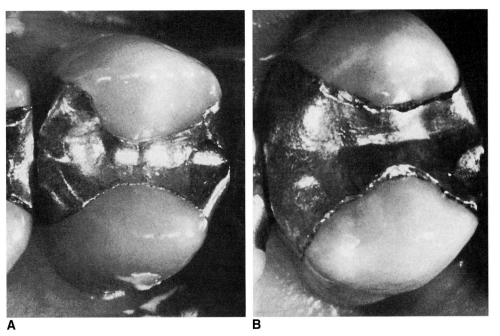

A   **B**

Fig. 17-14 Four-yr-old amalgam restorations. **A,** Amalgam placed with an alloy having minimal dynamic creep. **B,** Amalgam restoration of an alloy having a high creep value. (Courtesy of D.B. Mahler.)

However, for high-copper amalgams, creep is not necessarily a good predictor of marginal fracture. Many of these amalgams have creep rates of 0.4% (see Table 17-1) or less. It is prudent to select a commercial alloy that has a creep rate below the level of 3% specified in ANSI/ADA Specification No. 1. As tested by this specification, creep values of low-copper amalgams range between 0.8% and 8%. High-copper amalgams have much lower creep values, some even less than 0.1%. There are no data available that suggest that reducing the creep value below approximately 1% influences marginal breakdown.

Influence of Microstructure on Creep

The γ_1 phase has been found to exert a primary influence on low-copper amalgam creep rates. Creep rates increase with higher γ_1 volume fractions and decrease with larger γ_1 grain sizes. The presence of the γ_2 phase is also associated with higher creep rates. In addition to the absence of the γ_2 phase, the very low creep rates in single-composition high-copper amalgams may be associated with η rods, which act as barriers to deformation of the γ_1 phase.

Effect of Manipulative Variables on Creep

Those manipulative factors discussed previously that maximize strength also minimize creep rate for any given type of amalgam. Thus mercury/alloy ratios should be minimized and condensation pressure maximized for lathe-cut or admixed alloys, and careful attention should be paid to the timing of trituration and condensation.

CLINICAL PERFORMANCE OF AMALGAM RESTORATIONS

The exceptionally fine clinical performance of dental amalgam may be linked to its tendency to minimize marginal leakage. One of the greatest hazards associated with restoring teeth is the microleakage that may occur between the cavity walls and the restoration. With the exception of glass ionomer cement, no restorative material truly adheres to tooth structure; consequently, penetration of fluids and debris around the margins may be the greatest cause for secondary caries. At best, amalgam affords only a reasonably close adaptation to the walls of the prepared cavity. For this reason, cavity varnishes (see Chapter 16) are used to reduce the gross leakage that occurs around a new restoration. The use of dentin bonding agents with amalgam is another relatively new method to reduce microleakage. Clinical trials using the bonded-amalgam technique continue to show promise. Results after 2 to 5 yr appear to be equivalent to those for conventional amalgams. The long-term promise of this method is that it may allow more conservative cavity preparations with reduced mechanical retentive features.

The small amount of leakage under amalgam restorations is unique. If the restoration is properly inserted, leakage decreases as the restoration ages in the mouth. This may be caused by corrosion products that form along the interface between the tooth and the restoration, sealing the interface and thereby preventing leakage. The presence of calcium and phosphorus and the demineralization of tooth structures adjacent to the amalgam restoration also suggest a possible biological contribution to this corrosion process.

The ability to seal against microleakage is shared by both the low-copper amalgams and the newer high-copper amalgams. However, the accumulation of corrosion products is slower for the high-copper alloys.

Many amalgam restorations must be replaced because of problems, including secondary caries, gross fracture, "ditched" or fractured margins, and excessive tarnish and corrosion. The characteristics of an amalgam depend on its properties, which in turn depend on the alloy selected and how it is manipulated, as described in the previous sections. After placement, amalgams continue to undergo changes as a result of moisture contamination, corrosion, slow solid-state phase changes, and mechanical forces. The ultimate lifetime of an amalgam restoration is determined by a number of factors, including the material, the skill of the dentist and the assistant, and the patient's environment. The first two parameters are the dominant factors that control the amalgam performance during the early life of the restoration. As time proceeds, differences in the dynamics of the oral environment among patients contribute significantly to the variability of deterioration, particularly marginal ditching. Changes in the amalgam structure during clinical use and survival of amalgam restorations of various types are now discussed.

CRITICAL QUESTION

How can corrosion of an amalgam restoration lead to both positive and negative outcomes?

Tarnish and Corrosion

Amalgam restorations often tarnish and corrode in the oral environment. The degree of tarnish and the resulting discoloration appear to depend greatly on the individual's oral environment and, to a certain extent, on the particular alloy employed. Electrochemical studies indicate that some passivation offering partial protection against further corrosion occurs as a result of the tarnish process. A tendency toward tarnish, although perhaps unaesthetic, because of black silver sulfide, does not necessarily imply that active corrosion and early failure of a restoration will occur.

Active corrosion of a newly placed restoration occurs on the metal surface along the interface between the tooth and the restoration. The space between the alloy and the tooth permits the microleakage of electrolytes, and a classic concentration cell (crevice corrosion) process results. (See Chapter 3 for further details on corrosion processes.) The build-up of corrosion products gradually seals this space, making dental amalgam a self-sealing restoration.

The precise role of corrosion in the process of marginal breakdown has not been established. However, several theories have been developed relating the two phenomena. There is indirect evidence that the γ_2 phase is implicated in both marginal failure and active corrosion in traditional alloys, but such a correlation is not possible for high-copper alloys.

The most common corrosion products found with traditional amalgam alloys are oxides and chlorides of tin. These are found along the tooth-amalgam interface and within the bulk of older amalgam restorations, as shown in Figure 17-15. In the case of high-copper amalgams, many of the same products are found (Fig. 17-16).

Corrosion products containing copper can also be found in high-copper amalgams. However, the corrosion process is more limited because the η phase is less susceptible to corrosion than the γ_2 phase of traditional amalgams. Every effort should be made to produce a smooth, homogeneous surface on a restoration to minimize tarnish and corrosion, regardless of the alloy system used.

Whenever a gold restoration is placed in contact with an amalgam, corrosion of the amalgam can be expected as a result of the large differences in electromotive

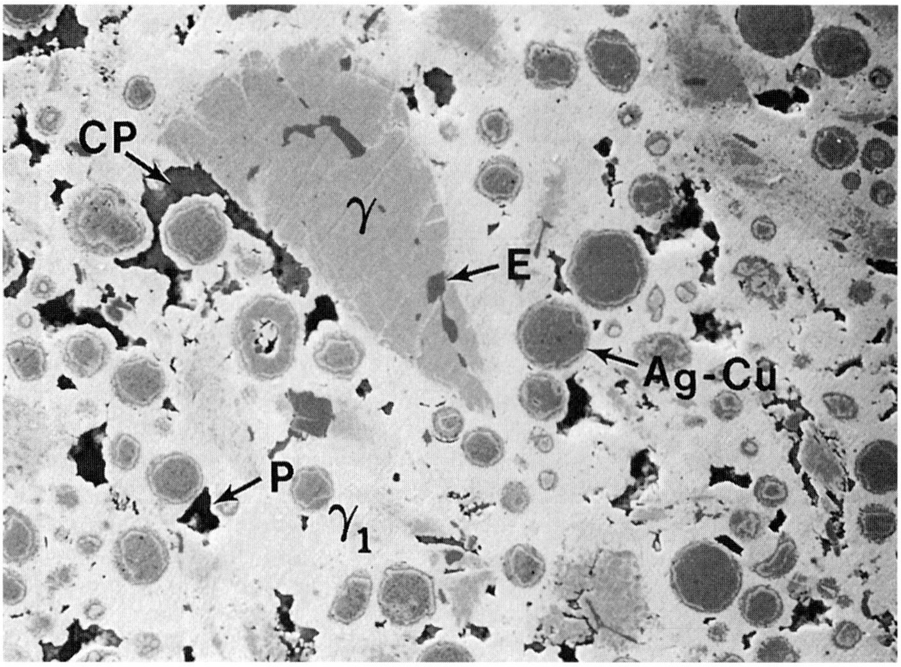

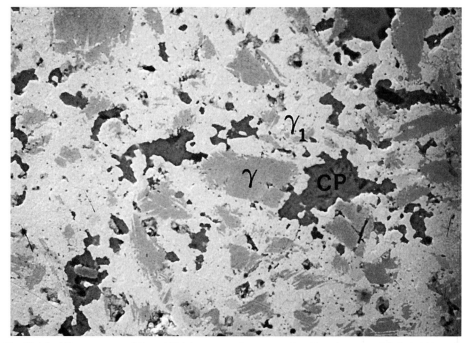

Fig. 17-15 Microstructure of 7-yr-old traditional amalgam alloy restoration. The various phases are marked. Note the extensive porosity **(P)** and the Sn-Cl corrosion product **(CP)** that has replaced the γ_2 area. (Courtesy of G.W. and S.J. Marshall.)

Fig. 17-16 Microstructure of 8-yr-old high-copper alloy restoration. The phases are labeled. Although some porosity is seen, it is less than that of the traditional alloy restoration seen in Figure 17-15, with fewer corrosion products **(CP).** (Courtesy of G.W. and S.J. Marshall.)

force (EMF) of the two materials. The corrosion process can liberate free mercury, which can contaminate and weaken the gold restoration. Biological effects such as galvanism can also result. Such a practice should be avoided.

A high-copper amalgam is cathodic with respect to a conventional amalgam. Thus concern has been expressed that if high-copper amalgam restorations were placed in the same mouth with existing restorations of low-copper amalgam, corrosion and failure would be accelerated in the latter. Clinical observations do not indicate accelerated corrosion in such situations. Laboratory models that are designed to monitor corrosion in adjacent restorations suggest that the current flow paths are such that electrochemical interaction between restorations is minimal.

Because the γ_2 phase is the most anodic of the phases present in set amalgam alloys, the high-copper amalgams, which virtually eliminate this phase, show improved laboratory corrosion behavior compared with traditional amalgams. However, as already noted, high mercury/alloy ratios can lead to the formation of γ_2 phase, even in amalgams produced from high-copper alloys, thus promoting corrosion.

Compositional Effects on the Survival of Amalgam Restorations

Although many factors may contribute to the deterioration of dental amalgams as noted in the preceding sections, the ultimate test is the long-term survival of the well-placed dental amalgam restoration. A number of clinical trials have attempted to determine differences in performance of dental amalgams based on amalgam type. Results of such long-term studies are illustrated in Figure 17-17.

In Figure 17-17, the survival of amalgam restorations are grouped into categories based on their content of copper and zinc. Modern high-copper amalgams with zinc (HCZ) have the best overall survival of nearly 90% after 12 yr. High-copper amalgams without zinc (HC) performed the next best, with survival rates of approximately 80%. The survival curves for these two groups of amalgams could be

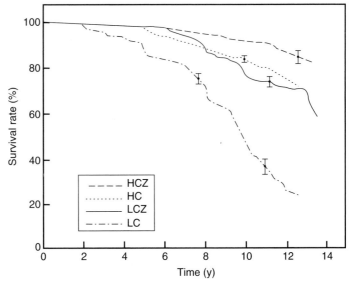

Fig. 17-17 Survival curves for amalgam restorations classified according to copper and zinc content. Both copper and zinc appear to provide protection to restorations. Thus many more high copper restorations containing zinc survived than low copper restorations without zinc in these clinical trials. (Courtesy H. Letzel, M. Van't Hof, S. Marshall, G.W. Marshall.)

distinguished only after approximately 8 yr, when the better survival of the high-copper systems that contain a small quantity of zinc became apparent. The next group includes the traditional low-copper amalgams with zinc (LCZ). The worst performance was exhibited by low-copper amalgams that were zinc-free. These systems exhibited failures in 50% of the restorations after only 10 yr. The reasons for the differences seen in survival are not completely clear. However, the combined and perhaps synergistic effects of the additional copper and zinc contents probably provide increased corrosion protection to the restorations. Additional survival data for amalgam and composite restorations are presented in Chapter 15.

CRITICAL QUESTION

What steps can be taken by a dentist to extend the survival time of amalgam restorations?

FACTORS AFFECTING THE SUCCESS OF AMALGAM RESTORATIONS

There are few alternative materials available that are as technique-insensitive as is dental amalgam. The most attractive direct-filling alternatives are the resin-based composites. However, compared with composites, amalgams have less technique-sensitivity, greater longevity, greater radiopacity, an appearance easily differentiated from tooth structure, and the ability to seal the marginal gap space over time. Compared with amalgam restorations, composite restorations are more aesthetic, more costly, require more time for placement, can be placed with less removal of tooth structure, are good thermal insulators, and do not cause galvanic effects.

A good modern dental amalgam alloy can be manipulated so that the restoration lasts, on the average, 12 to 15 yr. Approximately 90% of amalgam restorations are still functional after 10 yr (see Chapter 15). If the restoration is defective, the fault is most frequently associated with the dentist, auxiliary, or patient, and not with the material, although amalgam is a brittle material and must be manipulated with this deficiency in mind. The cavity preparation must be designed correctly, and the amalgam must be manipulated properly so that no part of the amalgam restoration is placed under excessive tensile stress. The manipulation aspects of amalgam are discussed in detail relative to the influence of technique on the physical properties and clinical success of these restorations.

Criteria involved in the selection of an alloy vary with each individual situation. Certainly, the first criterion is to make sure that the alloy meets the requirements of the ANSI/ADA Specification No. 1 or a similar specification.

The manipulative characteristics are extremely important and a matter of subjective preference. Matters such as rate of hardening, smoothness of the mix, ease of condensation, and ease of finishing vary with the alloy, the working speed, and choice of the operator. For example, lathe-cut amalgams have an entirely different feel during condensation than do spherical amalgams. It is essential that the alloy selected be one with which the dentist and the assistant are comfortable. The operator variable is a major factor affecting the clinical lifetime of the restoration. Use of alloys and techniques that encourage standardization in the manipulation and placement of the amalgam enhances the quality of the service. Another important factor is the delivery system provided by the manufacturer, including its convenience, expediency, and capability to reduce human variables. The alloy may be purchased in the form of either a powder, a pellet, or as preproportioned alloy with mercury in disposable capsules. For the first two types, the mercury must be obtained from a mercury dispenser, a device that is somewhat technique-sensitive. There are advantages and disadvantages to the use of preproportioned capsules that are discussed later. Nonetheless, the delivery system is an important consideration.

Obviously, the selection of one type of amalgam over others should be based on clinical performance or, lacking such information, on the physical properties. However, the initial analysis of properties should be compared with clinical performance as such data become available. This is especially necessary for alloy formulations that depart from traditional compositions and for which a consistent correlation between properties and performance has not yet been established.

Alloys of traditional composition are still available, and acceptable amalgam restorations can be obtained from many of these products. However, it is obvious that the newer high-copper alloy systems are the materials of choice. Improved physical properties, the elimination of the γ_2 phase, and the better corrosion resistance associated with these alloys generally lead to superior clinical performance.

There is only one requisite for dental mercury: purity. Common contaminating elements, such as arsenic, can lead to pulpal damage. Furthermore, a lack of purity may adversely affect the physical properties of the amalgam. It is unfortunate that terms such as *pure, redistilled,* and *triple distilled* do not indicate the chemical quality of the mercury.

The designation *U.S.P.* (United States Pharmacopoeia) ensures mercury of satisfactory purity with no surface contamination and less than 0.02% nonvolatile residue. This requirement is encompassed in the ANSI/ADA Specification No. 6 for dental mercury.

CRITICAL QUESTIONS

What is the ideal mercury alloy/ratio for an admixed amalgam and a spherical particle amalgam? What are the consequences of insufficient and excessive amounts of mercury on the amalgam restorations?

MERCURY/ALLOY RATIO

Historically, the only way to achieve smooth and plastic amalgam mixes was to use an amount of mercury considerably in excess of that desirable in the final restorations. Because of the deleterious effects of an excessive mercury content on the physical and mechanical properties of amalgam, manipulative procedures were employed to reduce the amount of mercury left in the restoration to an acceptable level.

For conventional mercury-added systems, two techniques were used for achieving mercury reduction in the final restoration. Initially, the removal of excess mercury was accomplished by squeezing or wringing the mixed amalgam in a squeeze cloth before insertion of the increments into the prepared cavity. Also, additional mercury-rich amalgam was worked to the top during condensation of each increment, and this excess was removed as the amalgam mix was built up to form a restoration. Although excellent restorations may be produced in this manner, the amount of mercury removed by the squeeze cloth and during condensation varied. Thus there was considerable chance for error. The most obvious method for reducing the mercury content of the restoration is to reduce the original mercury/alloy ratio. The present-day alloys are designed for manipulation with reduced mercury/alloy ratios. This method is known as the *minimal mercury technique* or the *Eames technique,* in recognition of the dentist who developed the concept. Sufficient mercury must be present in the original mix to provide a coherent and plastic mass after trituration;

however, the amount of mercury present must also be low enough so that the mercury content of the restoration is at an acceptable level without the need to remove an appreciable amount during condensation. The mercury content of the finished restoration should be comparable to that of the original mercury/alloy ratio, usually about 50 wt%, with lesser amounts (~42 wt%) being used with spherical alloys.

The obvious choice of method for placement of amalgam restorations with today's alloys is the minimal mercury technique, but manipulative procedures are still critical. The excellence of clinical restorations placed by this technique depends on proper manipulation, including proportioning of the mercury and alloy. Because the recommended amount of mercury is always the minimum amount required to produce a usable mix, proportioning of the two components must be exact. Trituration and condensation of the amalgam must be performed with equal care and attention to detail.

Proportioning

The amount of alloy and mercury to be used can be described as the mercury/alloy ratio, which signifies the parts by weight of mercury and of alloy to be used for the particular technique. For example, a mercury/alloy ratio of 6/5 indicates that 6 parts of mercury are to be used with 5 parts of alloy by weight. Sometimes instead of a mercury/alloy ratio, manufacturers' instructions specify the percentage of mercury by weight to be employed in the mix. A mix of amalgam prepared with a mercury/alloy ratio of 6:5 contains 54.5% mercury.

Of course, the recommended ratio varies for different alloy compositions, particle sizes, particle shapes, and heat treatments. The particular manipulative and condensation technique favored by the dentist can also be a factor in selecting the desired ratio. The recommended mercury/alloy ratios for most modern lathe-cut alloys is approximately 1:1, or 50% mercury, as noted earlier, although some may vary plus or minus a few percent. With spherical alloys, the recommended amount of mercury is closer to 42% because spherical particles have lower surface/volume ratios, requiring less mercury to completely wet the particles.

Regardless of the ratio, proportioning is critical for the minimum mercury alloys. If the mercury content is slightly low, the mix may be dry and grainy with insufficient matrix present to cohesively bond the mass. The use of too little mercury impairs the strength of high-copper amalgams as much as an excessive quantity of mercury. Corrosion resistance is also reduced.

A wide variety of mercury and alloy dispensers are available. The most common is the dispenser based on volumetric proportioning. Preweighed pellets or tablets are a more convenient method for correctly dispensing the alloy. The individual pellets are quite uniform in weight, provided that normal care is exercised in handling to avoid chipping the pellet. With preweighed pellets, all that is required is an accurate mercury dispenser.

As a liquid, mercury can be measured by volume without appreciable loss of accuracy. Standard deviations in weights of mercury dispensed as low as ±0.5% may be attained with a number of commercial mercury dispensers. However, precautions must still be exercised in their use. The dispenser should be held vertically to ensure consistent spills of mercury. Tilting the bottle at a 45-degree angle results in unreliable mercury/alloy ratios. The dispenser should be at least half full when it is used. If it is not, the weight of mercury dispensed may be erratic. Probably the most common cause of inaccurate delivery of the mercury is use of contaminated mercury that leads to entrapment of the contaminants in the reservoir and orifice of the device. If such variables are not controlled, variation in individual spills of mercury may amount to 3% or 4%. With the use of low mercury/alloy ratios, variations of this magnitude result in an unusable mix.

Disposable capsules containing preproportioned aliquots of mercury and alloy are now widely used. They contain alloy either in pellet form or as a preweighed portion of powder in conjunction with the appropriate quantity of mercury. To prevent any amalgamation from occurring during storage, the mercury and alloy are physically separated from each other. The older types of preproportioned capsules require activation before trituration, to allow the mercury to enter the compartment with the alloy. Some alloys are now available in *self-activating capsules,* which automatically release the mercury into the alloy chamber during the first few oscillations of the amalgamator. Although the preproportioned material is more expensive, it is convenient, eliminates the chance of mercury spills during proportioning, and should result in a reliable mercury/alloy ratio. At the same time, there is no opportunity to make minor adjustments in the mercury/alloy ratio to accommodate personal preference.

Regardless of the method used, the proper amount of mercury and alloy always must be proportioned before the start of trituration. The addition of mercury after trituration is contraindicated.

CRITICAL QUESTION

How should the optimal trituration time be determined for a given dental amalgam product?

MECHANICAL TRITURATION

Originally, the alloy and mercury were mixed, or *triturated,* by hand with a mortar and pestle. Today, however, mechanical amalgamation saves time and standardizes the procedure. In fact, it is probably impossible to employ hand trituration for mixing modern amalgams prepared with low mercury/alloy ratios.

The objective of trituration is to provide proper amalgamation of the mercury and alloy. The alloy particles are coated with a film of oxide, which is difficult for the mercury to penetrate. This film must be rubbed off in some manner so that a clean surface of alloy can come in contact with the mercury. The oxide layer is removed by abrasion when the alloy particles and mercury are triturated.

A large number of commercial brands of amalgamator are available. Two representative products are shown in Figure 17-18. The principle of operation is comparable for most of them. A capsule serves as a *mortar.* A cylindrical metal or plastic piston of smaller diameter than the capsule is inserted into the capsule, and this serves as the *pestle.* Capsules for disposable systems also usually contain an appropriate pestle.

The alloy and mercury are dispensed into the capsule, or if a disposable capsule system is being used, the capsule may require activation. When the capsule has been secured in the machine and it is turned on, the arms holding the capsule oscillate at high speed; thus trituration is accomplished. There is an automatic timer for controlling the length of the mixing time, and most modern amalgamators have two or more operating speeds. Multiple-speed amalgamators provide greater versatility, often permitting the amalgamator to be used for mixing other preproportioned materials, such as cements and composites. Some amalgam alloys and certain types of preproportioned capsule systems have specific recommendations for trituration speeds.

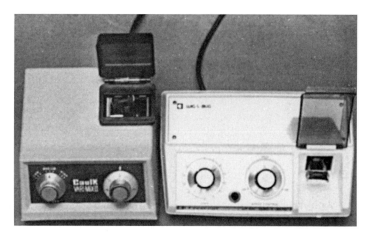

Fig. 17-18   Two representative commercial mechanical amalgamators.

New amalgamators must have hoods that cover the reciprocating arms holding the capsule, as shown in Figure 17-18. The purpose of the hood is to confine mercury that might escape into the room or to prevent a capsule from being accidentally ejected from the amalgamator during trituration.

Reusable capsules are available with a friction fit and screw-cap lids. With either type, it is important that the lid on the capsule fit tightly. If it does not, a fine mist of mercury will be sprayed out of the capsule during trituration, producing a risk for mercury inhalation. Loss of mercury can alter the mercury/alloy ratio to the extent that the mix is unusable. Capsule lids should be carefully checked before use, and any lids that appear to be loose should be discarded. Also, with long use, the fit may deteriorate. Disposable capsules should never be reused because leakage or fracture of the capsule is very probable.

A wide variety of capsule-pestle combinations are available. One type of capsule is of a one-piece construction such that no mercury is released during trituration. After trituration, the capsule is broken open by bending across a notched area. Pestles may be plastic or metal and come in a variety of sizes, shapes, and weights. In selecting a capsule-pestle combination, the size of the pestle is an important consideration. The diameter and length of the pestle should be considerably less than the comparable dimensions of the capsule. For example, the capsule-pestle combination shown in Figure 17-19, *A*, is acceptable from this standpoint. If the pestle is too large (Fig. 17-19, *B*), the resultant mix may not be homogeneous. When the pellet form of alloy is used, the pellet or a piece of it may become wedged between the wall of the capsule and the pestle and may not be completely broken up during mixing.

The pellets produced by different manufacturers differ to some extent by the ease with which they are reduced to powder. In instances in which pellets are difficult to break, the clinician should consider employing a small metal pestle rather than a plastic pestle of a lighter weight. Trituration of an alloy in a capsule without a pestle should be limited to those alloys for which that mode of mixing is specifically recommended.

An amalgamator should be used at the speed recommended by the alloy manufacturer. Some older amalgamators do not operate at a sufficient rate of speed to properly amalgamate high-copper alloys mixed with minimal mercury. Self-activating capsules are usually very sensitive to trituration speed. Regardless of the alloy or amalgamator used, no more than two pellets of alloy should be mixed in a capsule at one time.

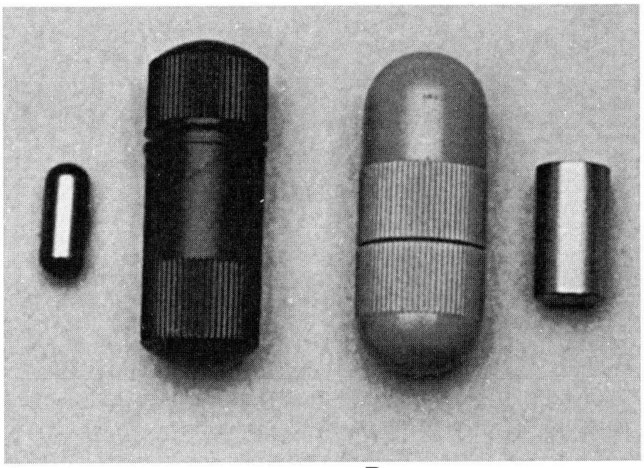

Fig. 17-19 Capsule and pestle combinations. **A,** Satisfactory size relationship between the capsule and pestle. **B,** An unsatisfactory pestle size.

A reusable capsule should be clean and free of previously mixed, hardened alloy. Scraping out hardened alloy usually produces scratches that compound the sticking problem in the future. In the long run, it is advisable to discard the capsule. This sticking problem can often be minimized by the following procedure: at the end of amalgamation, quickly remove the pestle from the capsule, replace the lid, reinsert the capsule in the amalgamator, turn it on for a second or two, and then remove it. This *mulling* process generally causes the mix to cohere so that it can be readily removed from the capsule.

No exact recommendations for mixing time can be given because of such factors as the wide variety of amalgamators, differences in speed and oscillating patterns, and capsule designs. The amount of work required for amalgamation of various alloys differs. Spherical alloys, for example, usually require less amalgamation time than do lathe-cut alloys. Also, a larger mix requires a slightly longer mixing time than a smaller one. Manufacturers' directions contain a time schedule for mixing the alloy. However, because of the speed variations among amalgamators, even among those of the same brand, this schedule should serve only as a rough guide.

An important factor to be decided by the dentist and assistant is the optimum amalgamation time required to attain a mix of correct consistency. A general rule is that for a given alloy and mercury/alloy ratio, increased trituration time and/or speed shortens the working and setting times. Alloys differ in the sensitivity to trituration time, as can be seen in Figure 17-20.

Consistency of the Mix

It is evident that the proper combination of the alloy and mercury is a prime manipulative consideration. At this stage, the composition of the final amalgam is largely determined, and the composition is a major determinant of the physical properties.

Provided that the same weights of alloy and mercury are used each time and are triturated by the same amalgamator, attainment of a proper mix can be controlled by timing the trituration. The proper time can be determined by observing the consistency of the mix. For example, the somewhat grainy mix shown in Figure 17-21 is undertriturated. Not only will the amalgam restoration made from this mix be weak, but also the rough surface left after carving of the granular amalgam increases the restoration's susceptibility to tarnish.

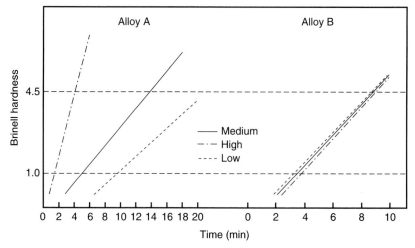

Fig. 17-20   Hardening data for two alloys mixed at low, medium, and high settings. Broken lines at 1.0 and 4.5 represent working and carving consistency, respectively. (From Brackett W.W., Swartz M.L., Moore B.K., and Clark H.E.: The influence of mixing speed on the setting rate of high-copper amalgam. J Am Dent Assoc 115[2]:289, 1987.)

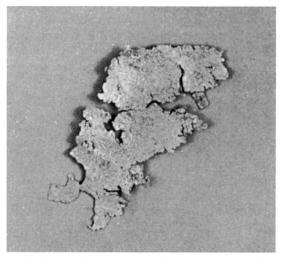

Fig. 17-21   Undertriturated mix of amalgam. Such a mix has low strength and poor resistance to corrosion.

If the trituration has produced an amalgam of the general appearance shown in Figure 17-22, the strength will approach the maximum value and the smooth carved surface will retain its luster longer after polishing. Such an amalgam mix may be warm (not hot) when it is removed from the capsule. This has no effect on the physical properties of the amalgam other than to shorten the working time somewhat. With experience, the proper consistency can be recognized, and the timing of the mix can be adjusted to attain it.

CRITICAL QUESTION

During the condensation of an amalgam, at what point should the triturated mixture be discarded and replaced by a new mixture?

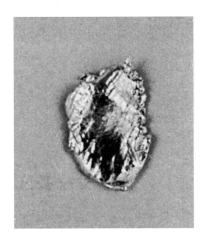

Fig. 17-22 Properly triturated amalgam having maximum properties.

CONDENSATION

The goal of condensation is to compact the alloy into the prepared cavity so that the greatest possible density is attained, with sufficient mercury present to ensure complete continuity of the matrix phase (Ag_2Hg_3) between the remaining alloy particles. If this goal is achieved, the strength of the amalgam is thereby increased, and creep is decreased. Also, mercury-rich amalgam must be brought to the top of each increment as it is being condensed, so that successive increments bond to each other. A major objective is to remove any excess mercury from each increment as it is worked to the top by the condensing procedure. With the minimum mercury technique, removal of the soft mushy material during condensation of the alloy is, of course, less critical. Under proper conditions of trituration and condensation, there is very little danger of removing too much mercury during condensation.

After the mix is made, condensation of the amalgam should be promptly initiated. As can be seen in Figure 17-23, the longer the time that elapses between mixing and condensation, the weaker the amalgam. In addition, the mercury content and creep of the amalgam are increased. Condensation of partially set material probably fractures and breaks up the matrix that has already formed. Also, when the alloy has lost a certain amount of plasticity, it is difficult to condense without producing internal voids and layering.

The loss in strength incurred depends on the hardening rate of amalgam. A fast-setting amalgam, such as that obtained for alloy *A* in Figure 17-23, is affected to a greater extent than the slower-setting alloy *B*. Most modern alloys mixed with minimal amounts of mercury harden with considerable speed. The working time is short, and the effects are analogous to those observed with alloy *A*. Therefore condensation should be as rapid as possible, and a fresh mix of amalgam should be made if condensation takes longer than 3 or 4 min.

The field of operation must be kept absolutely dry during condensation. The incorporation of the slightest moisture in a zinc-containing amalgam at this stage can result in a delayed expansion, as discussed previously, and associated problems such as corrosion and loss of strength. The ultimate result of moisture contamination is premature failure of the restoration.

Because of the nature of the operation, condensation is usually accomplished within four walls and a floor. One or more walls may consist of a thin sheet of stainless steel called a *matrix*. Condensation can be accomplished with either hand or mechanical instruments.

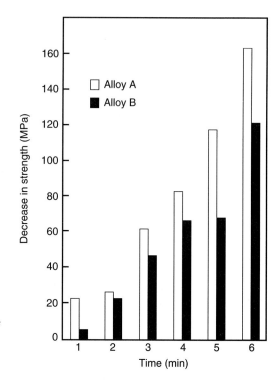

Fig. 17-23 The effect of the elapsed time between trituration and condensation on the strength of the hardened amalgam. The greater the elapsed time, the lower the strength.

Hand Condensation

The amalgam mixture should never be touched with bare hands because the freshly mixed alloy contains free mercury. Also, moisture on the surface of the skin is a source of contamination of the amalgam. However, because infection control requires that clinicians wear gloves, skin contact with mercury should not be a concern. The increments of alloy should be carried to and inserted in the prepared cavity by means of instruments such as small forceps or an amalgam carrier designed for that purpose.

Once the increment of amalgam is inserted into the cavity preparation, it should immediately be condensed with sufficient pressure to remove voids and to adapt the material to the walls. The condenser point, or face, is forced into the amalgam mass under hand pressure. Condensation is usually started at the center, and then the condenser point is stepped little by little toward the cavity walls. The force requirements depend on the shape of the alloy particle.

After condensation of an increment, the surface should be shiny in appearance. This indicates that there is sufficient mercury present at the surface to diffuse into the next increment so that each increment, as it is added, bonds to the preceding one. If this is not done and the increments do not bond, the restoration is laminated. Such a restoration is analogous to a stack of bricks with no mortar cementing them together. The restoration may subsequently fracture, probably when the matrix is removed. At best, it lacks homogeneity and will suffer severe corrosion.

Even with the minimal mercury techniques now in general use, it is probably desirable to remove some of the soft or mushy material that is brought to the surface of each increment. This step is far less critical than it was when the percentage of mercury recommended for the mix was far above the acceptable level for the final restoration.

The procedure of adding an increment, condensing it, adding another increment, and so forth is continued until the cavity is overfilled. Any mercury-rich material at the surface of the last increment, constituting the overfill, is removed when the restoration is carved.

If the cavity is large or, if for some reason, undue time is taken to complete condensation, another mix should be made just before the original one becomes unusable or loses its plasticity. This can easily be accomplished because mechanical mixing requires only a few seconds.

A well-condensed amalgam restoration can be achieved only if the mix has a proper consistency. A dry and grainy mix (see Fig. 17-21) has insufficient mercury and plasticity, as described previously, and a mix that is hard and hot to the touch has probably been mixed too long. In either case, condensation of the mix should not be attempted. Rather, a new mix should be prepared.

One of the most important factors in condensation is the size of amalgam increments carried into the cavity. The larger the piece, the more difficult it is to reduce the voids and to adapt the alloy to the cavity walls. However, when a large restoration is being produced, the goal is to maximize speed, and a large increment may be added to increase the time available for condensation. However, in general, relatively small increments of amalgam should be used throughout the condensation procedure to reduce void formation and to obtain maximum adaptation to the cavity. Likewise, sufficient condensation pressure must be used to force the alloy particles together, reduce voids, and work mercury to the surface to achieve bonding between the increments.

Condensation Pressure

The area of the condenser point, or face, and the force exerted on it by the operator govern the condensation pressure (force per unit area). When a given force is applied, the smaller the condenser, the greater the pressure exerted on the amalgam. For example, a thrust of 44 Newtons (N) (10 lb) exerted on a circular condenser point 2 mm in diameter results in a condensation pressure of 13.8 MPa (2000 psi). The same thrust applied to a condenser 3.5 mm in diameter produces a condensation pressure of only 4.6 MPa (667 psi). If the condenser point is too large, the operator cannot generate sufficient condensation pressure to condense the amalgam adequately and force it into retentive areas.

Although forces as great as 66.7 N (15 lb) are recommended for condensation, it is doubtful that forces of that magnitude are generally used. A study of the condensation forces applied by 30 practitioners showed that forces in the range of 13.3 to 17.8 N (3 to 4 lb) represent the average force employed. To ensure maximum density and adaptation to the cavity walls, the condensation force should be as great as the alloy will allow, consistent with patient comfort. It is doubtful that condenser points greater than 2 mm in diameter will provide adequate condensation of lathe-cut alloys.

One of the advantages of spherical amalgam alloys is that the strength properties tend to be less sensitive to condensation pressure. In fact, many of the spherical alloys have little "body" and offer only minimal resistance to the condensation force. In many instances, condensation becomes a matter of attaining good adaptation. When condensing these alloys, a large condenser can often be used. The potential disadvantages of a spherical alloy compared with an admixed alloy (lathe-cut and spherical particles) are the tendency for overhangs in proximal areas and weak proximal contacts.

The shape of the condenser points should conform to the area under condensation. For example, a round condenser point is ineffective adjacent to a corner or angle of a prepared cavity; a triangular or rectangular point is indicated in such an area. Points of various shapes are available to provide effective condensation.

Mechanical Condensation

The procedures and principles of mechanical condensation are the same as those for hand condensation, including the need to use small increments of amalgam. The only difference is that the condensation of the amalgam is performed by an automatic device. Various mechanisms are employed for these instruments. Some provide an impact type of force, whereas others use rapid vibration.

Whether the device is of the impact or vibratory type, less energy is needed than for hand condensation, and the operation may be less fatiguing to the dentist. Similar clinical results can be achieved using either hand or mechanical condensation. The method selected is usually based on the preference of the dentist.

CARVING AND FINISHING

After the amalgam has been condensed into the prepared cavity, the restoration is carved to reproduce the proper tooth anatomy. The objective of carving is to simulate the anatomy, rather than to reproduce extremely fine detail. If the carving is too deep, the bulk of amalgam, particularly at the marginal areas, is reduced. If this area is too thin, it may fracture under masticatory stress.

If the proper technique is followed, the amalgam should be ready for carving soon after completion of condensation; however, the carving should not be started until the amalgam is hard enough to offer resistance to the carving instrument. If the carving is started too soon, the amalgam may be so plastic that it may be pulled away from the margins, even by the sharpest carving instrument.

After carving is completed, the surface of the restoration should be smoothed. This may be accomplished by judiciously burnishing the surface and margins of the restoration. If the alloy is a reasonably fast-setting one, it should have achieved sufficient strength by this time to support firm, but not heavy, rubbing pressure.

Burnishing of the occlusal anatomy can be accomplished with a ball burnisher. A rigid, flat-bladed instrument is best used on smooth surfaces. Final smoothing can be concluded by rubbing the surface with a moist cotton pellet or by lightly smoothing the surface with a rubber polishing cup and an extremely fine polishing or prophylaxis paste. Burnishing has been a somewhat controversial subject, and its effect on marginal adaptation and hardness is not well defined. There is ample evidence that amalgam surfaces that have been burnished, or burnished and lightly polished, are much smoother than carved surfaces. Clinical data on performance of restorations support the desirability of burnishing the fast-setting, high-copper systems. Burnishing slow-setting alloys can damage the margins of the restoration. Undue pressure should not be exerted in burnishing, and heat generation should be avoided. Temperatures above 60° C (140° F) cause a significant release of mercury. The mercury-rich condition created at the margins results in accelerated corrosion, fracture, or both.

Regardless of alloy, trituration method, and condensation technique, the carved surface of the restoration is rough, as demonstrated by the dull surface of the restorations at the left *(A)* of Figure 17-24. The surfaces are covered with scratches, pits, and irregularities. Even though the restoration surfaces have been carefully finished by burnishing and smoothing, they are rough at the microscopic level. If these defects are not removed by further finishing after the

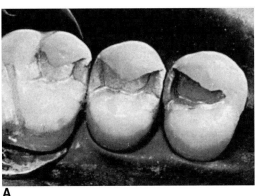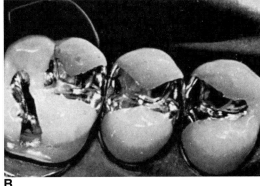

A **B**

Fig. 17-24 A, Amalgam restorations as they appear after carving. **B,** The same restorations after final finishing. (Courtesy of L.V. Hickey.)

amalgam is completely set, they can result in concentration cell type corrosion. The smooth surface on the restorations at the right *(B)* in Figure 17-24, produced by the final finishing procedure, is caused by the reduction in surface defects. Although final polishing is a traditional, logical, and accepted practice, it has not been demonstrated that polished amalgams restorations have longer service lives than unpolished amalgams.

As previously stated, the final finish of the restoration should not be done until the amalgam is fully set. It should be delayed for at least 24 hr after condensation, and preferably longer. The need for extremely high luster is questionable, but the metal surface should be smooth and uniform. The use of dry polishing powders and disks can easily raise the surface temperature above the 60° C (140° F) danger point. Thus a wet abrasive powder in a paste form should be used.

The polishing technique is a matter of personal preference, and textbooks on operative dentistry should be consulted. Essentially, diminishing grades (increased fineness) of abrasives should be used and heat production should be avoided. The restoration is not completed until its margins have been fully adjusted and its surfaces have been finely polished.

CLINICAL SIGNIFICANCE OF DIMENSIONAL CHANGE

After the amalgam is placed, a variety of changes occur at both the microstructural and the visual levels. Amalgams do deteriorate, and many are considered eventual failures. The leading causes for failures include (1) secondary caries, (2) marginal fracture, (3) bulk fracture, and (4) tooth fracture, as well as a variety of other factors. At the microstructural level, changes occur as a result of corrosion and tarnish, γ_1 to β_1 transformation, and stresses associated with mastication forces. All of these factors are probably interrelated. Thus the dentist can expect to observe such deterioration over extended periods, but the rate of failures should generally decrease as a result of improvement in alloys. Modern amalgams should have survival rates of at least 90% after 5 yr and 50% after 10 yr. Some amalgams are probably replaced prematurely for minor defects and because of uncertainty in diagnosis of early secondary caries. However, there are several types of dimensional instability that are under the direct control of the dentist.

CRITICAL QUESTION

A patient reports pain on chewing 1 day after an amalgam restoration has been placed. What are the most likely causes of this condition, and what are the best solutions?

Expansion

In an early survey of the causes for failures of amalgam restorations, 16.6% of a large group of defective restorations failed because of excessive expansion. There are several causes for excessive expansion of amalgam. One cause is insufficient trituration and condensation; another is the delayed expansion brought about by the contamination of the zinc-containing amalgam with moisture during trituration or condensation. The latter is unquestionably the principal cause of such failures.

Delayed expansion is probably caused by the internal pressure exerted by hydrogen gas that is one of the corrosion products between the zinc in the amalgam and the incorporated moisture. The large expansion begins 4 to 5 days following condensation. Thus a patient who complains of pain 1 day after a restoration is placed cannot be suffering the effects of delayed expansion caused by incorporation of moisture into the setting amalgam. The surface of the restoration should be examined for shiny abrasion marks that indicate the possibility of hyperocclusion. If this condition exists, the pain will disappear soon after the occlusion is properly adjusted. Another possibility is the development of cracks in the tooth that may have developed by removing too much remaining tooth structure and weakening the cusps. This situation may require replacement of the amalgam and *hooding* of the weakened cusp or cusps such as is done with a cast onlay restoration. It is also possible that the cracks are minor and do not threaten the integrity of the cusps or the vitality of the tooth. In this case, etching of the crack walls and bonding of the fissure may provide a sufficient interim solution. The last resort is to restore the tooth with an onlay or full crown to minimize the risk for fracture.

Delayed expansion of amalgam often causes intense pain. It is assumed that when an expansion of this magnitude occurs, the restoration may become wedged so tightly against the cavity walls that a pressure toward the pulp chamber results. Such pain may be experienced 10 to 12 days after the insertion of the restoration. If it is not removed, a contaminated amalgam restoration continues to expand, and the final result may be similar to the protruding restoration shown in Figure 17-25.

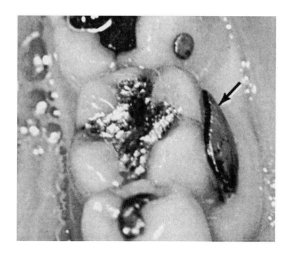

Fig. 17-25   A Class V amalgam restoration **(arrow)** that has failed because of excessive expansion. (Courtesy of J Osborne.)

Undoubtedly, moisture was incorporated into the amalgam mix because a dry field was not maintained. Excessive expansion and corrosion of the restoration have ensued, and the restoration extrudes out of the prepared cavity. Because the brittle amalgam margins are unsupported, they are susceptible to fracture, and marginal defects result. Leakage of the restoration can produce marginal discoloration, with further corrosion and pitting caused by the concentration cells formed.

Pitting and corrosion, regardless of the cause, definitely reduce the strength of the amalgam restoration. If this process proceeds far enough, the amalgam may become so pitted that it crumbles under stress.

Delayed expansion, occurring with moisture contamination of zinc-containing amalgams of either high or low copper content, is illustrated in Figure 17-26. At 20 wk, moisture-contaminated amalgam specimens prepared from both types of alloys (alloy A, low copper; and alloy B, high copper) had expanded far in excess of the same uncontaminated amalgams. The expansion of the alloys at 20 wk was also accompanied by a substantial reduction in strength (Fig. 17-27).

Contraction

It has been pointed out that undertrituration results in reduced strength and possibly undue expansion during hardening. It also is true that a slight contraction occurs with many modern amalgam alloys when they are properly triturated.

For many years, it was believed that a slight expansion of the amalgam during setting would result in a restoration that sealed the cavity against ingress of oral fluids. Laboratory tests indicate no difference in the sealing properties of expanding and con-

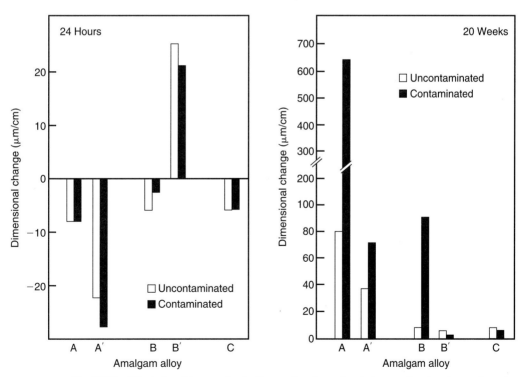

Fig. 17-26 Effect of moisture contamination on the dimensional change of various types of amalgam alloys. **A,** Zinc-containing low-copper lathe-cut alloy. **A',** Zinc-free low-copper lathe-cut alloy. **B,** Zinc-containing high-copper lathe-cut alloy. **B',** Zinc-free high-copper lathe-cut alloy. **C,** Zinc-free high-copper spherical alloy.

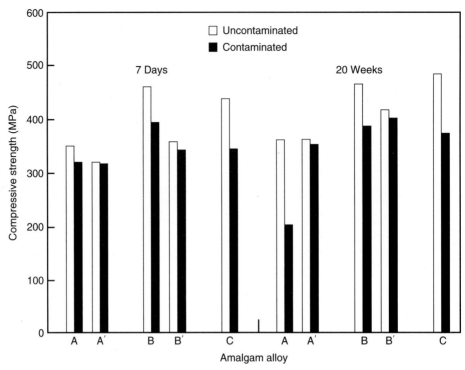

Fig. 17-27   Effect of moisture contamination on the compressive strength of various types of amalgam alloys. **A,** Zinc-containing low-copper lathe-cut alloy. **A',** Zinc-free low-copper lathe-cut alloy. **B,** Zinc-containing high-copper lathe-cut alloy. **B',** Zinc-free high-copper lathe-cut alloy. **C,** Zinc-free high-copper spherical alloy.

tracting alloys. Clinical studies of restorations placed with amalgams that contract 2 to 40 μm/cm failed to reveal a marginal contraction gap after several years.

It is very difficult to estimate whether an amalgam restoration in the mouth has contracted or expanded within the required 20 μm limits of such dimensional change. When it is recognized that the average human hair is 40 μm in diameter, it is virtually impossible to detect margins that may be open a few micrometers, either with the eye or with a dental instrument such as an explorer. For these reasons, the ANSI/ADA specification has been broadened in terms of the permissible dimensional change on hardening, as measured on an unrestricted specimen.

These observations should not be construed as a recommendation for a contracting amalgam. They merely emphasize that small contractions during hardening do not appear to be clinically significant.

Zinc-Free Alloys

As might be expected, the deleterious effects of moisture spurred interest in zinc-free alloys. Their use is certainly justified in those areas where it is virtually impossible to keep the operating region dry, such as the posterior teeth in the mouth of a child patient. In such cases, if a zinc-containing alloy is used, the dentist must sacrifice normal condensation procedures for the sake of speed. It is important that the restoration be placed before any moisture contamination occurs. For example, the condensation should be accomplished by filling the prepared cavity with a few large increments rather than with small increments, as previously recommended.

The use of zinc-free alloys provides some measure of safety in this regard, as was seen in Figures 17-26 and 17-27. When they are contaminated by moisture, the expansion at 20 wk of specimens of zinc-free alloys (A′, B′, and C) was not appreciably different from that of specimens prepared from the uncontaminated alloys. Also, at 20 wk, contaminated zinc-free alloys A′ and B′ showed virtually no reduction in strength. However, even though the spherical single composition high-copper alloy C contained no zinc, it suffered a loss in strength both at 24 hr and 20 wk when it was contaminated by moisture. Although the mechanism by which moisture reduces strength of alloys of this type has not been defined, it can be assumed that moisture present in the mix may interfere with the binding of the matrix. The present trend is toward reduction of the zinc content of alloys. Many of the spherical, single-composition, high-copper alloys are zinc-free, and although contaminated non-zinc alloys do not exhibit high expansion, the strength of some is reduced (Fig. 17-27).

Zinc was added primarily to aid in alloy manufacture, as discussed previously. There are no great differences in the mechanical properties of the two types of alloys. It is clear that zinc can have undesirable effects associated with delayed expansion. However, there is also evidence that in controlled clinical trials zinc-containing alloys have better marginal integrity and longer survival times than similar zinc-free alloys. This may be the result of preferential zinc corrosion leading to an early amalgam-tooth seal, which offers some advantage. Thus the influence of zinc on clinical performance still needs further clarification. Regardless of composition, moisture is to be avoided in the manipulation and placement of amalgam restorations or of any other restorative material.

CRITICAL QUESTION

A patient is concerned about the safety of amalgam restorations after hearing a news report on the toxicity of mercury. What quantifiable information can you provide to assure the patient that the levels of mercury vapor released from amalgam restorations are well below known threshold levels for mercury toxicity?

SIDE EFFECTS OF MERCURY

The amalgam restoration is possible only because of the unique characteristics of mercury. This metal provides the plastic mass that can be inserted and finished in the teeth, hardening to a structure that resists the rigors of the oral environment surprisingly well. However, it is also the element that so markedly influences the basic properties necessary to clinical services. The use of mercury in the oral environment has raised concerns regarding safety for more than 170 yr. Currently, several countries are phasing out the use of dental amalgam because of environmental concerns, as well as alleged side effects that may be sustained by patients who receive amalgam restorations. Although this topic cannot be covered thoroughly in this section, some aspects of the current controversy are discussed to place the issue in perspective relative to the safety of amalgam and other materials that may be considered as alternatives to amalgam. Additional information on biocompatibility or bioacceptance is given in Chapter 8. To understand the possible side effects of dental amalgam, the differences between allergy and toxicity must be discussed.

Allergy

Typically, allergic responses represent an antigen-antibody reaction marked by itching, rashes, sneezing, difficulty in breathing, swelling, or other symptoms. Contact dermatitis or Coombs' Type IV *hypersensitivity* reactions represent the most likely physiologic side effect to dental amalgam, but these reactions are experienced by less than 1% of the treated population. Allegations of signs and symptoms of amalgam toxicity have been made in recent years, causing some health care professionals to mistakenly conclude that certain patients were "hypersensitive" to mercury based on symptoms that mimicked those of various diseases such as multiple sclerosis, epilepsy, and arthritis. This misconception prompted a few dentists to request a dermatologic test for this hypersensitivity. Because the classic signs and symptoms of Type IV hypersensitivity are hyperemia, edema, vesicle formation, and itching, the term *hypersensitivity* was incorrectly applied in these cases. Inappropriate use of patch test kits with instructions for additional analyses of blood pressure, pulse rate, indigestion, blurred vision, headaches, irritability, fatigue, depression, and redness of the eyes has led to an erroneously high estimate of 25% positive responses in one report. To confirm suspicions of true hypersensitivity, especially when a reaction has been sustained for 2 wk or more, the patient should be referred to an allergist. A small percentage of people are allergic to mercury, just as a certain number of people are allergic to many other elements. When such a reaction has been documented by a dermatologist or allergist, an alternative material (e.g., a composite or ceramic) must be used unless the reaction is self-limiting (usually within two weeks). However, none of these materials has yet been proven to be *safer*, in all respects, than dental amalgam.

Toxicity

From its earliest use, mercury's possible side effects have been questioned. It is still sometimes conjectured that mercury toxicity from dental restorations is the cause of certain undiagnosed illnesses and that a real hazard may exist for the dentist or dental assistant when mercury vapor is inhaled during mixing, placement, and removal. In fact, less than 100 documented reports of mercury toxicity and allergy attributable to dental amalgam have been published over the past 60 yr in the scientific literature. Of these cases, most of the affected individuals were dentists or assistants (nurses) in a dental clinic. Few such cases have been reported during the past several decades, presumably because of improvements in encapsulation technology, capsule design, scrap storage methods, and the elimination of carpets and other mercury retention sites. The matter has again come to the fore with recent concern over mercury pollution of the environment. In some countries, amalgam particle collectors with efficiencies greater than 99% are required in dental clinics.

Undoubtedly, mercury penetrates from the restoration into tooth structure. An analysis of dentin underlying amalgam restorations reveals the presence of mercury, which in part may account for a subsequent discoloration of the tooth. Use of radioactive mercury in silver amalgam has also revealed that some mercury might even reach the pulp.

Small amounts of mercury are released during mastication. However, the possibility of toxic reactions in the patient from these traces of mercury penetrating the tooth or sensitization from mercury salts dissolving from the surface of the amalgam is slight. The danger has been evaluated in numerous studies.

The most significant contribution to mercury assimilation from dental amalgam is via the vapor phase. The patient's encounter with mercury vapor during insertion of the restoration is brief, and the total amount of mercury vapor released during function is far below the "no effect" level. The most reliable estimates suggest that mercury from dental amalgam does not contribute a significant amount to the total exposure of patients. In one study, patients with amalgam restorations were monitored with mercury vapor detectors over a 24-hr period, and the amount of vapor inhaled was calculated to be 1.7 μg per day. Three other studies have confirmed that the magnitude of vapor exposure for a patient with 8 to 10 amalgam restorations is in the range of 1.1 to 4.4 μg per day. The threshold value for workers in the mercury industry is 350 to 500 μg per day, depending on activity level, and is based on an exposure of 40 hr per week. Thus the toxicity threshold for patients receiving several amalgam restorations is far below this range of values established by the U.S. Federal government for occupational environments.

Dentists and their auxiliaries are exposed daily to the risk of mercury intoxication. Although metallic mercury can be absorbed through the skin or by ingestion, the primary risk to dental personnel is from inhalation. The maximum level of occupational exposure considered safe is 50 μg of mercury per cubic meter of air per day. This is actually an average value of instantaneous exposures over a standard work day. Mercury is volatile at room temperature and has a vapor pressure of 20 mg per cubic meter of air, about 400 times the maximum level that is considered acceptable. Mercury vapor has no color, odor, or taste, and cannot be readily detected by simple means at levels near the maximum safe exposure. Because liquid mercury is almost 14 times denser than water, a small spill can be significant. An eyedropper-sized drop of mercury contains enough mercury to saturate the air in an average operatory. The ADA has estimated that one dental office in 10 exceeded the maximum safe exposure level for mercury. However, only a few cases of serious mercury intoxication caused by dental exposure have ever been reported.

Mercury blood levels that were measured in one study indicated that the average level in patients with amalgam was 0.7 ng/mL compared with a value of 0.3 ng/mL for subjects with no amalgam. This difference was found to be statistically significant (P = 0.01). However, a study in Sweden demonstrated that one saltwater seafood meal per week raised average blood levels of mercury from 2.3 to 5.1 ng/mL, a seven-fold increase (2.8 ng/mL) compared with that associated with amalgam restorations (0.4 ng/mL). The normal daily intake of mercury is 15 μg from food, 1 μg from air, and 0.4 μg from water.

The potential hazards of mercury can be greatly reduced by attention to a few precautionary measures. The operatory should be well ventilated. All excess mercury, including waste, disposable capsules, and amalgam removed during condensation should be collected and stored in well-sealed containers. Proper disposal through reputable dental vendors is mandatory to prevent environmental pollution. Increasing legal attention is being focused on correct disposal of potentially hazardous waste materials, including dental amalgams and mercury. Amalgam scrap and materials contaminated with mercury or amalgam should not be incinerated or subjected to heat sterilization. If mercury is spilled, it must be cleaned up as soon as possible. It is extremely difficult to remove mercury from carpeting. Ordinary vacuum cleaners merely disperse the mercury further through the exhaust. Mercury suppressant powders are helpful, but these should be considered temporary measures. If mercury comes in contact with the skin, the skin should be washed with soap and water.

As noted earlier, the reusable capsule used with a mechanical amalgamator should have a tightly fitting cap to avoid mercury leakage. When grinding amalgam, a water spray and suction should be used. Eye protection, a disposable mask, and gloves are now standard requirements for dental practices.

The use of an ultrasonic amalgam condenser is not recommended. A spray of small mercury droplets has been observed surrounding the condenser tip during condensation. More detailed recommendations can be obtained by consulting the most recent reports of the ADA Council on Scientific Affairs.

An important part of a program for handling toxic materials is periodic monitoring of actual exposure levels. Current recommendations suggest that this procedure be conducted annually. Several techniques are available. Instruments can be used that yield a time-weighted average measurement for mercury exposure to sample the air in the operatory. Film badges are also available that can be worn by office personnel in a manner similar to radiation exposure badges. Biological determinations can be performed on office staff to measure mercury levels in blood or urine. The risk from mercury exposure to dental personnel cannot be ignored, but close adherence to simple hygiene procedures helps ensure a safe working environment.

Influence of Mercury Content on Quality of the Restoration

Mercury is very important to the physical behavior of the amalgam restoration. Analysis of clinical restorations indicates a wide variation in their mercury content. Characteristically, the mercury concentration is higher in the marginal areas. This is true regardless of the condensation method or the "dryness" of the increments used to build the restoration. Mercury analysis of a large number of restorations reveals that the mercury content of the marginal areas averaged between 2% to 3% higher than the bulk of the restoration. The higher mercury content at the margins is important because these areas are critical in terms of corrosion, fracture, and secondary caries.

Restorations that have an unduly high mercury content have been judged clinically unsatisfactory by visual examination. Such a relationship is to be expected in that a marked decrease in the strength of traditional silver-tin amalgams occurred at a mercury content of approximately 55% by weight, as noted. When clinical restorations were placed with a low-copper alloy containing various quantities of mercury, the restorations containing mercury in excess of 55% showed an appreciably higher incidence of marginal fracture and surface deterioration than did restorations that contained mercury in the 50% range. The higher the mercury content, the greater the incidence and severity of failure that occurred as the restorations aged.

Because high mercury content has the same effect on strength and creep of high-copper alloys as on the older low-copper amalgams, it is expected that high-copper amalgam restorations with an excessively high mercury content also will exhibit a greater incidence of marginal degradation. Certainly, if the mercury content is too high, the weaker and corrosion-susceptible γ_2 phase will be formed. Analysis of high-copper amalgam restorations, prepared with proper mercury/alloy ratios, has shown that after 7 yr, there is little or no change in overall mercury content of the restorations.

CRITICAL QUESTIONS

What variables affect marginal breakdown of amalgam restorations? Which of these factors are under the control of the dentist?

MARGINAL DETERIORATION

As has been repeatedly mentioned, one of the most common types of amalgam deterioration is the so-called "ditched" restoration shown in Figure 17-28. Although the ditching may not have progressed to the point at which secondary caries has developed, the restoration is unsightly, and further deterioration may be anticipated. Examination of clinical restorations has associated secondary caries with

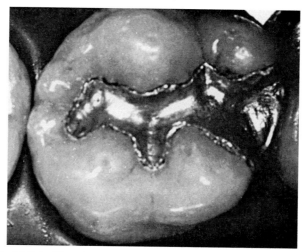

Fig. 17-28 A typical "ditched" amalgam restoration. (Courtesy of H.W. Gilmore.)

marginal discrepancies that exceeded 50 µm. Many such restorations are replaced as a preventive measure. However, the need to replace such restorations may be highly dependent on the oral hygiene status of the patient. Recent studies have shown that in a population with good oral hygiene, the incidence of secondary caries may be quite low even in the presence of severe marginal deterioration. Thus a more conservative approach to amalgam restoration replacement has been suggested.

Marginal gaps are often attributed to a contraction of amalgam, but as explained earlier, this is not likely. Instead, marginal breakdown of amalgam restorations may be caused by, or related to, several factors.

Improper Cavity Preparation or Finishing

If unsupported enamel is left at the marginal areas of the cavity preparation, the tooth structure itself may, in time, fracture. Thus the "ditched" amalgam may involve fracture of adjacent enamel as well as the amalgam.

Improper carving and finishing of the restoration and/or failure to remove a mercury-rich surface layer may leave a thin, weak ledge of amalgam extending over the enamel that will eventually fracture, leaving a ditched margin (Fig. 17-29). Such

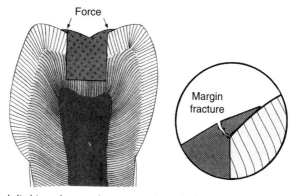

Fig. 17-29 Marginal ditching of an amalgam restoration. If a feather edge of the amalgam is left overlapping the enamel at the margin, or if a mercury-rich surface layer is not properly removed, the marginal extension will fracture under masticatory stress.

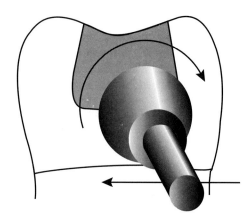

Fig. 17-30   Final finishing of an amalgam margin with a soft, unribbed prophylaxis cup and fine prophylaxis paste. The cup should be used with very light pressure to avoid flattening of anatomical contours.

thin extensions beyond the finish line of the tooth preparation are often difficult to detect and remove. One method is to finish the margins lightly with a soft, unribbed, prophylactic polishing cup and a fine, slightly moist prophylaxis paste. However, the cup should be tilted so that the edge rotates from amalgam to tooth as shown in Figure 17-30.

Excess Mercury

The effect of a high final mercury content on marginal deterioration has been discussed. Control of the mercury/alloy ratio, use of thorough trituration, and proper condensation reduce the possibility of such failures.

Creep

If the creep of the alloy is unduly high or if the manipulation is such that it tends to increase creep deformation, the potential for marginal breakdown is greatly enhanced. Certainly there is ample evidence that when other factors are controlled, the alloy used for the restoration is a highly significant factor in the incidence and severity of marginal failure of clinical restorations.

There appears to be little correlation between creep and marginal breakdown with alloys having creep values below 1%. However, when creep values are above this level, restorations made from higher-creep alloys generally experience greater marginal breakdown than do restorations of lower-creep alloys.

The absence of the corrosion-susceptible γ_2 phase in the microstructure of high-copper amalgams is assumed to be the principal factor responsible for the superior resistance of these alloys to marginal breakdown. If this assumption is correct, the property of creep is not an important property for the prediction of marginal breakdown in high-copper amalgams. However, creep is an important property of low-copper amalgams. Expansion of the amalgam from moisture contamination of a zinc-containing alloy can also cause this type of failure.

Thus several mechanisms, separately or working synergistically, may be responsible for marginal breakdown. At this time, the exact mechanism of marginal breakdown and these specific properties are still under study. However, it is advisable to select alloys that inherently have low creep and possess maximum resistance to corrosion.

REPAIRED AMALGAM RESTORATIONS

Occasionally when an amalgam restoration fails, as from marginal fracture, it is repaired. A new mix of amalgam is condensed against the remaining part of the existing restoration. Thus the strength of the bond between the new and the old amalgam is important.

The flexure strength of repaired amalgam is less than 50% of that of unrepaired amalgam. The bond is a source of weakness. Factors such as corrosion and saliva contamination at the interface present formidable barriers that interfere with bonding of the old and new amalgam.

Repair of amalgam restorations probably falls into the category of a hazardous procedure. Repair should be attempted only if the area involved is one that will not be subjected to high stresses or the two restoration parts are adequately supported and retained.

Another repair option for areas that exhibit minor marginal breakdown (i.e., gaps that are 250 µm in width) is to etch the enamel adjacent to the restoration and, after rinsing and drying the marginal gap area, sealing the gap with a dentin bonding adhesive. However, minimal scientific evidence is available to prove that this procedure can prevent secondary caries.

In conclusion, let us place the amalgam restoration in proper perspective. In Chapter 15, we saw that resin-based composites are now being used frequently in posterior Class II sites. Likewise, ceramic inlays and onlays are becoming popular in such situations (see Chapter 21). The principal advantage for the use of such materials compared with amalgam is their tooth-colored appearance.

However, amalgam still has several major advantages. It is far less technique-sensitive, more durable, and less costly than the current Class II composites. The time involved for placement of amalgam is less, and this is reflected in a lower fee charged to the patient. The wear resistance of amalgam is excellent, its abrasiveness against enamel is negligible, and corrosion tends to seal itself against leakage and bacterial invasion. Furthermore, bacteria do not tend to be as adherent to amalgam as to composite surfaces. Thus for situations in which aesthetics are not a prime consideration and for restorations that have large contact-bearing surfaces, dental amalgam is still considered the most reliable direct-filling material. In fact, amalgam still represents the material of choice for more than 50% of all Class II restorations.

SELECTED READINGS

Anusavice KJ: Quality Evaluation of Dental Restorations: Criteria for Placement and Replacement. Chicago, Quintessence Publishing Co, 1989.

Six chapters of the book written by various experts deal with clinical studies, methods of evaluation, and differences in diagnosis related to dental amalgam restorations. Evidence supporting a more conservative approach to replacement of the "ditched" amalgam restoration is presented.

Barbakow F, Gaberthuel T, Lutz F, and Schuepbach P: Maintenance of amalgam restorations. Quintessence Int 19:861, 1988.

A step-by-step procedure for recontouring, finishing, and polishing existing amalgam restorations. Proper selection of instruments is illustrated.

Bauer JG: A study of procedures for burnishing amalgam restorations. J Prosthet Dent 57:669-673, 1987.

This report describes the combined factors of time from end of trituration, burnishing force and number of burnishing strokes on margins, surface characteristics, and porosity for a high-copper admixed amalgam. Early times and minimal strokes gave the best results.

Browning WD, Johnson WW, and Gregory PN: Clinical performance of bonded amalgam restorations at 42 months. J Am Dent Assoc 131:607-611, 2000.

Two recent papers demonstrating the promise of bonded amalgams.

Dodes JE: The amalgam controversy. An evidence-based analysis. J Am Dent Assoc 132:348-56, 2001.

Authoritative studies consistently have found that amalgam restorations are safe and effective. This recent review of the literature further supports this conclusion.

Duke ES, Cochran MA, Moore BK, and Clark HE: Laboratory profiles of 30 high-copper amalgam alloys. J Am Dent Assoc 105:636, 1982.

The laboratory profiles identify the alloy systems and reflect the performance of the alloy. A classification for various types is presented.

Duperon DF, Nevile MD, and Kasloff Z: Clinical evaluation of corrosion resistance of conventional alloy, spherical-particle alloy, and dispersion-phase alloy. J Prosthet Dent 25:650, 1971.

Eames WB: Preparation and condensation of amalgam with a low mercury/alloy ratio. J Am Dent Assoc 58:78, 1959.

This technique revolutionized the procedure for constructing an amalgam restoration by use of minimal amounts of mercury in the original mix.

Fairhurst CW, and Ryge G: X-ray diffraction investigation of the Sn-Hg phase in dental amalgam. In: Mueller WM (ed): Advances in X-ray Analysis, Vol. 5. New York, Plenum Press, 1962.

Fédération Dentaire Internationale, Technical Report 33: Safety of dental amalgam. Int Dent 39:217, 1989.

This authoritative organization reviewed the literature on mercury toxicity and concluded that there is no documented scientific evidence to show adverse effects from mercury in amalgam restorations except in rare cases of mercury hypersensitivity.

Ferracane JL, Mafiana P, Cooper C, and Okabe T: Time-dependent dissolution of amalgams into saline solution. J Dent Res 66:1331, 1987.

The rate of dissolution of ions from amalgams into saline is low once the amalgam has set, probably inhibited by formation of a surface film.

Gale EN, Osborne JW, and Winchell PG: Fracture at the margins of amalgam as predicted creep, zinc content, and gamma-2 content. J Dent Res 61:678, 1982.

The findings suggested that equations based on in vitro data to predict marginal breakdown for alloys might not be predictive for non-γ_2 alloys.

Greener EH: Amalgam—yesterday, today, and tomorrow. Opera Dent 4:24, 1979.

An excellent review of the history of amalgam, the evolution of newer formulations, and citation of what the future may hold. Incidentally, some of these predictions have been prophetic.

Innes DBK, and Youdelis WV: Dispersion strengthened amalgams. Can Dent Assoc J 29:587, 1963.

The introduction of admix alloys via this research.

Klausner LH, Green TG, and Charbeneau GT: Placement and replacement of amalgam restorations. A challenge for the profession. J Oper Dent 12:105, 1987.

A national survey assessed factors underlying the placement and replacement of amalgam restorations. The reactions to questions such as expected length of service and reasons for failure are interesting, and a challenge to the profession is identified.

Leinfelder KF: Clinical evaluation of high-copper amalgam. Gen Dent March-April, 1983, p 105.

This review emphasizes that criteria in selecting an alloy include documented clinical studies, manipulative characteristics, physical properties, and quality control.

Letzel H, Vrijhoef MMA: The influence of polishing on the marginal integrity of amalgam restorations. J Oral Rehabil 11:89, 1984.

The effect of polishing on the marginal integrity of amalgam restorations continues to be a matter of some controversy, particularly with high-copper alloys. This study questions the necessity for polishing, at least in respect to marginal defects.

Letzel H, van't Hof MA, Vrijhoef MMA, et al: A controlled clinical study of amalgam restorations: Survival, failures, and causes of failure. Dent Mater 5:115, 1989.

Bulk fracture or fracture at the marginal ridge was reported as the leading mode of failure. It was suggested that further improvements in mechanical properties and corrosion resistance are needed.

Letzel, van't Hoff MA, Marshall GW, and Marshall SJ: The influence of amalgam alloy on the survival of amalgam restorations: A secondary analysis of multiple controlled clinical trials. J Dent Res 76:1787-1798, 1997.

An analysis of multiple clinical trials demonstrated the synergistic effects of copper and zinc content on the survival of amalgam restorations.

Lloyd CH, and Adamson M: The fracture toughness of amalgam. J Oral Rehab 12:59, 1985.

Admix high-copper products have higher fracture toughness than those of a single-component powder, attributed to differences in microstructures.

Mahler DB, and Van Eysden J: Dynamic creep of dental amalgam. J Dent Res 48:501, 1969.

The first suggestion that creep may be a major factor in marginal breakdown of amalgam restorations. Although modern alloys have low creep values, the test is a useful screening tool in selecting commercial alloys.

Mahler DB, Terkla LG, Van Eysden J, and Reisbick MH: Marginal fracture versus mechanical properties of amalgam. J Dent Res 49:1452, 1970.

The two independent studies showed clinical superiority for the admix alloy developed by Innes and Youdelis. These publications are classic, because they opened the vista of the high-copper alloy.

Mahler DB, Adey JD, and Van Eysden J: Quantitative microprobe analysis of amalgam. J Dent Res 54:218, 1975.

Mahler DB, Adey JD, and Marek M: Creep and corrosion of amalgam. J Dent Res 61:33, 1982.

Corrosion was directly related to the amount of γ_2 phase present, while creep was either high or low, depending on the absence or presence of γ_2.

Mahler DB, and Adey JD: Microprobe analysis of three high-copper amalgams. J Dent Res 63:921, 1984.

The composition and structure of three high-copper amalgams before and after their reaction were studied.

Mahler DB: Research on dental amalgam: 1982–1986. Adv Dent Res 2:71, 1988.

One of the premier authorities on amalgam traces the pertinent trends and literature over a 5-yr period. Excellent source reading and pertinent suggestions as to future avenues of meaningful research.

Marshall GW, Jr, Marshall SJ, Letzel H, and Vrijhoef MMA: Microstructures of Cu-rich amalgam restorations with moderate clinical deterioration. Dent Mater 3:135, 1987.

The large variations in porosity and corrosion products in clinically retrieved restorations are described. It also demonstrates a zinc-rich layer and other tin layers that form at the tooth-amalgam interface.

Marshall GW, Marshall SJ, and Letzel H: Mercury content of amalgam restorations. Gen Dent, Nov-Dec, 1989, p 473.

Amalgam restorations removed after prolonged clinical use contained nearly all the original mercury present, suggesting that mercury loss contributes only a minor amount to total daily dosage.

Marshall SJ, and Marshall GW: Dental amalgam: The materials. Adv Dent Res 6:94-99, 1992.

May KN, Wilder AD, and Leinfelder KF: Burnished amalgam restorations: A two-year clinical evaluation. J Prosthet Dent 49:193, 1983.

Clinical behavior of amalgam restorations found that precarved burnishing improved the marginal integrity of lathe-cut alloys. Coupled with postcarved burnishing, it was suggested as a viable substitute for conventional polishing.

Mitchell RJ, and Okabe T: Setting reactions in dental amalgam. Part 1. Phases and microstructures between one hour and one week. Crit Rev Biol Med 7:12-22, 1996.

Two recent reviews of setting reactions, microstructures of various amalgam types, and their properties as related to clinical performance.

Mjör IA: The safe and effective use of dental amalgam. Int Dent J 37:147, 1987.

Many pertinent matters related to the amalgam restoration are discussed in this review, including mercury toxicity, longevity of the restoration, common causes for failure, and certain properties that relate to performance.

Okabe T, Mitchell RJ, Butts MB, and Fairhurst CW: A study of high-copper amalgams. III. SEM observations of amalgamation of high-copper powders. J Dent Res 57:975, 1978.

Three publications representative of the literature that has defined the phases occurring in the setting reaction of the alloy and mercury, and the influence of parameters such as composition and particle configuration.

Özer L: The relation between gap size, microbial accumulation, and the structural features of natural caries in extracted teeth with class I amalgam restorations: A stereo- and polarized microscopic study. Tandlaegebladet 102 (NR6): 318, 1998.

Powell LV, Johnson GH, and Bales DJ: Effect of admixed indium on mercury vapor release from dental amalgam. J Dent Res 68:1231, 1989.

Addition of indium decreased the release of mercury by reducing the amount of mercury required to wet the alloy particle.

Rogers KD: Status of scrap (recyclable) dental amalgams as environmental health hazards or toxic substances. J Am Dent Assoc 119:159, 1989.

A review presenting available evidence to show amalgam scrap is not a toxic substance or environmental health hazard; it also covers portions of the literature that indicate intraoral amalgams do not present an adverse health hazard.

Sarkar NK, and Park JR: Mechanism of improved corrosion resistance of Zn-containing dental amalgams. J Dent Res 67:1312, 1988.

An in vitro study that may explain the mechanism of improved corrosion resistance of zinc-containing amalgams as compared with that of zinc-free alloys.

Schoonover IC, and Souder W: Corrosion of dental alloys. J Am Dent Assoc 28:1278, 1941.

The first suggestion of the potential for high-copper alloys, after which the subject lay dormant for several decades.

Staninec M, Eakle WS, Silverstein S, Marshall GW, and Artiga N: Bonded amalgam sealants: Two-year clinical results. J Am Dent Assoc 129:323-329, 1998.

Sutow EJ, Jones DW, and Hall GC: Correlation of dental amalgam crevice corrosion with clinical ratings. J Dent Res 68:82, 1989.

Marginal breakdown and the corrosion behavior of γ_2 and γ_2–free amalgams was studied in vitro. The methodology is of particular interest.

Swartz ML, and Phillips RW: In vitro studies on the marginal leakage of restorative materials. J Am Dent Assoc 62:141, 1961.

One of numerous studies demonstrating the reduction in microleakage as the amalgam restoration ages that is unique to restorative materials.

Vrihjoef MMA, Vermeersch AG, and Spanauf AJ: Dental Amalgam. Chicago, Quintessence Publishing Co, 1980.

A comprehensive treatment of the various factors involved in the design of amalgam alloys, their properties, and the parameters that influence clinical behavior. The lifetime of an amalgam is determined by the material, the dentist and assistant, and the patient.

18
Direct Filling Gold

Kenneth J. Anusavice

OUTLINE

KEY TERMS

Annealing—A controlled heating and cooling process designed to produce desired properties in a metal. (See *Key Terms* in Chapter 20 for additional details.)

Cohesive—Pertaining to the force of attraction of atoms or molecules of a single phase.

Cold welding—Process of plastically deforming a metal (usually at room temperature) accompanied by strain hardening.

Compaction (condensation)— Process of increasing the density of metal foil, pellets, or powder through compressive pressure.

Degassing—Process of removing gases (or other impurities) from a solid (or a liquid).

Desorption—Process of removing molecules that have attached to the surface of a solid by a physical or chemical action.

Ductile—Able to be elongated or thinned plastically without fracturing.

Malleable—Able to be hammered into thin sheets without fracturing.

Metallic bond—The primary interatomic attraction between metal atoms when they are sufficiently close to permit an interaction among the valence electrons.

Noncohesive—Pertaining to an inadequate force of attraction between molecules or atoms of a single phase.

Welding—Process of fusing two or more metal parts through the application of heat, pressure, or both, with or without a filler metal, to produce a localized union across an interface between the parts. (See Chapter 19 for additional details on heat-assisted welding.)

Work hardening—Process in which the hardness of a metal increases during cold working. This phenomenon, also called *strain hardening,* is usually accompanied by an increase in strength and hardness and a decrease in percent elongation. (See Chapters 19 and 20 for further details.)

Direct filling gold still represents the standard by which technique sensitivity of restorative materials is judged. A properly placed direct gold material can yield excellent, long-lasting restorations. On the other hand, improperly placed direct gold will result in poor-quality restorations that may be associated with excessive leakage, dislodgment, and postoperative sensitivity. Because of the very high demand for technical excellence and the recent increased demand for aesthetic restorations and prostheses, direct filling golds are used rarely in clinical practices. In fact few dental schools still teach the principles of gold foil, and state and regional boards do not require direct gold restorations as part of their licensure examinations. Nevertheless, it is important for dental students and practicing dentists to be knowledgeable about these materials so that clinical evaluations and decisions can be made relative to optimal rehabilitation of diseased, fractured, or restored teeth.

High quality direct-gold restorations can be ensured only when four principal conditions are satisfied: (1) the appropriate gold form is used for each specific clinical situation, (2) the material is used only where it is indicated, (3) a perfectly dry and clean field is provided, and (4) the material is properly manipulated with the correct instruments. Obviously, these conditions can only be satisfied if the clinician has acquired the necessary knowledge, skills, and experience. The cavity preparation is critically important since it must provide adequate access form, retention, adequate support, well-defined finish lines, and adequate pulp protection.

HISTORY OF GOLD FOIL USED AS A TOOTH-FILLING MATERIAL

The first evidence of gold foil used for jewelry may be traced to the Greek and Roman cultures that began about 3000 B.C. Historically, gold foil is the oldest of all the products described; it has been used for thousands of years. Gold jewelry was found in Sumerian, Babylonian, and Assyrian tombs built between 3000 and 2000 B.C. and later in Egyptian tombs built between 1570 and 1293 B.C.

Cavities in teeth have been filled since earliest times with a variety of materials, stone chips, turpentine resin, gum, metals, and ivory. Giovanni d'Arcoli recommended gold-leaf fillings in 1483, and his published work provided the first documented evidence of the use of gold foil for filling diseased teeth. The renowned physician Ambroise Paré (1510-1590) used lead or cork to fill teeth. In the 1700s, Pierre Fauchard (1678-1761), the father of modern dentistry, favored tin foil or lead cylinders. Philip Pfaff (1715-1767), dentist to Frederick the Great of Prussia (1712-1786), used gold foil to cap the pulp.

Gold leaf as a restorative material became popular in the United States in the early 19th century. Marcus Bull of Hartford, Connecticut, began producing beaten gold for dental applications in 1812. In 1853 sponge gold was introduced in the United States and England to replace gold leaf. This was followed by the **cohesive**, or adhesive, gold introduced by American dentist Robert A. Arthur in 1855.

PROPERTIES OF PURE GOLD

Few metals are used in the pure state for dental restorative purposes. Gold and titanium are the prominent exceptions. The purity of the gold products currently in use (99.99%) is higher than that used when it was first introduced as a restorative material. For direct filling restorations, gold has fallen in popularity considerably over the past four decades, but it has experienced a slight resurgence as a direct filling material in North America, Sweden, and Germany, in part because of environmental concerns about amalgam and the limitations of composites, glass ionomers, and ceramics. However, because of its technique sensitivity, metallic appearance, cost, and reduced emphasis in dental schools, it is likely that it will be used only with limited indications in the future.

Pure gold is the noblest of all dental metals, rarely tarnishing or corroding in the oral cavity. It is inactive chemically, and it is not affected by air, heat, moisture, or most solvents. It is the most **ductile** of all metals, as demonstrated by its ability for a 29-g (1-oz) cylinder to be drawn into a wire 100 km (62 miles) in length. It is the most **malleable** of metals, as shown by its ability to be rolled to a thickness of 0.00013 mm (0.13 μm), about one-third the thickness of the thinnest gold foil used in dentistry. Because gold is so malleable, it can be reduced in thickness almost to transparency. It is reduced by rolling to 25 μm (0.001 inch) or less. In its manufacture for dental use, 25 μm is the starting thickness for processing further to a submicron thickness.

Pure gold is extremely soft, but after cold working, its hardness (52 to 75 Vickers hardness number [HV]) is equivalent to and may exceed that of conventional Type I (soft) gold alloy (50 HV) in its softened state. After **work hardening**, its hardness approaches that of Type II gold alloy (90 HV). Although its percentage of elongation (ductility) decreases during cold working, it has a reasonably high value (12.8%) during condensation to allow sufficient lateral displacement to occur and to produce the wedging that is required to enhance retention. Because of these properties and certain other factors, pure gold is an almost ideal dental restorative material for permanently preserving tooth structure in nonaesthetic, low-stress areas. Its chief disadvantages are its metallic appearance, high thermal conductivity, and technical difficulties in forming a dense restoration. It has one of the highest densities of all elements (19.3 g/cm^3). The high density represents a drawback from an economic viewpoint because a greater mass of gold is required to restore a given volume of a prepared tooth compared with metals of lower densities.

The low hardness of pure gold would seem to contraindicate its use as a restorative material. However, its malleability and lack of surface oxide after **degassing** permit the condensation of a restoration directly in the cavity. During the condensation process, the strength of the gold is increased by cold working or work hardening. The lack of a surface oxide for gold and a few other metals allows **cold welding** to occur; that is, **welding** of increments together under pressure at mouth temperature rather than by melting, such as occurs commonly during the welding of metals.

Pieces of gold are placed in the prepared cavity and are cold-welded together under pressure applied by a suitable condensing instrument. This process is referred to as **compaction**, or **condensation**, and the gold restoration is built up into a coherent mass by this cold-welding technique. The cohesion results from **metallic bonding** between overlapping increments of gold under the pressure of compaction. This process requires the gold atoms to be forced into intimate contact with atoms in an adjacent segment and clearly indicates that impurity surface atoms, gaseous films, oily residues, or other intermediate contaminants must be avoided or eliminated before use.

FORMS OF DIRECT FILLING GOLD

Although the dental profession sometimes refers to direct filling golds (DFGs) or direct golds as *foils*, the products that are currently available may be divided into three categories: (1) foil (also known as *fibrous gold*), (2) electrolytic precipitate (also called *crystalline gold*), and (3) granular gold (also called *powdered gold*). The second type is misnamed as crystalline gold because all three types are crystalline metals.

The first two types have several subcategories or forms, as shown in the following classification:

I. Foil
  A. Sheet
    1. Cohesive
    2. Noncohesive
  B. Ropes
  C. Cylinders
  D. Laminated foil
  E. Platinized foil
II. Electrolytic precipitate (*crystalline gold*)
  A. Mat gold
  B. Mat foil (mat gold plus gold foil)
  C. Gold-calcium alloy
III. Granulated gold (*encapsulated gold powder*)

All three types have certain characteristics in common. All can be cold-welded. Furthermore, the efficacy of restorations made from these materials is adversely affected by improper handling, contamination, deviations from ideal cavity design principles, inefficient placement methods, and improper finishing techniques. With the exception of platinized foil and alloyed electrolytic precipitate, the chemical purity of most types of direct filling gold is 99.99% or higher.

GOLD FOIL

Sometimes called *fibrous gold*, gold foil is often provided in thicknesses as low as 0.6 μm. It is provided in sheets, pellets, cylinders, ropes, and partially precondensed laminates of varying thicknesses. Standard No. 4 gold foil is supplied in 100 × 100-mm (4 × 4-inch) sheets that weigh 4 grains (0.259 g) and are about 0.51 μm thick. The numbering system refers to the weight of a standard sheet, so it reflects the thickness as well. Thus No. 3 foil weighs 3 grains (0.194 g) and is about 0.38 μm thick. Other 100 × 100-mm gold foil sheets are available, including No. 20 (20 grains), No. 40 (40 grains), No. 60 (60 grains), and No. 90 (90 grains). The No. 3 foil is used in the electrolytic and powder products that are described later in this chapter. The surface of gold foil is shown in the scanning electron micrograph (SEM) image in Figure 18-1.

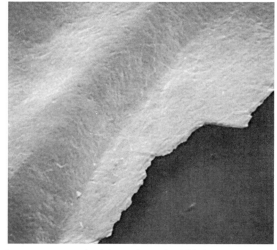

Fig. 18-1 Scanning electron micrograph of the surface of gold foil. (×750.) (Courtesy of C.E. Ingersoll.)

Cohesive and Noncohesive Gold

Although the forms of DFG can be supplied in both the cohesive and the **noncohesive** conditions, only the sheet foil is typically furnished in either of these two conditions. As previously noted, the ability of two gold surfaces to cohere by welding at oral temperature is dependent on an atomically clean surface. Gold, like most metals, attracts gases to its surface, and any adsorbed gas film prevents the intimate atomic contact required for cold welding. For this reason, the manufacturer can supply the foil to the dentist essentially free of surface contaminants and, therefore, inherently cohesive. Although some adsorption of gases may occur during storage, this type is referred to as *cohesive foil*.

However, most gold sheets are provided with an adsorbed protective gas film, such as ammonia. This substance minimizes adsorption of other less volatile substances and prevents premature cohesion of sheets or segments of sheets that may come into contact. The ammonia-treated foil is called *noncohesive foil*. The volatile film is readily removed by heating to restore the cohesive character of the foil.

Gold Foil Cylinders

This form is produced by rolling cut segments of No. 4 foils into a desired width, usually 3.2 mm, 4.8 mm, and 6.4 mm, around a modified No. 22 tapestry needle. An alternative method is to use No. 60 or No. 90 gold foil.

Preformed Gold Foils

Although in the past some dentists made their own ropes, cylinders, and laminates, cylinders and ropes are available in preformed shapes. Both are made from No. 4 foil that has been *carbonized* or *corrugated*. This form of gold foil is of historical interest because it was an outcome of the great Chicago fire of 1871. A dental dealer had some books of gold foil in a safe. After the fire, it was found that the paper between the sheets of foil had charred. However, the gold foil was unharmed, except that it had become corrugated because of the shriveling of the paper during carbonizing in the air-tight safe.

The ropes and cylinders are rolled in specific sizes and cut in various lengths to provide many sizes of increments for filling the prepared tooth cavity. The laminates are not available as preforms, but they can be made in a dental office by placing a number of sheets on top of one another and then cutting the laminate into pieces of a desired size.

Platinized Gold Foil

This form of gold foil is a laminated structure that can be produced in one of two ways: (1) two sheets of No. 4 pure gold foil and a layer of pure platinum foil sandwiched between them can be hammered until the thickness of a No. 4 sheet is obtained, and (2) layers of platinum and gold can be bonded together by a cladding process during the rolling operation and thus the *sandwich* is already welded together before the hammering procedure begins. This product is available only in No. 4 sheet form. The objective of adding platinum to the gold foil is to increase the hardness and wear resistance of restorations that are made from this material.

ELECTROLYTIC PRECIPITATE

Another form of gold for direct filling consists of microcrystalline gold powder formed by electrolytic precipitation (also called *crystalline*, *mat*, or *sponge*). It cannot be described as a foil because it is not formed by a thickness reduction process such as hammering and rolling. The powder, which consists of dendritic crystals approximately 0.1 mm in length, is formed into shapes by sintering at an elevated temperature well below the melting point of gold, which is 1063° C or 1945° F. Sintering causes interdiffusion between particles where they are in contact, so that the particles actually grow together (coalesce). An SEM image that illustrates the original dendritic structure of mat gold powder and the coalescence of particles resulting from interdiffusion is shown in Figure 18-2.

Mat Gold

Mat gold is an electrolytically precipitated crystalline form that is sandwiched between sheets of gold foil and formed into strips. These strips are cut by the dentist into the desired size. This form is often preferred for its ease in building up the internal bulk of the restoration because it can be more easily compacted within, and adapted to, the retentive portions of the prepared cavity. Because it is loosely packed, it is friable and contains numerous void spaces between particles. Therefore foil is generally recommended for the external surface of the restoration. Using this two-material technique, the mat is covered with a veneer of foil. The loosely packed crystalline form of the mat powder with its large surface area does not permit easy welding into a solid mass as does gold foil. Therefore there is a greater tendency for voids that may be seen as pits to form if mat gold is used on the surface of the restoration.

Alloyed Electrolytic Precipitate

One form of electrolytic precipitate is alloyed with calcium. The alloy is converted to a mat form by sintering at an elevated temperature. The calcium content of the finished product is about 0.1%. In this product, the granular gold, alloyed with a trace of calcium, is manufactured electrolytically. Its purpose is to produce stronger restorations by dispersion strengthening.

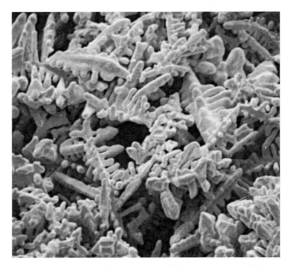

Fig. 18-2   Scanning electron micrograph of mat gold. (×750.) (Courtesy of C.E. Ingersoll.)

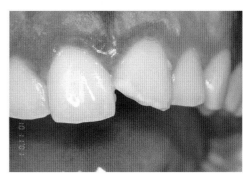

12 Hybrid composites have sufficient strength to restore fractured incisal edges. (Courtesy of Dr. William Rose.)

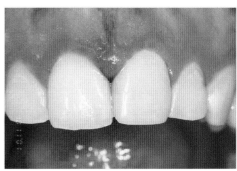

13 Class IV restoration made with a hybrid composite. (Courtesy of Dr. William Rose.)

14 Difficult access and poor manipulation usually results in open contacts for Class II composite restorations (proximal surface of second premolar tooth). This deficiency makes the tooth susceptible to food impaction and gingival trauma.

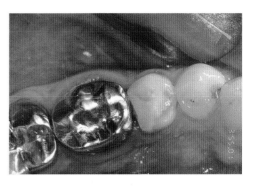

15 Composite allows conservative tooth preparation in the posterior area of a second premolar tooth.

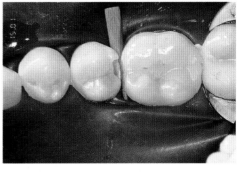

16 Use of a segmental matrix band is best for restoring proximal contacts with composite.

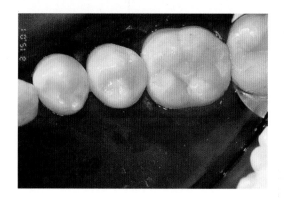

17 Class II composite restoration (DO in second premolar tooth).

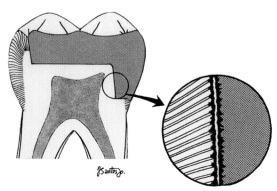

18 Diagram of the suggested mechanism through which a dental cement provides mechanical retention of a gold inlay. The cement penetrates into irregularities in the tooth structure and the casting. Upon hardening, these retentive sites aid in retaining the restoration in place. The enlargement shows fracture of these tiny cement projections and loss of retention, possibly resulting in dislodgement of the inlay. (From Phillips RW, Swartz ML, and Norman RD: Materials for the Practicing Dentist. St Louis, Mosby, 1969.)

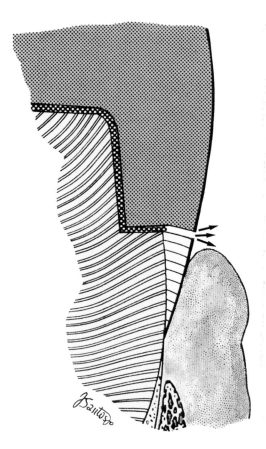

19 Loss of cement at the marginal area resulting from exposure to oral fluid.

Although compacted golds develop increased hardness and strength by cold working during compacting, a further increase in hardness can be achieved through the addition of other elements, such as palladium, platinum, indium, and silver, without affecting the handling properties.

GRANULAR (POWDERED) GOLD

Since the middle of the 19th century, chemically precipitated gold powders have been available in agglomerated form, but these agglomerates usually disintegrated when compaction was attempted. The first successful use of powdered gold was in the early 1960s, when the gold powder was enclosed in No. 3 gold foil. This form is supplied as irregularly shaped, precondensed pellets or clumps of particles that can be produced by comminution, chemical precipitation, or atomization from the molten state. Figure 18-3 illustrates a mixture of atomized and chemically precipitated gold powders after elimination of the wax binder and removal of the gold foil wrapper. The maximum particle size is about 74 μm (atomized), and the average is about 15 μm. The atomized and chemically precipitated powders are first mixed with a soft wax to form pellets. These wax-gold pellets are wrapped with foil. The resulting pellets are cylindrical and are available in several diameters and lengths.

Another type of granular gold, Goldent (originally by Morgan, Hastings Co, later by Williams Gold Refining Co Inc, Buffalo, NY), was introduced in the early 1960s. The individual particles or granules, averaging 15 μm, are gathered into masses of irregular shape ranging in size from 1 to 3 mm, lightly precondensed to facilitate handling. The masses are encased in an envelope of foil to make it easier to convey them to the cavity. The present form has some spherical atomized particles mixed with the granules to improve compacting properties.

REMOVAL OF SURFACE IMPURITIES

Heating (sometimes called **annealing**) to remove the volatile protective coating is accomplished by holding individual pellets over an open flame of pure alcohol or by placing a group of pellets or other gold form on a so-called *annealing plate* that is heated by electricity, gas, or a burning alcohol flame. The annealing

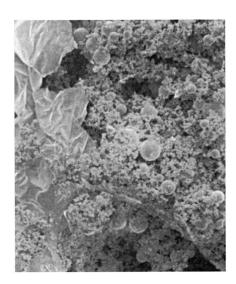

Fig. 18-3 With the wax burned away, the spherical atomized particles can be seen. The finer and rougher surface particles are the chemically precipitated portion. (×100.) (Courtesy of C.E. Ingersoll.)

temperature ranges from 650° to 700° C, depending on the selected method and the heating time.

The gold form is heated until it exhibits a dull red color. It is important not to underheat or overheat the gold segment. If the protective adsorbed layer is not driven off, the gold remains noncohesive and it will not bond to other desorbed segments.

With the exception of noncohesive golds, the DFGs are received by the dentist in a cohesive condition. During manufacture and packaging, these products are never handled manually, and there are various heating stages that remove gaseous surface contamination. However, during storage and packaging they are exposed to the atmosphere. Because gas can adsorb on the surface of the gold, it is necessary for the dentist or dental assistant to heat the foil or pellet immediately before it is carried into the prepared cavity. This step is commonly called *annealing, heat treatment,* or *degassing.* Although it is possible that a certain amount of recrystallization or stress relief may occur, these are unintentional because the primary purpose is to produce an atomically clean surface.

The gold is heated as a precautionary measure to remove any surface gases and to ensure a totally clean surface. Consequently, the term *annealing* is a misnomer. A more appropriate term would be **desorption**, because the objective is to remove adsorbed ammonia gas and other surface impurities.

Desorption is essential to the achievement of a cohesive mass. In the storage container, air (oxygen and nitrogen) is present. When the gold is not in the container, either in storage at the manufacturer's plant or in the dental office, other gases such as water vapor, sulfur dioxide, and ammonia are present as possible contaminants. If the dentist or assistant manipulates foil by hand, chamois finger tips should be worn to protect the gold from contamination. A totally dry cavity is mandatory throughout the compaction process to ensure complete cohesion.

From the foregoing discussion, it is obvious that decontamination of the gold surface is essential to ensure cohesion and to maximize the physical properties in the restoration. Proper desorption is a matter of heating long enough at a temperature that removes gases and, in the case of powdered gold, burns away the wax.

Underheating should be avoided because it does not adequately remove impurities. The result is incomplete cohesion because of the remaining impurities or carbon deposited by the flame. Overheating should be avoided because it leads to excessive sintering and, possibly, contamination from the tray, instruments, or flame. The result may be incomplete cohesion, embrittlement of the portion being heated, and poor compaction characteristics. Overheating can result from too long a time, even at a proper temperature, or from too high a temperature. However, heating times vary depending on the size and configuration of the gold segment. For example, powdered gold pellets may take 15 to 20 sec, whereas gold foil pellets and electrolytic gold pellets may require only 1 or 2 sec.

To determine the optimum temperature for removal of surface impurities, specimens were uniformly compacted from gold foil that had been heated for 5 min at various temperatures. The Brinell hardness numbers obtained are shown in Figure 18-4. The data indicate that temperatures below 315° C (600° F) are inadequate to attain optimum hardness of the compacted gold. The values were not significantly different in the temperature range between 315° C (600° F) and 760° C (1400° F).

It is not known whether these data are typical of other properties or for other forms of DFGs. The amount and form of DFG and the amount and type of surface contamination can influence the time-temperature combination needed to completely clean the surface. Aside from the purification of the gold surface, the total result of the heating process is not entirely known. Neither is it known what effect the structure or properties of the DFG have on the final properties of the restoration.

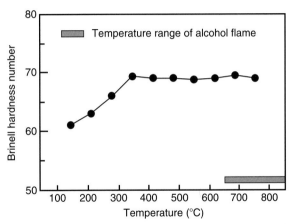

Fig. 18-4 Brinell hardness number of specimens prepared from gold foil that was heated to various temperatures for surface decontamination. The shaded area indicates the general temperature range produced by an open alcohol flame. (Modified from Hollenback GM, and Collard EW: J So Cal State Dent Assoc 29:280, 1961.)

As previously noted, the primary purpose of desorption (degassing) is to remove surface impurities. In practice, all but the powdered gold may be desorbed on a tray heated electrically. An alternative method is to pass each pellet through a well-adjusted alcohol flame. Powdered gold must be heated in a flame to ensure the complete burning away of the wax. When heating in bulk on a tray, an excessive amount of gold should be avoided, because the difficulties of prolonged heating, referred to earlier, can arise from repeated heating as well. Care should be taken to handle pieces with stainless steel wire points or similar instruments that will not contaminate the gold.

Problems that may cause incomplete tray desorption include adhesion of pellets, air currents that affect heating uniformity, heating an excessive amount of gold, excessive sintering, and greater exposure to contamination. The method of flame desorption consists of picking up each piece individually, heating it directly in the open flame, and placing it in the prepared cavity. Regardless of the type of direct gold that is used, flame desorption has occurred when the gold segment has exhibited a dull-red glow. Overheating causes the material to become stiffer, less ductile, and more difficult to condense. Underheating may lead to partial cohesiveness and subsequent peeling away of adjacent segments or layers.

The fuel for the flame may be alcohol or gas, but alcohol is preferred because there is less danger of contamination. The alcohol should be pure methanol or ethanol without colorants or other additives. Denatured alcohol can be used if the only other denaturant available is methanol. Some denaturants may be solid inorganic compounds or higher alcohol-containing residues that release smoke when they are burned. Advantages of flame desorption include the selection of a piece of appropriate size, desorption of only those pieces used, and reduced exposure to contamination.

COMPACTION OF DIRECT FILLING GOLD

Direct gold materials can yield conservative and long-lasting restorations. The technique for placing direct gold restorations is quite demanding, but the necessary skills can be acquired with minimal difficulty, although considerable practice is required. Two of the main processes that control the quality of the final direct gold restoration are welding and wedging. *Cold welding* refers to the process of forming atomic bonds between pellets, segments, or layers as a result of condensation.

Wedging refers to the pressurized adaptation of the gold form within the space between tooth structure walls or corners that have been slightly deformed elastically. Although a detailed account of the technique for insertion of DFG is not within the scope of this text, a brief description of foil compaction is given below.

Retention points are cut in the prepared cavity, and the first pieces of foil are wedged into these areas. Originally, compaction was accomplished by placing a condenser in contact with the foil and striking the other end of the condenser with a mallet. Subsequently, additional foil is welded to these pieces in the same manner. The compaction is continued, and the prepared cavity is gradually filled. This is one of several methods used for compaction.

The increments of gold must be of a proper size for insertion, and in the proper *atomically clean* condition for condensing or compacting. The first segment must be sufficiently large that it is secured by compacting it within the prepared cavity. The second and subsequent segments must cold-weld to each other; this will occur only if the surface is free of contaminants and moisture. Compaction of the gold segments will seal the cavity and be securely locked in place if the compacting force is applied in the appropriate direction and if it is of sufficient magnitude. If the force orientation is incorrect, the segment may loosen or become dislodged. A systematic stepping action must be performed, or the mass will become poorly condensed and it will be pitted and likely to fail.

Condensers

The condenser instruments can be straight, curved, angled, round, square, or rectangular, and the surface of the tip can be smooth or serrated. The tip can be flat-faced or convex-faced. Plastic flow of gold occurs over short distances under the face of the condenser. Areas not covered by the face of the condenser will remain porous.

The original foil condensers had a single pyramid-shaped face, but current instruments have a series of small pyramids or serrations on the face. These act as swaging tools that exert lateral force on their inclines, in addition to providing direct compressive forces as the load is applied to the condenser. They also tend to cut through the outer layers to allow air trapped below the surface to escape.

Each increment of gold must be carefully *stepped* by placing the condenser point in successive adjacent positions as the compacting force is applied. This permits each piece to be compacted over its entire surface so that voids are not bridged. The surface texture of condensed foil, seen in Figure 18-5, illustrates the variation in condensation effectiveness from one region to another. The densest structure occurs directly under the face of the condenser. To ensure dense masses in corners and at the junction between two walls, the line of force must be directed to bisect line angles and to trisect point angles. Loose or moderately compacted layers lie adjacent to, or below, the areas of greatest density. Thus the condenser should traverse the entire surface of each increment as nearly as possible.

Size of the Condenser Tip

The size of the condenser tip is an important factor in determining the effectiveness of compaction. The force distribution to the gold depends on the area of the point. For example, a given amount of force is distributed over four times as much area for a 2-mm-diameter tip as for a 1-mm tip. In other words, the pressure is four times as great with a 1-mm condenser as with a 2-mm condenser. Conversely, it takes four times as much force to fully compact the area under a 2-mm-diameter tip as it does for a 1-mm tip.

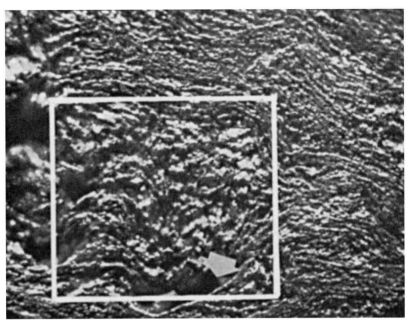

Fig. 18-5 A cross-section of compacted gold foil. A portion of loosely compacted foil is outlined by the rectangle, and the **arrow** indicates a void. The dense layers above the rectangle show good compaction directly under the face of the condenser. (From Hodson JT: Dent Progr 2:55, 1961.)

It follows that small condenser tips are indicated to achieve the desired compaction without using forces that might damage oral structures. The diameter of circular tips should be 0.5 to 1 mm. The lower limit is based on the tendency of the tip to penetrate an area of the condensed foil.

Pressure Application

In recent years, there has been a tendency to apply condensation pressure by hand, although this is often supplemented by a mallet. Using this method, gold foil and electrolytic gold are subjected to a direct thrust from the hand followed by use of a mallet. For powdered gold, in addition to direct thrusts, heavy hand pressure using a slight rocking motion is employed. Mechanical condensers are also available that provide a consistent force.

Compaction Method

The gold segments can be compacted by hand pressure alone, by hand pressure combined with a hand mallet, or by a mechanical device that is activated by a spring, pneumatic pressure, or electronically (using an electromallet). The direction of force application, the amount of applied pressure, and the compaction pattern are critically important factors that control the quality of the gold restoration.

For proximal surfaces, tooth separation is increased to provide space for the finishing strips. Care must be exercised when trimming with disks to avoid cutting into the surface of the tooth and to prevent injury of the adjoining soft tissues. For the final polishing procedure, a satin finish is preferable to a high gloss appearance since this surface will be more aesthetic because reflection of light will be reduced.

Condenser penetration should be less than the thickness of each increment that is compacted. The depth of the cold-welded mass is usually between 0.2 and

0.3 mm. The final density is controlled by the direction and the magnitude of the compaction force, and by the size and shape of the condenser tip.

The condenser tip must be stepped in a controlled overlapping pattern with the condenser tip placed approximately the distance of the tip radius away from the last area to be compacted. This method will ensure a homogeneous, dense mass, optimal flow of metal into vacant spaces, and complete sealing of the space between the gold and prepared cavity walls.

Porosity is likely to occur in all direct-gold restorations. Each type of gold requires a slight variation in technique to avoid either closed pores or open pores that intersect the surface. For mat gold, the best results are realized with condensers having a larger tip and a finer serration pattern. Powdered or granular pellets must be opened up in the cavity before compaction begins so that void formation will be minimized. These types of gold products tend to crumble as they are carried into the cavity, and they are difficult to manage. Some operators obtain a dense hard restoration using only mat or powdered gold; others find that if these forms are used, it is easer to obtain a better surface and polish if they apply a surface lamination of cohesive foil to the compacted mass of mat or powdered gold.

A small amount of excess material is provided to ensure proper contour and an adequate surface finish. The excess material is trimmed away with sharp gold knives and files of suitable shapes and sizes, and with abrasive disks, stones, and strips. Whenever the strips are used, cooling water spray must be applied to dissipate heat and reduce trauma to the pulpal tissue.

PHYSICAL PROPERTIES OF COMPACTED GOLD

The physical properties of the various forms of DFG and the influence of various methods of compacting have been reported extensively. It is difficult to compare data between studies because each investigation involves somewhat different conditions. However, some representative property values are listed in Table 18-1.

Table 18-1 Representative Physical Properties of Direct Filling Golds

Material and Technique	Transverse Strength		KHN	Apparent Density* (g/cm³)
	MPa	*psi*		
Mat gold				
Hand	161	23,000	52	14.3
Mechanical	169	24,100	62	14.7
Combined	169	24,100	53	14.5
Powdered gold				
Hand	165	23,600	55	14.4
Mechanical	155	22,200	64	14.5
Combined	190	27,100	58	14.9
Gold foil				
Hand	296	42,300	69	15.9
Mechanical	265	37,900	69	15.8
Combined	273	39,000	69	15.8
Mat gold and gold foil				
Hand	196	28,000	70	15.0
Mechanical	206	29,400	71	15.1
Combined	227	32,400	75	15.0

From Richter WA, and Cantwell KR: J Prosthet Dent 15:722, 1965.
KHN, Knoop hardness number.
*Density measured by dividing the weight of the specimen by its volume.

Transverse (bending) strength is chosen as being most representative of clinical applications. This strength is a reflection of three types of stress: compressive, tensile, and shear (see Chapter 4). Any failure can propagate from an area of weakness. In DFGs, the failure occurs usually from tensile stress because of incomplete cohesion. Bending strength represents an indirect indicator of cohesive strength.

Hardness may not be a valid measure of the effectiveness of a particular restorative material for its intended purpose of restoring the tooth. It may, however, indicate the overall quality of compacted gold; low hardness probably indicates the presence of porosity.

The density values shown in Table 18-1 are more properly called *apparent density* because they were determined by linear measurement. No allowance is made for voids. Without such voids, the maximum density should be 19.3 g/cm^3. It is evident from the table that true density is not achieved. The direct gold restoration may be characterized by nonuniform density (see Fig. 18-5). It is evident from this figure that deformation is limited to short distances that are confined to areas immediately below the condenser tip. Porosities are caused by lack of sufficient pressure to force the layers or crystals of gold into close enough contact to cause them to weld together. The greatest strength of compacted gold is in the densest (solid) area. The weakest part is the porous area, where layers or crystals are not closely compacted. Thus the maximum restoration strength is attained by minimizing the formation of internal voids.

Voids within the restoration surface (pits) increase the susceptibility to corrosion and deposition of plaque. Furthermore, voids at the restoration-tooth interface may be present to the extent that gross leakage and secondary caries may occur. However, one of the merits of properly compacted gold restorations is the small amount of leakage that takes place.

Apparently voids are inevitable, but they should be kept to a minimum, a factor that depends on the skill of the dentist. The size and shape of the condenser face, the dimensions of the prepared cavity, and the dynamics of the compacting process all influence the density of the compacted gold restoration.

The number of voids can be estimated by the apparent density of the restoration. The apparent density is the measured density, decreased from true density by the number of voids. The true density of pure gold is 19.3 g/cm^3. A survey of the apparent density of restorations placed by different operators using different forms of direct gold with varying techniques revealed values ranging from 16 to 19 g/cm^3. These results suggest that the theoretical density of a completely solid restoration is never achieved, regardless of the form of gold or the technique used.

The restorations made with the DFGs do not exhibit the high strength and hardness of those made with dental casting alloys (to be discussed in Chapter 19). Consequently, they cannot be used for large stress-bearing areas, such as a cast crown, nor can they withstand mastication stresses if they are used to restore a single cusp. Therefore the use of DFGs is generally limited to areas where they simply *fill* a space rather than serve as a high-stress–bearing region of a restored tooth. In addition, the present means of compacting DFGs provide little opportunity for producing large variations in the form or shape that can be constructed. Thus they are used principally for pits and small Class I restorations, for repair of casting margins, and for Class III and V restorations.

The transverse strength, hardness, and apparent density are evidently somewhat greater when gold foil is used alone or in combination with mat gold, as compared with the other forms. Such data seem to imply a somewhat better compaction of foil (and better cohesion). However, it is more probable that the dentist or dentists were more familiar with the use of foil than with the other forms.

There is no evidence that the differences in physical properties (shown in Table 18-1) among the various forms of gold, including the gold-calcium alloy, and the method of compaction, are clinically significant. The physical properties of the compacted gold (restoration) are probably more greatly influenced by the competence of the dentist in manipulating and placing the gold, as has been suggested.

THE DIRECT GOLD RESTORATION

The beginning of this chapter describes some of the fundamental requirements for placing direct gold restorations. Assuming that adequate training has been acquired and proper placement and finishing techniques are used, superb restorations can be produced. Shown in Figures 18-6, 18-7, and 18-8 are clinical examples of gold foil

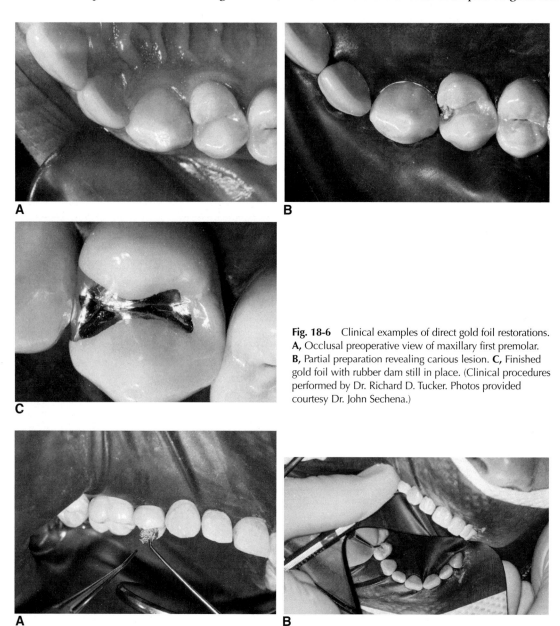

A

B

C

Fig. 18-6   Clinical examples of direct gold foil restorations. **A,** Occlusal preoperative view of maxillary first premolar. **B,** Partial preparation revealing carious lesion. **C,** Finished gold foil with rubber dam still in place. (Clinical procedures performed by Dr. Richard D. Tucker. Photos provided courtesy Dr. John Sechena.)

A

B

Fig. 18-7   Manipulation of gold foil. **A,** gold foil pellet on carrier and monoangle condenser ready to begin condensation procedure. **B,** Condensation of gold foil pellet with monoangle condenser. (Clinical procedures performed by Dr. Ralph G. Sternberg, and photos taken by Dr. Robert R. Murray. Photos provided courtesy of Dr. Richard D. Tucker, and Dr. John Sechena.)

restorations that were placed by members of the American Academy of Gold Foil Operators. Note that these restorations were placed under rubber dam isolation. The use of a rubber dam is essential to minimize the risk for contamination with saliva or water during placement.

Compared with other materials, properly inserted direct gold restorations provide a reasonably long clinical service. With the variety of forms that are now available and the modern equipment for manipulating and compacting the gold, the time involved in placing the restoration has been reduced. The concern for a possible damaging effect on the pulp has been disputed. Apparently, direct gold that is

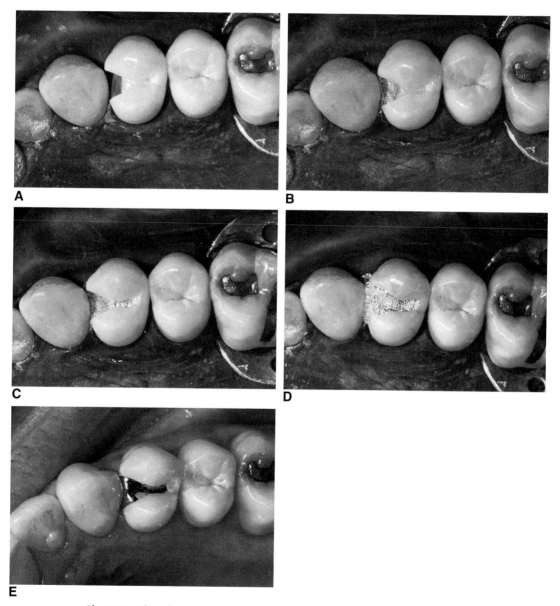

Fig. 18-8   Clinical examples of direct gold foil restorations. **A,** Class II MO tooth preparation maxillary first premolar. **B,** Buccal and lingual wall cylinders compacted and central noncohesive gold cylinder placed. **C,** Preparation half-filled with cohesive gold foil. **D,** Preparation filled with cohesive gold foil. **E,** Finished gold foil restoration after 1 week. (Clinical procedures performed by Richard D. Tucker. Photos provided courtesy of Dr. Richard D. Tucker and Dr. John Sechena.)

compacted properly into sound tooth structure produces only a minimal pulpal response.

However, the technical skill of the dentist is of paramount importance to success. A direct gold restoration of poor quality can prove to be one of the most inferior of all clinical restorations. The proper insertion of a direct gold restoration challenges the technical proficiency of the dentist as does no other type of restoration.

SELECTED READINGS

American Academy of Gold Foil Operators. http://www.goldfoil.org/archives/listing.htm. 1989 (Updated in 1991).

A comprehensive bibliography of references on gold foil.

Bauer JG: Microleakage of direct filling materials in class V restorations using thermal cycling. Quint Int 16:765, 1985; also, Welsh EL, Nuckles DB, and Hembree JH Jr: Microleakage of direct gold restorations: An in vivo study. J Prosthet Dent 51:33, 1984.

Two studies demonstrate that microleakage does occur with direct gold restorations, although the incidence is comparable to that of other restorative materials when the restorations are well placed. Thus the technique sensitivity of the material plays a major role in the quality of these restorations.

Baum L, Phillips RW, and Lund MR: Textbook of Operative Dentistry, ed 3. Philadelphia, WB Saunders, 1995.

A step-by-step coverage of the technical aspects of preparing and placing direct gold and finishing the restoration.

Birkett GH: Is there a future for gold foil? Oper Dent 20(2):41, 1995.

Carlson TJ, Naguib EA, Cochran MA, and Lund MR: Comparison of glass ionomer cements to repair cast restorations. Oper Dent 15(5):162-166, 1990.

Craig RG, Powers JM: Biocompatibility Testing of Dental Materials. In: Restorative Dental Materials, ed 11. St Louis, Mosby, 2002.

This review of the biocompatibility of restorative materials suggests that the placement of condensed gold restorations causes a moderate-to-severe pulpal inflammation 10 to 20 days postoperatively, but that after 35 days only a mild response remains, and reparative dentin may form under the restorations. Thus the use of direct gold is considered to be "biologically sound."

Hodson JT: Structure and properties of gold foil and mat gold. J Dent Res 42:575, 1963.

The data indicate that in clinical usage the theoretical density of direct gold is never attained.

Johansson G, Bergman M, et al: Human pulpal response to direct filling gold restorations, Scand J Dent Res 101(2):78-83, 1993.

In this clinical study, Class V restorations were prepared with Goldent, a powdered gold filling material. The following test groups were used: (A) cavity preparation, no filling, (B) cavity filled with Goldent only, (C) cavity lined with Tubulitec and filled with Goldent, (D) cavity with Goldent filling and sealed with IRM, and (E) positive and negative controls. The teeth were extracted after 1 to 200 days, and the pulpal response was histologically evaluated. The results revealed that when the cavity was filled with Goldent, pulpal reactions occurred, although the material itself (Group D) did not influence the pulpal tissue to any significant degree. The authors concluded that the Goldent material may not provide a marginal seal tight enough to prevent microleakage, allowing microorganisms to give rise to pulp damage and inflammation. In those cases in which the cavity had been isolated with Tubulitec liner before the gold restoration was made, the pulp was effectively protected from damage caused by microorganisms.

Lambert RL: Stopfgold: A new direct filling gold, Oper Dent 19(1):16-19, 1994.

A direct gold material, considerably different from other direct gold products, was introduced in 1989. The final restoration has a greater density than other forms of granular gold and has greater shear strength compared with gold foil.

Medina JE, Bridgeman RG, and Frazier KB: Compacted gold restorations. In: Clark's Clinical Dentistry, Vol 1, ed 2. Philadelphia, JB Lippincott, 1991.

An excellent review of the materials, tooth preparation requirements, placement techniques, and finishing techniques for Classes I, II, V, and VI restorations and for the repair of cast gold alloy restorations.

Richter WA, and Cantwell KR: A study of cohesive gold. J Prosthet Dent 15:722, 1965.

One of the most comprehensive surveys of the physical properties of various types of direct gold and compaction techniques.

Thomas JJ, Stanley HR, and Gilmore HW: Effect of gold foil condensation on human dental pulp. J Am Dent Assoc 78:788, 1969.

The compaction of direct gold does not produce a significant pulp response, as documented by this study.

Waikakul A, and Punwutikorn J: Clinical study of retrograde filling with gold leaf: Comparison with amalgam. Oral Surg Oral Med Oral Pathol. 71(2):228-231, 1991.

IV

INDIRECT RESTORATIVE AND PROSTHETIC MATERIALS

19

Dental Casting and Soldering Alloys

Kenneth J. Anusavice and Paul Cascone

OUTLINE

Historical Perspective on Dental Casting Alloys

Desirable Properties of Dental Casting Alloys

Classification of Dental Casting Alloys

Alloys for All-Metal and Resin-Veneered Metal Restorations

High Noble and Noble Alloys for Metal-Ceramic Prostheses

Base Metal Alloys for Cast Metal and Metal-Ceramic Prostheses

Biological Hazards and Precautions: Risks for Dental Laboratory Technicians

Guidelines for Selection and Use of Base Metals for Crown and Bridge Applications

Partial Denture Alloys and Guidelines for Selection

Alternatives to Cast Metal Technology

Soldering of Dental Alloys

Heat Sources for Soldering

Technique Considerations for Soldering

Radiographic Analysis of Solder Joint Quality

Laser Welding of Commercially Pure Titanium

Cast-Joining Process

KEY TERMS

Age hardening—Process of hardening certain alloys by controlled heating and cooling, which usually is associated with a phase change.

Antiflux—A substance such as graphite that prevents flow of molten solder on areas coated by the substance.

Base metal—A metal that readily oxidizes or dissolves to release ions.

Brazing—Process of building up a localized area with a filler metal or joining two or more metal parts by heating them to a temperature below their solidus temperature and filling the gap between them with a molten filler metal that has a liquidus temperature above 450° C (840° F). In comparison with welding, fusion of the metal surfaces does not usually occur during this process.

Cast-joining—Process of joining two components of a fixed partial denture by means of casting molten metal into an interlocking region between the invested components. This procedure is sometimes preferred for base metal alloys because of the technique sensitivity associated with brazing or soldering these alloys.

Cold working—Process of plastically deforming a metal (usually at room temperature) that is accompanied by strain hardening.

Coping—Metal substructure for a cast-metal or veneered-metal prosthesis.

KEY TERMS—cont'd

Copy milling—Process of cutting or grinding a desired shape to the same dimensions as a master pattern in a manner similar to that used for cutting a key blank from a master key.

Flux—Compound applied to metal surfaces that dissolves or prevents the formation of oxides and other undesirable substances that may reduce the quality or strength of a soldered or brazed area.

Investment—Refractory material used to form a mold cavity for cast metals or hot-pressed ceramics.

Liquidus temperature—Temperature at which an alloy begins to freeze on cooling or at which the metal is completely molten on heating.

Lost-wax technique—Process in which a wax pattern, prepared in the shape of missing tooth structure, is embedded in a casting investment and burned out to produce a mold cavity into which molten metal is cast.

Metal foil—A thin metal or alloy that can be plastically deformed to produce a coping for a metal-ceramic crown.

Noble metal—Gold and platinum group metals (platinum, palladium, rhodium, ruthenium, iridium, and osmium), which are highly resistant to oxidation and dissolution in inorganic acids. Gold and platinum do not oxidize at any temperature, rhodium has excellent oxidation resistance at all temperatures, osmium and ruthenium form volatile oxides, and palladium and iridium form oxides in the temperature ranges of 400° to 800° C and 600° to 1000° C, respectively.

Postsoldering—Process of brazing or soldering two or more metal components of a prosthesis after the metal substructure has been veneered with a ceramic.

Presoldering—Process of brazing or soldering two or more metal components of a prosthesis before a ceramic veneer is fired or hot-pressed on the structure.

Soldering—Process of building up a localized area with a filler metal or joining two or more metal components by heating them to a temperature below their solidus temperature and filling the gap between them using a molten metal with a liquidus temperature below 450° C (840° F). In comparison with welding, fusion of the joined alloy part(s) does not usually occur during this process. Bonding of the molten solder to the metal parts results from flow by capillary attraction between the parts without appreciably affecting the dimensions of the joined structure. In dentistry, many metals are joined by brazing, although the term *soldering* is commonly used.

Solidus temperature—Temperature at which an alloy becomes solid on cooling or at which the metal begins to melt on heating.

Strain hardening—Process in which the hardness of a metal increases during cold working. This phenomenon is usually accompanied by an increase in strength and a decrease in percentage elongation.

Welding—Process of fusing two or more metal parts through the application of heat, pressure, or both, with or without a filler metal, to produce a localized union across an interface between the parts.

HISTORICAL PERSPECTIVE ON DENTAL CASTING ALLOYS

The twentieth century generated substantially new changes to dental prosthetic materials. The major factors that are driving new developments are (1) economy—the new material performs the same function as the old material but at a lower cost; (2) performance—the new material performs better than the old product in some desirable way, such as ease of processing, improved handling characteristics, or increased fracture resistance; and (3) aesthetics—the new material provides a more aesthetic result, such as increased translucency. A brief description of the evolution of the currently marketed alloys is appropriate to understand the rationale for the development of the wide variety of alloy formulations. A summary of the major events in the evolution of dental casting alloys is shown in Table 19-1.

| Table 19-1 | Major Events in the Evolution of Dental Casting Alloys |||||

Event	Year	Economy	Performance	Aesthetics
Introduction of Lost-Wax Technique	1907	X	X	X
Replacement of Co-Cr for Gold in Removable Partial Dentures	1933	X		
Development of Resin Veneers for Gold Alloys	1950			X
Introduction of the Porcelain-Fused-to-Metal Technique	1959		X	X
Palladium-Based Alloys as Alternatives to Gold Alloys	1968	X		
Nickel-Based Alloys as Alternatives to Gold Alloys	1971	X		
Introduction of All-Ceramic Technologies	1980s			X
Gold Alloys as Alternatives to Palladium-Based Alloys	1999	X		

1905—The Lost-Wax Process

Taggart's presentation to the New York Odontological Group in 1907 on the fabrication of cast inlay restorations developed in 1905 often has been acknowledged as the first reported application of the **lost-wax technique** in dentistry. The inlay technique described by Taggart was an instant success. It soon led to the casting of inlays, onlays, crowns, fixed partial dentures (FPDs), and frameworks for removable partial dentures. Because pure gold did not have the physical properties required for producing durable restorations, existing jewelry alloys were quickly adopted. These gold alloys were further strengthened with additions of copper, silver, or platinum. Gold alloys were chosen because of their biocompatibility and ease of use.

1932—Classification of Gold-Based Casting Alloys

In 1932, the dental materials group at the National Bureau of Standards surveyed the alloys being used and classified them as Type I (Soft, Vickers hardness number [HV] between 50 and 90), Type II (Medium, HV between 90 and 120), Type III (Hard, HV between 120 and 150), and Type IV (Extra Hard, HV ≥150). This classification became the basis for American National Standards Institute/American Dental Association (ANSI/ADA) Specification No. 5 and later, ISO Standard 15592. Because of the multitude of casting alloys of diverse compositions and applications, it is extremely difficult to devise a universally acceptable classification system.

During this period, the results of some tarnish tests suggest that alloys with a gold content lower than 65% to 75% tarnished too readily for dental use. In the following years, several patents were issued for alloys containing palladium as a substitute for platinum. By 1948, the composition of dental noble alloys for cast metal restorations had become rather diverse. With these formulations, the tarnishing tendency of the original alloys apparently had disappeared. It is now known that, in gold alloys, palladium counteracts the tarnish potential of silver, allowing alloys with a lower gold content to be used successfully.

1933—Cobalt-Chromium Partial Denture Alloys

Base metal removable partial denture alloys were introduced in the 1930s. Since that time, both nickel-chromium and cobalt-chromium formulations have become increasingly popular compared with conventional Type IV gold alloys, which previously were the predominant metals used for such prostheses. The obvious advantages of the base metal alloys are their lighter weight, greater stiffness (elastic modulus), other beneficial mechanical properties, and reduced costs. For these reasons, nickel- and cobalt-based alloys have largely replaced **noble metal** alloys for removable partial dentures.

The success of the base metal alloys for constructing removable partial denture frameworks led to some early interest in using these same alloys to fabricate other types of restorations. However, intensive research into the characteristics of alloys for this purpose did not start until the 1970s, when new alloy development was stimulated by the rapidly escalating price of noble metals. Naturally, the track record of the nickel-chromium and cobalt-chromium partial denture alloys made them a logical choice for evaluation as probable alternatives for other dental applications. Likewise, by 1978 the price of gold was increasing so rapidly that attention was focused on the noble metal alloys—to reduce the noble metal content yet retain the advantages of the noble metals for dental use. The result was a series of new alloys, as described in the following sections.

1959—Porcelain-Fused-to-Metal Process

In the late 1950s, a breakthrough occurred in dental technology that was to influence significantly the fabrication of dental restorations. This was the successful veneering of a metal substructure with dental porcelain. Until that time, dental porcelain had a markedly lower coefficient of thermal expansion than did gold alloys. This thermal mismatch often led to cracking of the porcelain, which made it impossible to attain a bond between the two structural components. It was found that adding both platinum and palladium to gold lowered the coefficient of thermal expansion/contraction of the alloy sufficiently to ensure physical compatibility between the porcelain veneer and the metal substructure. (Undesirable differences in the thermal contraction of the alloy and porcelain may lead to dangerous stresses in porcelain when this composite structure is cooled, but generally similar coefficients of thermal expansion are assumed.) Weinstein et al (U.S. Patent No. 3052982) demonstrated that both the fusion temperature of palladium-based and gold-based alloys and the thermal expansion of the porcelains could be modified to produce thermally compatible metal-ceramic prostheses. The melting range of metal-ceramic alloys must be sufficiently high to permit firing of the porcelain onto the gold-based alloy without deforming the metal substructure. The first commercially successful alloy contained gold, platinum, and palladium. Development work in the 1960s improved the strength of the alloys, and research demonstrated that a chemical bond was responsible for porcelain adherence. The metal-ceramic systems that evolved from these advances are discussed in Chapter 21.

1971—The Gold Standard

The United States abandoned the gold standard in 1971. Gold then became a commodity freely traded on the open markets. As a result, the price of gold increased steadily over the next nine years. In response to the increasing price of gold, new dental alloys were introduced through the following changes:

1. In some alloys, gold was replaced with palladium.
2. In other alloys, palladium eliminated gold entirely.
3. Base metal alloys with nickel as the major element eliminated the exclusive need for noble metals.

1976—The Medical and Dental Devices Act

The 1976 Medical and Dental Devices Act in the United States placed the dental industry under the auspices of the FDA. Dental alloys for prosthetics were classified as passive implants. All materials on the market before 1976 were automatically *grandfathered* as acceptable for market distribution. Manufacturers were required to have a quality system in place, but no product standards were established.

1996—The European Medical Devices Directive

The European Union established that any imports of dental devices required a CE mark. A company needed to be compliant with an International Organization for Standardization standard (ISO 9000) and meet the requirements of the European Medical Device Directive. This performance standard went beyond the FDA requirements since no products were grandfathered and safety had to be demonstrated. Information and data on the development process were also required. Again, no specific product standards were established.

1998—The Clean Air Acts

To meet the requirements of reduced nitrogen and carbon monoxide emissions, automakers use palladium-containing catalytic converters. Each automobile requires about 1 troy oz of palladium. As new laws that required these devices went into effect, the demand for palladium soared sevenfold from 1993 to 1999. Supply could not meet the demand, and the price of palladium increased to new record highs (from $125 to over $1000 per troy oz in 2000). (Note that noble metals and silver are sold by the troy weight system. One troy oz equals 31.1 g, or 20 pennyweights.) At the same time the price of gold was trading during the decade below $300 per troy ounce. The result was an increased demand for gold-based dental alloys. The poor economy of 2001 decreased the demand for palladium and its price fell to a level comparable to that of platinum at $500 per troy ounce. In 2002, the price of palladium decreased further to a level comparable to that of gold in the $300 to $350 range.

DESIRABLE PROPERTIES OF DENTAL CASTING ALLOYS

All casting alloys must first be biocompatible and then exhibit sufficient physical and mechanical properties to ensure adequate function and structural durability over long periods of time. Depending on the primary purpose of the prosthesis, such as to restore function, enhance aesthetics, or maintain occlusion, the choice of casting alloy or metal is made by the dentist in collaboration with a qualified dental laboratory technician. The only nearly pure metal cast for dental applications is commercially pure titanium (often written as CP Ti). From a legal perspective, the dentist is primarily responsible for selecting an appropriate metal and prosthesis design, discussing the selection and alternative choices with the patient, and providing sufficient details on the design of the prosthesis to the dental laboratory technician to ensure clinical success.

From a standpoint of patient safety and to minimize the risk for medico-legal situations, it is highly important to understand the following clinically important requirements and properties of dental casting alloys:

Biocompatibility. The material must tolerate oral fluids and not release any harmful products into the oral environment.

Corrosion Resistance. As previously discussed in Chapter 3, corrosion is the physical dissolution of a material in an environment. Corrosion resistance is derived from the material components being either too noble to react in the oral environment (e.g., gold and palladium) or by the ability of one or more of the metallic elements to form an adherent passivating surface film, which inhibits any subsurface reaction (e.g., chromium in Ni-Cr and Co-Cr alloys and titanium in commercially pure titanium [CP Ti] and in Ti-6Al-4V alloy).

Tarnish Resistance. Tarnish is a thin film of a surface deposit or an interaction layer that is adherent to the metal surface (Chapter 3). These films are generally found on gold alloys with relatively high silver content or on silver alloys.

Allergenic Components in Casting Alloys. The concern for allergic reactions to dental materials gained momentum in the 1980s. Although some broad-based claims have been unsubstantiated, the subject is important from materials science and legal standpoints. Obviously, a restorative material should not cause adverse health consequences to a patient. Toxic materials are eliminated by regulation and sound business practices. Allergic reactions, however, are peculiar to the individual patient, and the practicing dentist has an obligation, morally and legally, to minimize this risk. The patient's "right-to-know" extends to having some knowledge of what is being placed into their bodies. Laws in some states are explicit in this respect. It is wise for the dentist to maintain a record of the material used for each restoration or prosthesis, as well as an understanding of any known allergies stated by the patient.

Aesthetics. Considerable controversy exists over the optimal balance among the properties of aesthetics, fit, abrasive potential, clinical survivability, and cost of cast-metal prostheses compared with direct-filling restorations, ceramic-based prostheses (all-ceramic and metal-ceramic), and resin-veneered prostheses.

Thermal Properties. For metal-ceramic restorations, the alloys or metals must have closely matching thermal expansion to be compatible with a given porcelain, and they must tolerate high processing temperatures.

Melting Range. The melting range of the alloys and metals for cast appliances must be low enough to form smooth surfaces with the mold wall of the casting **investment** (gypsum-bonded, phosphate-bonded, ethyl silicate-bonded, and other specialty types).

Compensation for Solidification. To achieve accurately fitting cast inlays, onlays, crowns and more complex frameworks or prostheses, compensation for casting shrinkage from the **solidus temperature** to room temperature must be achieved either through computer-generated oversized dies or through controlled mold expansion. In addition, the fit of a cemented prosthesis must be tailored to accommodate the layers of bonding adhesive (if used) and the luting cement.

Strength Requirements. The material must have sufficient strength for the application. For the full cast alloys the strength requirements increase as the number of tooth surfaces being replaced increases. Likewise, alloys for bridgework require higher strength than alloys for single crowns. Copings for metal-ceramic prostheses are finished in thin sections and require a sufficient elastic modulus (stiffness) to prevent excessive elastic deflection from functional forces, especially when used for long-span frameworks. The elastic moduli of many base metal alloys are considerably greater than those for other alloys, especially the gold-based alloys. Values for the elastic modulus of dental alloys are as follows: Co-Cr, 125 to 220 GPa; Ni-Cr, 145 to 190 GPa; CP Ti, 117; Pd-based alloys, 110 to 135 GPa; and Au-based alloys, 75 to 110 GPa.

Fabrication of Cast Prostheses and Frameworks. Assuming that a material meets the foregoing requirements, the ease with which a material is fabricated determines its ultimate commercial success. For example, the use of cobalt-chromium alloys rather than gold alloys for partial denture applications may require different casting investment products and casting equipment in order to produce high-quality restorations consistently. Selection of a suitable casting investment is a major problem when a dentist decides to use titanium for all-metal prostheses or as a metal-ceramic restorative material. Titanium is biocompatible and strong enough for these applications, but the ancillary products that are needed to produce consistent quality prostheses are limited in their capabilities.

Castability. To achieve accurate details in a cast framework or prosthesis, the molten metal must be able to wet the investment mold material very well (demonstrated by a sufficiently low contact angle) and flow into the most intricate regions of the mold without any appreciable interaction with the investment and without forming porosity within the surface or subsurface regions. The castability of some base metals is extremely challenging in this regard, because these alloys tend to readily form oxides or interact chemically with the mold wall during the casting process. In addition, these cast alloys tend to be more difficult to separate from the casting investment after cooling to room temperature.

Finishing of Cast Metal. Cutting, grinding, finishing, and polishing of some metals is quite demanding, and extra time is required to produce a satisfactory surface finish. Hardness, ductility (percent elongation), and ultimate strength are important properties in this regard. The hardness of an alloy is a good primary indicator of cutting and grinding difficulty, and this property varies widely among the current casting metals. For example, Co-Cr and Ni-Cr alloys are quite hard compared with other metals, as seen in the following listing of Vickers hardness numbers: Co-Cr, 450 to 650; Ni-Cr, 330 to 400; Ti-6Al-4V, 320; tooth enamel, 300 to 400; Type IV Au alloy, 250; Pd-based alloys, 235 to 400; CP Ti, 210 (bulk); Ag-Pd, 143 to 154; dentin, 60; and Type I Au alloy, 55.

Porcelain Bonding. To achieve a sound chemical bond to ceramic veneering materials, a substrate metal must be able to form a thin, adherent oxide, preferably one that is light in color so that it does not interfere with the aesthetic potential of the ceramic. The metal must have a thermal expansion/contraction coefficient that is closely matched to that of the porcelain. Stresses that develop in the ceramic adjacent to the metal/ceramic interface can enhance the fracture resistance of a metal-ceramic prosthesis (if the stresses are predominantly compressive in nature), or they can increase the susceptibility to crack formation (if they are predominantly tensile in nature).

Economic Considerations. The cost of metals used for single-unit prostheses or as frameworks for fixed or removable partial dentures is a function of the metal density and the cost per unit mass. For example, compared with a palladium alloy having a density of 11 g/cm^3, a gold alloy with a density of 18 g/cm^3 will cost 164% (18/11 × 100) more for the same volume and unit cost of metal.

Laboratory Costs. The metal cost is a major concern for the dental laboratory owner who must guarantee prices of prosthetic work for a certain period of time. Because of the fluctuating prices of noble metals over the past two decades, the cost of fabricating prostheses made form noble elements must be adjusted periodically to reflect these changes.

CLASSIFICATION OF DENTAL CASTING ALLOYS

This chapter presents a comparative evaluation of the positive and negative features of existing noble metal alloys and base metal alloys. As previously noted, the noble metals include gold, platinum, palladium, rhodium, ruthenium, iridium, and osmium. Virtually all noble alloys are based on gold or palladium as the principal noble metal by weight percentage. Several classification systems have been proposed to categorize the wide variety of commercial gold-based and palladium-based alloys. In 1984 the ADA proposed a simple classification for dental casting alloys. Three categories are described: high noble (HN), noble (N), and predominantly base metal (PB). This classification is presented in Box 19-1. Many manufacturers have adopted this classification to simplify communication between dentists and dental laboratory technologists. Some insurance companies use it as well to determine the cost of crown and bridge treatment. This system lacks the potential to discriminate among alloys within a given category (HN or N) that may have quite different properties.

The dental casting alloy classification is useful for estimating the relative cost of alloys, because the cost is dependent on the noble metal content as well as on the alloy density. It is also useful for identification of the billing code that is used for insurance reimbursement. Because insurance companies may pay more for high noble than for noble alloys or predominantly base metal alloys, it is important for

---

BOX 19-1
Alloy Classification of the American Dental Association (1984)

Alloy Type	Total Noble Metal Content
High Noble (HN)	Must contain ≥ 40 wt% Au and ≥ 60 wt% of noble metal elements (Au, Pt, Pd, Rh, Ru, Ir, Os)
Noble (N)	Must contain ≥ 25 wt% of noble metal elements (Au, Pt, Pd, Rh, Ru, Ir, Os)
Predominantly Base Metal (PB)	Contain < 25 wt% of noble metal elements

dentists to correctly identify the noble metal category of the alloy they are using (HN or N).

Several hundred brands of crowns and bridge alloys are currently available on the world market. Slightly more than half of these alloys are designed for all-metal crowns, FPDs, onlays, and inlays that are described according to ANSI/ADA Specification No. 5 (1997) as Types 1 through 4. In the past, this specification referred to gold-based alloys. Since 1989, ADA-approved casting alloys can have any composition, as long as they pass the tests for toxicity, tarnish, yield strength, and percent elongation. The mechanical property requirements for cast dental alloys required in ANSI/ADA Specification No. 5 are listed in Table 19-2. Note that the property requirements are generally specified for only the annealed condition (softened or quenched condition for gold casting alloys); requirements for the hardened condition are only stipulated for Type 4 alloys.

As stated previously, the proposed ISO 1562 Standard (2002) for casting gold alloys also classifies the four types of alloys according to their yield strength (proof stress at 0.2% offset) and specifies requirements for minimum proof stress and percent elongation for each type of alloy. These requirements are listed in Table 19-3. Although the properties for heat-treated specimens are not given in the table, it is assumed that the specimens are bench-cooled. If the manufacturer recommends a hardening heat treatment, all specimens will be subjected to this heat treatment before testing.

Alloys may be classified according to their composition, their dental use, or the relative level of stress that the metal prosthesis will sustain. For example, the ISO/DIS 1562 Standard for casting gold alloys lists in Table 19-3 the following four classes of gold alloys for all-metal prostheses or resin-veneered prostheses:

Type 1: Low strength—For castings subjected to very slight stress (e.g., inlays), the minimum yield strength (0.2% offset) is 80 MPa, and the minimum percent elongation is 18%.

Type 2: Medium strength—For castings subjected to moderate stress (e.g., inlays, onlays, and full crowns), the minimum yield strength (0.2% offset) is 180 MPa, and the minimum percent elongation is 10%.

Type 3: High strength—For castings subjected to high stress (e.g., onlays, thin **copings,** pontics, crowns, and saddles), the minimum yield strength (0.2% offset) is 270 MPa, and the minimum percent elongation is 5%.

Type 4: Extra-high strength—For castings subjected to very high stress (e.g., saddles, bars, clasps, thimbles, certain single units, and partial denture frameworks), the minimum yield strength (0.2% offset) is 360 MPa, and the minimum percent elongation is 3%.

| Table 19-2 | Mechanical Property Requirements in ANSI/ADA Specification No. 5 for Dental Casting Alloys (1997) |

| Alloy type | Yield strength (0.2% offset) | | | Elongation | |
| | Annealed | | Hardened | Annealed | Hardened |
	Minimum (MPa)	Maximum (MPa)	Minimum (MPa)	Minimum (%)	Minimum (%)
Type 1	80	180	—	18	—
Type 2	180	240	—	12	—
Type 3	240	—	—	12	—
Type 4	300	—	450	10	3

Table 19-3	Mechanical Property Requirements Proposed in ISO Draft International Standard 1562 for Casting Gold Alloys (2002)	
Alloy type	Minimum yield strength (0.2%) or proof stress of nonproportional elongation (MPa)	Minimum elongation after fracture (%)
Type 1	80	18
Type 2	180	10
Type 3	270	5
Type 4	360	3

Types 1 and 2 alloys are often referred to as *inlay alloys*. The development of modern direct and indirect tooth-colored filling materials has virtually eliminated the use of Types 1 and 2 gold alloys. Traditional Types 3 and 4 alloys are generally called *crown and bridge alloys*, although Type 4 alloys also are used occasionally for high-stress applications such as removable partial denture frameworks.

Over the past decade or so, base metal alloys have captured a significant share of the market. Introduced originally during the upward spiral of gold prices in the late 1970s and early 1980s, base metal alloys have been developed to the point where they are superior to high noble and noble alloys in several respects. Most removable partial denture frameworks have been made from base metal alloys for several decades, and about 40% of metal-ceramic prostheses are currently made from base metal alloys in the United States.

The principal cast metals and alloys used for all-metal (or resin-veneered metal) prostheses, metal-ceramic prostheses, and removable partial dentures are listed in Table 19-4. The alloys that are listed for metal-ceramic restorations can be used for all-metal (or resin-veneered) protheses, whereas the alloys for all-metal restorations should not be used for metal-ceramic restorations. The principal reasons that alloys for all-metal restorations cannot be used for metal-ceramic restorations are as follows: (1) The alloys may not form thin, stable oxide layers to promote atomic bonding to porcelain. (2) Their melting range may be too low to resist sag deformation or melting at porcelain-firing temperatures. (3) Their thermal contraction coefficients may not be close enough to those of commercial porcelains.

The descriptors *precious* and *semiprecious* should be avoided because they are imprecise terms; rather, the terms *high noble, noble,* and *predominantly base metal* should be used. As used by laboratory technicians, the term *semiprecious* generally refers to alloys that are based either on palladium or on silver. Alloys that contain at least 50 wt% of palladium include palladium-silver (Pd-Ag), palladium-copper-gallium (Pd-Cu-Ga), palladium-cobalt-gallium (Pd-Co-Ga), palladium-gallium-silver (Pd-Ga-Ag), palladium-gold (Pd-Au), and palladium-gold-silver (Pd-Au-Ag). Most of these alloys are classified as noble. The term *noble* can also apply to silver-palladium alloys if they contain at least 25% by weight of palladium and other noble metals. High noble and noble dental alloys are usually packaged and priced in 1, 2, and 20 pennyweight (dwt) lots.

Noble Metals

The periodic table of the elements (see Fig. 5-1) shows eight noble metals: gold, the platinum group metals (platinum, palladium, rhodium, ruthenium, iridium, osmium), and silver. However, as previously noted in Chapter 3, silver is more

Table 19-4	Classification of Casting Metals for Full-Metal and Metal-Ceramic Prostheses and Partial Dentures		

Metal type	All-Metal prostheses	Metal-Ceramic prostheses	Partial denture frameworks
High Noble (HN)	Au-Ag-Pd	Pure Au (99.7 wt%)	Au-Ag-Cu-Pd
	Au-Pd-Cu-Ag	Au-Pt-Pd	
	HN Metal-Ceramic Alloys	Au-Pd-Ag (5–12 wt% Ag)	
		Au-Pd-Ag (>12 wt% Ag)	
		Au-Pd	
Noble (N)	Ag-Pd-Au-Cu	Pd-Au	—
	Ag-Pd	Pd-Au-Ag	
	Noble Metal-Ceramic Alloys	Pd-Ag Pd-Cu-Ga	
		Pd-Ga-Ag	
Predominantly Base Metal (PB)	CP Ti Ti-Al-V	CP Ti Ti-Al-V	CP Ti Ti-Al-V
	Ni-Cr-Mo-Be	Ni-Cr-Mo-Be	Ni-Cr-Mo-Be
	Ni-Cr-Mo	Ni-Cr-Mo	Ni-Cr-Mo
	Co-Cr-Mo	Co-Cr-Mo	Co-Cr-Mo
	Co-Cr-W	Co-Cr-W	Co-Cr-W
	Cu-Al		

reactive in the oral cavity and is not considered a noble metal. Noble metals have traditionally been used for inlay, crown and bridge, and metal-ceramic alloys, by virtue of their tarnish and corrosion resistance. The term *noble metal* is relative. As discussed in the corrosion section of Chapter 3, the lower the position of an element in the standard electromotive force series, the more active it is. Conversely, the higher a metal is in the series, the more inert it is, and the greater is its nobility. Of the seven noble metals that are considered noble by dental standards, only gold, palladium, and platinum are currently of major importance in dental casting alloys.

Predominantly Base Metal Alloys

These alloys are based on more than 75 wt% of base metal elements or less than 25 wt% of noble metals. Base metals are invaluable components of dental casting alloys because of their low cost and their influence on weight, strength, stiffness, and oxide formation (which is required for bonding to porcelain). Compared with noble metals, base metals are more reactive with their environment. Cobalt- and nickel-based alloys derive their corrosion resistance from the passivating effect of chromium, as described in Chapter 3. Although these metals are still frequently referred to as *nonprecious* or *nonnoble*, the preferred designation is *predominantly base metal*. One reason for this designation is that some base metal alloys in the past have contained a minor amount of palladium, but because the properties of these alloys were controlled primarily by the base metals present, they should not have been classified as noble alloys. In this text, the terms *base metal* and *predominantly base metal* are used interchangeably, because noble metals are not currently included in most of the base metal alloys in use.

Karat and Fineness

Traditionally, the gold content of a dental alloy has been specified on the basis of karat or fineness. The karat system specifies the gold content of an alloy based on parts of gold per 24 parts of the alloy. For example, 24-karat gold is pure (100%) gold, whereas 22-karat gold (91.67% gold) is an alloy containing 22 parts pure gold and 2 parts of other metals.

Fineness is the unit that describes the gold content in noble metal alloys by the number of parts of gold per 1000 parts of alloy. For example, pure (100%) gold has a fineness of 1000, and a 650 fine alloy has a gold content of 65%. Thus the fineness rating is 10 times the gold percentage in an alloy. An 18-karat alloy that is three-fourths (75%) pure gold is 750 fine. *Fineness* is considered a more practical term than *karat*. The terms *karat* and *fineness* are rarely used to describe the gold content of current alloys. However, *fineness* is often used to identify gold alloy solders.

Identification of Alloys by Principal Elements

Alloys may also be classified based on the principal or most abundant element (e.g., a palladium-based alloy), or they may be named on the basis of the two or three most important elements (e.g., Ni-Cr or Ni-Cr-Be alloys). Casting alloys can be based on Au, Pd, Ag, Ni, Co, Cu, or Ti as the principal element. The properties of these alloys will be described in the following sections according to their use, that is, for all-metal, resin-veneered, and metal-ceramic prostheses, or for partial denture frameworks.

Because so many alternative alloy systems have emerged, it is necessary to discuss them in relation to their numerous applications. At the same time, an understanding of their composition is vital, in view of differences in formulations and the resulting properties. Thus the crown and bridge, metal-ceramic, and removable partial denture alloys are classified not only according to function but also according to their composition (principal element or elements). When an alloy is identified according to the elements it contains, the components are listed in decreasing order of concentration, with the largest constituent first followed by the second largest constituent. This is the basis for the general alloy classification given in Table 19-4 for all-metal restorations, metal-ceramic restorations, and removable partial denture frameworks. An exception to this rule is the identification of certain alloys by elements that significantly affect physical properties or that represent potential biocompatibility concerns, or both. For example, nickel-chromium-molybdenum-beryllium alloys are often designated as nickel-chromium-beryllium alloys because of the contributions of beryllium to the control of castability and surface oxidation at high temperatures and because of the relative toxicity potential of beryllium compared with other metals. Molybdenum (Mo) and tungsten (W) often exist in greater concentrations than beryllium to decrease the thermal coefficient of expansion. However, the concern for the biocompatibility of beryllium is a more important factor, and some research reports list these alloys as Ni-Cr-Be rather than Ni-Cr-Mo or Ni-Cr-Mo-Be.

ALLOYS FOR ALL-METAL AND RESIN-VENEERED RESTORATIONS

In 1927, the National Bureau of Standards (now the National Institute of Standards and Technology) established gold casting alloy Types I through IV according to

| Table 19-5 | Typical Compositions of Casting Alloys for Full-Metal, Resin-Veneered, and Metal-Ceramic Prostheses |

Alloy type	Classification	Elemental composition (wt%)				
		Au	Pd	Ag	Cu	Ga, In, and Zn
I	High Noble (Au-based)	83	0.5	10	6	Balance
II	High Noble (Au-based)	77	1	14	7	Balance
III	High Noble (Au-based)	75	3.5	11	9	Balance
III	Noble (Au-based)	46	6	39	8	Balance
III	Noble (Ag-based)	—	25	70	—	Balance
IV	High Noble (Au-based)	56	4	25	14	Balance
IV	Noble (Ag-based)	15	25	45	14	Balance
Metal-Ceramic	High Noble (Au-based)	52	38	—	—	Balance
Metal-Ceramic	Noble (Pd-based)	—	60	30	—	Balance
Metal-Ceramic	High Noble (Au-based)	88	7	1	—	Balance
Metal-Ceramic	Noble (Pd-based: High Pd)	0–6	74–88	0–10	0–15	Balance

dental function, with hardness increasing from Type I to Type IV. Typical compositions of these alloys are given in Table 19-5, in which the original convention of Roman numerals has been followed.

Heat Treatment of High Noble and Noble Metal Alloys

As previously discussed in Chapter 6, gold alloys can be significantly hardened if the alloy contains a sufficient amount of copper. Types I and II alloys usually do not harden, or they harden to a lesser degree than do the Types III and IV gold alloys. The actual mechanism of hardening is probably the result of several different solid-state transformations. Although the precise mechanism may be in doubt, the criteria for successful hardening are time and temperature. Type III and Type IV gold alloys that can be hardened (strengthened from the quenched as-cast condition) can, of course, also be softened. In metallurgical engineering terminology the softening heat treatment is referred to as a *solution heat treatment*. The hardening heat treatment is termed **age hardening.** The metallurgical basis for both heat treatments has been discussed in Chapter 6.

Softening Heat Treatment of Gold Casting Alloys

The casting is placed in an electric furnace for 10 min at a temperature of 700° C (1292° F), and then it is quenched in water. During this period, all intermediate phases are presumably changed to a disordered solid solution, and the rapid quenching prevents ordering from occurring during cooling. The tensile strength, proportional limit, and hardness are reduced by such a treatment, and the ductility is increased.

The softening heat treatment is indicated for structures that are to be ground, shaped, or otherwise **cold worked,** either in or out of the mouth. Although 700° C is an adequate average softening temperature, each alloy has its optimum temperature, and the manufacturer should specify the most favorable temperature and time.

Hardening Heat Treatment of Gold Casting Alloys

The age hardening or hardening heat treatment of dental alloys can be accomplished in several ways. One of the most practical hardening treatments is by soaking or aging the casting at a specific temperature for a definite time, usually 15 to 30 minutes, before it is water-quenched. The aging temperature depends on the alloy composition but is generally between 200° C (392° F) and 450° C (842° F). The proper time and temperature are specified by the manufacturer.

Ideally, before the alloy is given an age-hardening treatment, it should be subjected to a softening heat treatment to relieve all **strain hardening** and to start the hardening treatment with the alloy as a disordered solid solution. Otherwise, there will not be proper control of the hardening process, because the increase in strength, proportional limit, and hardness and the reduction in ductility are controlled by the amount of possible solid-state transformations. The transformations, in turn, are controlled by the temperature and time of the age-hardening treatment.

Because the proportional limit is increased during age hardening, a considerable increase in the modulus of resilience can be expected. The hardening heat treatment is indicated for metallic partial dentures, saddles, FPDs, and other similar structures. For small structures, such as inlays, a hardening treatment is not usually employed.

The yield strength, the proportional limit, and the elastic limit are all measures of essentially the same property, that is, the stress at which plastic deformation begins or at which a very limited amount of plastic deformation has occurred. Additional details about these properties are given in Chapter 4. These properties reflect the relative capacity of an alloy (and hence the cast prosthesis) to withstand mechanical stresses induced by an applied load without permanent deformation. In general, the yield strength increases when progressing from Type I to Type IV alloys. Age hardening substantially increases the yield strength (in one case by nearly 100%).

The hardness values for noble metal alloys correlate quite well with their yield strengths. Traditionally, hardness has been used for indicating the suitability of an alloy for a given type of clinical application.

Elongation (percent) is a measure of ductility as the amount of permanent tensile elongation that an alloy can undergo before fracture. A reasonable amount of such elongation is essential if the clinical application requires some permanent deformation of the as-cast structure, such as is needed for clasp and margin adjustment and for burnishing. Age hardening reduces the percent elongation, in some cases very significantly. Alloys with low elongation are relatively brittle materials and fracture readily if loaded beyond the proportional limit or yield strength.

Casting Shrinkage

As noted in Chapter 12, all metals and alloys of practical dental interest shrink when they change from the liquid to the solid state. As will be seen, this consideration is important in the dental casting procedure. For example, if the mold for an inlay is an accurate reproduction of the missing tooth structure, the cast gold inlay will be too small by the amount of its casting shrinkage.

The shrinkage occurs in three stages: (1) the thermal contraction of the liquid metal between the temperature to which it is heated and the **liquidus temperature;** (2) the contraction of the metal inherent in its change from the liquid to the solid state; and (3) the thermal contraction of the solid metal that occurs on further cooling to room temperature.

The first-mentioned contraction is probably of no consequence; because as the liquid metal contracts in the mold with a properly designed sprue system more molten metal can flow into the mold to compensate for such a shrinkage. The casting technique, described in Chapter 12, allows for such flow of molten metal. The relative solidification shrinkage of various alloys cast as smooth cylinders is listed in Box 19-2.

The values for the casting shrinkage differ for the various alloys, presumably because of differences in their composition. For example, platinum, palladium, and copper are effective in reducing the casting shrinkage of an alloy. The casting shrinkage of pure gold closely approaches that of its maximal linear thermal contraction.

In general, the casting shrinkage values given in Box 19-2 are less than their linear thermal contraction values, even though the casting shrinkage as obtained includes both the solidification shrinkage and the thermal contraction from the solidification temperature to room temperature. This seemingly anomalous condition can be accounted for by logical assumptions: (1) When the mold becomes filled with molten metal, the metal starts to solidify at the walls of the mold, because the temperature of the mold is less than that of the bulk molten metal. (2) During initial cooling, the first layer of metal to solidify against the walls of the mold is weak, and it tends to adhere to the mold until it gains sufficient strength as it cools to pull away. When the metal is sufficiently strong to contract independently of the mold, it shrinks thermally until it reaches room temperature. (3) There may be constraints by the mold on the metal contraction during cooling, because of the typical complex geometry of dental castings.

The thermal shrinkage of the first weak solidified layer is initially prevented by its mechanical adhesion to the walls of the mold. During this period, it is actually stretched because of its interlocking with the investment material, which has a lower thermal contraction coefficient. Thus any contraction occurring during solidification

BOX 19-2
Linear Solidification Shrinkage of Casting Alloys

Alloy Type	Casting Shrinkage (%)
Type I (Au-based)	1.56
Type II (Au-based)	1.37
Type III (Au-based)	1.42
Type IV (Ni-Cr–based)	2.30
Type IV (Co-Cr–based)	2.30

can be eliminated, particularly with a well-designed sprue system that feeds new liquid metal to the sites undergoing solidification. Also, part of the total thermal contraction can be eliminated, with the result that the observed casting shrinkage is less than might be expected on the basis of the possible stages of the shrinkage.

Because the thermal contraction as the alloy cools to room temperature dominates the casting shrinkage, the higher melting alloys tend to exhibit greater shrinkage. This must be compensated for in the casting technique if good fit is to be obtained.

Remelting Previously Cast Metal

When fusing an alloy to prepare a casting, a dental laboratory will typically use new metal ingots, and they may also add metal sprues that were removed from previous castings. The accepted guideline is that 50% new alloy should be used with previously melted alloy. A carefully controlled study on a low-gold Type III alloy found significant decreases in yield strength and percentage elongation for specimens that consisted entirely of metal that had been previously melted one time and two times, although there were no significant changes in tensile strength. The prevalence of casting defects increased with the number of times that the alloy was melted. There is no established limit on the number of times that previously cast metal can be reused along with 50% new alloy and still yield clinically acceptable castings of adequate strength and long-term in vivo performance.

Silver-Palladium Alloys

Silver-palladium alloys are white and predominantly silver in composition but have substantial amounts of palladium (at least 25%) that provide nobility and promote tarnish resistance. They may or may not contain copper and a small amount of gold. Casting temperatures are in the range of the yellow gold alloys. The copper-free Ag-Pd alloys may contain 70% to 72% silver and 25% palladium and may have physical properties similar to those for a Type III gold alloy. Other silver-based alloys might contain roughly 60% silver, 25% palladium, and as much as 15% or more copper and may have properties more like a Type IV gold alloy. Despite early reports of poor castability, the Ag-Pd alloys can produce acceptable castings. The major limitation of Ag-Pd alloys in general, and the Ag-Pd-Cu alloys in particular, is their greater potential for tarnish and corrosion. They should not be confused with Pd-Ag alloys that are designed for metal-ceramic restorations.

Because of the increasing interest in aesthetics by dental patients, all-metal restorations have been used less frequently during the past decade. The use of metal-ceramic restorations in posterior sites has increased relative to the use of all-metal crowns and onlays. Because most crown and bridge restorations in posterior teeth are based on metal-ceramic systems, the alloys for these prostheses are discussed more completely.

The compositions of representative high noble and noble alloys (including the Ag-Pd alloys) for all-metal restorations (Type I to Type IV) and metal-ceramic restorations are given in Table 19-5.

Nickel-Chromium and Cobalt-Chromium Alloys

Nickel-chromium and cobalt-chromium alloys are described in more detail in the sections on metal-ceramic prostheses and partial dentures. They are rarely used for all-metal restorations.

Titanium and Titanium Alloys

The use of commercially pure titanium (CP Ti) and titanium alloys increased significantly over the last two decades of the twentieth century. These metals can be used for all-metal and metal-ceramic prostheses, as well as for implants and removable partial denture frameworks. Titanium is considered the most biocompatible metal used for dental prostheses. Because of the unique properties of titanium, and especially its biocompatibility, it does not fall within the classification of base metals. It is worthy of a separate class of metals.

According to the American Society for Testing and Materials (ASTM), there are five unalloyed grades of CP Ti (Grades 1–4, and Grade 7), based on the concentration of oxygen (0.18 wt% to 0.40 wt%) and iron (0.2 wt% to 0.5 wt%). Other impurities include nitrogen (0.03 wt% to 0.05 wt%), carbon (0.1 wt%), and hydrogen (0.015 wt%). Grade 1 CP Ti is the purest and softest form. It has a moderately high tensile strength (Grade 1 CP Ti, 240 MPa; Grade 4 CP Ti, 515 MPa), moderately high stiffness (elastic modulus, 117 GPa), low density (4.51 g/cm^3), and low thermal expansion coefficient (9.4 × 10^{-6}/°C). The elastic modulus of CP Ti is comparable to that of tooth enamel and noble alloys, but it is lower than that of other base metals. As discussed in Chapter 3, CP Ti is very resistant to tarnish and corrosion. The corrosion protection is derived from a thin (10 nm) passivating oxide film that forms spontaneously. However, because the oxidation rate of titanium increases markedly above 900° C, it is desirable to use ultralow-fusing porcelains (sintering temperature less than 850° C) for titanium-ceramic prostheses. A porcelain sintering temperature below 800° C is desirable to minimize oxidation and to avoid the conversion of alpha phase to the higher-temperature beta phase discussed in the following.

Titanium has a high melting point (1668° C), and a special casting machine with arc-melting capability and an argon atmosphere is typically used, along with a compatible casting investment, to ensure acceptable castability. Because of reaction with the investment, a very hard so-called α case having a thickness of approximately 150 μm forms at the surface of cast dental titanium alloys.

For cast CP Ti, the HV increases from a bulk value of nearly 200 to approximately 650 at a depth of 25 μm below the surface, and special tools are required in the dental laboratory for finishing and adjusting CP Ti castings. Because of the presence of the α case, special surface modifications of cast titanium, using caustic NaOH-based solutions or silicon nitride coatings, have been employed to improve the bond between cast CP Ti and dental porcelain.

Titanium has the highest melting temperature of all metals used for metal-ceramic prostheses and is highly resistant to sag deformation of metal frameworks at porcelain sintering temperatures. This high melting point is accompanied by a relatively low thermal expansion coefficient, and special low-expansion dental porcelains are necessary for bonding to titanium.

Commercially pure titanium undergoes an allotropic transformation from a hexagonal close-packed crystal structure (α phase) at 885° C to a body-centered crystal structure (β phase). Four possible types of titanium alloys can be produced: α, near-α, α–β, and β. A β alloy will form no β phase on cooling. A near-α phase alloy will form limited β phase on cooling. An α–β alloy will contain α phase at room temperature and may contain retained β phase and/or transformed β phase. A β alloy will retain the β phase on cooling, and it can precipitate other phases as well during heat treatment. Vanadium, which has a bcc structure, is one of the alloying elements that is isomorphous with the β phase and is a β phase stabilizer, that is, causing the transformation from β phase to α phase to occur at lower temperatures on cooling. Aluminum, which is an α phase stabilizer (i.e., causing the transformation of α phase to β phase to occur at a higher temperature on heating), is included in α and near-α alloys. Aluminum, tin, and zirconium are soluble in both the α and β phases. The most widely used titanium alloy in dentistry and for general commercial applications is Ti-6Al-4V, which is an α–β alloy. Although this alloy has greater strength than CP Ti, it is not as attractive from a biocompatibility point of view because of some concerns about health hazards from the slow release of aluminum and vanadium atoms in vivo.

Aluminum Bronze Alloy

One alloy based on copper as the major element has been approved previously by the ADA. However, because of its susceptibility to tarnish and corrosion, this status of acceptance was subsequently withdrawn. Although bronze is traditionally defined as a copper-rich, copper-tin (Cu-Sn) alloy with or without other elements such as zinc and phosphorus, there exist essentially two-component (binary), three-component (ternary), and four-component (quaternary) bronze alloys that contain no tin, such as aluminum bronze (copper-aluminum [Cu-Al]), silicon bronze (copper-silicon [Cu-Si]), and beryllium bronze (copper-beryllium [Cu-Be]). The aluminum bronze family of alloys may contain between 81 wt% and 88 wt% copper, 7 wt% to 11 wt% aluminum, 2 wt% to 4 wt% nickel, and 1 wt% to 4 wt% iron. No long-term clinical data are available on this aluminum bronze dental alloy. There is a potential for copper alloys to react with sulfur to form copper sulfide, which may tarnish the surface of this alloy in the same manner that silver sulfide darkens the surface of gold-base or silver-base alloys that contain a significant silver content.

CRITICAL QUESTION

How do alloys for all-metal prostheses differ from those required for metal-ceramic prostheses?

HIGH NOBLE AND NOBLE ALLOYS FOR METAL-CERAMIC PROSTHESES

The chief objection to the use of dental porcelain as a restorative material is its low strength under tensile and shear stress conditions. Although porcelain can resist compressive stresses with reasonable success, the substructure design should not include shapes in which significant tensile stresses are produced during loading.

A method by which this disadvantage can be minimized is to bond the porcelain directly to a cast alloy substructure made to fit the prepared tooth. If a strong bond is attained between the porcelain veneer and the metal, the porcelain veneer is usually well supported during loading of the prosthesis. Thus the risk for brittle fracture can be avoided or, at least, minimized.

To fabricate this restoration, a metal substructure is waxed, cast, finished, and heat treated (oxidized). A thin layer of opaque porcelain is fused to the oxidized metal surface to establish the porcelain-metal bond and mask the color of the substructure. Then dentin and enamel porcelains, sometimes referred to as *body and incisal porcelains,* are fused to the opaque porcelain, shaped, stained to improve the aesthetic appearance, and glazed.

The original metal-ceramic alloys contained 88% gold and were much too soft for stress-bearing restorations such as fixed partial dentures. Because there was no evidence of a chemical bond between these alloys and dental porcelain, mechanical retention and undercuts were used to prevent detachment of the ceramic veneer. Bond strength tests were developed in which predominantly shear or tensile stress was concentrated at the porcelain-metal interface. It was found that the bond strength of the porcelain to this type of alloy was less than the cohesive strength of the porcelain itself. This meant that if a failure occurred in the metal-ceramic prosthesis, it would most probably arise at the metal-porcelain interface. By adding less than 1% of oxide-forming elements such as iron, indium, and tin to this high–gold-content alloy, the porcelain metal bond strength was improved by a factor of 3. Iron also increases the proportional limit and strength of the alloy by forming an $FePt_3$ precipitate with platinum.

The 1% addition of base metals to the gold, palladium, and platinum alloy was sufficient to produce a slight oxide film on the surface of the substructure to achieve a porcelain-metal bond strength level that surpassed the cohesive strength of the porcelain. This new type of alloy, with small amounts of base metals added, became the standard for metal-ceramic prostheses. In response to economic pressures, other gold- and palladium-based metal-ceramic alloys emerged. In time, base metals were also developed for this same purpose.

Despite the large number of alloys possessing the technical capability to bond to dental porcelain, they can be arranged in the previously described classification based on alloy composition. As shown in Box 19-1, metal-ceramic alloys fall into one of the three general categories—high noble, noble, or predominantly base metal—and are arranged according to composition. Using this approach, alloys with similar compositions, physical properties, and handling characteristics can be grouped together.

In spite of vastly different chemical compositions, all the alloys described in the following according to their principal chemical elements share at least three common features: (1) They have the potential to bond to dental porcelain. (2) They possess coefficients of thermal contraction compatible with those of dental porcelains. (3) Their solidus temperature is sufficiently high to permit the application of low-fusing porcelains. The integrity and longevity of that bond are dependent on a multitude of factors, as described in Chapter 21.

The coefficients of thermal expansion (CTE) tend to have a reciprocal relationship with the melting points of alloys (because of an inverse dependence on the relative strength of interatomic bonding), as well as the melting range of alloys; that is, the higher the melting temperature of a metal, the lower its CTE. This fact is important in formulating metal-ceramic alloys for different dental porcelains. Metal-ceramic alloys are also often referred to as *porcelain fused to metal* (PFM) or *ceramometal alloys*. The preferred descriptive term is *metal-ceramic*, followed by *porcelain-fused-to-metal*, even though the latter involves sintering of porcelain, rather than fusion. Likewise, the preferred acronyms are PFM or MC, rather than other acronyms such as PBM (porcelain bonded to metal) and PTM (porcelain to metal).

As previously noted, alloys for metal-ceramic bonding have several unique requirements that do not apply to all-metal products. These alloys must have a thermal expansion/contraction coefficient that is comparable to or slightly greater than that of the veneering porcelain, and they must also have a sufficiently high melting range to avoid sag deformation or melting during sintering of porcelain veneers. Shown in Figure 19-1 is a schematic illustration of sag deformation in a fixed partial denture (FPD) framework. To avoid this potential problem, a sag-resistant alloy should be used. Your laboratory technician or alloy manufacturer will provide expert advice about choices. If sag deformation has occurred during firing of porcelain, this problem can be corrected by the laboratory technician in one of three

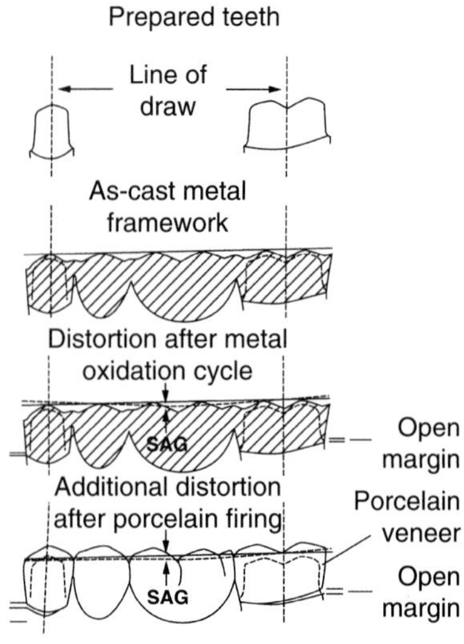

Fig. 19-1 Sag deformation in a fixed partial denture (FPD) framework.

ways: (1) The FPD can be sectioned and soldered to obtain an acceptable fit on the prepared dies. (2) **Cast-joining** of the bridge sections can be performed. This process entails placing undercut slots in the walls of the sectioned pieces for mechanical retention, indexing the units, waxing and spruing, investing and burning out the wax or resin, and casting new metal into the sectioned area. (3) A remake of the cast structure with a sag-resistant alloy (Groups III–X in Table 19-6 and all base metal alloys) is also an option. In this case, the laboratory technician should rewax the framework and increase the thickness of the interproximal connectors in an incisal-gingival or occlusal-gingival direction. The technician should also attempt to support the recast or soldered framework at an intermediate point along the length of the span during firing.

Gold-platinum-palladium alloys are ideally suited for single units or short-span FPDs when aesthetics and biocompatibility are primary concerns. Typical yellow and white gold alloy products are listed in Table 19-6. These alloys range in gold content from approximately 50% to 88%. Oxidizable elements such as Sn, In or Fe are included in each alloy to promote adherence to porcelain. However, because of their sag potential, the use of these alloys must be limited to crowns and three-unit FPDs.

Gold-Palladium-Silver Alloys (Low Silver Content)

Gold-palladium-silver alloys (Group III in Table 19-6), which contain 5% to 11.99% Ag are economical alternatives to the Au-Pt-Pd or Au-Pd-Pt alloys. Their excellent resistance to tarnish and corrosion and relative freedom from technique sensitivity associated with porcelain bonding and thermal contraction differences have contributed to their long-term success. The principal disadvantage of this alloy group is the potential for porcelain discoloration when silver vapor is released and deposited on the porcelain surface.

Gold-Palladium-Silver Alloys (High Silver Content)

Gold alloys that contain 12% Ag or more (Group IV in Table 19-6) account for approximately 20% of the current alloy market. These include Au-Pd-Ag, Pd-Au-Ag, and Pd-Ag alloys. The Au-Pd alloys with high silver contents (12% to 22%) have been popular alternatives to the higher gold content alloys for many years despite

Table 19-6 Compositions of Representative High Noble (HN)* and Noble (N)† Alloys for Metal-Ceramic Prostheses

Typical products	Supplier	Principal elements (wt%)							
		Au	Pt	Pd	Ag	Cu	Co	Ga	Sn, Zn, and In
I. Au-Pt-Pd or Au-Pd-Pt (0% to 4.99% Ag)	SMG-3 (Dentsply Ceramco)	81	6	11	—	—	—	—	Bal.
	Jelenko "O" (Heraeus-Kulzer)	87	4.5	6	1	—	—	—	Bal.
	Argedent Y86 (Argen)	86	10	2	—	—	—	—	Bal.
II. Au-Pt-Ag/Au-Pd-Ag (9% to 10% Ag)	Degunorm (Dentsply Ceramco)	74	9	—	9	—	—	—	Bal.
	Argedent 62 (Argen)	62	—	24	9	—	—	—	Bal.
III. Au-Pd-Ag (5% to 11.99% Ag)	Argedent 75 (Argen)	75	—	12	10	—	—	—	2.8
	Rx Sp CG (Pentron Lab Tech.)	75	—	13	10	—	—	—	Bal.
IV. Au-Pd-Ag (12% Ag or more)	Aspire (Dentsply Ceramco)	52	—	26	17	—	—	—	Bal.
	Cameo (Heraeus-Kulzer)	52.5	—	27	16	—	—	—	Bal.
V. Au-Pd (No Ag)	Olympia (Heraeus-Kulzer)	51.5	—	38	—	—	—	1.5	Bal.
	Lodestar (Ivoclar Vivadent)	52	—	37	—	—	—	—	Bal.
	Argedent 65SF (Argen)	65	—	26	—	—	—	—	Bal.
VI. Pd-Au (No Ag)	Olympia II (Heraeus-Kulzer)	35	—	57	—	—	—	5	2.8
	Argedent 35SF (Argen)	35	—	57	—	—	—	5	3.0
VII. Pd-Au-Ag or Pd-Ag-Au	SWCG (Pentron Lab Tech)	32	3	42	14	—	—	—	Bal.
	Pegasus (Sterngold)	5	—	74	6.5	—	—	—	Bal.
VIII. Pd-Ag	Jelstar (Heraeus-Kulzer)	—	—	60	28	—	—	—	12
	Will-Ceram W-1 (Ivoclar Vivadent)	—	—	54	38	—	—	—	Bal.
IX. Pd-Cu-Ga	Liberty (Heraeus-Kulzer)	2	—	75	—	10	—	5.5	Bal.
	Spartan Plus (Ivoclar Vivadent)	—	—	75	—	10	—	9	Bal.
X. Pd-Ga-Ag	Argebond 80 (Argen)	—	—	80	5	—	—	6.3	Bal.
	Argelite 85 (Argen)	—	—	85	1.2	—	—	10	Bal.

Bal., Balance.

*Alloys in Groups I through V are HN alloys according to the classification of the American Dental Association.

†Alloys in Groups VI through IX are N alloys.

their potential for porcelain discoloration. These alloys are white-colored and are used primarily for their lower cost and comparable physical properties. The commonly used alloys in this group contain between 39% and 53% Au and 25% to 35% Pd. A typical alloy in this group may have a Vickers hardness of 220, a yield strength of 421 MPa (61,000 psi), an elongation value of 10%, and a yield strength of 552 MPa (80,000 psi). Compared with a Ni-Cr-Be alloy that has a HV of 350, a gold alloy should be easier to grind and polish based on its lower hardness.

The burnishing potential of alloys is difficult to compare. An elongation of 20% or more for either alloy combined with lower yield strength facilitates the burnishing process. Some researchers believe that burnishability of alloys may be compared by dividing the elongation by the product of yield strength and hardness.

This would indicate that the gold alloy would be easier to burnish. A practical comparison of mechanical properties to predict handling characteristics is difficult. The extremely high hardness of most base metal alloys renders these alloys difficult to cut, grind, and polish. From a clinician's point of view, the lower hardness and greater ductility of most noble alloys are major advantages compared with base metal alloys.

Although the noble metal alloys have lower values of modulus of elasticity compared with base metal alloys, this is not considered a major disadvantage if proper framework connector geometries are employed. When thin connectors and long-span frameworks are considered, the lower values of elastic modulus for the noble metal alloys would be disadvantageous since comparable intraoral forces would produce higher bending displacements, which could cause porcelain cracking.

The potential for porcelain discoloration is greatest with alloy Groups IV, VII, and VIII in Table 19-6, which have the highest silver contents. Exceptions include alloys that contain less than 8% Ag, such as Shasta (Wilkinson). The factors that intensify the porcelain color changes because of the release of silver were identified previously. In general, it is advisable to avoid these types of alloys when using lighter shades and ceramic products that are sensitive to silver discoloration.

Because of the addition of higher palladium concentrations in Au-Pd-Ag alloys, the melting ranges are raised above those of the Au-Pt-Pd alloys. Thus it would be expected that resistance to creep deformation (sag) would be improved at elevated temperatures.

Gold-Palladium Alloys

The first alloy of the gold-palladium type (Group V alloy in Table 19-6), Olympia (Heraeus Kulzer), was introduced in 1977 by J.F. Jelenko & Co. This alloy was designed to overcome the porcelain discoloration effect (because it is silver-free) and also to provide an alloy with a lower thermal contraction coefficient than that of either the Au-Pd-Ag or Pd-Ag alloys. These latter two types of alloys have thermal expansion or contraction coefficients that are considered too high for use with certain porcelains. A slight thermal contraction mismatch (produced with a higher contraction of the metal) is recommended to develop compressive hoop and axial stresses in porcelain, which are protective in nature (Fig. 19-2). However, significantly higher mismatches (with a much higher thermal contraction coefficient for the metal) may lead to porcelain cracking or metal-ceramic bond failure because of the development of tensile stress, which exceeds the tensile strength of porcelain or the strength of the metal-ceramic bond. It is unlikely that high compressive hoop (circumferential) stresses are responsible for failure of these systems since the compressive strength of dental porcelain is very high. A more plausible cause of incompatibility failure is the development of radial tensile stresses that exceed the tensile strength of porcelain.

When used with compatible porcelains, Au-Pd alloys are considered nearly ideal compared with other noble metal alloys, since these alloys contain no silver and their surface oxide is virtually indiscernible. Thus the aesthetic capability of metal-ceramic prostheses made with Au-Pd (silver-free) alloys is comparable to that obtained with Au-Pt-Pd alloys. The sag resistance of these alloys is somewhat better than that of Au-Pt-Pd alloys. Their castability, corrosion resistance, and adherence to porcelain are excellent. Typical alloys of this type have a HV of about 200, a yield strength of 570 MPa (83,000 psi), and an elongation of approximately 20%. The gold content of Au-Pd alloys ranges from 45% to 52%, and the palladium content varies between 37% and 45%. Examples of this alloy are given in Table 19-6 (Type V alloy). Oxidizing elements include indium and tin. With a specific gravity of

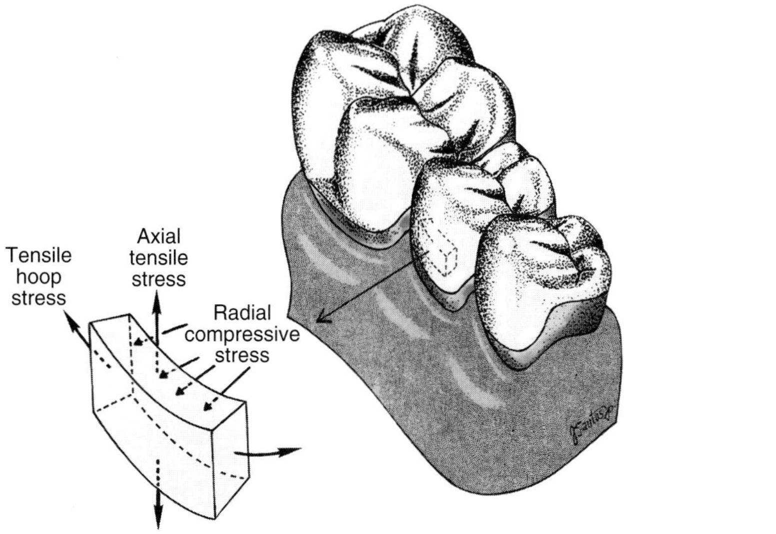

Fig. 19-2 Residual stress in the porcelain veneer of a metal-ceramic crown for a case in which the coefficient of thermal contraction for the porcelain is greater than that for the metal. See also color plate.

approximately 13.5, these alloys are moderately priced. All of these alloys are white in color.

Palladium-Gold Alloys

Relatively few products of the palladium-gold alloy type (Group VI in Table 19-6) are available in the current dental marketplace, because their popularity has been diminished by the recent price volatility of palladium. These Pd-Au alloys are free of silver, as are the Au-Pd alloys. Therefore they do not contribute to porcelain discoloration. Little data are available on their laboratory and clinical performance. Their physical properties are generally similar to those of the Au-Pd alloys. Information related to the thermal compatibility with commercial porcelain products has not yet been reported in the dental literature.

Palladium-Gold-Silver Alloys

The palladium-gold-silver alloy group is similar to the Au-Pd-Ag types of alloys in their potential for porcelain discoloration. Examples are listed as Group VII alloys in Table 19-6. These alloys have gold contents ranging from 5% to 32% and silver contents varying between 6.5% and 14%. One would expect the potential for porcelain discoloration to be greater for the higher silver-content alloys in this group. These alloys have a range of thermal contraction coefficients that increase with an increase in silver content.

Palladium-Silver Alloys

The palladium-silver alloy type (Group VIII in Table 19-6) was introduced to the U.S. market in 1974 as the first gold-free noble alloy available for metal-ceramic restorations. These alloys, like all Pd-based products, have been occasionally called *semiprecious*. As stated previously, this term should not be used, because it cannot be precisely defined and because it tends to encourage the association of many dissimilar alloys in the same group.

The compositions of Pd-Ag alloys fall within a narrow range of 53% to 61% Pd and 28% to 40% Ag. Tin and/or indium are usually added to increase alloy hardness and to promote oxide formation and adequate bonding to porcelain. A proper balance is needed to maintain a reasonably low casting temperature and a compatible coefficient of thermal contraction. The replacement of gold by palladium raises the melting range but lowers the contraction coefficient of an alloy. Increasing the silver content tends to lower the melting range and increases the contraction coefficient. In Chapter 6 it was noted that the microstructures of various commercial Pd-Ag alloys can differ substantially at the submicron level when examined with the transmission electron microscope, where the composition and morphology of the precipitates observed depend on the specific proportions of the secondary elements in the alloys. These precipitates account for differences in mechanical properties and corrosion behavior of the commercial Pd-Ag alloys.

Because of their high silver content compared with that of gold-based alloys, the silver discoloration effect is most severe for these alloys. Gold metal conditioners or ceramic coating agents may minimize this effect. However, many of today's porcelains are formulated to minimize or eliminate this problem. Nonetheless, one should proceed with caution when light shades are desired. Except for posterior restorations, experience should be gained with isolated single-unit restorations before proceeding with the fabrication of FPDs.

The low specific gravity of these alloys (10.7 to 11.1), combined with their low intrinsic cost, make them attractive as economical alternatives to the gold-based alloys. Some of the alloys in this class with lower silver contents (approximately 28%) are easier to burnish compared with other noble metal alloys. An alloy with a HV of 170 to 180, a yield strength of about 460 MPa (67,000 psi), and an elongation value of 25% should be readily burnishable. Alloys of this type are easy to grind and polish.

Adherence to porcelain is considered to be acceptable for most of the Pd-Ag alloys. However, one study indicates that some of these alloys may form internal rather than external oxides. Instead of the formation of the desired external oxide, Pd-Ag nodules may develop on the surface (Fig. 19-3), which enhance retention of porcelain by

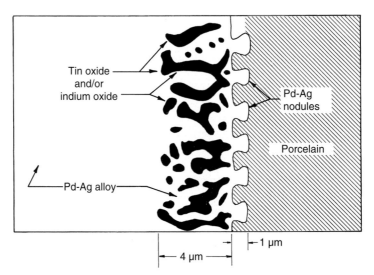

Fig. 19-3 Internal oxide formation and creep-induced nodule formation in a Pd-Ag alloy for metal-ceramic restorations.

mechanical rather than chemical bonding. However, this condition has apparently not produced a significant number of debonding failures to warrant concern.

The thermal compatibility of these alloys is generally good except with certain low-expansion porcelains. As is true for all alloys, one should consult with the alloy manufacturer to determine which porcelains may be incompatible with a given alloy.

Palladium-Copper-Gallium Alloys

Palladium-copper-gallium alloys (Group IX in Table 19-6) date from the 1983 patent for the Option alloy (Ney), and these alloys were very popular in the 1990s. No clinical reports of adverse events have been reported for Pd-Cu-Ga alloys. However, the price volatility of palladium in the early 2000s required dentists to use other alloys. Compared with a price of $117 per troy oz in November 1996, the price of palladium rose to $1090 per troy oz in January 2001. In December 2002, the price had declined to $222 per troy oz.

The clinician should be aware of the potential effect on aesthetics of the dark brown or black oxide formed during oxidation and subsequent porcelain firing cycles. X-ray diffraction and x-ray photoelectron spectroscopy studies have established the compositions of the oxide layers on these alloys, and the dark color correlates with the oxide species present. Care should be taken by the technician to mask this oxide completely with opaque porcelain and to eliminate the unaesthetic dark band that develops at metal-porcelain junctions. It is also important to ensure that a brown rather than a black oxide is formed on the metal surface during the oxidation treatment. Because of the potential aesthetic problems associated with these alloys, they have not been well accepted in dental practices.

Compositional differences for the Pd-Cu-Ga alloys result in a wide range of mechanical properties: yield strengths ranging from approximately 520 MPa to over 1200 MPa (75,000 psi to over 170,000 psi), percentage elongation at fracture ranging from approximately 7% to 30%, and HV ranging from approximately 265 to over 400. The HVs for some of the original Pd-Cu-Ga alloys are as high as those of some base metal alloys. Thus these alloys would appear to have a poor potential for burnishing except when the marginal areas are relatively thin. However, laboratory technicians report that most of these alloys are easier to handle than base metal alloys, and careful composition control by manufacturers has resulted in Pd-Cu-Ga alloys with HVs substantially lower than 300. Although thermal incompatibility is not considered to be a major concern, distortion of ultrathin metal copings (0.1 mm) has been reported. Despite concerns from earlier research about sag deformation, dimensional changes of high-palladium alloy crowns during fabrication of metal-ceramic restorations should not be a significant problem with appropriate control of dental laboratory procedures. The major portion of the dimensional changes occurs during the initial oxidation step for these alloys and as a result of excessive sandblasting pressure and/or time.

Palladium-Gallium-Silver

Palladium-gallium-silver alloys (Group X in Table 19-6), the most recent of the noble metal alloys, were introduced because they tend to have a slightly lighter-colored oxide than the Pd-Cu alloys and they are thermally compatible with lower expansion porcelains. Compared with most Pd-based alloys, Pd-Cu-Ga alloys have a lower hardness; this property enhances the ability of clinicians to adjust the cast alloy in the dental laboratory and at chair-side. The oxide, which is required for bonding to porcelain, is relatively dark, but it is somewhat lighter than those of the Pd-Cu-Ga and Pd-Co-Ga alloys. The silver content is generally relatively low (5 wt% to 8 wt% in most cases) and is usually inadequate to cause significant porcelain *greening*. Caution should be exercised in their initial use until clinical data are available. Little information is available on metal-ceramic bond strength or thermal compatibility. Pd-Ga-Ag alloys generally have relatively low thermal contraction coefficients and are expected to be more compatible with lower expansion porcelains. To ensure against unnecessary clinical failures, the clinician should select alloys certified as acceptable by the ADA or ISO. Furthermore, the clinician should ask the alloy manufacturer to provide a list (in writing if possible) of the porcelain products with which the selected alloy is compatible.

Discoloration of Porcelain by Silver

The mechanism of porcelain discoloration is not clearly understood. It is believed that the colloidal dispersion of silver atoms entering body and incisal porcelain or the glazed surface from vapor transport or surface diffusion may cause color changes, including green, yellow-green, yellow-orange, orange, and brown hues. The term *greening* is generally applied to this discoloration phenomenon.

Porcelains with higher sodium contents are believed to exhibit a more intense discoloration because of more rapid silver diffusion in sodium-containing glass. This hypothesis is based on observations of greater discoloration in lighter shades of porcelain and in porcelains with lower opacifier contents and higher sodium concentrations.

Although this phenomenon is called *greening*, yellowish tones may also occur in the discolored areas of ceramic. The intensity of discoloration (chroma) usually increases near the cervical region, because surface diffusion of silver from the marginal metal provides a higher localized silver concentration. Tuccillo and Cascone have speculated that silver in the form of a silver oxide gas also vaporizes from the alloy and deposits in cooler areas of the furnace. During subsequent heating and cooling cycles, silver vaporizes and condenses on the restoration and again on the cooler areas of furnace walls. Since the silver gas is more active near the alloy surface, absorption into the surface of porcelain occurs. This phenomenon further explains the more intense discoloration that is often observed near metal-porcelain finish lines.

Certain porcelains are resistant to silver discoloration. The mechanism proposed to explain this difference is the silver ionization by porcelains with high oxygen potential. Since the principal discoloration effect is believed to result from the presence of neutral silver atoms rather than silver ions, conversion of silver oxide to silver ions by porcelains with a higher affinity for oxygen would minimize this effect.

The extent of porcelain discoloration is most severe for higher silver-content alloys, lighter shades, multiple firing procedures, higher temperatures, body porcelain in direct contact with the alloy, vacuum firing cycles, and certain brands of porcelains. At least two suppliers of commercial porcelains claim that their porcelain products, Will-Ceram (Ivoclar Vivadent, Amherst, NY)and Pencraft (Pentron Corp., Wallingford, CT), are resistant to discoloration when used with alloys containing up to 38% silver.

Greening may occur even when porcelains are fired on silver-free alloys. This is attributed to vaporization of silver from the walls of contaminated furnaces. First, a graphite block should be employed routinely to maintain a reducing atmosphere near the alloy. A reducing atmosphere inhibits the formation of silver oxide. This chemical form of silver facilitates the vaporization potential of silver. The graphite block, however, is not effective in removing silver from the walls of a furnace that has been heavily contaminated with silver.

Two types of metal coating agents may be used to reduce porcelain discoloration effects. A pure gold film can be fired on a metal substrate to reduce the surface silver concentration. This technique lowers the silver content at the alloy surface as a result of diffusion of gold atoms into the alloy during the oxidation cycle and thereby reduces the concentration of silver atoms available for evaporation from the surface at elevated temperatures. A ceramic conditioner can also be fired on the metal surface as a barrier between the alloy and porcelain. However, in either case an additional procedural step is required. Neither of these precautions is recommended, because an extra layer may reduce the metal-porcelain bond strength. Instead it is more desirable to either use an ultralow-fusing porcelain or a nongreening porcelain.

The Au-Pd-Ag alloys, which contain between 5% and 12% Ag, are more susceptible to porcelain discoloration than are the alloys with lower silver concentrations in the 5% to 8% range (Au-Pt-Pd or Au-Pd-Pt). Compared with the first two alloy types given in Table 19-6, the Au-Pd-Ag alloys exhibit comparable castability, bond strength to porcelain, burnishability, solder joint quality, and corrosion resistance. The sag resistance of long-span frameworks is somewhat better than that of the higher–gold-content alloys.

Thermal Compatibility and Incompatibility of Metal-Ceramic Systems

Thermal compatibility refers to the ability of a metal and its veneering porcelain to contract at similar rates (thermal expansion coefficient of metal, α_M, is comparable in magnitude with the thermal expansion coefficient of porcelain, α_p) during cooling from the ceramic sintering temperature (>871° C or 1600° F) for low-fusing porcelain and <871° C for ultralow-fusing porcelain). If the combination of metal and porcelain is compatible, the transient tensile stresses that develop during cooling are insufficient to cause immediate cracking of porcelain or delayed cracking after cooling to room temperature. Clinical success of porcelain-veneered restorations also depends on acceptable adherence, framework or coping fit (marginal adaptation), aesthetics, and the absence of high residual tensile stress. (The instantaneous stress at a given temperature during the cooling cycle is termed *transient stress.* The stress distribution, which exists at room temperature, is called the *residual stress.*) While adherence to porcelain is a critical factor, the number of clinical failures attributable to poor adherence of the metal-ceramic restorations (fabricated with gold-based alloys) is believed to be low. Of greater concern are delayed cracks that develop in the porcelain, leading to premature failure of metal-ceramic prostheses. This type of failure is presumably caused by the interaction of moisture and relatively high residual tensile stresses within porcelain at the conclusion of the glazing cycle. Delayed failure of this type is attributed to stress corrosion. Superimposed tensile stresses resulting from intraoral forces may result in later crack propagation and possible porcelain delamination.

Shown in Figure 19-4 is an illustration of the additive effects of tangential tensile stress (+20 MPa) induced in the porcelain veneer by intraoral forces and residual tangential compressive stress (−40 MPa) produced by thermal contraction differences for the case in which $\alpha_M > \alpha_p$. Thus the result is −20 MPa of tangential compressive stress. In this case the force is applied on the facial surface of a mandibular incisor crown, which has been fabricated with a compatible metal-ceramic system. Note that the residual compressive stress in the axial or tangential direction actually increases the *effective* tensile strength of porcelain, since this net compressive stress

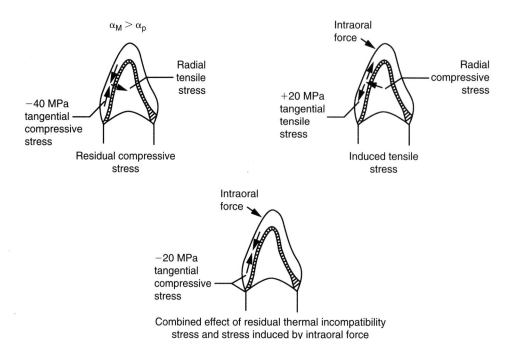

Fig. 19-4   Combined effect of residual metal/ceramic incompatibility stress and intraorally induced stresses. **A,** Thermally compatible metal-ceramic system $\alpha_M > \alpha_p$, in which a residual compressive tangential stress of -40 MPa results in the ceramic veneer. An induced intraoral tensile stress of $+20$ MPa results in a combined stress of -20 MPa. **B,** Thermally incompatible metal-ceramic system $\alpha_p > \alpha_M$, in which a residual incompatibility tensile stress of $+40$ MPa is produced in the ceramic veneer. An induced intraoral tensile stress of $+20$ MPa results in a combined stress of $+60$ MPa and the formation of a crack within the ceramic.

(−20 MPa) must first be overcome before tensile stress can develop by the applied intraoral force on the facial surface of porcelain. Note that the stress state in the porcelain veneer is more complex than that shown in this figure. There are three components of stress; the circumferential or hoop stress is not shown. Shown in Figure 19-4 are two of the other components: the axial or tangential compressive stress that acts parallel to the long axis of the crown, and the radial tensile stress that is oriented toward the center of the crown and perpendicular to the facial surface, causing the metal to pull away from the porcelain.

Incompatibility stresses are either transient or residual in nature. Ideally, the thermal contraction mismatch between alloy and porcelain should be small. Stresses begin to develop because of a difference in thermal coefficients between metal and porcelain ($\alpha_M - \alpha_p$) as a prosthesis is cooled below the glass transition temperature of the porcelain. For today's porcelains, this temperature lies within the range of 500° C to 650° C. If the porcelain has a much larger coefficient of contraction ($\alpha_p \gg \alpha_M$) than that of the metal (α_M) between this temperature and room temperature, the tensile strength of porcelain may be exceeded because of large tensile hoop stresses causing crack propagation in the porcelain veneer. Note that although axial tensile and hoop (not shown) tensile stresses are generated as a result of the mismatch in α values, a radial compressive stress results at the interface, which may effectively increase the bond strength. For the compatible system shown in Figure 19-4, *A*, (i.e., $\alpha_M > \alpha_p$), radial tensile stress develops and the axial and hoop stresses are compressive in nature.

It is also possible to develop failure level stresses near the metal-porcelain interface when the contraction coefficient of the porcelain is much lower than that of the metal ($\alpha_p \ll \alpha_M$). Although compressive hoop stress develops in the porcelain, tensile radial stress develops in porcelain next to the interface, as shown in Figure 19-4. If, upon cooling of the metal-ceramic prosthesis, this stress component exceeds the tensile strength of the porcelain, failure may be experienced at some temperature between the glass transition temperature (Tg) and room temperature. Even though the transient stress at any point has not caused visible crack formation, microscopic cracks may exist that will propagate later to cause porcelain failure. Moreover, under this circumstance of $\alpha_p \ll \alpha_M$, a high residual stress state will remain in the porcelain structure when the prosthesis is delivered to the dentist by the laboratory technician. To minimize subsequent clinical failures caused by stress corrosion or residual stress combined with that produced from intraoral forces, the dentist, in consultation with the laboratory technician or the alloy manufacturer, should select only those systems that are known to be compatible. (Internet addresses are easily found for technical support from the major dental casting alloy manufacturers.)

Because there are no standardized laboratory tests that can predict residual stress compatibility of metal-ceramic systems, one must rely on feedback from dental alloy or porcelain suppliers who obtain case report information on failed prostheses that were prepared under a wide variety of laboratory conditions.

Although not all prostheses prepared with incompatible systems fail by visible crack formation under ideal laboratory conditions, those that do not fail may sustain high residual tensile or shear stresses. Since the tensile strength (50 MPa) and shear strength (130 MPa) of typical dental porcelains are relatively low compared with their compressive strength (350 MPa), premature failure under superimposed intraoral tensile or shear stresses may be a primary cause of restoration failure. Porcelains that are more compatible with dental alloys generally have slightly lower thermal expansion and contraction coefficients compared with those of the alloys. In fact, it may be desirable to develop small compressive stresses in the porcelain to minimize clinical failure. However, radial tensile stresses near the interface may occur simultaneously with the compressive hoop stress.

Although a metal-ceramic system may be considered compatible under normal conditions, a significant number of prostheses may be fabricated under less than ideal conditions. Incompatibility failures may result with compatible (or incompatible) systems when atypical cooling rates, excessive porcelain-metal thickness ratios, and improper framework or coping geometries are used, or when the number of firing cycles exceeds the number recommended by the porcelain manufacturers. Excessive firing is known to cause an increase in the contraction coefficient of some porcelains because of structural changes in the leucite phase, the principal crystal present in the glassy matrix. Leucite, which has the chemical formula $K_2O \cdot Al_2O_3 \cdot 4SiO_2$, is the principal high-expansion microstructural component of dental porcelains, and its presence may cause large increases in the contraction coefficient of porcelain when more than five firing cycles are necessary. Some of the programmable porcelain furnaces are used with much faster firing rates and slower cooling rates than were possible with conventional, manually operated furnaces. The temperature distribution in vertical-muffle furnaces may also be different than that in manually operated horizontal-muffle furnaces. Larger porcelain-metal thickness ratios are believed to be associated with higher residual tensile stresses in porcelain. This situation may arise when a dental laboratory technician decides to maintain a minimum metal thickness for economy purposes. Also, the presence of small acute external angles on the incisal edges of metal copings may act as stress raisers that amplify the magnitude of tensile stresses in these areas even though the average residual tensile stress in low.

One of the more controversial issues regarding compatibility of metal-ceramic systems is whether marginal opening of single-unit copings or generalized distortion of frameworks can result from the generation of high transient stresses in the alloy because of a thermal contraction mismatch. Several studies have provided evidence that the marginal gap change is greatest after the oxidation cycle, as previously noted for the high-palladium alloys. The results of these studies indicate that metal-ceramic thermal incompatibility stresses are not the primary cause of marginal or generalized distortion of castings. In fact, sandblasting the internal surface of the metal coping to remove the oxide layer is a possible cause of such metal distortion. Care should be taken to limit the time for sandblasting and to apply a minimal sandblasting pressure to minimize distortion of metal margins.

Alloys for Ultralow-Fusing Porcelains

Porcelain developments have focused on improving the lifelike (aesthetic) qualities of the materials. As a result the sintering temperatures of some newer ultralow-fusing porcelains are now below 850° C. The lower fusing temperature has benefited the high-gold alloys that sometimes suffer from poor sag resistance during porcelain firing.

Less Abrasive Porcelains

A new type of porcelain was introduced in the mid-1980s. These materials contain a glass phase and very small crystal particles. They are generally less abrasive to opposing teeth and are sintered at a lower temperature than conventional porcelains. They also have a higher thermal expansion coefficient than conventional porcelains and must accordingly be more closely matched to the thermal expansion coefficients of the cast alloys to be used in metal-ceramic prostheses.

Partial Denture Alloys

The majority of removable partial denture frameworks are made from alloys based primarily on nickel, cobalt, or titanium as the principal metal component. Nickel is a malleable, ductile, silver-colored transition element with atomic number 28 and a melting point of about 1450° C. Cobalt is a silver-colored transition element with atomic number 27, having a melting point of about 1500° C and little ductility at room temperature. All cobalt-based and nickel-based alloys contain chromium to prevent corrosion and tarnish. The passivation mechanism of the alloy occurs through a thin surface layer of chromium oxide (Cr_2O_3). Most Co-Cr alloys contain molybdenum (Co-Cr-Mo), and some may contain nickel (Co-Cr-Ni). Some Ni-Cr alloys contain beryllium (Be), which lowers the melting point to improve castability. Frameworks may also be made from CP Ti and Ti-6Al-4V. The most biocompatible metal for frameworks is CP Ti.

Physical Properties of High Noble and Noble Alloys

Important physical properties of alloys for all-metal and metal-ceramic restorations are provided in Table 19-7. Similar listings of properties are generally available for the alloys of any particular manufacturer. The melting range sets the basis for the casting temperature. The upper limit of the range is the liquidus. To this value, 75° C to 150° C (approximately 167° F to 302° F) should be added to obtain the proper casting temperature. In normal dental laboratory practice, when a torch is used to melt the metal, the optimum casting temperature is judged visually when the molten metal has sufficient fluidity to respond to movement of the torch. With modern centrifugal casting machines that use induction melting, the desired casting temperature can be set by the operator. The lower limit of the melting range can similarly be used to estimate maximum **soldering** temperatures.

The metal-ceramic alloys must have a high melting range so that the metal is solid well above the porcelain sintering temperature to minimize distortion (sag) of the casting during porcelain application. On the other hand, the Type I to Type IV gold-based alloys for all-metal restorations must have considerably lower fusion temperatures if they are to be cast with conventional equipment and if gypsum investments are used. The width of the melting range is also of interest, since the wider the melting range, the greater the tendency for coring during solidification (Chapter 6).

The lost-wax method of casting that is used for the fabrication of crowns involves filling a fixed volume of an alloy. Alloys, however, are sold by weight. For an equivalent weight of alloy, more crowns can be made with an alloy of a lower density, because less weight of metal is needed to fill the same volume. The specific volume (cm^3/g), which is the reciprocal of density (g/cm^3), is an indication of the volume of the metal (cm^3) that can be cast from a mass (g) of the metal. The range of specific gravities (10.6 to 18.3 g/cm^3 for the noble metal-ceramic alloys) indicates that considerably more equivalent castings (approximately 72%) can be made from the lowest-density alloy in the table than from the one with the highest density.

CRITICAL QUESTION

What are the advantages and drawbacks of base metal alloys compared with high noble or noble alloys for metal-ceramic restorations?

Table 19-7	Physical Properties of Some Modern Noble Metal Dental Alloys

Alloy type	Main elements	Melting range	Density (g/cm^3)	Yield strength‡		Hardness (VHN)	Percent elongation
				(MPa)	(psi)		
I	High noble	943–960° C (1730–1760° F)	16.6	103	(15,000)	80	36
II	High noble	924–960° C (1695–1760° F)	15.9	186	(27,000)	101	38
III	High noble	924–960° C (1710–1760° F)	15.5	207 H275	(30,000) (H40,000)	121 H182	39 H19
	Noble	843–916° C (1550–1680° F)	12.8	241 H586	(35,000) (H85,000)	138 H231	30 H13
	Ag-Pd noble	1021–1099° C (1870–2010° F)	10.6	262 H323	(38,000) (H47,000)	143 H154	10 H8
IV	High noble	921–943° C (1690–1720° F)	15.2	275 H493	(40,000) (H71,500)	149 H264	35 H7
	High noble	871–932° C (1600–1710° F)	13.6	372 H720	(54,000) (H104,500)	186 H254	38 H2
	Noble	930–1021° C (1705–1870° F)	11.3	434 H586	(63,000) (H85,000)	180 H270	10 H6
Metal-ceramic	*High noble	1271–1304° C (2320–2380° F)	13.5	572	(83,000)	220	20
	Noble	1232–1304° C (2250–2380° F)	10.7	462	(67,000)	189	20
	†High noble	1149–1177° C (2100–2150° F)	18.3	450	(65,300)	182	5
	Noble	1155–1302° C (2111–2375° F)	10.6–11.5	476–685	(68,000–95,000)	235–270	10–34

HV, Vickers hardness number.
*White colored.
†Yellow colored.
‡H, Age-hardened condition. Other values are for the quenched (softened) condition.

BASE METAL ALLOYS FOR CAST METAL AND METAL-CERAMIC PROSTHESES

A survey of 1000 dental laboratory owners in 1978 revealed that only 29% of these laboratories were using Ni-Cr or Co-Cr alloys for cast metal or metal-ceramic restorations. By 1981, the percentage of laboratories using these base metal alloys increased to 70%, because of the unstable price of noble metals during this period. Most of these dental laboratories indicated a preference for Ni-Cr alloys over Co-Cr alloys. The percentage of base metal use in dentistry decreased between 1981 and 1995. Although the increased acceptance of these alloys during this period was greatly influenced by the rapidly fluctuating international cost of gold and other noble metals, the subsequent decline in the cost of noble metals has had a small effect on reversing this trend. The Ni-Cr-Be alloys have retained their popularity despite the potential toxicity of beryllium and the

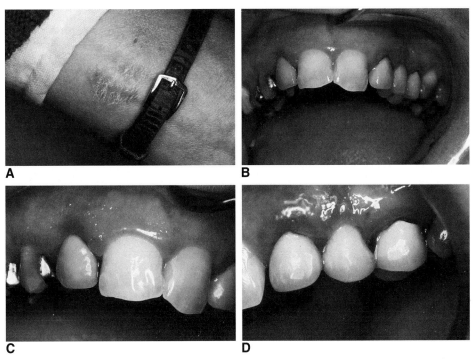

Fig. 19-5 Allergy to nickel alloy. **A,** Eczematous type reaction to metal watch buckle. **B,** Potential allergy to nickel-based alloys used for metal-ceramic crowns on FPD (**B** and **C**) and single crown (**D**). See also color plate.

allergenic potential of nickel. In some regional areas, an increase in the use of palladium alloys has been observed.

This section has been prepared to provide a critical assessment of the risks and benefits of base metal alloys when compared with gold-based or palladium-based alloys for metal-ceramic prostheses. One might inquire why the Ni-Cr and Ni-Cr-Be alloys retain their popularity despite the known toxicity of beryllium as well as the allergenic potential of nickel. Shown in Figure 19-5 are examples of potential nickel allergies on the hand of an individual who has had frequent exposure to nickel metal.

There are several reasons for the use of nickel-chromium alloys in dentistry:

1. Nickel is combined with chromium to form a highly corrosion resistant alloy.
2. Ni-Cr alloys became popular in the early 1980s as low cost metals ($2 to $3 per conventional avoirdupois ounce) when the price of gold rose to more than $500 per troy ounce. Because metal-ceramic restorations made with Ni-Cr-Be alloys have exhibited high success rates from the mid-1980s to the present, many dentists have continued to use these alloys.
3. Alloys such as Ticonium 100 have been used in removable partial denture frameworks for many years with few reports of allergic reactions. However, it is believed that palatal epithelium may be more resistant to allergic reactions (contact dermatitis) than gingival sulcular epithelium.
4. The Ni-Cr and Ni-Cr-Be alloys are relatively inexpensive compared with high noble or noble alloys. The price of nickel-based alloys is stable, unlike the price of palladium-based alloys.

5. Although beryllium is a toxic metal, dentists and patients should not be affected because the main risk occurs primarily in the vapor form, which is a concern for technicians who melt and cast large quantities of Ni-Cr-Be alloys without adequate ventilation or fume hoods in the melting area.

6. Nickel alloys have excellent mechanical properties, such as high elastic modulus (stiffness), high hardness, and a reasonably high elongation (ductility).

Since the development of cobalt-chromium alloys for cast dental appliances in 1928 and the subsequent introduction of nickel-chromium and nickel-cobalt-chromium alloys in later years, base metal alloys have demonstrated widespread acceptance in the United States as the predominant choice for the fabrication of removable partial denture frameworks. Compared with Type IV gold alloys, cobalt-based alloys and nickel-based alloys feature lower cost, lower density, higher modulus of elasticity, higher hardness, and comparable clinical resistance to tarnish and corrosion. However, a comparison between nickel-based alloys and noble metal alloys designed for metal-ceramic crowns and fixed partial dentures (FPD) is more complex. Relatively small compositional differences or certain base metal additions such as beryllium, silicon, boron, and aluminum produce significant changes in base metal alloy microstructures and properties, which could affect the bond strength of ceramics to the metal oxide layer that is required to achieve chemical bonding.

The majority of nickel-chromium alloys for crowns and FPD prostheses contain 61 wt% to 81 wt% nickel, 11 wt% to 27 wt% chromium and 2 wt% to 4 wt% molybdenum. These alloys may also contain one or more of the following elements: aluminum, beryllium, boron, carbon, cobalt, copper, cerium, gallium, iron, manganese, niobium, silicon, tin, titanium, and zirconium. The cobalt-chromium alloys typically contain 53 wt% to 67 wt% cobalt, 25 wt% to 32 wt% chromium, and 2 wt% to 6 wt% molybdenum, which could affect the metal-ceramic bond strength.

BIOLOGICAL HAZARDS AND PRECAUTIONS: RISKS FOR DENTAL LABORATORY TECHNICIANS

Laboratory technicians may be exposed occasionally or routinely to excessively high concentrations of beryllium and nickel dust and beryllium vapor. Although the beryllium concentration in dental alloys rarely exceeds 2% by weight, the amount of beryllium vapor released into the breathing space during the melting of nickel-chromium-beryllium alloys may be significant over an extended period of time. Actually, the potential hazards of beryllium should be based on its atomic concentration rather than its weight concentration in an alloy. One can demonstrate that an alloy which contains 80% Ni, 11.4% Cr, 5% Mo, 1.8% Fe, and 1.8% Be on a weight basis contains 73.3% Ni, 11.8% Cr, 2.6% Mo, 1.6% Fe, and 10.7% Be on an atomic basis. Thus toxicity considerations for beryllium should be based on the atomic concentration (approximately 11 at%) rather than the weight percentage (1.8 wt%). The vapor pressure of pure beryllium is approximately 0.1 torr (mm Hg) at an assumed casting temperature of 1370° C. Comparable vapor pressures for chromium, nickel, and molybdenum are 5×10^{-3} torr, 8×10^{-4} torr, and 3×10^{-11} torr, respectively.

The risk for beryllium vapor exposure is greatest for dental technicians during alloy melting, especially in the absence of an adequate exhaust and filtration system. The Occupational Health and Safety Administration (OSHA) specifies that exposure to beryllium dust in air should be limited to a particulate beryllium concentration of 2 $\mu g/m^3$ of air (both respirable and nonrespirable particles) determined from an 8-h time-weighted average. The allowable maximum concentration is 5 $\mu g/m^3$ (not to be exceeded for a 15-min period). For a minimum duration of 30 min, a maximum ceiling concentration of 25 $\mu g/m^3$ is allowed. The National Institute for

Occupational Safety and Health (NIOSH) recommends a limit of 0.5 µg/m^3 based on a 130-min sample. Moffa et al (1973) reported that high levels of beryllium were accumulating during finishing and polishing when a local exhaust system was not used. When an exhaust system was used, the concentration of beryllium in the breathing zone was reduced to levels considered safe by the authors. Workers exposed to moderately high concentrations of beryllium dust over a short period of time, or prolonged exposure to low concentrations, may experience signs and symptoms representing acute disease states. Physiological responses vary from contact dermatitis to severe chemical pneumonitis, which can be fatal. The chronic disease state is characterized by symptoms persisting for more than 1 year, with the onset of symptoms separated by a period of years from the time of exposure. Symptoms range from coughing, chest pain, and general weakness to pulmonary dysfunction.

Airborne levels of beryllium can be controlled with a local exhaust system. However, one should not conclude that melting and grinding of Ni-Cr alloys without beryllium and grinding of other dental materials pose no major risk to the health of laboratory technicians. Good ventilation and exhaust facilities should be employed whenever any material is ground. The dental profession should investigate methods to minimize such risks.

Potential Patient Hazards

Of greater concern to dental patients is the intraoral exposure to nickel, especially for patients with a known allergy to this element. Dermatitis resulting from contact with nickel solutions was described as early as 1889. Inhalation, ingestion, and dermal contact of nickel or nickel-containing alloys are common, because nickel is found in environmental sources such as air, soil, and food, as well as in man-made objects such as coins, kitchen utensils, and jewelry. The concentration of nickel in the air is generally relatively low, except where environmental pollution conditions exist as a result of nickel processing operations or burning of fossil fuels.

In 1982, Moffa et al reported that, for patients between the ages of 24 and 44 who possessed a fixed nickel alloy prosthesis, 9.7% of the females and 0.8% of the males experienced a positive reaction to 2.5% nickel sulfate. The nickel hypersensitivity incidence for all age groups was 4.5% for females and 1.5% for males. Of the positive reactions to nickel, female patients with pierced ears accounted for 90% of the total. None of the males with pierced ears exhibited positive reactions. No correlation was found between the incidence of nickel sensitivity and the presence of intraoral nickel alloy prostheses. These results are consistent with the findings of Vreeburg et al (1984) who concluded that the oral exposure of nickel and chromium to guinea pigs via a fixed appliance or the dietary intake of these elements as metallic powder or salts did not induce an allergic reaction to these metals. Even more significant is their observation that subsequent attempts to elicit an allergic response in previously exposed animals generally failed, whereas nonexposed animals exhibited a higher incidence of hypersensitive responses.

Because of concerns over the carcinogenic potential of nickel, NIOSH has recommended that OSHA adopt a standard to limit employee exposure to inorganic nickel in the laboratory or office to 15 µg/m^3 (air), determined as a time-weighted average (TWA) concentration for up to a 10-h work shift (40-h work week). The existing OSHA standard specifies an 8-h TWA concentration limit of 1000 µg/m^3 or 1 mg/m^3 of nickel and nickel compounds. This limit is of the same magnitude as the standard established in Japan but is 100 times higher than the 10 µg/m^3 limit specified in Sweden.

It appears that the potential carcinogenic risks of nickel are unlikely to be a factor for dental patients and dentists, as compared with dental technicians. Because of a far greater time-weighted exposure to nickel and beryllium dust and vapor, dental technicians should be provided with adequate protection facilities so that such risks are minimized.

To minimize exposure of metallic dust to patients and dentists during metal-grinding operations, a high-speed evacuation system should be used when such procedures are performed intraorally. Patients should be informed of the potential allergic effects of nickel exposure, and a thorough medical history should be taken to determine whether the patient is at risk for exhibiting an allergic reaction to nickel. As a conservative approach, the dentist should adopt the policy that evidence of a previous allergic response to any alloy should be sufficient grounds to bar the use of nickel-based alloys.

GUIDELINES FOR SELECTION AND USE OF BASE METALS FOR CROWN AND BRIDGE APPLICATIONS

The main advantages of certain high noble alloys are their biocompatibility and their yellow color. This hue tends to yield a warmer, more aesthetic result, and no blue or gray line occurs subgingivally, as sometimes results from the use of white-colored metals such as white gold alloys, nickel-based alloys, and cobalt-based alloys.

Several questions should be addressed whenever the dentist considers the use of a nickel-based alloy as an alternative or replacement for a time-tested gold-based alloy: (1) Is there any evidence to show that the alloy is technique-sensitive with respect to castability, adherence to porcelain, thermal compatibility with porcelain, porcelain discoloration potential, or solderability? (2) Do the advantageous properties and financial benefits outweigh the potential biological hazards? (3) How many years of proven success has the laboratory technician had with this alloy? (4) How long has the alloy been available to the dental profession? (5) Has the alloy been classified as acceptable according to ISO standards or the acceptance program established by the ADA Council on Scientific Affairs for alloys used to fabricate dental restorative and prosthetic devices?

Before attempting to answer these questions, the dentist should recognize that no alloy is ideal in all respects. Compared with other alloys for metal-ceramic prostheses, base metal alloys generally have higher hardness and elastic modulus (stiffness) values and are more sag-resistant at elevated temperatures, but they may be more difficult to cast and presolder than gold-palladium or palladium-silver alloys. Some claims have been made that base metal alloys are, in general, more technique-sensitive than well-established noble metal alloys. It is well known that **presoldering** of nickel-chromium alloys with a high degree of reliability requires considerable experience. A survey by the National Association of Dental Laboratories indicated that only 46% of the laboratory owners surveyed were satisfied with the soldering performance of these alloys. The ability to obtain acceptable-fitting base metal castings represents a challenge to technicians and may require special procedures to adequately compensate for their higher solidification shrinkage. Another potential disadvantage of some nickel-based or cobalt-based alloys is their potential for porcelain delamination as a result of separation of a poorly adherent oxide layer from the metal substrate. In addition, relatively small differences in composition may produce wide variations in metal-ceramic bond strength.

Examples of the three most common types of base metal alloys for metal-ceramic prostheses and their properties are given in Tables 19-8 through 19-11.

Compositions of the three elements listed in each case fall within a narrow range; other elements may produce considerable variations in castability, corrosion resistance, and solder joint strength and quality. Using a mesh screen pattern as a castability monitor, Whitlock et al (1985) measured percent castability values of fourteen metal-ceramic alloys, including four nickel-chromium-beryllium alloys, several nickel-based alloys without beryllium, and three gold-based alloys. Castability (percentage completion of the mesh screen pattern) values ranged from approximately 43% to 92% for the alloys with beryllium. The nickel alloys without beryllium demonstrated castability values varying from approximately 10% to 67%.

Table 19-8 — Typical Base Metal Alloys Used for Metal-Ceramic Prostheses

Alloy name	Composition (wt%)									
	Ni	Co	Cr	Mo	Be	W	Ru	Al	Ga	Other
Rexillium III (Pentron Lab Tech)	76	–	14	6	2	–	–	2	–	–
Neptune (Pentron Lab Tech)	63	–	22	9	–	–	–	–	–	Balance
Litecast (Ivoclar Vivadent)	68.5	–	15.5	14	–	–	–	1	–	Balance
Pisces Plus (Ivoclar Vivadent)	61.5	–	22	–	–	11.2	–	2.3	–	Balance
Genesis II (Heraeus Kulzer)	–	53	27	–	–	10	3	–	3	Balance
Novarex (Pentron Lab Tech)	–	52	25	–	–	14	–	1	8	–

Table 19-9 — Physical and Mechanical Properties of Base Metal Alloys and a Gold Alloy for Metal-Ceramic Prostheses*

Property	A	B	C	D	E	F	Gold alloy
TENSILE STRENGTH							
MPa	1150	1140	1360	660	540	703	490
ksi	167	165	197	95.7	78.3	102	71.1
YIELD STRENGTH							
MPa	591	782	838	360	260	543	400
ksi	85.7	113	122	52.2	37.7	78.7	58.0
MODULUS OF ELASTICITY							
GPa	207	190	210	193	154	208	88
10^3 ksi	30.0	27.6	30.5	28.0	22.3	30.2	12.8
Percent Elongation	23.9	11.6	18.0	27.9	27.3	2.3	9.1
Vickers Hardness	293	348	357	211	175	316	161
Density (g/cm^3)	8.1	8.0	7.9	8.0	8.7	8.3	18.3
BOND STRENGTH TO PORCELAIN							
MPa	97.9	51.0	87.6	70.3	80.7	106	111
ksi	142	74.0	12.7	10.2	11.7	15.4	16.1

*See compositions in Table 19-10.
Modified from Moffa JP: Physical and Mechanical Properties of Gold and Base Metal Alloys. In: Alternatives to Gold Alloys in Dentistry, DHEW Publication No. (NIH) 77-1227, 1977.

The beryllium-containing alloys as a group did not demonstrate overall superiority to the non–beryllium-containing alloys, although the highest castability value of the 14 alloys tested was exhibited by a nickel-chromium-beryllium alloy. Because induction melting equipment was used in this study, some of the variability in castability may have been caused by differences in the amount of superheating beyond the liquidus temperature (resulting from differences in emissivity values for the alloys, which were measured by an optical pyrometer). Another factor might be the differences in emissivity from nonoxidized and oxidized surfaces of the molten nickel-based alloys.

The subject of castability is controversial, since some researchers claim that all alloys will theoretically produce complete castings under optimum burnout, melting, and casting conditions. The point to be made here, however, is that generalized statements on the superiority of beryllium-containing or nonberyllium-containing alloys should not be made without appropriate supporting research data and statistical analyses.

Table 19-10   Composition of Base Metal Alloys for Metal Ceramic Restorations

Element	A	B	C	D	E	F
Nickel	80.75	79.67	78.51	68.96	80.86	68.75
Chromium	12.58	13.24	19.47	16.54	11.93	19.57
Iron	0.34	0.11	0.43	0.37	0.20	0.38
Aluminum	3.42	3.87	0.21	4.15	2.95	—
Molybdenum	1.53	1.52	—	5.10	1.87	4.22
Silicon	0.29	0.30	1.10	0.83	0.18	2.72
Beryllium	0.57	0.65	—	—	1.55	—
Copper	0.15	—	—	—	0.13	1.54
Manganese	0.13	0.12	—	3.05	0.14	1.24
Cobalt	—	—	—	0.42	—	—
Tin	—	—	—	—	—	1.25

Adapted from Physical and Mechanical Properties of Gold and Base Metal Alloys in Moffa JP, Alternatives to Gold Alloys in Dentistry, DHEW Publication No. (NIH) 77–1227, 1977.

Table 19-11   Comparative Properties of High Noble Alloys and Base Metals for Metal-Ceramic Prostheses

Property	High noble alloy	Co-Cr	Ni-Cr-Be	CP Ti
Biocompatibility	Excellent	Excellent	Fair	Excellent
Density	14 g/cm^3	7.5 g/cm^3	8.7 g/cm^3	4.5 g/cm^3
Elastic Modulus (Stiffness)	90 GPa	145–220 GPa	207 GPa	103 GPa
Sag Resistance	Poor to excellent	Excellent	Excellent	Good
Technique Sensitivity	Minimal	Moderately high	Moderately high	Extremely high
Bond to Porcelain	Excellent	Fair	Good to excellent	Fair
Metal Cost	High	Low	Low	Low*

*The dental laboratory costs for fabricating metal-ceramic prostheses are high for CP Ti, and the number of dental laboratories with this capability is limited.

The creep (sag deformation) resistance of nickel-based alloys at porcelain firing temperatures is considered to be far superior to the resistance of gold-based and palladium-based alloys under the same conditions. One study revealed that under an applied bending stress of 19.6 MPa, the relative creep rates (measured as mid-span deflection rates) of cast metal strips at 1000° C were approximately 1.8 mm/min for a palladium-copper-gallium alloy, 1.1 mm/min for a gold-palladium alloy, 0.9 mm/min for a gold-palladium-silver alloy, and 0.6 mm/min for a nickel-chromium-beryllium alloy. The higher creep values indicate that greater distortion of long-span frameworks is more likely to result at elevated temperatures unless special precautions are taken by the dental technician.

The tarnish and corrosion resistance of base metal alloys containing nickel is of principal concern because of the allergic potential of nickel and nickel compounds. Little information is available on the influence of corrosion products, which form under in vivo conditions.

The bond strength values of nickel-chromium and cobalt-chromium alloys to porcelain as determined from in vitro studies have not generally been shown to be superior or inferior to those for noble metal alloys. Furthermore, clinical studies have not demonstrated a difference in the failure incidence between metal-ceramic restorations made from base metal alloys and those fabricated from noble metal alloys. However, some research indicates that certain characteristics of the oxide layer that forms on these alloys during preoxidation and porcelain firing cycles may adversely affect the bond strength of metal-ceramic restorations. An oxide layer that is nonadherent to the alloy substrate is susceptible to delamination under relatively low stresses. Contrary to previous theories for noble dental alloys, the thickness of this oxide layer or wettability of the oxide layer by porcelain may not be as important in the control of metal-ceramic adherence to base metal alloys as the adherence of the oxide layer to the metal substrate.

For the laboratory technician to produce the optimum metal oxide characteristics, the instructions from the manufacturer must be followed precisely. However, some instructions are relatively imprecise. For example, some alloys require a light sandblasting procedure after the metal oxide is formed during the initial oxidation step (sometimes incorrectly termed *degassing* by dental laboratory personnel). Although a 50 µm aluminum oxide abrasive is generally recommended, the purity level is not usually specified. The use of more economical, lower-purity aluminum oxide abrasives by dental technicians could contaminate the metal surface and subsequently affect the integrity of the metal-ceramic adherence zone. The ability of a laboratory technician to discriminate light from moderate grit-blasting to remove these surface oxides is one example of the technique sensitivity of base metal alloys. Other procedures that may be more technique-sensitive than those for noble metal alloys include the determination of the proper casting temperature and the judgment of the proper flow-point of solder during the presoldering process.

The thermal contraction differential between base metal alloys and dental porcelains may, under certain conditions, contribute to high levels of stress in porcelain, which could induce cracking of porcelain or delayed failure. Although the thermal expansion and contraction values of base metal alloys generally fall within the range of noble metal alloys, porcelain cracking occasionally results when the thermal expansion and contraction differences between metal and porcelain are excessive.

Perhaps the greatest disadvantage of nickel-based alloys is the variability in quality and strength of presoldered connectors. Flexure tests of presoldered specimens reveal relatively brittle fracture patterns, which typically propagate within the solder. Tensile tests have demonstrated both intrasolder and interfacial types of failure.

The principal defects within the solder alloy are voids, localized shrinkage porosity, and **flux** inclusions. Beryllium-containing alloys are generally more difficult to solder, and specimens of these alloys contain relatively high concentrations of voids within the solder joint.

To circumvent the uncertainties and variations associated with presoldering procedures, some dental technicians prefer to avoid the soldering process by using a cast-joining procedure instead. A pontic is cut diagonally in half, and each half is prepared with large undercut channels. After each half of the bridge is stabilized on an occlusal index, the undercut areas are waxed to full contour, sprued, invested, burned out, and cast with new metal. This process is known as *cast-joining*. No clinical research has been performed to identify the adequacy of this approach. However, it should be noted that the two components are retained by mechanical interlocking effects and the excessive displacement of these regions will likely cause porcelain fracture.

The elastic modulus of base metal alloys is as much as two times greater than the values for some of the more popular noble metal alloys. To take advantage of this property, some clinicians have proposed that the coping thickness in veneered areas can be reduced from the minimum thickness of 0.3 mm that is recommended for noble metal alloys to a uniform thickness of 0.1 mm. Theoretically, the cross-section area of cast interproximal connectors can be reduced from 4–8 mm^2 to 1–2 mm^2 when base metal alloys are used. These drastic changes in procedure should be analyzed by controlled research studies before such procedures are adopted for clinical practice. Jones (1983) has criticized this approach on the basis that the deflection of a base metal alloy beam will be greater than that of a gold alloy beam if the former is reduced in thickness by 50%, even though its modulus of elasticity is higher. The deflection of a cantilever beam is inversely proportional to t^{3}E, where t is the beam thickness in the plane of bending and E is the elastic modulus. Jones concluded that the connector thickness can be reduced by only 16% when the elastic modulus is doubled. Furthermore, a reduction of the coping thickness from 0.3 mm to 0.1 mm is likely to increase the risk for porcelain fracture because of the increased flexibility of the coping. However, a recent study based on finite element stress analysis of stresses induced in anterior PFM crowns under intra-oral forces indicates that a reduction of base metal coping thickness (in veneered areas) from 0.3 to 0.1 mm has only a slight effect on porcelain stresses.

The mechanical properties of nickel-based alloys for fixed prosthodontics are known to vary considerably. Asgar et al (1968) reported that the 0.2% offset yield strength of 14 nickel-based alloys ranged from 310 MPa to 828 MPa in the as-cast condition. After a heat-treatment process, the yield strength decreased to between 241 MPa and 724 MPa. The hardness values of these 14 alloys were comparable. These authors also reported lower modulus of elastic values, for example, 152 GPa for some of these base metal alloys after heat treatment. In comparison, the modulus of elasticity for some palladium-silver alloys approximately 117 GPa.

In general, the high hardness and high strength of these base metal alloys contribute to certain difficulties in clinical practice. Grinding and polishing of fixed restorations to achieve proper occlusion occasionally requires more time at chairside. Removal of defective restorations may also require more time. Repair of crowns with fractured porcelain veneers, which may be simply performed on noble metal substrates using pin-retained facings or metal-ceramic onlays, is more difficult to accomplish when the failed restoration has a framework cast with nickel-based or cobalt-based alloys. Such difficulties may partially offset the economic advantage of these alloys.

Despite the widespread use of nickel-based alloys for metal-ceramic restorations, claims for the safety of these alloys have not yet been universally accepted. The allergenic effects of nickel on dental patients and the potential toxic effects of nickel and beryllium on laboratory technicians continue to cause concern within the dental profession. The systemic response to metallic nickel and nickel compounds due to intraoral corrosion and dissolution of nickel-based restorations over extended periods of time have not been studied adequately. The dental profession may be overgeneralizing the relative safety of nickel alloys because of the lack of allergy-induced intraoral lesions observed in private practices. Additional animal studies are needed to characterize the acute and chronic toxicities of nickel compounds that may occur in dental prostheses. In addition to the risks associated with nickel, the potential for dermatological and systemic effects that may result from patient and personnel exposure to cobalt alloys should not be overlooked.

Although allergic reactions are of some concern, the toxicity potential of cobalt-chromium alloys appears to be insignificant. Little research has been performed to determine the carcinogenic potential of nickel on dental laboratory technicians. In addition, animal and human studies are needed to determine the effect of nickel and beryllium exposure on the reproductive system. In the interim period, specific equipment and facilities that minimize dust and vapor exposure to dental technicians should be used. This would reduce airborne concentrations of nickel and beryllium in commercial dental laboratories and dental offices and also minimize the exposure of personnel to airborne debris from noble metal alloys, amalgams, porcelains, and other dental materials.

CRITICAL QUESTION

What three questions should be asked when using a commercial dental laboratory for the first time?

To ensure the safety of patients, dentists, dental office staff, and dental technicians, manufacturers and laboratory managers should identify alloys and alloy components used in the fabrication of prosthetic devices in terms of elements that may adversely affect the health of individuals (e.g., nickel, chromium, cobalt, and beryllium). Dentists and administrators of dental laboratories are encouraged to inform employees who work as technicians regarding the need to avoid inhalation exposure to dusts and vapors from alloys. Practitioners are encouraged to document in patient records the content and specific brand names of alloys used in restorative materials. Health histories should include documentation of patients sensitive to metals. Patch testing for sensitivity to metals should not be performed by dentists but by professionals trained in the administration and interpretation of these tests. Practitioners are encouraged to report case histories of adverse reactions to metals and other biomaterials to the American Dental Association or other national professional organizations.

Before selecting a base metal alloy for practice, the dentist should ask the technician three basic questions to ensure that the selection is being approached from a conservative point of view. These questions are as follows:

1. What is the brand name of the porcelain, the alloy, and the alloy type you are using?

The response to this question will allow you to classify the alloy (e.g., Ni-Cr, Ni-Cr-Be or Co-Cr) and determine whether the product has been tested and accepted according to the testing standards of national or international standards organizations (ADA, ISO, BSI, etc.). The porcelain brand name must be known to determine whether a compatible system is being used. A telephone call to the laboratory manager should answer this question.

2. *How long have you been using the alloy, and what are the main problems you have experienced?*

If the alloy-porcelain system has been used for less than 3 years, limited information will be available on the clinical performance of the alloy in metal-ceramic prostheses. If the technician mentions porcelain debonding or crack formation as the major problem, the dentist should find another laboratory or a more reliable product.

3. *Have you had any difficulty in soldering, cast-joining, or bonding porcelain to the alloy used for metal-ceramic prostheses?*

If difficulties have been experienced, the dentist should determine whether they have been satisfactorily resolved. If problems still persist, every effort should be made to shift to a laboratory and/or materials system that has at least 3 years of proven success in all aspects of use for the indicated purposes of the material system.

CRITICAL QUESTION

What are the advantages and drawbacks for selection of a base metal casting alloy, rather than a noble metal casting alloy, for a metal-ceramic prosthesis?

PARTIAL DENTURE ALLOYS AND GUIDELINES FOR SELECTION

Summarized in Table 19-12 are the properties of nickel-based and cobalt-based partial denture alloys compared with high noble alloys, CP Ti, and Ti-6V-4Al alloy. The main advantage of CP Ti is its biocompatibility. Titanium is believed to be the most biocompatible of all metals. However, titanium is quite technique-sensitive when casting, bonding to porcelain, and soldering. As noted previously, special (relatively expensive) machines are required for casting titanium, in which arc melting and casting in an argon atmosphere are typically employed.

Previously, it was noted that the base metal alloys in widespread use for removable partial denture frameworks are Co-Cr, Ni-Cr, and Co-Cr-Ni. Beryllium is added to the compositions of some nickel-based alloys to reduce their liquidus

Table 19-12	Mechanical Properties of Removable Partial Denture Alloys				
Metal type	Yield strength (MPa/ksi)	Tensile strength (MPa/ksi)	Elongation (%)	Hardness (HV)	Elastic modulus (GPa/ksi × 10³)
Co-Cr* (A)	710/103	870/120	1.6	432	224/32.4
Ni-Cr * (B)	690/100	800/116	3.8	300	182/26.4
Co-Cr-Ni* (C)	470/68	685/99	8.0	264	198/28.7
Fe-Cr* (D)	703/102	841/122	9	309	202/29.3
Type IV Gold[†]	493/71.5	776/112	7	264	90/13
CP Ti	344/50	345/50	13	210	103/14.9
Ti-6V-4Al	870/126	925/134	5	320	117/17

(A, B, C, and D: Data from Morris HF et al: J Prosthet Dent 41:388, 1979.)
*Bench cooled in investment after casting.
[†]Age-hardened.

temperature and facilitate casting of the metal. The mechanical properties of representative Co-Cr, Ni-Cr, and Fe-Cr alloys given in Table 19-12 reflect relatively high elastic moduli. This property suggests that the thickness of partial denture frameworks can be thinner than those for Type IV gold, CP Ti, and Ti-6V-4Al alloy. The ductility of CP Ti is significantly greater than that of the six alloys. The lower yield strength and tensile strength and higher percentage elongation of CP Ti suggest that cast clasps may be more easily adjusted. Mechanical properties of more recently introduced Co-Cr and Ni-Cr alloys have been reported in the article by Bridgeport et al (1993) listed in the Selected Readings section.

As noted, the advantages of these cobalt-based and nickel-based alloys are their high elastic modulus (compared with the hardened Type IV gold alloys that were formerly used for removable partial denture frameworks) and their low unit metal cost. Particular concerns are the higher hardness of some alloys compared with tooth enamel, which can cause in vivo wear, as well as the need for special finishing equipment in the dental laboratory and the tendency of these alloys to undergo rapid work hardening.

When adjusting clasps on the cast framework, caution should be taken by the dental laboratory technician or the clinician to avoid fracture, even with those partial denture alloys that exhibit higher values of percent elongation. The rapid work hardening is associated with the complex microstructures of these alloys, which arise from their complex elemental compositions. Because of the absence of known grain-refining elements, the as-cast microstructures are dendritic, with facile pathways for crack propagation. Morris and Asgar (1975) (see Table 19-12) found that heat treatment was ineffective in generally improving the mechanical properties of these alloys, which are recommended for clinical use in the as-cast condition.

It is very important for the dentist to select a dental laboratory with a technician who is highly experienced in fabricating partial denture frameworks. Because of their high melting points, these alloys are induction-melted and cast using phosphate-bonded or silicate-bonded investments, as recommended by the manufacturer, and they exhibit high casting shrinkage with a potential for casting defects. The Ni-Cr and Co-Cr-Ni alloys were found by Bridgeport et al (1993) to have higher mean values of elongation than the Co-Cr alloys, but studies are needed to determine whether the former alloy types exhibit better long-term clinical performance.

CRITICAL QUESTIONS

What factors must be considered by the dental laboratory and dentist for the preparation and adjustment of partial denture frameworks cast from base metal alloys? What are the merits and drawbacks for the use of alternative techniques to casting for dental alloys?

ALTERNATIVES TO CAST METAL TECHNOLOGY

Cast metals are used in dental laboratories to produce inlays, onlays, crowns, conventional all-metal fixed partial dentures (FPDs), metal-ceramic FPDs, resin-bonded FPDs, endodontic posts, and frameworks for removable partial dentures. The metals must exhibit (1) biocompatibility, (2) ease of melting, (3) minimal reactivity with the mold (investment) material, (4) excellent castability, (5) little solidification shrinkage, (6) sound brazed (or soldered) connectors, (7) acceptable polishability, (8) good wear resistance, (9) high yield strength and fatigue resistance, (10) acceptable sag resistance (metal-ceramic alloys), and (11) excellent tarnish and corrosion resistance. Generally, conventional Type II and III gold alloys represent the standards against which the performance of other casting alloys are judged.

Four other technologies are currently available to avoid the challenges and cost associated with the metal-casting process. These include: (1) sintering (or diffusion bonding) of burnished **metal foil,** (2) CAD-CAM processing of metal blocks, (3) **copy milling** of metal blocks, and (4) electroforming of metal copings.

Sintering of Burnished Foil

The most commonly used commercial foil system (Captek; Precious Metals Co Inc, Altamonte Springs, FL) requires three pairs of materials to form composite metal structures: (1) Captek P and Captek G, which are used to fabricate crown copings and fixed partial denture abutments; (2) Capcon and Capfil, which are used to connect copings; and (3) Captek Repair paste and Capfil, which are used to add material to Captek structures. Captek copings contain 88.2 wt% Au, 9.0 wt% platinum-group metals (including 4 wt% Pt), and 2.8 wt% Ag. The copings are made with a thickness of 0.25 mm for anterior crowns and 0.35 mm for posterior crowns. The inner and outer gold-rich layers are approximately 25 μm in thickness, and the middle layer is made of a gold-platinum metal. The Captek P layer is adapted first to the die and fired at a temperature of 1075° C. During this firing cycle, the adhesive and binders are eliminated, and the Pd and Pt particles become interconnected by sintering to form a three-dimensional network of capillary channels. Captek G is applied over the Captek P coping, the former containing 97 wt% gold plus binders. The Captek G metal is drawn by capillary action into the network structure of the Captek P coping vacated by the adhesive binder. Captek G is provided in two thicknesses, one for anterior copings and one for posterior copings. A 0.35-mm–thick layer of porcelain is applied to the coping, which may or may not require the Capbond bonding agent.

The main advantage of Captek crowns is the very low metal thickness that can be achieved, which ensures minimal tooth reduction or improved aesthetics compared with conventional metal-ceramic crowns made with cast metal copings. For example, the metal margin of a Captek coping can be ground to a thickness of 50 μm, and the total thickness of metal and porcelain can be as low as 0.3 mm, although optimal aesthetics dictates that anterior crown thicknesses of 0.7 to 1.0 mm are indicated. Posterior crown thicknesses should be a minimum of 1.2 mm to resist fracture.

CAD-CAM Processing

Directly placed restorations can be made of direct-filling gold Dental amalgam, an acid-base cement, or a polymer resin-based composite. Indirect restorations use cast alloys, sintered ceramics, or polymerized resins. These processes restrict the range of materials that can be used. CAD-CAM (computer-aided design and computer-aided machining) systems provide an alternative method to produce metal, ceramic, or composite restorations without the need for processes that require two or more patient appointments for a given type of restoration or prosthesis. For example, CAD-CAM technology allows a technician or dentist to use higher quality ceramics, which have been produced under nearly ideal conditions. Such materials exhibit several improved properties compared with conventional sintered or hot-pressed ceramics.

This processing method was developed in the early 1980s to produce ceramic inlays and crowns during one chair-side appointment. Although CAD-CAM processing of metal crowns and other prostheses is not commonly used, the basic process is important to understand because many products in the future will be fabricated using this technology. As an alternative to the metal-casting process, the metal can be milled or ground from a metal block using a CAD-CAM process or by electrolytic or electrical discharge removal of metal. The following description focuses on the former option, since it is the most widely used technology. A CAD-CAM system electronically or digitally records surface coordinates of the prepared tooth and stores these retrieved data in the memory of a computer. The image data can be retrieved immediately to mill or grind a metal, ceramic, or composite prosthesis by computer control from a solid block of the chosen material. Within minutes, the prosthesis can be fabricated and placed in a prepared tooth and bonded or cemented in the mouth of the patient in a period ranging from 10 min to 1 hr.

The optical scanning procedure eliminates the need for an impression. An advantage of ceramics is that homogeneous, high-quality materials with minimal porosity and other typical defects are designed for CAD-CAM application. The computer-controlled milling machine can then be used to perform the milling or grinding for fabrication of a ceramic prosthesis within a few minutes. The CAD-CAM technique could also be used to prepare prostheses from CP Ti or Ti-6Al-4V alloy that would not contain bulk casting defects or the hard alpha (α) case found near the surface of cast titanium prostheses.

Copy Milling

This process is based on the principle of tracing the surface of a pattern that is then replicated from a blank of ceramic, composite, or metal that is ground, cut, or milled by a rotating wheel whose motion is controlled by a link through the tracing device. The process is similar to that associated with cutting a key blank using a tracing of a master key. One commercial system of this type (Celay; Mikrona Technologies, Spreitenbach, Switzerland) has been in use since 1991. The pattern to be traced is made from a blue-colored resin-based composite (Celay-Tech; 3M ESPE).

Electroforming

A master cast of the prepared tooth (teeth) is prepared and coated with a special die spacer to facilitate separation of the duplicating material. The dies are duplicated with a gypsum product that has a setting expansion of 0.1% to 0.2%. After applying a conductive silver layer to its surface, the die is connected to a plating head and connected to a power source and then placed in a plating solution. After a sufficiently thick layer of gold or other metal is deposited, the gypsum is removed and the coping is sandblasted. The coping is then coated with a bonding agent during the wash bake, and subsequent ceramic layers are condensed and sintered in a conventional way.

CRITICAL QUESTION

What are the differences among soldering, brazing, and welding?

SOLDERING OF DENTAL ALLOYS
Substrate Metal for Soldering

Metal-joining operations are usually divided into three categories: **brazing,** soldering, and **welding.** The definitions seem remarkably similar. The primary difference between soldering and brazing is that brazing requires a heating temperature above 450° C (840° F) but below the solidus temperature of the substrate metal(s). The difference between these two processes and welding is that welding may not require a filler metal and the metal surfaces to be joined will fuse locally. For dental applications the term *soldering* is commonly used to describe the build-up of a contact area or the joining of two metal parts, such as components of a fixed partial denture or an intraoral appliance. The soldering process involves the substrate metal(s) to be joined, a filler metal (usually called *solder*), a flux, and a heat source. All are equally important, and the role of each must be taken into consideration to solder metal components successfully. Some of the terms and definitions listed in the *Key Terms* section are modified versions of those provided in the *Metals Handbook, Desk Edition* (1992). The terms and definitions that follow serve as a reference to differentiate among brazing, soldering, and welding. Because the liquidus temperature of the filler metal is the only difference between the terms *brazing* and *soldering*, the term *soldering* is used subsequently as a general term to describe both processes.

The substrate metal, sometimes known as the *basis metal*, is the original pure metal or alloy that is prepared for joining to another substrate metal or alloy. Before casting became the popular method of producing metal prosthetic structures, many appliances were constructed by forming shapes from wrought plate and wire and then soldering these pieces together to produce the required configuration.

Dental casting alloys that can be soldered or welded include gold-based, silver-based, palladium-based, nickel-based, cobalt-based, and titanium-based alloys, as well as commercially pure titanium. Note that the principles for soldering or welding are the same for any substrate metal. However, this does not mean that the ease of soldering or welding is the same for any substrate metal. Thus the individual who performs the soldering or welding procedure should have considerable knowledge about the optimal procedure for cleaning the surfaces to allow intimate contact with molten filler metal, the most compatible filler metal to be used, and the heating temperature that will ensure adequate flow of filler metal or fusion of adjacent surfaces if welding is performed.

The composition of the substrate metal determines its melting range. As previously noted, the soldering should take place below the solidus temperature of the substrate metal(s). The composition of the substrate metal determines the oxide that forms on the surface during heating, and, if used, a flux must be able to reduce this oxide, inhibit further oxidation, or facilitate its removal. The composition and cleanliness of the substrate metal and the temperature to which it is heated determine the wettability of the substrate by the molten solder alloy. The solder chosen must wet the metal at as low a contact angle as possible to ensure wetting of the joint area. To prevent flow onto adjacent areas, an **antiflux** such as rouge mixed with chloroform can be painted on the areas before heating the assembly.

The manufacturer or supplier is responsible for providing explicit instructions for eliminating the oxide layer during the joining process. The instructions for every alloy should also include a recommendation for the appropriate filler metal (solder) and flux. For alloys that will be bonded to porcelain, this recommendation should include filler metals for both prefiring (presolder) and postfiring (postsolder), and the appropriate flux for the substrate alloy. As stated earlier in this chapter, the technical term for joining metals before firing of the veneering ceramic layers is *presoldering* (or *prebrazing*), and the technical term for joining metals after the veneering process is **postsoldering** (or *postbrazing*).

CRITICAL QUESTION

What materials and methods can be used to enhance or restrict the flow of solder?

Soldering Flux

The Latin word *flux* means "flow." Soldering filler metals are designed to melt, wet the surface(s) of the part(s) to be joined, and flow across clean metal surfaces; they cannot wet oxidized surfaces without the use of a flux. The purpose of a flux is to eliminate any oxide coating on the substrate metal surface when the filler metal is molten and ready to flow into place. Fluxes may be divided into the following three types, according to their primary purpose:

(Type I) Surface protection—Covers the metal surface and prevents access to oxygen so that no oxides can form.

(Type II) Reducing agent—Reduces any oxides present and exposes clean metal.

(Type III) Solvent—Dissolves any oxides present and carries them away.

The composition of most commercial fluxes is formulated to accomplish two or three of these purposes. Fluxes have temperature ranges for optimum activity in breaking down oxides. Thus a flux that is designed for presoldering may not do well for postsoldering, and vice versa. For instance, a borax flux is usually too fluid to remain in place for presoldering, and a fluoride flux may not have sufficient chemical activity at the lower postsoldering temperatures. In addition, fluoride-containing fluxes are likely to attack the porcelain if they are used for postsoldering.

Fluxes for use with noble metal alloys are generally based on boric or borate compounds such as boric acid, boric anhydride, and borax. They act as protective fluxes (Type I) by forming a low-temperature glass. They are also reducing fluxes (Type II) for low-stability oxides such as copper oxide.

Because the oxides that form on base metal alloys are more stable, fluoride fluxes (Type III) are used to dissolve chromium, nickel, and cobalt oxides. They usually contain borates as glass formers (protective), and the fluoride dissolves any metal oxide with which it comes in contact, acting as a solvent.

The flux may be used by painting it on the substrate metal at the junction of the pieces to be joined, or it may be fused onto the surface of the filler metal strip. One product is furnished as a filler metal in a tubular form, and the flux is contained inside the tube. This type is called *prefluxed solder*.

Whatever technique is used, it is of primary importance to minimize the amount of flux used. Excess flux may become entrapped within the filler metal and cause a weakened joint. Residual flux that is covered with porcelain can cause discoloration and bubbling of the porcelain. Flux, when combined with metal oxides, forms a glass during the soldering process that is difficult to remove completely. A two-step method for removing residual glass from some metals is to sandblast the joint immediately after removal from the investment with alumina abrasive particles and to follow by boiling in water for about 5 minutes.

Soldering (Brazing) Filler Metal

Soldering filler metal compositions are as diverse as the compositions of the substrate metals. The filler metal must be compatible with the oxide-free substrate metal, but it does not necessarily have a similar composition. Compatibility consists of three primary properties: (1) sufficiently low flow temperature; (2) ability to wet the substrate metal; and (3) sufficient fluidity at the flow temperature. Other properties that should be considered include an acceptable color and adequate hardness, strength, and tarnish and corrosion resistance.

Flow temperature is that temperature at which the filler metal wets and flows on the substrate metal and produces a bond. It is not related to any physical property of the alloy, such as the liquidus temperature. The flow temperature of the filler metal is usually higher than its liquidus temperature. The flow temperature of a filler metal varies, depending on the combination of substrate metal, flux, and ambient atmosphere. This temperature should be specified by the filler metal manufacturer and is one of the requirements of a standard established by the International Organization for Standardization (ISO 9333). This standard also provides a method for its determination.

The flow temperature of the filler metal should be lower than the solidus temperature of the metals being joined. A general rule is that the flow temperature of the filler metal should be at least 55.6° C (100° F) lower than the solidus temperature of the substrate metal. For a presoldered alloy substrate that will be veneered with porcelain, a higher–melting-range solder is usually needed to avoid remelting the solder when the porcelain is fired and to prevent sag deformation of a bridge framework during subsequent porcelain firing.

Wetting of the substrate metal by the filler metal is essential to produce a bond. The wetting phenomenon is discussed in Chapter 2. Wetting may be understood by comparing the placement of a drop of water on a piece of wax and on a piece of soap. The drop of water "balls up" on the wax and contacts the wax over a smaller area. On the soap, it spreads as far as the amount of water allows. The water wets the soap, whereas it does not wet the wax.

Similarly, if pure silver is melted on nickel or nickel-based alloys, it stands up in a ball, as seen on the right side of Figure 19-6. In contrast, when pure silver is melted on gold and palladium-silver alloys, it spreads over the surface. However, spreading of a molten metal does not occur if an oxide layer is present on the surface of the substrate metal, because oxides have poor wettability characteristics.

When two different substrate metals are joined through the use of a filler metal, such as a cast gold alloy crown to a bridge made of a Pd-Ag alloy, the filler metal

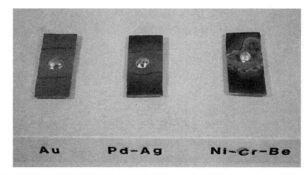

Fig. 19-6   Pure silver melted on three different alloys. It wets the gold (Au) alloy and palladium-silver (Pd-Ag) alloy but does not flow onto the surface of the base metal (Ni-Cr-Be) alloy. (Courtesy of C.E. Ingersoll.)

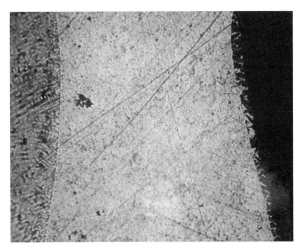

Fig. 19-7 Joining of two different substrate metals with the filler metal **(in center)**. **Left,** Good bonding with no alloying between the filler metal and substrate metal. **Right,** A nodular region of alloying that has occurred at the interface between the filler metal and another substrate alloy, which is not distinct in this micrograph. (Courtesy of C.E. Ingersoll.)

represents a compromise. If the flow temperature of the filler metal is close to or above the solidus of either substrate metal, alloying can take place through a welding process. Figure 19-7 shows such a soldered joint. Two different substrate metals are joined. In this case, the interface between the filler metal and substrate metal is represented by a sharply defined plane. If the substrate metal has melted at the joint surface, the interface region is indistinct because of alloying or an interaction layer (nodular area to the right of the solder boundary) that has formed between the substrate metal and filler metal. Diffusion of filler atoms into the substrate metal and diffusion of substrate metal atoms into the soldering metal are controlled by temperature and time. Alloying can take place by diffusion if the temperature remains sufficiently high for a sufficiently long time. An alloy formed through diffusion can have properties different from those of both the solder and the substrate metal. As shown in Figure 19-8, for a nickel-based alloy with a gold solder, the resultant

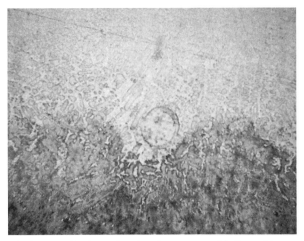

Fig. 19-8 Micrograph showing alloying at interface between a gold-alloy solder metal and a base metal substrate. ×100. (Courtesy of C.E. Ingersoll.)

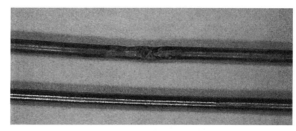

Fig. 19-9   A sag test in which soldering (brazing) of a nickel-based alloy with a gold-based soldering alloy **(top)** produced a gold-nickel diffusion zone. The soldered rod has sagged as compared with the nonsoldered rod **(bottom).** (Courtesy of C.E. Ingersoll.)

diffusion process can form an alloy of gold and nickel that can begin to melt at 950° C (1740° F). Such an alloy could then melt during the firing of porcelain if the soldered metals are used in a metal-ceramic prosthesis. The result of this process is distortion of the prosthesis, as demonstrated for a soldered bar at the top of Figure 19-9. For this reason, gold-based filler metals should not be used as a presolder for base metal alloys.

CRITICAL QUESTIONS

Which type of torch gas should be used for soldering noble alloys? Why can't all torch gasses be used?

HEAT SOURCES FOR SOLDERING
Flame Temperature

The heat source is an important part of the soldering process. The most common instrument for the application of heat is a gas-air or gas-oxygen torch, and the type of torch should be chosen according to the fuel being used. There is a tendency to choose fuel based on its flame temperature, but the flame temperature tells only half the story. Although an alloy cannot be melted if its melting range is higher than the flame temperature, all the gases shown in Table 19-13 potentially have flame temperatures high enough to melt any dental casting alloy currently in use. The flame must provide enough heat to raise the temperature of both the substrate metal and the filler metal to the soldering temperature (the flow temperature of the filler metal). One must also compensate for heat loss to the surroundings. Thermal energy is derived from the heat of combustion of the fuel, and the heat content is measured in calories per cubic meter or British thermal units (BTU) per cubic foot of the fuel. The lower the heat content of the fuel, the more cubic feet of fuel must

Table 19-13	Fuel Gas Characteristics			
	Flame temperature		Heat content	
Fuel (with oxygen)	**° C**	**° F**	**kcal/m³**	**(BTU/ft³)**
Hydrogen	2660	4820	2362	275
Natural gas	2680	4855	8898	1000
Propane	2850	5160	21221	2385
Acetylene	3140	5685	12884	1448

be burned to provide the required total heat. A lower heat content of fuel requires a longer period for heating to the desired temperature and is associated with more danger of oxidation during the soldering process.

Hydrogen

The low heat content value for hydrogen indicates that heating would be slow when it is used as a fuel. The loss of heat to the air, to the soldering investment, and to the other parts of the casting might be enough to take up all of the heat generated by the flame. Using hydrogen, it is impossible to bring the joining area of a large bridge up to the proper temperature required for presoldering.

Natural Gas

The heat content of natural gas is about four times that of hydrogen gas and can be expected to raise the temperature of the soldered joint four times as fast. However, the value in this instance is an average value for dry natural gas. The gas that is normally available is nonuniform in composition and frequently has water vapor in it. Water vapor cools the flame and uses some of the heat content of the gas. This explains why some technicians have had trouble with this fuel when melting alloys for the casting process.

Acetylene

Acetylene has the highest flame temperature, and its heat content is greater than that of either hydrogen or natural gas. However, certain problems are associated with acetylene. The variation in temperature from one part of the flame to another may be more than 100° C. With this variation, the positioning of the torch is critical to ensure that the proper zone of the flame is used. Acetylene is also a chemically unstable gas, and it decomposes readily to carbon and hydrogen. Carbon can be incorporated into both nickel and palladium alloys, resulting in adverse effects on mechanical properties of these alloys and porosity in the porcelain. Hydrogen can be taken up by palladium-based alloys, potentially resulting in increased casting porosity. Improper adjustment of the flame may extinguish the torch with an associated release of carbon from the torch tip. Only individuals with extensive experience with this gas should consider its use for metal joining procedures.

Propane

Of the fuel gases listed in Table 19-13, the best choice is propane. It has a good flame temperature, and its heat content is the highest of the readily available gases. Butane, which is more readily available in some parts of the world, has a similar flame temperature and a similar heat content. Both propane and butane have the advantage of being relatively pure compounds; therefore they are uniform in quality, virtually water-free, and clean-burning (provided that the torch flame is properly adjusted).

Oven (Furnace) Soldering

For oven soldering, a furnace should be chosen with enough wattage to provide the heat required to raise the temperature of the filler metal to its flow point. The furnace will also provide a high-temperature environment, so less heat is lost to other parts of the bridge or to the ambient atmosphere than with torch soldering.

The success of furnace soldering depends on the heat transmission from the heating elements to the substrate metals. For maximum success in furnace soldering, the person performing the soldering process should be familiar with the three modes of heat transmission: convection (transmission by means of air currents), conduction (transmission by conductance through the furnace structure), and radiant heat (transmission by radiation from the heating coils).

Before the metal substrate that will be soldered is placed into the oven, a uniform coating of a paste flux should be applied to the surface to be soldered. Care should be taken to avoid the use of an excessive amount of flux, because some residue may be incorporated into the solder joint, thereby weakening the structure.

CRITICAL QUESTION

How can one best assess whether the quality of a solder joint is acceptable?

TECHNIQUE CONSIDERATIONS FOR SOLDERING

Operator skill, an important element of successful soldering, is a combination of psychomotor ability, knowledge of soldering principles, technique, and experience. This skill is especially important in torch soldering.

Except for the joining of two bridge units, soldering is generally an emergency procedure to repair a metal appliance that may exhibit casting defects, an inadequate proximal contact area, or distortion that occurred during previous fabrication procedures. Technicians may experience problems simply because they do not solder metals routinely, and because skill cannot be maintained, particularly in torch soldering, without practice. The problem is amplified when alloys of titanium, nickel, or cobalt are involved because of the difficulty in removing the surface oxide(s).

Technical Procedures

The soldering technique involves several critical steps: (1) cleaning and preparing the surfaces to be joined, (2) assembling the parts to be joined, (3) preparing and fluxing the gap surfaces between the parts, (4) maintaining the proper position of the parts during the procedure, (5) controlling the proper temperature, and (6) controlling the time to ensure adequate flow of solder and complete filling of the solder joint.

Gap. The optimum gap between parts of substrate metal to be joined has never been defined. If the gap is too great, the joint strength will be controlled by the strength of the filler metal. If the gap is too narrow, the strength will probably be limited by flux inclusions, porosity caused by incomplete flow of the filler metal, or both. Inclusions or porosity can lead to distortion if any heating, such as porcelain application, takes place after the soldering operation.

The two bars shown in Figure 19-10 are of the same nickel-based alloy. They were cut in the same manner and prepared for soldering exactly in the same way except for the gap. The gap for the upper bar was 1.0 mm, whereas the gap for the lower bar was 0.3 mm. Both bars were soldered with the same filler metal. The upper bar

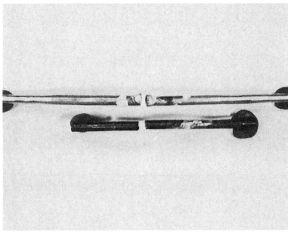

Fig. 19-10 The upper bar was soldered with an excessive gap. When it was tested to failure under tension, the failure occurred in the filler metal. The lower bar, with a proper gap, failed in the substrate metal. (Courtesy of CE Ingersoll.)

failed in the filler metal. The lower bar failed in the substrate metal even though the tensile strength of the substrate metal was greater than that of the filler metal.

Flame. The flame can be divided into four zones as shown in Figure 19-11, and the portion of the flame used to heat the soldering assembly is at the tip of the reducing zone, because this produces the most efficient burning process and the most heat. An improperly adjusted torch or improperly positioned flame can lead to oxidation of the substrate or filler metal and may result in a poor solder joint. It is also possible to introduce carbon into substrate and filler metal by using the unburned gas portion of the flame. To prevent oxide formation, the technician should not remove the flame once it has been applied to the joint area until the soldering process has been completed. The flame provides protection from oxidation, especially at the soldering temperature.

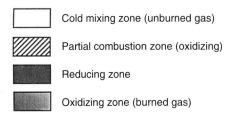

Cold mixing zone (unburned gas)

Partial combustion zone (oxidizing)

Reducing zone

Oxidizing zone (burned gas)

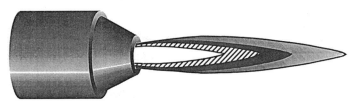

Fig. 19-11 Mixing, combustion, reducing, and unburned gas zones in a propane-oxygen torch flame.

Temperature. The optimal temperature required to solder an area should be the lowest temperature sufficient to produce a sound solder joint. The flame or furnace chamber should provide enough heat to the substrate metal to reach the flow temperature of the filler metal. Thus the substrate metal will be hot enough to melt the filler metal as soon as the filler metal contacts the area to be joined.

Higher temperatures of the substrate metal increase the possibility of diffusion between substrate metal and filler metal. Lower temperatures of the substrate metal do not allow the filler metal to wet the substrate metal, and thus no bonding will occur.

Time. The flame should be maintained in place until the filler metal has flowed completely into the connection and a moment longer to allow the flux or oxide to separate from the fluid filler metal. This longer time increases the possibility of diffusion between substrate metal and filler metal, while a shorter time increases the possibility of incomplete filling of the joint and of flux inclusion in the joint. Both of these conditions result in weaker solder joints.

RADIOGRAPHIC ANALYSIS OF SOLDER JOINT QUALITY

When a fixed partial denture is delivered to a dental office from the dental laboratory, the processing history of the prosthesis is usually unknown to the dentist. Of particular importance is the need to identify whether the fixed partial denture was cast in one piece or whether it was soldered or cast-joined. The flexural strength of a joined metal structure decreases in the following order: cast structure, soldered structure, cast-joined structure. If it is certain that the fixed partial denture was cast in one piece, there should be little concern for its fracture potential. If the structure was soldered at one site, the fracture resistance will be decreased, especially when the joint is positioned more posterior in the fixed partial denture. If the framework was cast-joined (see the following section), the structure should be carefully examined for evidence of defects and for potential mechanical displacement during bending under a manually applied flexural load in one's hands. If any noticeable displacement can be detected, the fixed partial denture should be discarded or returned to the laboratory.

For either the soldered or cast-joined structures, as well as the cast connection, a radiographic examination of the joined area can be performed. The simplest method is to lay the structure on an unexposed piece of intraoral radiographic film and expose the film with an x-ray beam, using an accelerating voltage of 90 kV and a current of 10 mA for 1 s. Another film should be exposed after rotating the fixed partial denture at a 90-degree angle to the initial orientation. Shown in Figure 19-12 are radiographic images of a metal-ceramic framework. One can clearly see the radiolucent voids at the buccal and lingual aspects of the posterior presoldered connector, whereas the cast metal in the other embrasure area is sound.

LASER WELDING OF COMMERCIALLY PURE TITANIUM

Commercially pure titanium (CP Ti) that is used in dentistry for crowns, FPDs, and partial denture frameworks is a highly reactive metal in air. The thin oxide film that forms instantaneously on a cleaned surface converts this metal from an active to a passive state. At temperatures used for soldering procedures, the thickness of the titanium oxide layer increases and may spontaneously debond from the parent metal surface at temperatures exceeding 850° C. Thus the process of soldering this

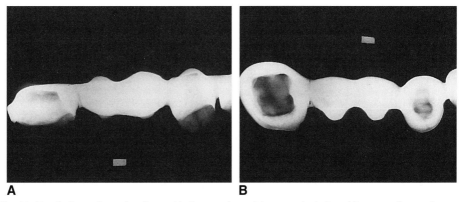

Fig. 19-12 A, Buccolingual radiographic image of metal framework designed for a metal-ceramic fixed partial denture (bridge). **B,** Occlusogingival view. Note the radiolucencies at the buccal and lingual aspects of the posterior soldered connector **(A).**

metal using traditional torch-soldering or oven-soldering procedures is technique-sensitive, and the quality of the soldered joint is quite variable.

To effectively join titanium components of dental crowns, FPDs, and partial denture frameworks, the technician can perform laser welding and plasma welding in an argon gas atmosphere. Since laser welding is associated with a lower thermal influence on the parts being joined than is plasma welding, it is the preferred method for dental applications. An advantage of welding is that the joint will be composed of the same pure titanium as the substrate components, thereby preserving the excellent biocompatibility potential of CP Ti and avoiding the risk for galvanic corrosion effects within the prosthesis.

A few commercial laser welding units are available for joining CP Ti. These are usually based on a pulsed high-power neodymium laser with a very high power density. The first successful units of this type include the Dentaurum Dental-Laser DL 2002 (Dentaurum, Pforzheim, Germany), the Haas Laser LKS (Haas-Laser GmbH, Schramberg, Germany), and the Heraeus Haas Laser 44 P (Heraeus Kulzer GmbH, Hanau, Germany). The units consist of a small type of "glove box" that contains the laser tip, an argon gas source, and a stereomicroscope with lens crosshairs for precise alignment of the laser beam with the CP Ti components. The maximum penetration depth of these laser welding units is 2.5 mm. Since only a small amount of heat is generated, the parts could be hand-held during the welding procedure. Welding can also be performed close to ceramic or polymeric veneers without causing damage to these materials.

CAST-JOINING PROCESS

Because of the technique sensitivity of soldering predominantly base metal alloys and the variation in solder-joint quality associated with presoldering of these alloys, the cast-joining technique (see *Key Terms*) was proposed by Weiss and Munyon (1980) as an alternative method for joining cast components of a fixed partial denture. Cast-joined components are held together purely by mechanical retention (Fig. 19-13). Because of this situation, a bridge with poorly adapted cast secondary metal within the cast-joined area will exhibit greater displacement when a bending force is manually applied. Under this condition, a porcelain veneer over this region is likely to fracture. Thus a radiographic examination should be made of all metal frameworks to minimize this risk.

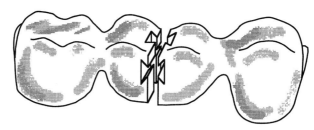

Fig. 19-13   Mechanical interlocking design of a cast-joined framework for a metal-ceramic fixed partial denture (bridge).

SELECTED READINGS

Agarwal DP, and Ingersoll CE: High-temperature soldering alloy. US Patent No. 4399096, 1983.

A particularly important patent, because it involved the development of a palladium-silver-nickel soldering filler metal for presoldering.

American Dental Association: Classification system for cast alloys. J Am Dent Assoc, 109:766, 1984.

Established a system for classifying casting alloys as high noble, noble, or predominantly base metal.

Anusavice KJ, Shen C, Hashinger D, and Twiggs SW: Interactive effect of flexure stress on PFM alloy creep rate. J Dent Res 64:1094, 1985.

This article compares the flexural creep behavior of several representative metal-ceramic alloy types available at the time. Two different creep regimens are described: high-temperature, low-stress sag from the mass of the prosthesis and lower-temperature, high-stress sag from incompatibility in the thermal contraction of the metal and ceramic.

Anusavice KJ, Okabe T, Galloway SE, Hoyt DJ, and Morse PK: Flexure test evaluation of presoldered base metal alloys. J Prosthet Dent 54:507, 1985.

Wide variability in the strength of brazed joints in Ni-Cr-Mo-Be and Ni-Cr-Mo alloys was reported. The strength of the brazed joint ranged from 20% to 90% of that of a solid bar of the same metals and was not affected by gap widths of 0.25 or 0.51 mm.

Anusavice KJ, and Shafagh I: Inert gas presoldering of nickel-chromium alloys. J Prosthet Dent 55:3137, 1986.

An argon gas environment did not improve the strength of presoldered joint strength of nickel-chromium-molybdenum and nickel-chromium-molybdenum-beryllium alloys. Most of the fractures appeared to originate within the solder filler alloy. Entrapped flux particles and gases were the most likely cause of these failures.

Anusavice KJ, and Carroll JE: Effect of incompatibility stress on the fit of metal-ceramic crowns. J Dent Res 66:1341, 1987.

The results of this study suggest that thermal incompatibility stress resulting from a mismatch in thermal contraction coefficients may not be a significant cause of metal distortion.

Asgar K, and Allan FC: Microstructure and physical properties of alloys for partial denture castings. J Dent Res 47(2):189, 1968.

Baran GR: The metallurgy of Ni-Cr alloys for fixed prosthodontics. J Prosthet Dent 50:639, 1983.

A classic article that contains an extensive presentation of alloy compositions, mechanical properties, microstructures, and clinically relevant considerations for the use of these alloys.

Bergman M, Bergman B, and Soremark R: Tissue accumulation of nickel released due to electrochemical corrosion of non-precious dental casting alloy. J Oral Rehab 7:325, 1980.

Brantley WA, Cai Z, Carr AB, and Mitchell JC: Metallurgical structures of as-cast and heat-treated high-palladium dental alloys. Cells Mater 3:103, 1993.

This study describes how the microstructures of these alloys can be explained from a materials science viewpoint in terms of their compositions and the rapid solidification conditions for dental casting.

Brantley WA, Cai Z, Papazoglou E, Mitchell JC, Kerber SJ, Mann GP, and Barr TL: X-ray diffraction studies of oxidized high-palladium alloys. Dent Mater 12:333, 1996.

This study revealed the extremely complex structure of the internal oxide layers on the high-palladium dental alloys and the profound effect of surface preparation on the oxide phases found in these layers.

Bridgeport DA, Brantley WA, and Herman PF: Cobalt-chromium and nickel-chromium alloys for removable prosthodontics, Part 1. Mechanical properties of as-cast alloys. J Prosthod 2:144, 1993.

This article presents more recent measurements of the mechanical properties of partial denture alloys and contains noteworthy SEM photographs of the fracture surfaces.

Brune D, and Beltesbrekke H: Dust in dental laboratories. Part 1. Types and levels in specific operations. J Prosthet Dent 43:687, 1980.

Cai Z, Bunce N, Nunn ME, and Okabe T: Porcelain adherence to dental cast CP titanium: Effects of surface modifications. Biomaterials 22:979, 2001.

This recent article provides an explanation of the need to perform surface modifications on cast CP titanium to improve the porcelain adherence.

Cai Z, Chu X, Bradway SD, Papazoglou E, and Brantley WA: On the biocompatibility of high-palladium dental alloys. Cells Mater 5:357, 1995.

This review article provides an extensive discussion of the potential for palladium allergy that has been reported for certain palladium dental casting alloys.

DeHoff PH, Anusavice KJ, Evans J, and Wilson HR: Effectiveness of cast-joined structures. Int J Prosthodont 3:550, 1990.

A study of the load transfer effectiveness of five cast-joined connector designs. Compared with a solid nickel-chromium alloy bar, the percentage of effectiveness in sustaining an applied bending load ranged from 4.4% to 21.3%.

DeHoff PH, and Anusavice KJ: Viscoelastic stress analysis of thermally compatible and incompatible metal-ceramic systems. Dent Mater 14:237, 1998.

A theoretical and experimental analysis of stress development in ceramic veneers resulting from mismatches in the thermal expansion/contraction coefficients between metals and ceramic veneers.

Doremus RH: Optical properties of small silver particles. J Chem Phys 42:414, 1965.

This paper provides background information on the possible mechanisms for silver discoloration of certain dental ceramics.

Fairhurst CW, Anusavice KJ, Hashinger DT, Ringle RD, and Twiggs SW: Thermal expansion of dental alloys and porcelains. J Biomed Mat Res 14:435, 1980.

Fasbinder DJ: Restorative material options for CAD/CAM restorations. Compendium 23:911, 2002.

Glendenning WE: Allergy to cobalt in metal denture as a cause of hand dermatitis. Contact Dermatitis 10:225, 1971.

Hawbolt EB, MacEntee MI, and Zahel JI: The tensile strength and appearance of solder joints in three base metal alloys made with high and low temperature solders. J Prosthet Dent 50:362, 1983.

Hinman RW, LyndeTA, Pelleu GB Jr, and Gaugler RW: Factors affecting airborne beryllium in dental spaces. J Prosthet Dent 33:210, 1975.

Hinman RW, Tesk JA, Whitlock RP, Parry EE, and Durkowski JS: A technique for characterizing coating behavior of dental alloys. J Dent Res 64(2):134, 1985.

Huget EF, and Cutright DE: Potential hazards in military dental practice. Military Med 143:718, 1978.

Jones DW: The strength and strengthening mechanisms of dental ceramics. In: McLean JW (ed): Dental Ceramics, Proceedings of the First International Symposium on Ceramics. Chicago, 1983, Quintessence Publishing Co, pp 83-141.

Kaylakie WG, and Brukl CE: Comparative tensile strengths of nonnoble dental alloy solders. J Prosthet Dent 53:455, 1985.

Tensile strengths are given and failure sites of a large number of base metal solders are described. In addition, various soldering technique variables were studied, and a radiographic method for evaluating soldered joints was described.

Kerber SJ, Barr TL, Mann GP, Brantley WA, Papazoglou E, and Mitchell JC: The complementary nature of x-ray photoelectron spectroscopy and angle-resolved x-ray diffraction. Part II. Analysis of oxides on dental alloys. J Mater Eng Perform 7:334, 1998.

Combined use of these two techniques revealed information about the oxide layers on high-palladium alloys that could not be obtained by conventional x-ray diffraction. The difference in growth mechanisms for the oxide layers may account for the differences found in porcelain adhesion.

Mackert JR Jr, Parry EE, Hashinger DT, and Fairhurst CW: Measurement of oxide adherence to dental alloys for porcelain. J Dent Res 63:1335, 1984.

Mackert JR Jr, Ringle RD, and Fairhurst CW: High-temperature behavior of a Pd-Ag alloy for porcelain. J Dent Res 52:1229, 1983.

The results of this study indicated that internal oxidation and the associated formation of nodules on the surface of a Pd-Ag alloy rather than external oxidation may occur in spite of the inclusion of oxidizable elements in the alloy.

McLaren EA, and Sorensen JA: High-strength alumina crowns and fixed partial dentures generated by copy-milling technology, Quint Dent Technol 18:31, 1995.

As an alternative to casting metal or sintering, hot-pressing, or CAM of ceramics, copy milling can be used as one of four alternative processing methods. This issue of Quint Dent Technol offers explanations of copy milling, sintered foil, and electro-forming methods. (See also references to articles by Shoher and Whiteman and by Traini.)

Metals Handbook, Desk Edition: Metals Park, OH, American Society for Metals, 1992.

An excellent reference book for metallurgical terms and the properties of pure metals and alloys.

Moffa JP, Guckes AD, Okawa MT, and Lilly GE: An evaluation of nonprecious alloys for use with porcelain veneers. Part II. Industrial safety and biocompatibility. J Prosthet Dent 30:432, 1973.

This article provides quantitative information about the levels of beryllium produced during the finishing and polishing of cast base metal dental alloys.

Moffa JP, and Jenkins WA: Status report on base-metal crown and bridge alloys, J Am Dent Assoc 89:652, 1974.

Moffa JP: Biological effects of nickel-containing dental alloys. Council on Dental Materials, Instruments, and Equipment, J Am Dent Assoc 104:50, 1982.

Moffa JP: Biocompatibility of nickel based dental alloys, CDAJ 12: 45, 1984.

Monday JL, and Asgar K: Tensile strength comparison of presoldered and postsoldered joints. J Prosthet Dent 55:23, 1986.

No significant differences in the tensile strength of presoldered and postsoldered joints were found when the same technique was used. Torch soldering yielded significantly stronger joints than the vacuum oven technique employed.

Morris HF, and Asgar K: Physical properties and microstructure of four new commercial partial denture alloys. J Prosthet Dent 33(1):36, 1975.

Morris HF: Properties of cobalt-chromium metal ceramic alloys after heat treatment. J Prosthet Dent 62:426, 1989.

Okabe T, Ohkubo C, Watanabe I, Okuno O, and Takada Y: The present status of dental titanium casting. J Metals 50(9):24, 1998.

This review article also provides important references for the historical development of casting titanium for dental applications.

Papazoglou E, Brantley WA, and Johnston WM: Evaluation of high-temperature distortion of high-palladium metal-ceramic crowns. J Prosthet Dent 85:133, 2001.

Experiments that simulated the steps in the preparation of single metal-ceramic crowns suggest that these alloys pose no clinically significant problems with dimensional changes, provided appropriate dental laboratory procedures are followed.

Papazoglou E, Brantley WA, Carr AB, and Johnston WM: Porcelain adherence to high-palladium alloys. J Prosthet Dent 70:386, 1993.

Papazoglou E, and Brantley WA: Porcelain adherence vs force to failure for palladium-gallium alloys: A critique of metal-ceramic bond testing. Dent Mater 14:112, 1998.

This and the previous article describe two currently used methods to evaluate the metal-ceramic bond. No correlation was found between these methods for a series of Pd-Ga-Ag alloys bonded to the same porcelain.

Papazoglou E, Brantley WA, Johnston WM, and Carr AB: Effects of dental laboratory processing variables and in vitro testing medium on the porcelain adherence of high-palladium casting alloys. J Prosthet Dent 79:514, 1998.

This article describes the effects of recasting old alloy, stripping and rebonding porcelain, an alternative oxidation cycle, and artificial saliva on the porcelain adherence to several palladium alloys.

Papazoglou E, Wu Q, Brantley WA, Mitchell JC, and Meyrick G: Comparison of mechanical properties for equiaxed fine-grained and dendritic high-palladium alloys. J Mater Sci: Mater Med 11:601, 2000.

This article provides a detailed explanation of the laboratory measurement of mechanical properties and discusses how simulated porcelain firing changes the properties of as-cast Pd-Cu-Ga and Pd-Ga-Ag alloys. SEM observations of fracture surfaces and microstructures are presented, and the role of casting porosity is reported.

Peltonen L: Nickel sensitivity in the general population. Contact Dermatitis 5:27, 1979.

Rasmussen EJ, Goodkind RJ, and Gerberich WW: An investigation of tensile strength of dental solder joints. J Prosthet Dent 41:418, 1979.

Higher strengths were reported for Type III gold alloy as gap distance was increased, but that trend was not noted for a gold-palladium alloy. These and other observations are partially explained in terms of the competing effects of yield strength, wettability, and voids at the various gap distances.

Reisbick MH, and Brantley WA: Mechanical property and microstructural variations for recast low-gold alloy. Int J Prosthodont 8:346, 1995.

Significant decreases in yield strength and percentage elongation were observed for recasting the alloy but not in tensile strength. The number of casting defects increased with the number of times the alloy was remelted.

Rogers OW: The gold solder–gold alloy interface. Aust Dent J 22:168, 1977.

A discrete study of the diffusion mechanics at the grain boundaries of the substrate gold alloy and gold alloy soldering filler.

Shillingburg HT, Hobo S, and Fisher DW: Preparation, design and margin distortion in porcelain-fused-to-metal restorations. J Prosthet Dent, 29:276, 1973.

The results of this study suggested that thermal incompatibility stresses were likely to cause margin distortion in metal-ceramic crowns. However, subsequent studies support other potential mechanisms, including the effect of excessive sandblasting time and/or pressure.

Shoher I, and Whiteman A: Captek: A new capillary casting technology for ceramometal restorations, Quint Dent Technol 18:9, 1995.

Togaya T, Suzuki M, Tsutsumi S, and Ida K: An application of pure titanium to the metal porcelain system, Dent Mater J 2:210, 1983.

This paper highlights the potential of porcelain bonding to CP Ti and the importance of matched expansion coefficients of metal and porcelain on the bond strength of the bonded metal-ceramic specimens.

Traini T: Electroforming technology for ceramometal restorations, Quint Dent Technol 18:21, 1995.

Tuccillo J, and Cascone P: Private communication, 2003.

Vreeburg KJ, de Groot K, von Blomberg M, and Scheper RJ: Induction of immunological tolerance by oral administration of nickel and chromium. J Dent Res 63:124, 1984.

This highly important article describes the effects of oral administration of nickel and chromium to guinea pigs.

Weiss PA, and Munyon RE: Repairs, corrections, and additions to ceramo-metal frameworks. II. Quint Dent Technol 7:45, 1980.

Cast-joining is proposed as an alternative to soldering of cast metal components of a fixed partial denture.

Wu Q, Brantley WA, Mitchell JC, Vermilyea SG, Xiao J, and Guo W: Heat-treatment behavior of high-palladium dental alloys. Cells Mater 7:161, 1997.

A Pd-Cu-Ga alloy with much lower Vickers hardness is described, along with the complex metallurgical behavior of several alloys during heat treatments at temperatures within the range for porcelain firing cycles.

20

Wrought Alloys

William A. Brantley

KEY TERMS

Annealing—Controlled heating and cooling process designed to produce desired properties in a metal. The annealing process usually is intended to soften metals, to increase their plastic deformation potential, to stabilize shape, and to increase machinability (see *stress relief*).

Brittle fracture—Rupture of a solid structure with little or no fractographic evidence of plastic deformation.

Dislocation—Imperfection in the crystalline arrangement of atoms consisting of either an extra partial plane of atoms (edge dislocation), a spiral distortion of normally parallel atom planes (screw dislocation), or a combination of the two types.

Ductile fracture—Rupture of a solid structure that results in measurable plastic deformation.

Grain growth—Increase in the mean crystal size of a polycrystalline metal produced by a heat-treatment process.

Grain refinement—Process of reducing the crystal (grain) size in a solid metal by adding an element or compound to the molten metal and cooling at a prescribed rate.

Interstitial atom—Imperfection in a crystal lattice consisting of an extra atom located between the adjacent atoms in normal lattice sites.

Point defect—Lattice imperfection of atomic size in three dimensions, such as a vacancy, divacancy, trivacancy, or interstitial atom.

Precipitation hardening—Process of strengthening and hardening a metal by precipitating a phase or constituent from a saturated solid solution.

Recovery—Stage of heat treatment that results in the partial or total regaining of properties of a metal that were altered by work hardening (cold working), without a change in the grain structure.

Recrystallization—Process of forming new stress-free crystals in a work-hardened metal through a controlled heat-treatment process.

KEY TERMS—cont'd

Recrystallization temperature—Lowest temperature at which total recrystallization of a work-hardened structure occurs within a specific period (usually 1 hr).

Springback—Amount of elastic strain that a metal can recover when loaded to and unloaded from its yield strength (important for orthodontic wires).

Strain hardening—Increase in strength and hardness and decrease in ductility of a metal that is caused by plastic deformation below the recrystallization temperature; also called *work hardening*.

Stress relief—Reduction or elimination of residual stresses by heat treatment.

Superelasticity—Ability of certain nickel-titanium alloys to undergo extensive deformation resulting from a stress-assisted phase transformation, with the reverse transformation occurring on unloading; called *pseudoelasticity* in engineering materials science.

Vacancy—Imperfection in a crystal lattice consisting of an unoccupied atom site.

Working range—Maximum amount of elastic strain that an orthodontic wire can sustain before it plastically deforms.

Wrought metal—Cold-worked metal that has been plastically deformed to alter the shape of the structure and certain mechanical properties (strength, hardness, and ductility).

DEFORMATION OF METALS
Introduction to Wrought Alloys and Orthodontic Wires

Wrought base metal alloys are used for orthodontic wires, clasps for removable partial dentures, root canal files and reamers, crowns in pediatric dentistry, and surgical instruments. The metallurgy of these alloys is relatively complex. The primary alloy used for orthodontic wire is stainless steel, and a variety of endodontic instruments are fabricated from this alloy. Stainless steel crowns are used in pediatric dentistry, and stainless steel cutting instruments are important for oral surgery. Other major wrought alloys used for orthodontic, removable partial denture, and endodontic applications include cobalt-chromium-nickel, nickel-titanium, and beta-titanium. There is also limited use of wrought noble metal alloys for dental applications, and wrought commercially pure (CP) titanium is used for some dental implants. Before considering each of these systems in detail, a brief discussion of the manufacture of wires and their use in orthodontics illustrates many of the concepts involved for wrought alloys.

Wires are used by orthodontists for correcting displacements of teeth from proper occlusion, as well as by prosthodontists and general practitioners for retention and stabilization of removable partial dentures. A round wire is made by drawing a cast alloy through a series of dies, with intermediate heat treatments to eliminate effects of severe work hardening (discussed later) between drawing steps. Orthodontic wires with rectangular or square cross-sections are fabricated by rolling round wires, using a Turk's head apparatus that consists of pairs of rollers. Many accessory dental materials and instruments are fabricated from cast alloys that have been rolled to form sheet or rod, drawn into wire or tubing, or forged (plastically deformed by a die under compressive force, usually at an elevated temperature) into a finished shape. Of the many metallic articles encountered in everyday life, most are **wrought metal** and not castings. (In this chapter, the terms *metal* and *alloy* are frequently used interchangeably. When the discussion specifically refers to pure metals, this distinction is noted.)

Whenever a casting is permanently deformed in any manner, it is considered a wrought metal. A wrought alloy exhibits properties and a microstructure that are not associated with the same alloy when cast. For example, the differences are so marked that dentists should assess benefits and limitations of cast and wrought clasps for removable partial dentures before proceeding with their selection and use. It is highly important to be knowledgeable about the effects on properties of cast alloy prostheses when adjustments are made by plastic deformation.

Orthodontic wires are formed into various configurations or appliances to apply forces to teeth and move them into a more desirable alignment. The force system that develops is determined by the appliance design and wire alloy composition. For a given design and elastic deflection of the wire, the force applied to the tooth is proportional to the elastic modulus (E) of the wire. Low, constant forces are biologically desirable, although a threshold force level is necessary for tooth movement. Large elastic deflections are clinically desirable for orthodontic wires, and the maximum elastic deflection is called the **working range.** From Chapter 4, it follows that the maximum elastic deflection for tensile loading is given by the quotient of the proportional limit (PL) and E. (Because the bending deformation used by orthodontists involves tensile and compressive strains parallel to the wire axis, these concepts for tensile loading are applicable.) Clinicians usually activate orthodontic wires (other than the nickel-titanium wires to be discussed later) somewhat into the permanent deformation range. Consequently, the practical working range is considered to be the elastic strain at the yield strength (YS) of the wire, namely the quotient of YS and E. This important property (YS/E) is termed **springback.**

Other properties of orthodontic wires are also clinically important. A ductile wire can be formed into various shapes, although there are applications that do not require permanent bends. Ease of joining is important, and most wires can be either brazed (soldered) or welded together. Orthodontic alloys must also have excellent corrosion resistance in the oral environment, which is highly important for biocompatibility as well as for appliance durability. Finally, the cost of the wires is a significant factor for the orthodontic office. Although the nickel-titanium and beta-titanium wires are much more expensive than the stainless steel and cobalt-chromium-nickel wires, the two titanium-containing wires have unique properties that account for their widespread clinical selection, as is discussed later in this chapter.

In Chapter 4 on mechanical properties, the principles of elastic and plastic deformation were described. For example, when an applied tensile force is small so that stress is below the proportional limit, the separation between metal atoms is increased a very small amount from the equilibrium interatomic spacing in the crystal structure. When this force is removed, the interatomic separation returns to the equilibrium value. However, once the PL is exceeded during the application of a sufficiently strong force, permanent deformation begins for most metals, characterized by irreversible changes in the structure on the atomic scale. (Alloys with a substantial amount of eutectic microstructural constituent, as well as dental amalgams, undergo **brittle fracture,** rather than significant permanent deformation, as noted in Chapters 6 and 17.) Only the elastic strain that also takes place when a metal is loaded beyond the PL can be recovered. As the induced stress continues to increase beyond the PL, the interatomic separation continues to increase, and eventually fracture of the metal occurs. A detailed description of the fracture processes at the atomic level is complex and beyond the scope of this book.

CRITICAL QUESTION

Why does the inherent ductility of a particular pure metal depend on its crystal structure?

Theoretical and Actual Shear Strengths of Metals

An atomic model illustrating permanent deformation of a perfect metal subjected to an applied shear stress is illustrated in Figure 20-1. Notice that the deformation or slip process requires the simultaneous displacement of the entire plane of *A* atoms relative to the plane of *B* atoms. If the elastic modulus in shear for a given metal is known, this model can be used to calculate the maximum theoretical shear strength. However, Table 20-1 shows that such theoretical shear strengths (applicable to perfect single crystals) for copper and iron are approximately 40 times higher than the values measured for the bulk polycrystalline metals. For BeO and SiC, which are ceramic materials in which the interatomic bonding is a combination of covalent and ionic mechanisms, Table 20-1 shows that the calculated theoretical shear strengths are approximately 80 and 190 times the values obtained for polycrystalline materials. Values of shear strength approaching the theoretical values are found only when measurements are made on whisker specimens, which are very thin single crystals of pure materials having high perfection.

The key difference between whiskers and bulk polycrystalline specimens of the same material is the presence of *structural imperfections* at the atomic level in the bulk material. Single-crystal filaments, approximately 2.5 mm in diameter, have been

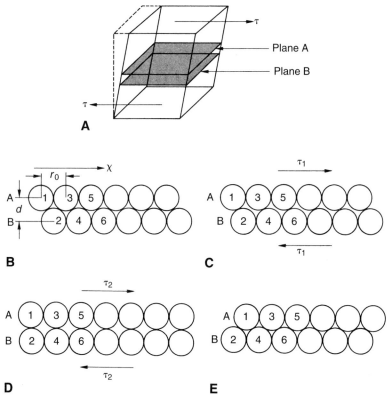

Fig. 20-1   Slip between adjacent planes of atoms. **A,** A solid subjected to a shear stress. Planes *A* and *B* are adjacent. **B,** The configuration of planes *A* and *B* when the solid is not stressed. **C,** Application of a shear stress τ_1 causes plane *A* to move with respect to plane *B*. **D,** Increasing the shear stress to τ_2 increases the relative lateral displacement of the two planes. This configuration corresponds to the state of maximum stored elastic energy. **E,** The two planes have been displaced by one interatomic distance r_o, shown in **B,** with respect to each other. This configuration will be maintained if the load is removed. If the shear stress (τ_2) remains, the planes will continue to slip past each other. (From Eisenstadt MM: *Introduction to Mechanical Properties of Materials,* New York, Macmillan Publishing Company, 1971.)

Table 20-1	Theoretical and Observed Shear Strength			
Material	Shear modulus (GPa)	Observed ultimate shear strength (Polycrystalline) (MPa)	Calculated ultimate shear strength (GPa)	Observed ultimate shear strength (Whisker)* (GPa)
Copper	48	220	7.7	2.1
Iron	80	290	12.4	9.5
Nickel	76	480	—	2.7
Al_2O_3	170	—	12.1	14.6
BeO	140	280 (Tension)	21.7	9.2
SiC	200	170 (Tension)	32.3	14.6

(From: Eisenstadt M: Introduction to Mechanical Properties of Materials, Upper Saddle River, NJ, Prentice-Hall, Inc, 1971.)
*The shape of the whiskers is not conducive to shear testing. The tabulated values were calculated from tensile strength data given by Broutman IJ, and Krock RH: Modern Composite Materials, Reading, MA, Addison-Wesley, 1967.

used as reinforcing agents in commercial composite materials, and their use has been investigated for other dental applications.

Point Defects

It was previously noted in Chapter 5 that crystallization from starting nuclei during solidification of a metal does not occur in a regular fashion, that is, atomic plane by atomic plane. Instead, growth is likely to be more random, with some positions in the crystal structure left vacant and other positions in which atoms are located interstitially between neighboring atoms in normal lattice positions.

Point defects in the crystal structure have all three dimensions of atomic size; three types of these defects are diagrammed in Figure 20-2. A **vacancy** or vacant atom site in a crystalline lattice may occur at a single site in the atomic arrangement, as shown in Figure 20-2, *A*, and two vacancies may condense as a *divacancy*, as shown in Figure 20-2, *B*; *trivacancies* may also exist. An interstitial atom is illustrated in Figure 20-2, *C*. Vacancies and other point defects are equilibrium defects, and a crystalline material that is in equilibrium contains a certain number of these defects at a given temperature. Although there is a local increase in internal energy around the site of a given type of point defect, there is also a compensating entropy contribution from these point defects. The equilibrium concentration of each type of

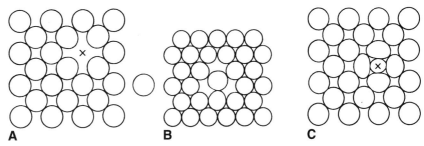

Fig. 20-2 Point defects. **A,** Vacancy. **B,** Divacancy (two missing atoms). **C,** Interstitial (extra atom). (From Van Vlack LH: Elements of Materials Science, ed 4. Reading, MA, Addison-Wesley Publishing Co, 1980.)

point defect increases exponentially with temperature. The most important point defects are vacancies, which provide the principal mechanism for atomic diffusion in crystalline materials.

Dislocations

The chief difference in mechanical properties between a perfect single crystal and a polycrystalline metal is associated with the presence of **dislocations** in the latter. These line defects have two dimensions at the atomic level, but the third dimension is at a more macroscopic level.

The simplest type of dislocation, known as an edge dislocation, is illustrated diagrammatically in Figure 20-3, *A*, for a simple cubic structure. Note that the atomic arrangement is regular except for the one vertical plane of atoms that is discontinuous. The edge dislocation (represented by ⊥) is located at the edge of the half plane. The formation of dislocations creates localized strain at the atomic level in the metal structure and requires significant internal energy, which is not compensated by their

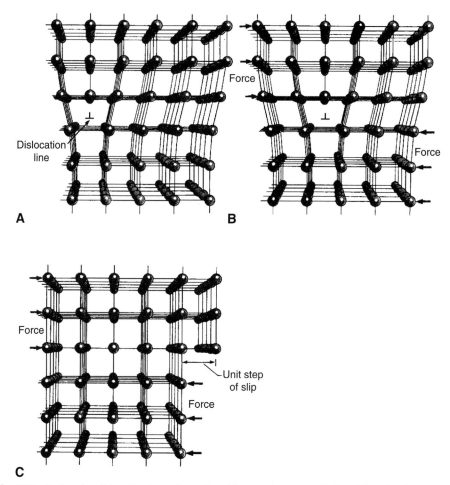

Fig. 20-3   A, An edge dislocation in a schematic cubic crystal structure. **B,** The dislocation has moved one interatomic distance along the slip plane under the action of the shearing force indicated by the arrows. **C,** The dislocation has reached the edge of the crystal, and a unit amount of slip has been produced. (From Guy AG: Elements of Physical Metallurgy, ed 2. Reading, MA, Addison-Wesley Publishing Co, 1959.)

entropy contributions. Hence dislocations are not equilibrium crystal defects, in contrast to point defects, and a metal attempts to rid itself of dislocations when heated to elevated temperatures.

If a sufficiently large shear stress is applied across the top and bottom faces of the metal crystal in Figure 20-3, *A*, the bonds in the row of atoms adjacent to the dislocation are broken and new bonds with the next row are established, resulting in movement of the dislocation by one interatomic distance, as indicated in Figure 20-3, *B*. Continued application of this shear stress causes similar movements of one interatomic distance until the dislocation reaches the boundary of the crystal. The plane along which an edge dislocation moves is known as a *slip plane*. As Figure 20-3, *C*, illustrates, the result of this dislocation movement across the crystal is that the atomic planes on one side of the slip plane have been displaced one interatomic spacing (one unit of slip) with respect to the atomic planes on the other side of the slip plane. The crystallographic direction in which the atomic planes have experienced this displacement is termed the *slip direction,* and the combination of a slip plane and a slip direction is termed a *slip system.*

The dominant slip planes for edge dislocations in metals are characteristic for each crystal structure and are the most densely packed atomic planes, which have the largest interplanar separation. Note that the inherent ability of a metal to deform permanently generally depends on the number of slip systems associated with the crystal structure. For example, the face-centered cubic (fcc) structure has the largest number of slip systems, and metals with this crystal structure, such as copper, gold, nickel, palladium, platinum, and silver, are highly ductile. The hexagonal close-packed (hcp) structure has relatively few slip systems, and zinc, which has this crystal structure, is relatively brittle. The body-centered cubic (bcc) structure has a potentially large number of slip systems, but fewer than the number for the fcc structure, and metals with this crystal structure have intermediate levels of ductility.

Vast numbers of dislocations must move across slip planes to achieve practical levels of permanent strain in metals, often in excess of 10%. Moreover, the application of sufficiently high tensile or compressive stress also causes movement of dislocations because a shear stress component acts on slip planes.

When Figure 20-3 is compared with Figure 20-1, it is evident that much less shear stress is required for permanent deformation of the metal crystal containing the edge dislocation because only one row of atomic bonds is broken at a time, compared with the perfect crystal in which all rows of bonds across two atomic planes must be simultaneously broken for the shear deformation to occur. This accounts for the difference in Table 20-1 between the values of theoretical shear strength for a dislocation-free metal whisker and a polycrystalline metal containing dislocations. The PL for a metal generally corresponds to the onset of significant movement of dislocations, which provides the mechanism for permanent deformation.

In addition to edge dislocations, there are other types of dislocations of more complex geometry, and their movement along slip planes in response to sufficiently high stress yields permanent deformation in a manner analogous to that in Figure 20-3. Evidence of slip can be viewed in the optical microscope for metals that have been polished and etched, and then permanently deformed. The slip lines in Figure 20-4 correspond to slip planes in which large numbers of dislocations exited the metal, causing surface offsets that scattered the light used for observation.

It should be evident from Figure 20-3 that dislocations can exist only in materials that have a crystalline structure, that is, an atomic arrangement that has long-range periodicity in three dimensions. Dislocations cannot exist in materials with noncrystalline structures, such as dental ceramic and polymeric materials. Other mechanisms applicable to polymers are required for the permanent deformation of

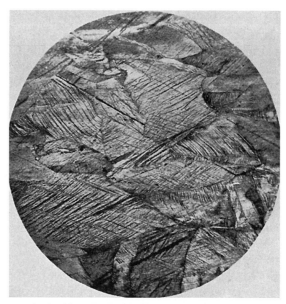

Fig. 20-4 Photomicrograph of cold-worked gold, showing deformed grains and slip lines at surface offsets where dislocations have exited their slip planes. (×100.) (Courtesy of S.D. Tylman.)

elastomeric impression materials and some glass-ionomer cements. The absence of dislocation movement accounts for the brittle character of dental porcelains, composite resins, and most dental cements, as well as dental amalgams.

CRITICAL QUESTION

What fundamental strengthening mechanisms available for alloys are not possible for pure metals?

Strengthening Mechanisms Involving Dislocations

From Figure 20-3, one can deduce that there is little hindrance to the movement of an edge dislocation along its slip plane in the absence of other defects in the atomic arrangement or obstacles such as precipitates. In reality, this is largely true, although there is a relatively small inherent barrier to dislocation movement (called the *Peierls stress*) imposed by the bonds associated with the arrangement of atoms in a given crystal structure.

However, the movement of dislocations in response to sufficiently high stress can be impeded in several major ways, which provide methods for strengthening metals and alloys:

1. The atomic arrangement in the vicinity of foreign atoms (a solid solution) is locally distorted, whether the solute atom is larger or smaller than the atoms of the solvent metal, as noted in Chapter 6. Although the detailed mechanisms for solid solution strengthening are rather complex, the reader will intuitively appreciate that the movement of dislocations along slip planes will be impeded by the presence of such solute atoms. This is the basis for solid solution strengthening of alloys.

2. Grain boundaries block the movement of dislocations because, as noted in Chapter 5, a given slip plane is discontinuous at a grain boundary. Thus

dislocations pile up at grain boundaries, eventually creating a substantial local stress that causes dislocation movement in adjacent grains and continuing the process of permanent deformation. It follows that the PL and YS for a metal is increased as a result of a decrease in grain size because there is more grain boundary area per unit volume to impede dislocation motion. This is the mechanism for **grain refinement** strengthening and is applicable to both pure metals and alloys. In Chapter 5, it is noted that the yield strength of a metal varies inversely with the square root of grain size (Hall-Petch equation).

3. Precipitates also impede movement of dislocations, resulting in **precipitation hardening** of alloys, but the mechanisms are also complex.

   a. Very small (submicroscopic) precipitates can be coherent. The atomic bonds are continuous across the interface with the solid solution matrix; such precipitates provide highly effective strengthening because of the localized distortion in the atomic arrangement. Because the precipitate and matrix have the same crystal structure, dislocations can move through and shear coherent precipitates.

   b. Large precipitates, notably those with a crystal structure different from that of the solid solution matrix, are incoherent, in which interatomic bonds are not continuous across the interface. (The intermediate case of semicoherent precipitates exists, in which some interatomic bonds are continuous across the interface.) Analogous to the situation with grain boundaries, dislocations cannot move through incoherent precipitates, but instead form dislocation loops of increasing size around these particles. The mechanism of order hardening, discussed in Chapter 6, can be considered as similar to the standard precipitation hardening for alloys. However, dislocation movement through an ordered region is much more complex than through a disordered substitutional solid solution, and the reader should consult the appropriate references at the end of Chapter 6 for details.

4. Substantial permanent deformation by cold working creates vast numbers of dislocations within metals at sources whose nature is beyond the scope of this book. (*Cold working* is defined as mechanical deformation below the **recrystallization temperature,** discussed later, in contrast to the forging operations that are performed industrially at elevated temperatures to create metal items of the desired shapes.) These dislocations interact with each other, mutually impeding their movements. The increased stress required for further dislocation movement to achieve continued permanent deformation provides the basis for work hardening or **strain hardening** of the metal.

In addition, substantial permanent deformation creates vast numbers of point defects, which has important consequences when a cold-worked metal is subjected to heat treatment, as discussed later. Cold working can significantly alter the shapes of grains and, in the limit of a wire, the grains are severely elongated parallel to the wire axis. When a polished and etched wrought alloy is viewed in the optical microscope it resembles closely spaced strands of spaghetti.

Practical examples of cold work and strain hardening at room temperature are very familiar. For example, when a wire is bent back and forth beyond the proportional limit, eventually fracture occurs after extensive permanent deformation. A second example is the flattening of a nail with a hammer: the first few blows are quite effective but later blows are much less effective, until finally no further deformation takes place and the nail cracks or fractures. The same phenomenon can occur when a patient bends a clasp back and forth several times to relieve discomfort caused by a removable partial denture and fracture of the clasp occurs.

From the preceding relationship between impeding the movement of dislocations and the strengthening of metals, it follows that the hardness, strength, and proportional limit are increased with strain hardening and the other strengthening mechanisms just described, whereas the ductility is decreased. The corrosion resistance is also decreased for a permanently deformed metal because the dislocations produce localized regions of strain at the atomic level, which have higher energy than atomic arrangements in the undeformed metal. In general, the elastic modulus of a metallic material remains largely unchanged as a result of cold working; an exception is stainless steel orthodontic wire, which is discussed later in this chapter.

The changes in mechanical properties of a metal that can be produced by strain hardening often serve as the basis of a practical method in dentistry to achieve the desired levels of these properties. For example, in Chapter 18 it is noted that strain hardening during condensation of direct filling gold is necessary to provide proper strength and hardness for the restoration. Likewise, stainless steel wires used in dentistry are very dependent on their wrought metal characteristics to produce a suitable level of yield strength for clinical applications.

It is instructive to examine the effects of severe cold working on the grain structure of an important practical copper-zinc alloy (brass). This is shown in the first row of photomicrographs (longitudinal sections) at the top of Figure 20-5, in which rolling of the metal took place in the plane perpendicular to the plane of these photomicrographs. It can be observed that the thinner the specimen, as designated above each photomicrograph, the flatter or thinner each grain appears to be. Although brass was used in this example, the same effect appears in wrought gold alloys. For the extreme example of a wire, the grains are elongated parallel to the wire axis and resemble strands of spaghetti in a photomicrograph showing a longitudinal section.

An interesting effect of cold working or strain hardening of metals is the tendency for preferred (crystallographic) orientation in the distorted grain structure, which results in anisotropic (direction-dependent) mechanical properties. The slip planes tend to become aligned with the shear planes of the deformation process. For example, the strength of a rolled sheet of metal is usually greater in the transverse direction than in the direction of rolling. The mechanical properties of an orthodontic wire are also different if measured parallel and perpendicular to the wire axis.

Twinning

An alternative mode of permanent deformation in metals is *twinning*, in which there are small atomic movements on either side of a twinning plane that result in the atoms having a mirror relationship, as shown in Figure 20-6. In metals that have relatively few slip systems, twinning is favored over dislocation movement; this mechanism is also favored at high strain rates and at low temperatures. Twinning has significance for deformation of α-titanium alloys, which are highly important for some dental implants and also of interest for cast restorations. In α-titanium the (c/a) ratio involving the lattice parameter (a) in the basal plane and the lattice parameter (c) in the perpendicular direction to the basal plane (see Figure 2-14) is slightly less than the ideal value of 1.633 for the hcp structure. This deviation results in additional slip planes and the tendency to readily undergo twinning. Twinning is also the mechanism for reversible transformation between the austenitic and martensitic structures in nickel-titanium orthodontic wires, which has considerable clinical significance.

Original annealed metal thickness	Cold rolled to thickness				
0.110" No. 9 B. & S. GA.	0.100" No. 10 B. & S. GA.	0.090" No. 11 B. & S. GA.	0.080" No. 12 B. & S. GA.	0.070" No. 13 B. & S. GA.	0.060" No. 14 B. & S. GA.

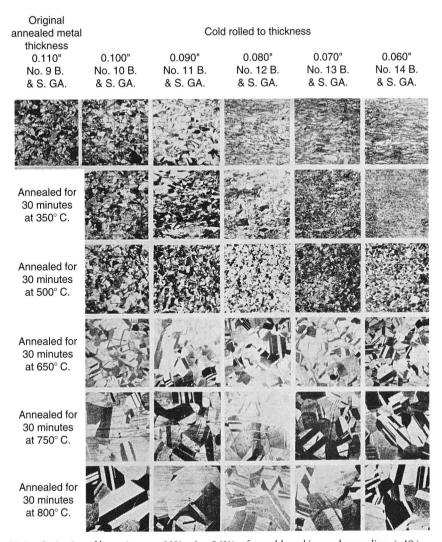

Annealed for 30 minutes at 350° C.

Annealed for 30 minutes at 500° C.

Annealed for 30 minutes at 650° C.

Annealed for 30 minutes at 750° C.

Annealed for 30 minutes at 800° C.

Fig. 20-5 Grain size of brass (copper 66%, zinc 34%), after cold working and annealing. (×40.) (Prepared by L.H. DeWald.)

Fracture

If cold work is continued, a heavily deformed metal eventually fractures. However, as previously noted, the stress required for fracture is much less in the polycrystalline metal than is expected theoretically. The microcracks that act as sites of fracture initiation can arise from multiple causes, including an accumulation of dislocations or strain incompatibility at boundaries between two different microstructural phases.

Alloys undergo brittle fracture or **ductile fracture,** depending on a variety of factors, such as composition, microstructure, temperature, and strain rate. For example, the alloy may contain multiple phases or phases with certain crystal structures, which greatly limit the movement of dislocations. At low temperatures and high strain rates (rates of loading) there may be less dislocation movement to relieve localized stress concentrations associated with microcracks. This mechanism also results in an increase in the observed tensile strength of the metal.

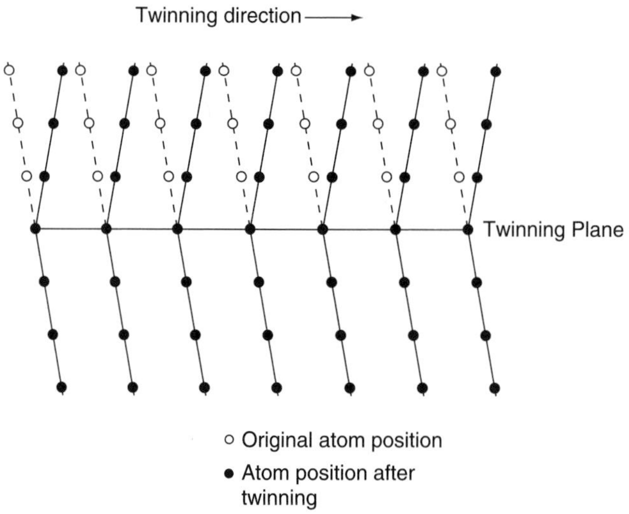

Twinning direction ⟶

Twinning Plane

○ Original atom position
● Atom position after twinning

Fig. 20-6 Schematic illustration of twinning in a metal. The atoms on either side of the twinning plane have a mirror relationship.

In Chapter 5 an example of a brittle fracture surface was shown for a cast base metal for removable partial denture frameworks, which was associated with its dendritic microstructure. Figure 20-7 illustrates the appearance of a brittle fracture surface for a carbon steel rotary endodontic instrument subjected to torsional loading. In contrast, Figure 20-8 presents a ductile fracture surface for a gold casting alloy specimen that had been loaded to failure in tension. The ductile fracture surfaces of metals are characterized by a dimpled rupture morphology, in which failure has occurred because of the coalescence of microvoids that typically form at impurity particles during the later stages of permanent deformation. The dimpled rupture pattern maps the local stress field, and has characteristic appearances for bending and torsional fracture surfaces of rotary endodontic instruments fabricated from stainless steel.

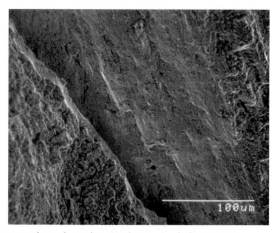

Fig. 20-7 Brittle fracture surface of a carbon steel rotary endodontic instrument subjected to counterclockwise torsional loading. (×500.) (From Luebke NH, Brantley WA, Sabri ZI, and Luebke JH: Physical dimensions, torsional performance, and metallurgical properties of rotary endodontic instruments. III. Peeso drills. J Endod 18:13, 1992.)

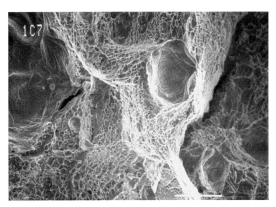

Fig. 20-8 Ductile fracture surface of a cast gold alloy specimen that was loaded to failure in tension, illustrating the appearance of dimpled rupture. The overall topography of the fracture surface indicates the grain size of the alloy, and casting porosity can also be seen. (×2000, with scale bar length of 10 µm.) (From Reisbick MH, and Brantley WA: Mechanical property and microstructural variations for recast low-gold alloy. Int J Prosthodont 8:346, 1995.)

Careful observation of photomicrographs of fracture surfaces often indicates whether the fracture was *transgranular,* in which crack propagation was across the grains, or *intergranular,* in which crack propagation occurred predominantly at the grain boundaries. The dominant fracture mode depends on factors such as the inherent ductility of the matrix phase of the alloy, the presence of secondary phases, the rate of loading, and the temperature. The secondary phases may be relatively weak or brittle, and the location of such phases within the grains or at the grain boundaries are also important factors. When a ductile alloy is loaded to failure in tension, there is substantial necking down (narrowing of the specimin diameter) before fracture, which does not occur for a brittle alloy.

CRITICAL QUESTION

Why must recrystallization be avoided when orthodontic wires are given a **stress-relief** *heat treatment after manipulation to minimize fracture during placement?*

EFFECTS OF ANNEALING COLD-WORKED METAL

The effects associated with cold working—for example, strain hardening, decreased ductility, and distorted grains—can be reversed simply by heating the metal to an appropriate elevated temperature. This process is called **annealing.** The more severe the degree of cold working, the more rapidly the effects can be reversed by annealing.

Annealing can take place in three successive stages: **recovery, recrystallization,** and **grain growth.** The effects of each of these stages on the tensile strength and ductility of a metal are shown in Figure 20-9. The microstructural changes that accompany annealing were previously shown in Figure 20-5. The benefits of annealing depend on the melting range of the alloy and the annealing temperature that is used. Annealing is a relative process; the higher the melting point of the metal, the higher is the temperature needed for annealing. A rule of thumb is to use a temperature that is approximately half the melting point of a pure metal or the fusion temperature of an alloy on the absolute temperature scale (° K).

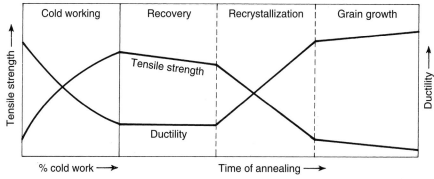

Fig. 20-9   Tensile strength and ductility of a metal as a function of the percentage of cold work and annealing time. Tensile strength increases, and ductility decreases during cold working. These properties change only slightly during recovery. During recrystallization, tensile strength decreases and ductility increases rapidly. Only slight changes occur during grain growth. (From Richman MH: Introduction to the Science of Metals. Waltham, MA, Blaisdell Publishing Co, 1967.)

Recovery

In the recovery stage the properties of the cold-worked metal begin to disappear before any significant changes are observed under microscopic examination. As can be seen in Figure 20-9, there is a very slight decrease in tensile strength and no change in ductility during recovery. Although not shown, there is a rather pronounced decrease in electrical resistivity during recovery, and there is a decrease in dislocation density with rearrangement of the dislocations into lower-energy configurations. Also, a cold-worked metal contains residual stresses, and relaxation of these stresses during machining frequently results in warping of a cold-worked metal; this tendency for warping during machining disappears if the residual stresses are eliminated by heat treatment in the temperature range in which recovery occurs.

Orthodontic appliances fabricated by bending wires are often subjected to a stress-relief anneal before their placement. This heat treatment stabilizes the configuration of an appliance and allows an accurate determination of the force that an appliance will be able to deliver in the mouth. Elimination of residual stresses in an appliance also reduces the likelihood of fracture during clinical adjustments. It is essential that this heat treatment be performed in the recovery temperature range and not at higher temperatures, at which recrystallization occurs.

Recrystallization

When a severely cold-worked metal is annealed, recrystallization occurs after the recovery stage. This involves a radical change in the microstructure, as seen in Figure 20-5. The old, deformed grains disappear completely and are replaced by new strain-free grains. These new grains nucleate in the most severely cold-worked regions in the metal, and their grain boundary migration consumes the original cold-worked structure. After completion of recrystallization, the metal essentially attains its original soft and ductile condition (see Fig. 20-9). It can now be appreciated why recrystallization must be avoided during the stress-relief heat treatment of orthodontic appliances. The wrought microstructure that provides the desirable levels of mechanical properties is replaced by a microstructure containing equiaxed grains, and the alloy is relatively soft and has greatly decreased resilience. If a metal is not sufficiently coldworked, recrystallization does not occur during annealing. An excellent example that has been reported for this level of cold work is the typical clinical adjustment of a removable partial denture clasp.

Grain Growth

The average grain size of the recrystallized structure depends on the initial number of nuclei. The more severe the cold working, the greater the number of such nuclei, and the grain size for the recrystallized metal can range from fine to fairly coarse.

If the recrystallized metal is further annealed, grain growth, illustrated in Figure 20-5, occurs in such a way to minimize the grain boundary area (energy), with large grains consuming small grains. Grain growth does not proceed indefinitely to yield a single crystal, but rather ceases after a coarse grain structure is produced. Although prolonged annealing of a wrought alloy produces coarse grains, it was noted in Chapter 6 that the grain size of a cast alloy, which is determined by the casting temperature of the alloy and the mold temperature, is not affected by prolonged annealing near the solidus temperature (homogenization heat treatment). This is because the impurity atoms or secondary phases that are found at the grain boundaries or dendrites of cast alloys after solidification (Chapter 5) immobilize the grain boundaries and prevent their migration during annealing.

Previously, it was noted that the dislocation mechanism for permanent deformation provides the explanation for the increases in strength and hardness of an alloy and the decrease in ductility as the grain size becomes smaller. In contrast, with a sufficiently large grain size, particularly in a dental appliance with a small thickness, a large grain may have an orientation in which the resolved shear stress results in a low proportional limit and substantial local permanent deformation. Figure 20-10 shows that the catastrophic fracture of a cast 9.5-mm–diameter gold alloy rod occurred in one grain that occupied the entire cross-section.

Cast Structure Versus Wrought Structure

Generally, all metals and alloys are produced from castings. Castings can be machined, forged, drawn, extruded, or mechanically worked in some manner to provide the required article or appliance, thereby becoming a wrought metal. Most dental restorations and prostheses are cast and not wrought, and thus the factors that affect the grain size of the casting (alloy composition, presence and concentration of grain-refining elements, and difference between casting and mold

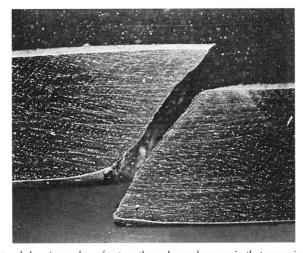

Fig. 20-10 A cast rod showing a shear fracture through one large grain that occupied the entire cross-sectional area of the rod. Although ductility was high, fracture occurred because of a high stress concentration. (×24.)

temperatures) are very important. However, if the dentist bends a cast removable partial denture clasp arm or burnishes a cast crown margin during adjustment, the structure may be cold worked sufficiently to convert the as-cast microstructure to a microstructure partially having the properties of a wrought metal.

In dental applications in which certain wrought alloys are used (e.g., orthodontic bands and wires, appliances in pediatric dentistry, and removable partial denture clasp arms), the strength and fracture resistance of the wrought alloy is significantly reduced by annealing in the temperature range at which recrystallization occurs. Prolonged heating of stainless steel to high temperatures can markedly reduce its corrosion resistance, and this concern is an important consideration during soldering operations for stainless steel orthodontic appliances. Also, before heating any instrument such as a rubber dam clamp (retainer) or a metal matrix band, the dentist should consider the possibility that it might be ruined by grain growth or by other microstructural changes.

CRITICAL QUESTION

What are the differences in the martensitic structures that form in plain carbon steels and austenitic stainless steels?

CARBON STEELS

As has been pointed out, stainless steels are the major alloys used in orthodontics, and these alloys have many other applications in dentistry. The metallurgy and terminology of stainless steels are intimately connected to the simpler binary iron-carbon system and to carbon steels. Therefore a brief outline of the iron-carbon system and carbon steels is presented. Currently, these extremely important industrial alloys have relatively limited use in dentistry. However, stainless steels have demonstrated superior performance for curettes and endodontic instruments compared with carbon steel instruments.

Plain carbon steels are iron-carbon binary alloys that contain less than approximately 2.1% carbon. (All alloy compositions in this chapter are expressed in weight percentage.) The starting point for understanding their metallurgy is the Fe-Fe_3C phase diagram, and the interested reader should consult the textbook by Brick, Pense, and Gordon listed in the Selected Readings section. The major classes of carbon steels are based on three possible crystal structures that can occur for the iron-carbon alloys. *Ferrite* is a bcc phase, stable to temperatures not exceeding 912° C and containing carbon atoms in interstitial sites between the iron atoms. *Austenite* is an fcc phase, stable between 912° C and 1394° C, in which carbon atoms are also located interstitially between the iron atoms. The carbon atoms are larger than the interstitial sites in the bcc and fcc structures of pure iron, so substantial local distortion exists in either atomic arrangement of iron near a carbon atom. The greater size of the interstitial sites in austenite accounts for the considerable difference in maximum solid solubility of carbon, approximately 0.02% in ferrite and 2.1% in austenite. All plain carbon steels have the single-phase austenitic structure at an elevated temperature; iron-carbon alloys that contain higher percentages (up to approximately 4%) of carbon are cast irons.

When a plain carbon steel containing 0.8% carbon is cooled slowly in the austenitic phase, it undergoes a solid-state eutectoid transformation at 723° C to yield a microstructural constituent referred to as *pearlite*, which consists of alternating fine-scale lamellae of ferrite and iron carbide (Fe_3C), called *cementite* or simply *carbide.* The Fe_3C phase has an orthorhombic crystal structure and is much harder and more rigid than austenite or ferrite. (The eutectoid transformation is analogous to the eutectic transformation previously described in Chapter 6. In this case a solid phase, rather than a liquid phase, transforms to two other solid phases.) Except for alloys with very low percentages of carbon, the microstructures at room temperature for slowly cooled plain carbon steels containing less than 0.8% carbon consists of ferrite and pearlite, whereas slow cooling of plain carbon steels containing more than 0.8% carbon yields much harder alloys with microstructures consisting of cementite and pearlite.

These transformations from austenite require substantial elemental diffusion and, if austenite is cooled very rapidly (quenched), it undergoes spontaneous, diffusionless transformation to a body-centered tetragonal (bct) structure called *martensite.* The arrangement of the iron atoms in martensite is highly distorted by the carbon atoms, resulting in a very hard, strong, brittle alloy.

The formation of martensite is an important strengthening mechanism for carbon steels. The cutting edges of carbon steel instruments are ordinarily martensitic because the high hardness of this structure allows the grinding of a sharp edge that is retained in use. Martensite is a metastable phase and decomposes to form ferrite and carbide when heated at elevated temperatures. The hardness of carbon steel is reduced by the *tempering* process, but this is balanced by an increase in toughness that is of considerable practical importance. That Japanese Samurai swords have temper lines is historically significant.

The metallurgy of industrial carbon steels is highly interesting and complex because a wide variety of alloying elements are employed to yield appropriate properties for a large number of applications. The interested reader should consult the textbook by Brick, Pense, and Gordon for additional information.

STAINLESS STEELS
Background

When approximately 12% to 30% chromium is added to iron, the alloy is commonly called *stainless steel.* Elements other than iron, carbon, and chromium may be present, resulting in a wide variation in composition and properties of the stainless steels. For example, room temperature yield strengths may range from approximately 200 megapascals (MPa) to more than 1700 MPa.

As noted in Chapters 3 and 5, the resistance of stainless steels to tarnish and corrosion is associated with the passivating effect of chromium. A very thin, transparent, adherent layer of Cr_2O_3 forms on the surface of stainless steel when it is exposed to an oxidizing atmosphere such as room air, and this protective layer provides a barrier to oxygen diffusion and other corrosive environments, and prevents further corrosion of the underlying alloy. If the oxide layer is ruptured by mechanical or chemical means, only a temporary loss of protection against corrosion occurs, and the passivating oxide layer eventually forms again in an oxidizing environment.

There are three major types of stainless steels, classified on the basis of the previously described crystal structures formed by the iron atoms. This classification, with approximate compositions, is provided in Table 20-2.

Ferritic Stainless Steels

These alloys are designated as American Iron and Steel Institute (AISI) Series 400 stainless steels. This series number is shared with the martensitic stainless steels. The ferritic stainless steels provide good corrosion resistance at low cost, provided

Table 20-2	Composition (Weight Percentage) of Three Types of Stainless Steel*		
Type of stainless steel (crystal structure formed by iron atoms)	Chromium	Nickel	Carbon
Ferritic (bcc)	11.5–27.0	0	0.20 max
Austenitic (fcc)	16.0–26.0	7.0–22.0	0.25 max
Martensitic (bct)	11.5–17.0	0–2.5	0.15–1.20

*Silicon, phosphorus, sulfur, manganese, tantalum, and niobium may also be present in small amounts. The balance is iron. *bcc,* Body-centered cubic; *fcc,* Face-centered cubic; *bct,* Body-centered tetragonal.

that high strength is not required. Because temperature change induces no phase change in the solid state, these stainless steels are not hardenable by heat treatment. Also, ferritic stainless steels are not readily work-hardenable. Consequently, although these stainless steels have numerous industrial uses, they have little application in dentistry.

Martensitic Stainless Steels

As previously noted, martensitic stainless steels share the AISI Series 400 designation with the ferritic stainless steels. They can be heat treated in the same manner as plain carbon steels, with similar results. Because of their high strength and hardness, martensitic stainless steels are used for surgical and cutting instruments.

The yield strength of a high-carbon martensitic stainless steel may range from approximately 500 MPa in the annealed condition up to nearly 1900 MPa in the hardened (quenched and tempered) state. The corresponding hardness ranges from a Brinell hardness number of approximately 230 to 600.

Corrosion resistance of the martensitic stainless steels is less than that of the two other major types and is reduced further following hardening heat treatment. Such heat treatment decreases the ductility, which may be only 2% for a high-carbon martensitic stainless steel.

Austenitic Stainless Steels

The austenitic stainless steels are the most corrosion-resistant alloys of the three major types and are the stainless steels used for orthodontic wires, endodontic instruments, and crowns in pediatric dentistry. The austenitic structure for the AISI Series 300 stainless steels is achieved by the addition of nickel to the iron-chromium-carbon composition. (The lower-cost AISI Series 200 austenitic stainless steels substitute manganese and nitrogen for nickel and are not used for dental applications.) Type 302 stainless steel is a basic alloy, containing 17% to 19% chromium, 8% to 10% nickel, and a maximum of 0.15% carbon. Type 304 stainless steel has a similar composition of 18% to 20% chromium and 8% to 12% nickel, along with a maximum carbon content of 0.08%. Both 302 and 304 stainless steel are often given the general designation of *18-8 stainless steel,* based on the percentages of chromium and nickel in their composition, and are the types most commonly used in orthodontic stainless steel wires and bands. Type 316L (low carbon) contains 10% to 14% nickel, 2% to 3% molybdenum, 16% to 18% chromium, and 0.03% maximum carbon, and is the stainless steel ordinarily employed for implants. All of the preceding stainless steel alloys contain 2% manganese.

Austenitic stainless steel is preferable to ferritic stainless steel for dental applications because, in addition to reasonable cost, it possesses the following excellent combination of properties:

- Greater ductility and ability to undergo more cold work without fracturing
- Substantial strengthening during cold working (some transformation to a martensite phase)
- Greater ease of welding
- Ability to overcome sensitization (discussed in the following section)
- Less critical grain growth
- Comparative ease in forming

X-ray diffraction analyses of as-received austenitic stainless steel orthodontic wires has shown that these wires may not have a completely austenitic single-phase (γ phase) with an fcc crystal structure. The austenite phase in 18-8 stainless steels is metastable, and cold working creates a bcc martensite structure (termed α' to distinguish it from the α phase designation used for the bcc ferrite structure). Formation of the duplex ($\gamma + \alpha'$) structure in as-received wires depends on both the orthodontic wire product and the cross-section dimensions of the wire. The major factors appear to be the carbon content of the stainless steel alloy and the sequence of proprietary intermediate heat treatments given by the manufacturer during the wire processing.

CORROSION RESISTANCE AND PROPERTIES OF AUSTENITIC STAINLESS STEEL
Sensitization

Austenitic stainless steel may lose its resistance to corrosion if it is heated between approximately 400° C and 900° C, the exact temperature depending on its carbon content. Such temperatures are within the range used by the orthodontist for soldering and welding. The decrease in corrosion resistance is caused by the precipitation of chromium-iron carbide at the grain boundaries at these high temperatures. The small carbon atoms rapidly diffuse to the grain boundary regions to combine with the chromium and iron atoms in solid solution and form $(CrFe)_4C$, resulting in loss of the corrosion resistance provided by chromium. Formation of $(CrFe)_4C$ is most rapid at 650° C. Below this temperature the diffusion rate for carbon is slower, whereas decomposition of $(CrFe)_4C$ occurs at higher temperatures. Corrosion resistance is reduced in regions adjacent to the grain boundaries in which the chromium level is depleted below that necessary for protection (approximately 12%). The stainless steel becomes susceptible to intergranular corrosion, and partial disintegration of the weakened alloy may result.

Two methods can be used to minimize sensitization when austenitic stainless steel is heated into this problematic elevated temperature range. One method is to reduce the carbon content of the steel to an extent that such carbide precipitation cannot occur, but this remedy is not economically feasible. On the other hand, if the stainless steel is severely cold worked and heated within the sensitization temperature range, the chromium-iron carbides instead precipitate at dislocations, which are located on slip planes within the bulk grains. As a result, the carbides are more uniformly distributed throughout the alloy, rather than forming a network of grain boundary precipitates. Fortunately, the manufacturing process for orthodontic stainless steel wires should provide some resistance to intergranular corrosion by this mechanism because the final wires still possess substantial strain hardening, despite the intermediate heat treatments performed at different stages during the wire-drawing sequence.

Stabilization

The method employed most successfully in industrial practice to prevent the sensitization of austenitic stainless steels at elevated temperatures is the introduction of one or two elements that form carbide precipitates in preference to chromium, such as niobium or titanium plus tantalum. Stainless steels that have been treated in this manner are said to be stabilized. However, this method does not appear to be used for stainless steel orthodontic wires, presumably because of the additional cost.

General Causes of Corrosion

As previously noted, the function of chromium in stainless steel is to prevent corrosion of the bulk alloy by oxidation. Stainless steel is highly prone to oxidation, but the passive surface oxide film blocks significant oxygen diffusion to the underlying alloy. With respect to prevention of electrolytic (electrochemical) corrosion, the situation is somewhat analogous to that for dental amalgam, which is discussed in Chapter 17.

From Chapter 3 it follows that any surface inhomogeneity in the surface of a metal is a potential source of tarnish or corrosion. Severe strain hardening may also produce localized anodic regions in the presence of an electrolyte such as saliva. Because of the likelihood of in vivo deposits, any site of surface roughness on a metal may result in a concentration cell that causes localized corrosion. A stainless steel orthodontic appliance should be polished so that it remains cleaner and less susceptible to tarnish or corrosion during use, as well as for patient comfort.

A common cause of the corrosion of stainless steel is the incorporation of bits of carbon steel or a similar metal in its surface. For example, if a stainless steel wire is manipulated carelessly with carbon steel pliers, it is possible that some of the carbon steel from the pliers may become embedded in the stainless steel. Or, if the stainless steel appliance is abraded or cut with a carbon steel bur or similar steel tool, some of the carbon steel from the tool may also become embedded in the stainless steel. Such a situation results in an electrochemical cell that may cause considerable corrosion in vivo.

Brazed or soldered joints (Chapter 19) in orthodontic appliances can also form galvanic couples in vivo. In addition, as pointed out in Chapter 3, austenitic stainless steels are susceptible to attack by solutions containing chlorine. Chlorine-containing cleansers should not be used to clean removable appliances fabricated from stainless steel.

Mechanical Properties

Approximate values of the mechanical properties for a stainless steel orthodontic wire are presented in Table 20-3, in which the elastic modulus is 180 gigapascals (GPa), the 0.2% offset yield strength is 1600 MPa, and the ultimate tensile strength is 2100 MPa. Strength and hardness may increase with a decrease in cross-section dimensions, because of the increased cold work required for forming the smaller wires. (The lack of such changes for certain sizes of the same stainless steel wire product is the result of intermediate heat treatments during wire drawing.) As previously noted, the substantial cold working during fabrication of the stainless steel wires contributes a major proportion of their strength values.

Although the tensile strength at which the wire fractures is of metallurgical interest, this property has no clinical significance. The elastic modulus, which determines

		Yield strength	Ultimate	Number of 90-degree cold
	Modulus of	(0.2% offset)	tensile strength	bends without
Alloy	elasticity (GPa)	(GPa)	(GPa)	fracture*
Stainless steel	179	1.6	2.1	5
Cobalt-chromium-nickel	184	1.4	1.7	8
Nickel-titanium	41	0.43	1.5	2
Beta-titanium	72	0.93	1.3	4

Table 20-3 Mechanical Properties of Orthodontic Wires

* Formerly required in ANSI/ADA Specification No. 32 for orthodontic wires.

the alloy contribution to the orthodontic force delivery from a wire segment, is of paramount clinical importance, as is the yield strength, which determines the practical limit of the elastic working range. Although there was formerly a requirement in American National Standards Institute/American Dental Association (ANSI/ADA) Specification No. 32 for orthodontic wires not containing precious metals on the number of 90-degree cold bends that could be performed before fracture, this requirement has been eliminated from the current specification. Nevertheless, the relative number of such cold bends indicates the comparative formability (ability to be permanently deformed into complex shapes) of the major orthodontic wire alloys.

The previously mentioned phase change from the metastable austenitic (γ) phase to the α' martensitic phase during manufacture of the stainless steel wires can be readily demonstrated because the bcc structures (ferrite and martensite) are ferromagnetic at room temperature, whereas austenite is nonmagnetic. Because the martensite phase has a lower elastic modulus than the austenite phase, there is a reduction in the modulus of elasticity for stainless steel orthodontic wires in which the work hardening effects have not been eliminated by heat treatment. For example, the elastic modulus can decrease from approximately 200 GPa for fully annealed austenitic stainless steel to 150 GPa after extensive cold working. This presents no problem clinically because stainless steel orthodontic wires have a very high elastic modulus relative to the titanium-containing wires to be discussed later. Concomitantly, extensive cold working can increase the yield strength to approximately 1100 MPa from a value of 275 MPa for the fully annealed stainless steel. Presumably, the strengthening is associated with work hardening of the α' martensitic phase, but definitive studies have not been performed on stainless steel orthodontic wires to verify this hypothesis.

It is unfortunate that a stainless steel orthodontic wire can become fully annealed, resulting in a recrystallized microstructure, in a few seconds at temperatures from 700° C to 800°C, which lie within the soldering and welding temperature range. The yield strength of the wire and thus the range of elastic deformation (working range) necessary for a satisfactory orthodontic appliance are greatly reduced after such annealing. This result is a decided clinical disadvantage. This disadvantage can be minimized by using low-fusing solders, and by confining the time for soldering and welding procedures to a minimum. Any softening that occurs under such conditions of heating can be remedied considerably by the strain hardening incurred in subsequent clinical operations, such as contouring and polishing.

Recovery Heat Treatment

An increase in the elastic properties of a stainless steel wire can be obtained by heating to temperatures between approximately 400° C and 500° C after it has been cold-worked. This stress-relief heat treatment promotes the recovery annealing stage, which removes residual stresses introduced during manipulation of the wire, and thus stabilizes the shape of the appliance. This is important clinically because such residual stresses might cause fracture when the appliance is being adjusted by the clinician for the patient.

A study of the heat treatment effects on straight segments of austenitic stainless steel orthodontic wires with a range of cross-section dimensions from two manufacturers revealed increases of up to 10% for the modulus of resilience in tension. Springback improved from a range of 0.0060 to 0.0094 for the as-received wires to a range of 0.0065 to 0.0099 after heat treatment. For certain cross-section sizes of one product, heat treatment eliminated the α' martensitic phase found in the as-received wires, yielding an entirely single-phase austenitic (γ) structure.

Braided and Twisted Wires

Very small-diameter stainless steel wires have been braided or twisted together by manufacturers to form larger multistranded wires for clinical orthodontics. The separate strands may be as small as 0.178 mm (0.007 inch) in diameter, and the final intertwined wires may have round or rectangular cross-sections with dimensions between 0.406 mm and 0.635 mm (0.016 and 0.025 inch). Figure 20-11 shows the magnified appearance of two such wires. Although the bending mechanics analysis for multistranded orthodontic wires is complex, it can be appreciated that these wires are composite beams of individual strands that are very flexible. Consequently, the braided or twisted wires are able to sustain large elastic deflections in bending, and these wires apply much lower forces for a given deflection, compared with solid stainless steel wires with the same cross-section dimensions.

CRITICAL QUESTION

What failure processes might be observed clinically for soldered joints and welded joints in stainless steel orthodontic appliances?

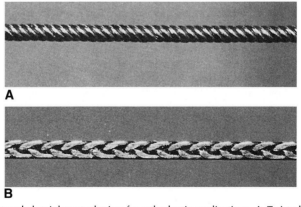

Fig. 20-11   Multistranded stainless steel wires for orthodontic applications. **A,** Twisted form with overall diameter of 0.44 mm. **B,** Braided form with overall dimensions of 0.44 mm × 0.63 mm. (Courtesy of J.Y. Morton and J. Goldberg.)

SOLDERING AND WELDING OF STAINLESS STEEL

Solders (Brazing Materials)

It is important that the stainless steel wire not be heated to an excessively high temperature to minimize carbide precipitation and prevent substantial softening of the wire so that its usefulness is lost. The requirement of a low-temperature soldering (brazing) technique generally rules out any of the gold soldering (brazing) materials normally employed with gold alloy wires because their melting ranges (difference between liquidus and solidus temperature, as described in Chapter 6) are typically too high. Instead, silver solders are used. As noted in the Chapter 19, the term *soldering* is preferred rather than *brazing* for such joining processes because of its common usage in dentistry.

Silver solders are alloys of silver, copper, and zinc to which elements such as tin and indium may be added to lower the fusion temperature and improve solderability. Although such solders corrode in use because they are anodic to stainless steel, this effect in clinical orthodontic appliances is not too objectionable. These appliances are temporary structures, usually not worn in the mouth for more than 6 to 30 months, and frequent inspections by the orthodontist are necessary.

The soldering temperatures for orthodontic silver solders are typically between approximately 620° C and 665° C. A small melting range is an important characteristic of the solder materials used for the freehand soldering practiced by orthodontists. In freehand soldering, the joint metal should harden promptly when the work is removed from the flame. Otherwise, the operator may inadvertently move the work before the soldering material has completely solidified, and the joint will be weakened.

Soldering Fluxes

In addition to the usual reducing and cleaning agents described in Chapter 19, a flux used for soldering stainless steel also contains a fluoride to dissolve the passivating surface film formed by chromium. The solder will not wet the metal when such a film is present. Potassium fluoride is one of the most active chemicals in this respect. The flux is similar to that recommended for gold soldering in Chapter 19, with the exception of the addition of potassium fluoride. Boric acid is used in a greater ratio to borax than in the flux for gold soldering, because it lowers the fusion temperature.

Technical Considerations for Soldering

The freehand soldering of stainless steel is not greatly different from that of gold soldering described in the previous chapter. A needlelike, nonluminous, gas-air flame may be used. The thinner the diameter of the flame, the less the metal surrounding the joint is annealed. The work should be located about 3 mm inward from the tip of the blue cone, in the reducing zone of the flame. The soldering procedure should be observed in a shadow, against a black background, so that the temperature can be judged by the color of the work. The color should never exceed a dull red.

Before soldering, the parts should be tack-welded for alignment during the soldering procedure. Then flux should be applied, and the heavier-gauge part should be heated first. Flux must cover all of the areas to be soldered before heat is applied. As soon as the flux fuses, the solder alloy should be added and heating continued until the metal flows around the joint. After the metal has flowed, the work should be immediately removed from the heat and quenched in water. From the preceding

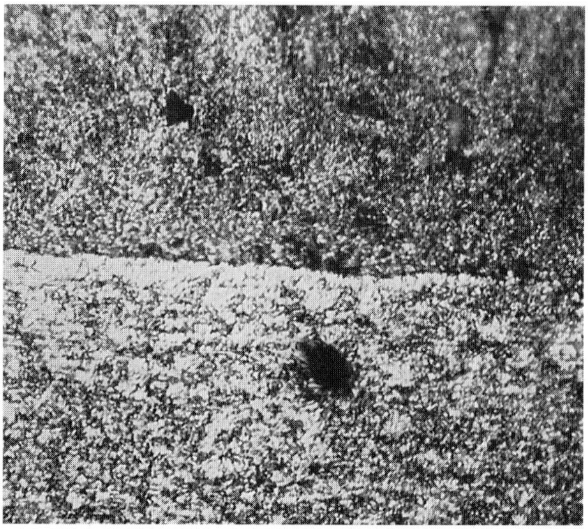

Fig. 20-12 Photomicrograph of a soldered joint between a stainless steel orthodontic wire and a silver solder. (×800.)

discussion about sensitization of austenitic stainless steels, it should be evident that the objective during soldering is to use as little heat for as short a time as possible.

In addition to the conventional gas-air torch, a number of other techniques can be used to supply the heat for soldering. These include a hydrogen-oxygen torch, electric resistance heating, and indirect heating using an intermediary brass wire. Gas-air and hydrogen-oxygen torch heating have been shown to produce comparable joints in terms of strength.

A photomicrograph of a cross-section of a stainless steel wire/silver solder junction is shown in Figure 20-12. Although intimate contact between the two metals is seen at this moderate magnification, research has indicated that no measurable amount of atomic diffusion occurs at the interface and that the bond is strictly mechanical. The absence of appreciable diffusion during the brief periods of soldering is plausible. The tensile strength of a good silver solder joint can exceed that of the bulk alloy used for silver soldering. Interfacial constraint between the thin layer of solder alloy and the stronger wire might account for the higher strength of the solder joint, but further research is necessary to verify this hypothesis.

Welding

Although soldering of stainless steel orthodontic wires is not uncommon, flat structures such as bands and brackets are usually joined by welding. The spot (electrical resistance) welding apparatus produces a large electric current that is forced by the electrode to flow through a limited area (spot) on the overlapped materials to be welded. The interfacial resistance of the materials to the current flow produces intense localized heating and fusion of the overlapped metals. No solder is employed. Ideally, melting is confined to the junction area and can be observed metallographically in cross-section as a region of resolidified alloy with a distinctive cast microstructure. The grain structure of the surrounding wrought alloy should not be affected, but stress exists at the interface of the cast and wrought structures, which would be one likely path of joint failure if this were to occur. The strength of the welded joint decreases with an increase in the area of recrystallization of the adjacent wrought structure, and the joint strength increases with the area of the weld.

The welded joint is susceptible to corrosion, primarily because of the loss of passivation resulting from chromium-iron carbide precipitation at the elevated temperatures associated with welding. The tendency for corrosion is also increased because of the localized stress at the interface between the weld area and the surrounding wrought structure.

COBALT-CHROMIUM-NICKEL ALLOYS
Composition and Mechanical Properties

Cobalt-chromium-nickel alloys drawn into wire were first marketed for use in orthodontic appliances during the 1950s. These alloys were originally developed for use as watch springs (Elgiloy), and a representative composition is 40% cobalt, 20% chromium, 15% nickel, 15.8% iron, 7% molybdenum, 2% manganese, 0.16% carbon, and 0.04% beryllium. The metallurgy of Elgiloy is complex, and its composition bears some resemblance to a cobalt-chromium-nickel casting alloy for removable partial denture frameworks. Although the latter alloy contains higher percentages of cobalt and chromium, it contains only a small amount of iron and no beryllium. Elgiloy has excellent resistance to tarnish and corrosion in the oral environment, and can be subjected to the same welding and soldering procedures used for stainless steel wires.

One manufacturer offers Elgiloy wires in four different tempers (soft, ductile, semiresilient, and resilient), which are color-coded for the clinician's convenience. The most widely used is the soft temper (Elgiloy Blue), which is easily manipulated and then heat treated to achieve increased resilience; other tempers are also responsive to heat treatment. The resulting changes in mechanical properties are associated with precipitation reactions. Clinicians can easily perform heat treatment using an electrical resistance welding apparatus and a special paste provided by the manufacturer to indicate the optimum period of time. Alternatively, furnace heat treatment at approximately 480° C and 7 to 12 min can be employed.

Heat treatment of straight segments of Elgiloy Blue orthodontic wires with several cross-section dimensions increase the elastic modulus in tension from a range of 160 to 190 GPa for as-received wires to a range of 180 to 210 GPa for heat-treated wires. The springback, which varies between 0.0045 and 0.0065 for the as-received wires, increased to a range of 0.0054 to 0.0074 after heat treatment. Other studies have shown that significant increases in the elastic properties of stainless steel and Elgiloy Blue wires are also obtained when orthodontic loop configurations (rather than straight as-received wire specimens) are subjected to heat treatment.

Mechanical properties for the different tempers of Elgiloy orthodontic wires are similar to those for certain stainless steel wires because these latter wires are available in a range of properties. Representative property values for an Elgiloy orthodontic wire are provided in Table 20-3. Because of their nearly identical values of elastic modulus, the orthodontic force delivery for Elgiloy Blue and stainless steel orthodontic wires is essentially the same. In the as-received condition, the Elgiloy Blue wires have a soft feel because of their much lower values of yield strength compared with the more resilient stainless steel wires.

Large-diameter Elgiloy Blue wires have also been fabricated into quad-helix appliances similar to those used for slow maxillary expansion in pediatric dentistry, and their in vitro force delivery for elastic activation was compared with that for appliances fabricated from stainless steel wires of the same diameter. As would be anticipated from their essentially equal values of elastic modulus, there was no significant difference in force delivery for the two wire alloys. Expected significant differences occurred in force delivery as a function of wire diameter and appliance size.

NICKEL-TITANIUM ALLOYS

A nickel-titanium orthodontic wire alloy was first introduced commercially (Nitinol, 3M Unitek, Monrovia, CA) during the 1970s, following research by Andreasen and his colleagues. This wire alloy had significantly different mechanical properties from the stainless steel and Elgiloy orthodontic wires (see Table 20-3), notably much lower elastic modulus and much wider elastic working range. The alloy name "Nitinol" originally came from the two elements *ni*ckel and *ti*tanium, and the *N*aval *O*rdinance *L*aboratory where these alloys were first developed by Buehler and associates.

Mechanical Properties

Approximate mechanical properties for Nitinol wire are 40 GPa for elastic modulus, 430 MPa for 0.2% offset yield strength, and 1500 MPa for tensile strength. Placement of permanent bends by the clinician in Nitinol wires is difficult because of their high resilience, as evidenced by the small number of 90-degree cold bends before fracture (see Table 20-3). Tensile tests in which wires were loaded to failure showed that Nitinol has high ductility, and its capability of undergoing substantial work hardening is evident from the considerably higher tensile strength compared with its yield strength. The very low elastic modulus of Nitinol (approximately one-fourth that of stainless steel and Elgiloy) results in very low orthodontic forces when compared with similarly constructed and activated appliances from these other two alloys, and the springback (YS/E) or elastic range available for tooth movement is much greater for Nitinol.

CRITICAL QUESTION

What are the clinical advantages of a shape-memory nickel-titanium orthodontic wire, compared with a stainless steel orthodontic wire?

Orthodontic Wire Alloys: Composition, Superelasticity, and Shape Memory

The nickel-titanium alloys used in dentistry are based on the equiatomic intermetallic compound NiTi, which contains 55 wt% nickel because of the differing atomic weights of nickel and titanium. Orthodontic wire alloys contain small amounts of other elements, such as cobalt, copper, and chromium. The microstructure consists predominantly of NiTi, but small precipitates, which can be oxide phases because of the alloy reactivity with the atmospheric environment during wire processing, are also observed. The NiTi intermetallic compound can exist in different crystal structures. The austenitic NiTi phase has a complex ordered bcc (cesium chloride) structure, and the martensitic NiTi phase has been reported to have a distorted monoclinic, triclinic, or hexagonal structure. The names *austenitic* and *martensitic* for these different crystallographic forms of NiTi have been taken from the metallurgical terminology for carbon steel and stainless steel.

Transformation between the austenitic and martensitic forms of NiTi can be induced by both temperature and stress. Austenitic NiTi is the high-temperature, low-stress form, and martensitic NiTi is the low-temperature, high-stress form. Transformation occurs by a twinning process, which is reversible below the elastic limit. There are also changes in volume and electrical resistivity. In addition, a third form of NiTi, called the *R phase* (because of its rhombohedral crystal structure), appears as an intermediate phase during the transformation between martensitic NiTi and austenitic NiTi. The NiTi phase relationships in orthodontic wires have been studied in detail by x-ray diffraction and differential scanning calorimetry, and a summary of these studies is provided in the referenced textbook on orthodontic materials in the Selected Readings.

The original Nitinol wire is made from a predominantly heavily work-hardened martensitic alloy and has a Vickers hardness of approximately 430. In the mid 1980s nickel-titanium orthodontic wires possessing **superelasticity** (termed *pseudoelasticity* in engineering materials science) were introduced commercially. In contrast to the original *(nonsuperelastic)* Nitinol wire, as-received superelastic wires contain substantial austenitic NiTi structure at room temperature or body temperature (37° C).

A schematic illustration of superelastic behavior for an orthodontic wire specimen in bending is shown in Figure 20-13. Segment *a–b* corresponds to the initial elastic deformation of the wire, followed by segment *b–c*, where the austenitic NiTi structure transforms to the martensitic NiTi structure. After the transformation is completed at point *c* (typically at approximately 10% strain), plastic deformation and further elastic deformation occur with increasing stress (or bending moment) along segment *c–d*. During unloading, this sequence of events is reversed, with segment *d–e* corresponding to loss of elastic strain in the martensitic NiTi structure, followed by a transformation back to the austenitic NiTi structure along segment *e–f*, and finally loss of elastic strain in the austenitic NiTi structure as the stress or bending moment decreases to zero. A small amount of permanent angular deflection remains in the wire, because of the permanent deformation in segment *c–d*. For tensile loading and unloading of the wire specimen, segments *b–c* and *e–f* are parallel to each other because stress is uniform over the cross-section. Superelastic behavior is desirable clinically, because very low and nearly constant forces for tooth movement are provided by the wire during unloading (deactivation).

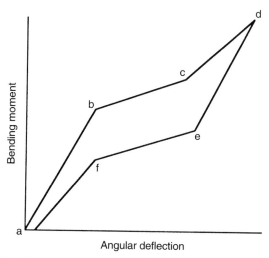

Fig. 20-13 Schematic bending movement versus angular deflection curve for a nickel-titanium orthodontic wire, showing the regions of superelasticity: *b–c* during loading (activation) and *e–f* during unloading (deactivation). Such behavior imparts a large working range to the archwire. Region *c–d* corresponds to permanent deformation during loading, and *d–e* corresponds to initial unloading of the permanently deformed archwire. Regions *b–c* and *e–f* correspond to the forward and reverse directions, respectively, of the stress-induced transformation between the low-stress austenitic and high-stress martensitic structures. (Courtesy of J. Goldberg.)

In the early 1990s new nickel-titanium orthodontic wires possessing true *shape memory* in the oral environment were introduced. Manufacturers can achieve the shape memory effect by first establishing a shape when the alloy is heated at a temperature near 480° C. If the appliance, such as an orthodontic archwire, is then manipulated by the clinician and placed into brackets bonded to malpositioned teeth, exposure of the wire to the lower transformation temperature (approximately body temperature) causes the archwire to return to its original shape (the passive configuration) and thereby promote tooth movement. Differential scanning calorimetric analyses of shape memory nickel-titanium wires show that the transformation from the martensitic NiTi structure to the austenitic NiTi structure on heating from very low temperatures is completed below 37° C, whereas temperatures higher than that of the oral environment are required for complete transformation to the austenitic NiTi structure in the superelastic wires.

The shape memory wires have superior springback to the superelastic and nonsuperelastic nickel-titanium wires and, in principle, are the most desirable nickel-titanium orthodontic wires for clinical use. In the mid 1990s one manufacturer introduced new copper-containing nickel-titanium orthodontic wires that are available in three different variants, corresponding to the approximate *austenite-finish* temperature (27° C, 35° C, or 40° C) at which transformation to the entirely austenitic NiTi structure is completed.

The preceding discussions show that a wide variety of nickel-titanium orthodontic wires are currently available. Manufacturers are able to control the percentages of martensitic and austenitic NiTi phases in these wires, as well as the phase transformation temperatures, by a variety of strategies, such as the amount of cold work and annealing temperatures during wire processing and the alloy composition, where cobalt, copper, and chromium have been incorporated in various products. Despite their advantages of very low elastic modulus and high springback (very wide elastic working range), the nickel-titanium orthodontic wires have some disadvantages. As noted previously, they are difficult to form into clinical shapes, and they have to be joined by mechanical crimping because the alloy can be neither soldered nor welded. In addition, nickel-titanium orthodontic wires have relatively rough surfaces, which result in high values of archwire-bracket friction that can potentially prolong the time needed for clinical treatment.

Nickel-Titanium Endodontic Instruments

Following a pioneering study by Walia and associates published in the late 1980s, there has been considerable interest in nickel-titanium instruments for endodontics. Whereas the small nickel-titanium hand files in the original study were fabricated from the nonsuperelastic Nitinol orthodontic alloy, the superelastic property is more desirable for the nickel-titanium endodontic instruments. In particular, within the upper superelastic plateau region (see segment *b–c* in Fig. 20-13), the markedly increased strain for a small increase in bending stress facilitates adaptation of the instrument along a sharply curving root canal, thereby minimizing the risk for perforation of the root. Recent differential scanning calorimetric analyses have confirmed that the alloys for the two most popular nickel-titanium rotary endodontic instruments are in the superelastic condition, with the austenite-finish temperature being approximately 25° C.

The nickel-titanium endodontic instruments must be fabricated by machining the starting wire blanks, in contrast to stainless steel endodontic instruments in which a special apparatus is used to twist the tapered starting wire blank. The edges of the cutting flutes on some nickel-titanium instruments are characterized by

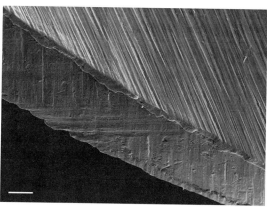

Fig. 20-14 Photomicrograph of a nickel-titanium rotary endodontic instrument, showing permanent deformation at the edges of the flutes (rollover) and other surface defects that resulted from the machining process used for fabrication. (Courtesy of S.B. Alapati.)

substantial permanent deformation (which is called *rollover*), as shown in Figure 20-14. Scanning electron microscope observations suggest that fracture of nickel-titanium endodontic instruments during laboratory torsional testing takes place at surface flaws introduced during manufacturing. The nickel-titanium alloy may be inherently notch-sensitive, because the coexisting austenitic and martensitic NiTi phases have very different crystal structures. Future developments of nickel-titanium endodontic instruments with improved resistance to failure under clinical conditions are anticipated.

CRITICAL QUESTION

What is a potential clinical disadvantage of an orthodontic wire fabricated from α-titanium?

BETA-TITANIUM ALLOYS

Crystallographic Forms of Titanium and Titanium Alloys

Like the stainless steel and nickel-titanium orthodontic wires, pure titanium has different crystallographic (polymorphic or allotropic) forms at high and low temperatures. At temperatures below 885° C, the stable form is α-titanium, which has the hcp crystal structure, whereas at higher temperatures the stable form is β-titanium, which has the bcc structure. The elastic modulus and yield strength at room temperature for α-titanium are approximately 110 GPa and 40 MPa, respectively.

Certain elements, such as aluminum, carbon, oxygen, and nitrogen, stabilize the α-titanium structure, that is, raise the temperature for transformation to β-titanium. Other elements, such as vanadium, molybdenum, and tantalum, stabilize the β-titanium structure, that is, extend the β-titanium phase field or region of stability and thus lower the temperature for transformation to α-titanium. The Ti-6Al-4V alloy, which contains 90% titanium, 6% aluminum, and 4% vanadium (wt%), is popular for dental implants and has received attention for cast restorations. This alloy has a duplex microstructure, containing both the α-titanium and β-titanium phases, which can be varied substantially with appropriate heat treatment. Although Ti-6Al-4V can exhibit a yield strength as high as 960 MPa, this alloy has not been used for commercial orthodontic wires, perhaps because of difficulties in fabrication and lower formability compared with the β-titanium wires. Comparing the clinically relevant fatigue (cyclic loading) properties for dental implants (Chapter 23), Ti-6Al-4V has superior fatigue strength relative to that of CP titanium, when manufacturers employ appropriate heat treatment strategies to control the morphologies of the α-titanium and β-titanium phases.

Following research by Burstone and Goldberg, commercial β-titanium wires with an approximate composition of 79% titanium, 11% molybdenum, 6% zirconium, and 4% tin were introduced around 1980. The addition of molybdenum stabilizes the bcc β-titanium structure to room temperature, yielding an alloy of high formability. This commercial alloy (Ormco, Glendora, CA) has the trade name of TMA (titanium-molybdenum alloy). Recently, with the expiration of the patent for the TMA product, two other manufacturers (GAC, Islandia, New York; 3M Unitek) have introduced a different β-titanium orthodontic wire products (Resolve and Beta III Titanium, respectively).

Mechanical Properties of Beta-Titanium Wires

Beta-titanium orthodontic wires (TMA product) have an elastic modulus of approximately 70 GPa and 0.2% offset yield strength between approximately 860 and 1200 MPa (see Table 20-3), which provide favorable clinical properties. The elastic modulus for β-titanium wires is intermediate between the values for stainless steel and Elgiloy wires and that for Nitinol wires. The springback (YS/E) for β-titanium wires is much greater than that for the stainless steel and Elgiloy wires and very similar to that for the Nitinol wires. The β-titanium wires can be highly cold-worked, and because of the bcc structure of the β-phase, the wires have high formability (comparable to that of austenitic stainless steel). Thus they can be readily bent into various orthodontic configurations. Although tensile tests have shown that there are no significant differences in the elastic modulus and yield strength for the TMA and Resolve β-titanium wire products, transmission electron microscopic examination has revealed differences in the morphology of precipitates in the wires, suggesting differences in the processing procedures used by the two manufacturers.

There have been anecdotal reports that some batches of the TMA β-titanium wires are susceptible during clinical manipulation, but definitive experiments to verify this apparently occasional problematic behavior have not been performed. Because of the high reactivity of titanium, careful control of the original cast ingot quality, the atmosphere, and other processing parameters during wire drawing is essential. This is also true for manufacturing of the nickel-titanium orthodontic wires. Although heat treatments can be performed to alter the mechanical properties of β-titanium wires, these wires should not be heat treated by the clinician.

Welding

The β-titanium wires are the only major orthodontic wire alloy type considered to possess true weldability, and clinically satisfactory joints can be made by electrical resistance welding. Such joints need not be reinforced with solder, which is necessary with welded joints for stainless steel and Elgiloy wires. A weld made with insufficient heat will fail at the interface between the wires, whereas overheating may cause a failure adjacent to the joint. Figure 20-15 is a cross-section of a

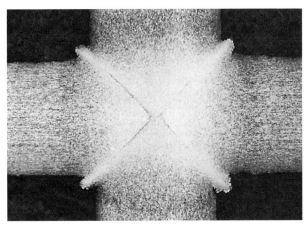

Fig. 20-15 Photomicrograph of a weld joint between two 0.43 × 0.63 mm beta-titanium orthodontic wires, showing minimum distortion of the original cold-worked microstructure. (Courtesy of T.C. Labenski and A.J. Goldberg.)

welded β-titanium joint, showing minimum distortion of the original cold-worked structure.

Corrosion Resistance

Because of a passive TiO_2 surface film, which is analogous to the Cr_2O_3 film on stainless steel and Elgiloy, titanium and its alloys generally have excellent corrosion resistance and environmental stability. (Research has shown that a TiO_2 passive film that contains minimal amounts of nickel is also present on the nickel-titanium alloys.) These features have stimulated the general use of titanium alloys in chemical processing, as well as in biomedical applications, such as heart valves and hip implants, besides orthodontic appliances. There has been some concern about biocompatibility of orthodontic wires containing nickel, which may cause localized tissue irritation in some patients, and it should be noted that β-titanium is the only major orthodontic wire alloy that is nickel-free.

The surface roughness of the TMA wires is much greater than that for the stainless steel and Elgiloy wires, which is expected to significantly affect in vivo archwire-bracket friction, in a similar manner to that with the nickel-titanium archwires. Scanning electron microscope observations suggest that the surface roughness originates from adherence of the titanium in both wire alloys to the dies or rollers used in wire processing. During orthodontic treatment, not only do the rough archwire surfaces increase sliding friction, but also the archwire alloy may cold weld locally to the metal bracket.

Manufacturers have developed nitrogen ion-implantation techniques to decrease the bracket friction for nickel-titanium and beta-titanium orthodontic wires. A recent clinical study revealed that there were no significant differences for the rate of space closure when ion-implanted TMA, conventional TMA (not ion-implanted), and stainless steel wires were used. In contrast, an earlier study reported significant differences for in vitro tooth movement with ion-implanted TMA and nickel-titanium wires, compared with wires of both alloys that were not ion-implanted. Additional research is needed to unambiguously assess the clinical efficacy of these ion-implanted wires.

OTHER WROUGHT ALLOYS

Noble Metals

Noble metal wires are still occasionally employed in the construction of removable partial denture clasps and orthodontic appliances, as well as retention pins for restorations and endodontic posts. Wire clasps for removable partial dentures may be attached by soldering, casting the framework to the wire, or embedding a portion of the wire in the resin denture base. Wrought clasps have superior flexibility and strength, compared with cast clasps of the same composition, because of the elimination of many casting defects and the strain hardening caused by extensive cold working. Wrought clasps were highly popular in the past for removable partial denture frameworks because the limited ductility and rapid work hardening of the available base metal alloys frequently resulted in fracture during adjustments of cast clasps. Current dental laboratory technicians tend to cast the entire removable partial denture framework with the clasps, because of improvements in ductility of the base metal alloys (Chapter 19).

Formerly, ANSI/ADA Specification No. 7 was based on two types of high noble or noble gold alloy wires, but this specification has now been withdrawn. Nonetheless, it is instructive to briefly consider the two types of wires, composition limits of which are given in Table 20-4, because manufacturers may still offer wires with similar compositions. Properties of the noble alloy wires in Table 20-4 are given in Table 20-5. Type I gold alloy wires were stronger, had higher fusion temperatures, and contained at least 75% gold, platinum, and palladium; Type II wires contained at least 65% gold, platinum, and palladium. The elastic moduli of these gold alloy wires are approximately 100 to 120 GPa, which are slightly higher than the values for gold casting alloys, but considerably lower than the values for the base metal casting alloys for removable partial denture frameworks. The elastic modulus for the gold alloy wires increases by approximately 5% following hardening heat treatment.

The composition limits for these two types of gold alloy wires resemble the compositions of traditional Type IV gold casting alloys (see Chapter 19), although the wires typically contain less gold. The gold alloy wires can contain nickel. The generally much greater percentages of platinum provide the high fusion temperatures needed for clinical use. The roles of the elements other than nickel in these wires are the same as for the gold casting alloys. Copper provides the capability of additional strengthening by the ordering transformation with gold. Nickel also provides additional strengthening, but the amount is limited to avoid reduction in tarnish resistance and interference with age hardening. Heat treatments to strengthen or soften the wrought alloys are identical to those for gold casting alloys.

Platinum-gold-palladium (P-G-P) wires are marketed for endodontic posts and for clasps to which a removable partial denture framework can be cast. Table 20-5 shows that the high fusion temperature (hence high recrystallization temperature) of P-G-P wire would be especially useful for casting a removable partial denture

Table 20-4	Composition Limits of Principal Elements in Some High-Strength Wires				
Wire Type	**Gold**	**Platinum**	**Palladium**	**Silver**	**Copper**
P-G-P	25–30	40–50	25–30	—	16–17
P-S-C	—	0–1	42–44	38–41	—

P-G-P, platinum-gold-palladium; *P-S-C*, palladium-silver-copper.
(From Lyman T: Metals Handbook: Properties and Selection of Metals, ed 8, Vol 1. Metals Park, OH, 1964.

Table 20-5 Physical Properties of Wires

Wire type	Yield strength oven-cooled (min) (MPa)	Tensile strength oven-cooled (min) (MPa)	Elongation quenched (min) (%)	Elongation oven-cooled (min) (%)	Fusion temperature (min) (°C)
Formerly ANSI/ADA Type I	860	930	15	4	960
Formerly ANSI/ADA Type II	690	860	15	2	870

Wire	Type proportional limit (MPa)	Tensile strength (MPa)	Minimum elongation		Minimum fusion temperature (°C)
			Quenched (%)	Oven cooled (%)	
P-G-P	550–1030*	860–1240*	14–15	—	1500–1530
P-S-C	690–790†	960–1070†	16–24	8–15	1040–1080

(Data from Dentists Desk Reference: Materials, Instruments and Equipment, ed 1. Metals and Alloys: Precious Metal Wrought Wire. Chicago, American Dental Association, 1981; Lyman T: Metals Handbook, ed 8, Vol 1. Properties and Selection of Metals. Metals Park, OH, American Society for Metals, 1964.)
*Quenched (alloy does not age harden); †hardened.
P-G-P, platinum-gold-palladium; *P-S-C*, palladium-silver-copper.

framework to this alloy. Palladium-silver-copper (P-S-C) wires have also been considered to be useful for dental applications. The composition and property ranges of P-S-C wires are listed in Tables 20-4 and 20-5. The fusion temperatures for these wires are higher than those for the gold alloy wires, but they are considerably lower than the fusion temperatures (and recrystallization temperatures) for the P-G-P wires. The fusion temperature of P-G-P wires is increased because of platinum and palladium.

Other Wrought Base Metal Alloys

In addition to the wrought base metal alloys summarized earlier in this chapter, cobalt-chromium alloys are available for partial denture clasps. For example, a cobalt-chromium-tungsten-nickel wire (Ticonium) has a yield strength of approximately 920 MPa, a tensile strength of nearly 1400 MPa, and a percent elongation of 19%. This wrought alloy is not heat treatable and is designed for use with the lower-fusing nickel-chromium-beryllium casting alloy from the manufacturer. All of these wrought base metal alloys have complex compositions and strengthening mechanisms.

Wrought base metal alloys are also used for retention pins in large direct restorations (dental amalgam, composite resin, and glass ionomer). The main alloy is 18-8 stainless steel, but titanium and titanium alloy pins have also been employed. Compared with stainless steel, the titanium and titanium alloys have values of elastic modulus that more closely match the moduli of the direct restorative materials and also have superior corrosion resistance and biocompatibility.

SELECTED READINGS

Andreasen GF, and Morrow RE: Laboratory and clinical analyses of Nitinol wire. Am J Orthod 73:143, 1978.
  This classic article describes the laboratory properties and clinical uses of the first commercially available nickel-titanium orthodontic wire.

Asgharnia MK, and Brantley WA: Comparison of bending and tension tests for orthodontic wires. Am J Orthod 89:228, 1986.
  A complete set of bending and tensile data for various sizes of the four common orthodontic archwire alloys.

Brantley WA: Orthodontic wires. In: Brantley WA, and Eliades T: Orthodontic Wires: Scientific and Clinical Aspects. Stuttgart, Germany, Thieme, 2001.

This comprehensive chapter on orthodontic wires contains an extensive discussion of x-ray diffraction and differential scanning calorimetric analyses of nickel-titanium wires.

Brantley WA, Luebke NH, Luebke FL, and Mitchell JC: Performance of engine-driven rotary endodontic instruments with a superimposed bending deflection: V. Gates Glidden and Peeso drills. J Endod 20:241, 1994.

A series of articles that describe the effects of torsion, bending and bending fatigue on stainless steel rotary instruments. The micrographs are of particular interest.

Brick RM, Pense AW, and Gordon RB: Structure and Properties of Engineering Materials, ed 4. New York, McGraw-Hill, 1977.

An undergraduate engineering textbook that discusses carbon steels, stainless steels, titanium alloys, and deformation and strengthening mechanisms for metals.

Bryant ST, Thompson SA, al-Omari MA, and Dummer PM: Shaping ability of ProFile rotary nickel-titanium instruments with ISO sized tips in simulated root canals: Part 1. Int Endod J 1998; 31:275-281. Part 2. Int Endod J. 1998; 31:282-289.

This research group has published several articles that evaluate the ability of a variety of rotary endodontic instruments to shape root canals.

Burstone CJ: Application of bioengineering to clinical orthodontics. In: Graber TM, Vanarsdall RL (eds): Orthodontics: Current Principles and Techniques, ed 3. St Louis, Mosby, 2000.

The application of mechanics to clinical orthodontics is described. The relationship among alloy properties, wire geometry, and appliance force systems is also explained.

Burstone CJ, and Goldberg AJ: Beta titanium: A new orthodontic alloy. Am J Orthod 77:121, 1980.

This classic article was concurrent with the introduction of the beta-titanium orthodontic wires and presents clinical applications, as well as a brief review of the other wire alloys.

Burstone CJ, and Goldberg AJ: Maximum forces and deflections from orthodontic appliances. Am J Orthod 84:95, 1983.

Maximum properties of various orthodontic wire sizes and alloys are presented and related to theoretically predicted values, assuming complete elastic behavior.

Dieter GE: Mechanical Metallurgy, ed 3. New York, McGraw-Hill, 1986.

An undergraduate engineering textbook that contains highly readable descriptions of strengthening mechanisms, fracture processes, and mechanical testing for metals.

Duerig TW, Melton KN, Stöckel D, and Wayman CM (eds): Engineering Aspects of Shape Memory Alloys. London, Butterworth-Heinemann, 1990.

A highly readable account of the shape memory phenomenon and shape memory alloys. A variety of dental and medical applications for shape memory alloys are discussed.

Kusy RP, and Greenberg AR: Effects of composition and cross section on the elastic properties of orthodontic archwires. Angle Orthod 51:325, 1981.

A comprehensive derivation of the effects of wire shape, wire size, and alloy type on the strength, stiffness, and range properties in the elastic region.

Miura R, Mogi M, Ohura Y, and Hamanaka H: The superelastic property of the Japanese Ni-Ti alloy wire for use in orthodontics. Am J Orthod Dentofacial Orthop 90:1, 1986.

A classic article that first described the metallurgy, mechanical properties, and clinical applications of nickel-titanium orthodontic wires possessing superelastic characteristics.

Parr JG, and Hanson A: An Introduction to Stainless Steel. Metals Park, OH, American Society for Metals, 1971.

A useful review of the applications, metallurgy, mechanical properties, and corrosion principles for stainless steel.

Sarkar NK, Redmond W, Schwaninger B, and Goldberg AJ: The chloride corrosion behavior of four orthodontic wires. J Oral Rehabil 10:121, 1983.

A classic article that presents the in vitro cyclic potentiodynamic polarization of stainless steel, cobalt-chromium-nickel, beta-titanium, and nickel-titanium orthodontic wires.

Thompson SA: An overview of nickel-titanium alloys used in dentistry. Int Endod J 33:297, 2000.

A recent review article that describes the shape memory effect and the manufacture of nickel-titanium endodontic instruments.

Walia H, Brantley WA, and Gerstein H: An initial investigation of the bending and torsional properties of Nitinol root canal files. J Endod 14:346, 1988.

The original article that stimulated the interest of the endodontic profession and manufacturers in the use of nickel-titanium root canal instruments.

21
Dental Ceramics

Kenneth J. Anusavice

OUTLINE

What Are Ceramics?

History of Dental Ceramics

Classification of Dental Ceramics

Ceramic Processing Methods

Metal-Ceramic Prostheses

Ceramic Prostheses

Methods of Strengthening Ceramics

Abrasiveness of Dental Ceramics

Clinical Performance of Ceramic Prostheses

Porcelain Denture Teeth

Factors Affecting the Color of Ceramics

Chemical Attack of Glass-Phase Ceramics by Acidulated Phosphate Fluoride

Criteria for Selection and Use of Dental Ceramics

KEY TERMS

Alumina core—A ceramic containing sufficient crystalline alumina (Al_2O_3) to achieve adequate strength and opacity when used for producing the core structure of ceramic prostheses.

Aluminous porcelain—A ceramic composed of a glass matrix phase and at least 35 vol% Al_2O_3.

Body porcelain (also dentin or gingival porcelain)—A veneering ceramic for ceramic or metal-ceramic prostheses.

CAD-CAM ceramic—A ceramic that is formulated for the production of the whole or part of an all-ceramic prosthesis through the use of a computer-aided design and computer-aided manufacturing process.

Castable ceramic—A glass or other ceramic specially formulated to be cast into a refractory mold to produce a core coping or core framework for a ceramic prosthesis.

Ceramic—An inorganic compound with nonmetallic properties typically composed of metallic (or semimetallic) and nonmetallic elements (e.g., Al_2O_3, CaO, and Si_3N_4).

Copy-milling—The process of cutting or grinding a structure using a device that traces the surface of a master metal, ceramic, or polymer pattern and transfers the traced spatial positions to a cutting station where a blank is cut or ground in a manner similar to a key-cutting procedure.

Core ceramic—An opaque dental ceramic material that provides sufficient strength, toughness, and stiffness to support overlying layers of veneering ceramics.

KEY TERMS—cont'd

Dental ceramic—An inorganic compound with nonmetallic properties typically consisting of oxygen and one or more metallic or semimetallic elements (e.g., aluminum, calcium, lithium, magnesium, potassium, silicon, sodium, tin, titanium, and zirconium) that is formulated to produce the whole or part of a ceramic-based dental prosthesis.

Feldspathic porcelain—A ceramic composed of a glass matrix phase and one or more crystalline phases (such as leucite, $K_2O \cdot Al_2O_3 \cdot 4SiO_2$).

Glass—An inorganic nonmetallic compound that lacks a crystalline structure.

Glass-ceramic—A ceramic consisting of a glass matrix phase and at least one crystal phase that is produced by the controlled crystallization of the glass.

Glass-infiltrated ceramic—A minimally sintered core ceramic with a porous structure that has been densified by the capillary inflow of a molten glass.

Glaze ceramic—A specially formulated ceramic powder that, when mixed with a liquid, applied to a ceramic surface, and heated to an appropriate temperature for a sufficient time, forms a smooth glassy layer on a dental ceramic surface (see **natural glaze**).

Green state—A term referring to an as-pressed condition before sintering.

Metal-ceramic prosthesis—A partial crown, full crown, or fixed partial denture made with a metal substrate to which porcelain is bonded for aesthetic enhancement via an intermediate metal oxide layer. The terms *porcelain-fused-to-metal* (PFM), *porcelain-bonded-to-metal* (PBM), *porcelain-to-metal* (PTM), and *ceramometal* are also used to describe these prostheses, but *metal-ceramic* is the preferred term.

Natural glaze—A vitrified layer that forms on the surface of a dental ceramic containing a glass phase when the ceramic is heated to a glazing temperature for a specified time.

Overglaze—The surface coating of glass formed by fusing a thin layer of glass powder (see **glaze ceramic**) that matures at a lower temperature than that associated with the ceramic substrate.

Pressable ceramic (hot-pressed ceramic)—A ceramic that can be heated to a specified temperature and forced under pressure to fill a cavity in a refractory mold.

Shoulder porcelain—A ceramic that is formulated to be sintered at the cervical area of a metal-ceramic crown to produce an aesthetic and fracture-resistant butt-joint margin.

Sintering—The process of heating closely packed particles to a specified temperature (below the melting point of the main component) to densify and strengthen a structure as a result of bonding, diffusion, and flow phenomena.

Slip casting—A process used to form "green" ceramic shapes by applying a slurry of ceramic particles and water or a special liquid to a porous substrate (such as a die material), thereby allowing capillary action to remove water and densify the mass of deposited particles.

Spinel—A crystalline mineral composed of mixed oxides such as $MgAl_2O_4$ ($MgO \cdot Al_2O_3$). Also spelled *spinelle*.

Stain ceramic—A mixture of one or more pigmented metal oxides and a low-fusing glass that can modify the shade of the ceramic-based restoration when it is dispersed in an aqueous slurry or monomer medium, applied to the surface of porcelain or other dental ceramic, and heated to its vitrification temperature for a specific time.

Thermal compatibility—A condition of low transient and residual tensile stress in ceramic adjacent to a metal or ceramic core that is associated with a small difference in the thermal contraction coefficients between the core material and the veneering ceramic.

CRITICAL QUESTIONS

Which mechanical property is most indicative of a ceramic's susceptibility to fracture in the presence of surface flaws? How does transformation toughening increase the resistance to such fractures? Why is pure zirconia not useful as a dental ceramic?

Restorative and prosthetic materials used currently in dentistry can be grouped into one of four categories: (1) metals, (2) polymers, (3) composites, and (4) **ceramics.**

Dental prosthetic alloys are characterized by their high tensile strength, toughness, hardness, resistance to abrasion, fracture resistance, elasticity, ductility, and fatigue resistance. Polymers are generally inferior in most of these properties, highlighted by their potential for brittle fracture. Compared with dental alloys, composites are also susceptible to brittle fracture, although they are far superior in their potential to produce superb aesthetic restorations. Other advantages are their thermal and electrical insulation ability.

Ceramics are very susceptible to fracture when they are exposed to tensile or flexural stresses. Compared with ceramics, alloys used in dentistry are generally very strong and resistant to fracture when subjected to different types of stresses. Ceramics can be classified in one of four categories: (1) silicate ceramics, (2) oxide ceramics, (3) nonoxide ceramics, and (4) **glass-ceramics.** Silicate ceramics are characterized by an amorphous **glass** phase with a porous structure. The main components are SiO_2 with small additions of crystalline Al_2O_3, MgO, ZrO_2, and/or other oxides. Dental porcelains fall into this category.

Oxide ceramics contain a principal crystalline phase (e.g., Al_2O_3, MgO, ThO_2, or ZrO_2) with either no glass phase or a small content of glass phase. Zirconia is of major dental importance because of its high fracture toughness. Pure ZrO_2 is not a useful **dental ceramic** because cracks occur during **sintering** as a result of a phase transformation from the tetragonal to the monoclinic structure. This transformation can be fully or partially suppressed by the addition of certain other oxides such as MgO, Y_2O_3, CaO, and CeO. One of the more recent ceramic materials for dental prostheses is ZrO_2 fully stabilized with yttria (Y_2O_3); this is sometimes designated as Y-CSZ. Multicomponent or mixed oxide structures may also be useful for dental applications. Three examples of this class of ceramics include $MgO \cdot Al_2O_3$ **(spinel)**, $3Al_2O_3 \cdot 2SiO_2$ (mullite), and $Al_2O_3 \cdot TiO_2$ (Al_2TiO_5 or aluminum titanate). The spinel structure is used in a **glass-infiltrated ceramic** (In-Ceram Spinell) when greater translucency is required compared with glass-infiltrated alumina or zirconia.

Nonoxide ceramics are impractical for use in dentistry; the reasons for their impracticality vary but usually involve either their high processing temperatures, complex processing methods, or unaesthetic color and opacity. Such ceramics include borides (TiB_2, ZrB_2), carbides (B_4C, SiC, TiC, WC), nitrides (AlN, BN, Si_3N_4, TiN), selenide ($ZnSe$), silicide ($MoSi_2$), sialon (Si_3N_4 with Al_2O_3), and syalon (Si_3N_4 with Al_2O_3 and Y_2O_3).

WHAT ARE CERAMICS?

Dental ceramics may consist primarily of glasses, porcelains, glass-ceramics, or highly crystalline structures. Dental ceramics exhibit chemical, mechanical, physical, and thermal properties that distinguish them from other materials such as metals and acrylic resins. The properties of ceramics are customized for dental applications by precise control of the type and amount of the components used in their production. Ceramics are more resistant to corrosion than plastics, and metals are much tougher than either ceramics or plastics. Ceramics generally do not react with most liquids, gases, alkalis, and acids. Ceramics also remain stable over long time periods. Dental ceramics exhibit fair to excellent flexure strength and fracture toughness. One of the strongest ceramics, zirconium dioxide, has a flexure strength similar to that of steel, although the fracture toughness of steel is far greater than that of zirconia. Although ceramics are strong, temperature-resistant, and resilient, these materials are brittle and may fracture when flexed or when quickly heated and cooled. Most dental ceramics are compounds of oxygen with lighter metals or semimetals (metalloids) that have some properties of metals and nonmetals, but they are generally nonmetallic in nature. Typical compositions of **feldspathic porcelains** and an aluminous core porcelain are provided in Table 21-1.

Glass-ceramics are partially crystallized glasses that are produced by nucleation and growth of crystals in the glass matrix phase. An example of such a product that has been used in dentistry is Dicor glass-ceramic, which was based on the growth of tetrasilicic fluormica crystals in a glass matrix. This material was originally supplied as glass ingots (containing a nucleating agent) that were melted and cast into a refractory mold and subsequently processed thermally to produce the crystal phase. Casting of glass forms is no longer applied for producing dental prostheses, although certain glass-ceramics have been used for CAD-CAM processing systems.

Dental ceramics are nonmetallic, inorganic structures, primarily containing compounds of oxygen with one or more metallic or semimetallic elements (aluminum, calcium, lithium, magnesium, phosphorus, potassium, silicon, sodium, titanium, and zirconium). Ceramic structures composed of a single element are rare. The diamond structure is a major ceramic of this type and the unit cell consists of carbon atoms, each one sharing an electron with each of four surrounding carbon atoms. This structure is bonded by strong covalent forces, which result in a high elastic modulus, high temperature stability in an oxygen-free environment (up to at least 3700° C), and the highest hardness of any natural material.

| Table 21-1 | Typical Compositions of Some Dental Porcelains |

| Component | Low-fusing vacuum porcelain | | | Metal-ceramic porcelain | | |
| | | | | Low-fusing | | Ultralow-fusing* |
	Aluminous core	Dentin	Enamel	Dentin	Enamel	Dentin
SiO_2	35.0	66.5	64.7	59.2	63.5	60–70
Al_2O_3	53.8	13.5	13.9	18.5	18.9	5–10
CaO	1.1	2.1	1.8	—	—	1.0–3.0
Na_2O	2.8	4.2	4.8	4.8	5.0	10–15
K_2O	4.2	7.1	7.5	11.8	12.3	10–15
B_2O_3	3.2	6.6	7.3	4.6	0.1	0–1.0
ZnO	—	—	—	0.6	0.1	—
ZrO_2	—	—	—	0.4	0.1	0–1.0
Other	—	—	—	—	—	BaO, Y_2O_3: 0–0.2
						SnO_2: 0–0.2
						Li_2O: 0–1.0
						F: 0–1.0
						Sb_2O_3: 0–1.0
						CeO_2: 0–0.2
						TiO_2: 1–3
Firing temperature (°C)	980	980	950	900	900	650–700

Modified from Yamada H and Grenoble P: Dental Porcelain—State of the Art, Proceedings, University of Southern California, 1977, p 26.
*Duceram LFC: Modified from Kappert HF, and Krah MK, Keramiken—eine Übersicht, Quintessenz Zahntech 27(6):668-704, 2001.

Many dental ceramics contain a crystal phase and a glass phase based on the silica structure. This structure is characterized by a Si-O tetrahedron in which a Si^{4+} cation is positioned at the center of a tetrahedron with O^- anions at each of the four corners. The resulting structure is not close-packed, and it has both covalent and ionic characteristics. The SiO_4 tetrahedra are linked together by sharing their corners.

Dentists have searched for the ideal restorative material for many years. Although direct restorative materials such as amalgam, composites, and cements have been used with reasonably good success during the past several decades, they are not ideal for large restorations or for fixed partial dentures (FPDs). For many single-unit restorations aesthetic results are critically important. In this regard the restorative material should maintain its surface quality and aesthetic characteristics over an extended period of time, preferably for the lifetime of the patient. Dental ceramics are attractive because of their biocompatibility, long-term color stability, wear resistance, and their ability to be formed into precise shapes, although in some cases they require costly processing equipment and specialized training.

Dentists and their laboratory technicians must understand the benefits and limitations of the properties of dental ceramics and their design requirements to minimize the risk for catastrophic fractures that require costly repairs or replacements and which cause patients to make potentially unnecessary return visits to the dental office. This chapter focuses on these properties and highlights processing and design factors that play a major role in ensuring long-term clinical success of ceramic-based prostheses. Although other ceramic products and processing methods will be introduced in the future, the principles for selection and use of ceramics based on the properties and microstructural characteristics of these ceramics and the fundamental concepts of prosthesis design will endure.

Most ceramics are characterized by their refractory nature, high hardness, susceptibility to brittle fracture at relatively low stresses (relatively low tensile strength and essentially zero percent elongation), and chemical inertness. For dental applications a hardness of a ceramic less than that of enamel and an easily polishable surface are desirable to minimize the wear damage that can be produced on enamel by the ceramic surface. A **glazed ceramic** surface is generally considered beneficial by increasing the fracture resistance and reducing the potential abrasiveness of ceramic surfaces. The strength values of glazed and nonglazed porcelains are given in Table 21-2.

The susceptibility of ceramics to brittle fracture is a drawback, particularly when flaws and tensile stress coexist in the same region of a ceramic restoration. Chemical inertness is an important characteristic because it ensures that the surface of dental

Table 21-2	Flexural Strength of Glazed and Nonglazed Medium-Fusing Dental Porcelain and Aluminous Porcelain		
Type	Firing environment	Surface condition	Flexural strength (MPa)
Feldspathic porcelain	Air	Ground	75.8
	Air	Glazed	141.0
	Vacuum	Ground	79.6
	Vacuum	Glazed	132.0
Aluminous porcelain	Air	Ground	136.0
	Air	Glazed	139.0

Modified from McLean JW, and Hughes TH: The reinforcement of dental porcelain with ceramic oxides. Br Dent J, 119:251, 1965.

restorations does not release potentially harmful elements and it reduces the risk for surface roughening and susceptibility to bacterial adhesion over time. Two other important attributes of dental ceramics are their potential for matching the appearance of natural teeth and their insulating properties (low thermal conductivity, thermal diffusivity, and electrical conductivity). Because the metal atoms transfer their outermost electrons to the nonmetallic atoms and thereby stabilize their highly mobile electrons, ceramics are excellent thermal and electrical insulators.

CRITICAL QUESTION

Which technological developments have significantly improved the quality and properties of ceramic and metal-ceramic prostheses?

HISTORY OF DENTAL CERAMICS

During the Stone Age more than 10,000 years ago, ceramics were important materials, and they have retained their importance in human societies ever since. Craftsmen of this era used rocks that could be shaped into tools and artifacts by a process called *flaking*, in which stone chips could be fractured away from surfaces of hard, fine-grained, or amorphous rocks including chert, flint, ignimbrite, indurated shale, lava, obsidian, quartz, and silicified limestone. In approximately 700 B.C. the Etruscans made teeth of ivory and bone that were held in place by a gold framework. Animal bone and ivory from the hippopotamus or elephant were used for many years thereafter. Later, human teeth sold by the poor and teeth obtained from the dead were used, but dentists generally disliked this option.

The first porcelain tooth material was patented in 1789 by a French dentist (de Chemant) in collaboration with a French pharmacist (Duchateau). The product, an improved version of "mineral paste teeth" that was produced in 1774 by Duchateau, was introduced in England soon thereafter by de Chemant. However, this baked compound was not used to produce individual teeth because there was no effective way at that time to attach the teeth to a denture base material.

In 1808, Fonzi, an Italian dentist, invented a "terrometallic" porcelain tooth that was held in place by a platinum pin or frame. Planteau, a French dentist, introduced porcelain teeth to the United States in 1817, and Peale, an artist, developed a baking process in Philadelphia for these teeth in 1822. Commercial production of these teeth began in 1825 by Stockton. In England, Ash developed an improved version of the porcelain tooth in 1837. In Germany, Pfaff developed a technique to make impressions of the mouth using plaster of Paris in 1756, but it was not until 1839 that the invention of vulcanized rubber allowed porcelain denture teeth to be used effectively in a denture base. In 1844, the nephew of Stockton founded the S.S. White Company, and this led to further refinement of the design and the mass production of porcelain denture teeth.

Dr. Charles Land introduced one of the first ceramic crowns to dentistry in 1903. Land, who was the grandfather of aviator Charles Lindbergh, described a technique for fabricating ceramic crowns using a platinum foil matrix and high-fusing feldspathic porcelain. These crowns exhibited excellent aesthetics, but the low flexural strength of porcelain resulted in a high incidence of failures.

Since then, feldspathic porcelains with reliable chemical bonding have been used in metal-ceramic prostheses for more than 35 years. A schematic illustration of a cross-section of a metal-ceramic crown is shown in Figure 21-1. Unfortunately,

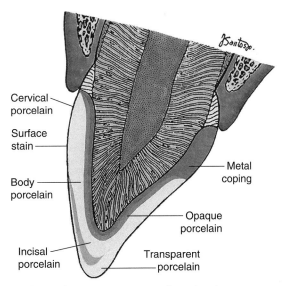

Cervical porcelain

Surface stain

Body porcelain

Incisal porcelain

Metal coping

Opaque porcelain

Transparent porcelain

Fig. 21-1 Cross-section of a metal-ceramic crown. See also color plate.

feldspathic porcelains have been too weak to use reliably in the construction of all-ceramic crowns without a cast-metal core or metal-foil coping. Furthermore, their firing shrinkage causes significant discrepancies in fit and adaptation of margins unless correction bakes are made.

Two of the most important breakthroughs responsible for the long-standing superb aesthetic performance and clinical survivability of metal-ceramic restorations are the patents of Weinstein and Weinstein (1962) and Weinstein et al (1962). One of these patents described the formulations of feldspathic porcelain that allowed systematic control of the sintering temperature and thermal expansion coefficient. The other patent described the components that could be used to produce alloys that bonded chemically to and were thermally compatible with feldspathic porcelains. The first commercial porcelain was developed by Vita Zahnfabrik in about 1963. Although the first Vita porcelain products were known for their aesthetic properties, the subsequent introduction of the more versatile Ceramco porcelain led to thermal expansion behavior that allowed this porcelain to be used safely with a wider variety of alloys.

A significant improvement in the fracture resistance of porcelain crowns was reported by McLean and Hughes in 1965 when a dental aluminous **core ceramic** consisting of a glass matrix containing between 40 and 50 wt% Al_2O_3 was used. Because of inadequate translucency (opaque, chalky-white appearance) of the **aluminous porcelain** core material, a veneer of feldspathic porcelain was required to achieve acceptable aesthetics. The flexural strength (modulus of rupture) of the core material was approximately 131 MPa. McLean (1979) reported a low 5-year failure rate of only 2% for anterior crowns but an unacceptably high failure rate of 15% when aluminous porcelain was used for molar crowns. Furthermore, because of the large sintering shrinkage (approximately 15%–20%) of the aluminous porcelain core material at its high firing temperature, and the use of a 20- to 25-μm–thick platinum foil, excellent marginal adaptation was difficult to achieve except by highly skilled laboratory technicians. Because of its relatively high fracture rate in posterior sites, the principal indication for use of aluminous porcelain crowns is the restoration of maxillary anterior crowns when aesthetics is of paramount importance and when no other ceramic product is available.

Since the introduction of aluminous porcelain crowns in the early 1900s and the methods to produce durable metal-ceramic crowns in the 1960s, improvements in both the composition of ceramics and the method of forming the ceramic core of ceramic crowns have greatly enhanced our ability to produce more accurate and fracture-resistant crowns made entirely of ceramic material.

Recent developments for metal-ceramics such as opalescent porcelain, specialized internal staining techniques, greening-resistant porcelains, and porcelain shoulder margins have significantly enhanced the overall appearance of metal-ceramic crowns and bridges and the clinical survivability of these prostheses. Improvement in all-ceramic systems developed by controlled crystallization of a glass (Dicor) was demonstrated by Adair and Grossman (1984). This glass was melted and cast into a refractory mold and subsequently crystallized to form the Dicor glass-ceramic that contained tetrasilicic fluormica crystals in a glass matrix. A further development was the introduction of a machinable glass-ceramic version (Dicor MGC), which has a tetrasilicic fluormica crystal volume of approximately 70%. In the early 1990s a pressable glass-ceramic (IPS Empress) containing approximately 34 vol% leucite was introduced that provided a strength and marginal adaptation similar to those of Dicor glass-ceramic but required no specialized crystallization treatment. Neither of these materials was indicated for producing FPDs. Subsequently, a more fracture-resistant, pressable glass-ceramic (IPS Empress2) containing approximately 70 vol% of lithia disilicate crystals was introduced in the late 1990s. This product could be used for 3-unit FPDs up to the second premolar. The fracture toughness of IPS Empress2 glass-ceramic ($3.3\ \mathrm{MPa \cdot m^{1/2}}$) is 2.5 times greater than that of the IPS Empress glass-ceramic ($1.3\ \mathrm{MPa \cdot m^{1/2}}$).

These improvements in both the composition of ceramics and the method of forming the core of an all-ceramic crown have greatly enhanced our ability to produce more accurate and fracture-resistant ceramic crowns made entirely of ceramic. Significant progress has been made toward the goal of developing less abrasive veneering ceramics. In 1992 Duceram LFC (low-fusing ceramic) was marketed as an ultralow-fusing ceramic with three unique features: First, Duceram LFC is a hydrothermal glass in which water is incorporated into the silicate glass structure to produce nonbridging hydroxyl groups that disrupt the glass network, thereby decreasing the glass transition temperature, viscosity, and firing temperature and increasing the thermal expansion coefficient to allow its use as a veneer for certain low-expansion metals. Second, these types of ceramics are also claimed to be "self-healing" through a process of forming a 1-μm–thick hydrothermal layer along the ceramic surface. Third, the extremely small size of the crystal particles (400 to 500 nm) enhances the opalescence of the ceramic by reflecting blue light hues from the surface and yellow hues from the interior of the ceramic. Other ultralow-fusing ceramics (sintering temperatures below 850° C), now commonly referred to as *low-fusing ceramics*, have been introduced as veneering glasses. Some of these veneering ceramics are claimed to be kinder to opposing tooth enamel either because they are predominantly a glass phase material or because they contain very small crystal particles.

This chapter describes the ceramics used for metal-ceramic prostheses; the new generation of ceramics, including Cercon, Lava, In-Ceram Zirconia, IPS Empress2, and Procera AllCeram used for ceramic prostheses; and some of the previously used products that dentists may observe in their dental practices. Soon after IPS Empress2 was introduced, stronger, tougher, and more fracture resistant ceramics were developed, including Procera AllCeram, a dry-pressed, milled, and sintered **alumina core** ceramic; In-Ceram Alumina, a glass-infiltrated alumina core ceramic; In-Ceram Zirconia, a glass-infiltrated zirconia-alumina core ceramic; Lava, a partially sintered or fully sintered zirconia core ingot that is formed by a true CAD-CAM process (by scanning dies without the need for a wax pattern); and Cercon, a presintered zirconia ceramic that is milled to an enlarged size in the **green state** based on scanning of a wax pattern. It is also possible to scan prepared teeth and mill a prosthesis using the Cerec system (Sirona Corporation). The Cerec 1 system was introduced in the mid-1980s, and improvements in software and hardware led to the Cerec 2 and Cerec 3 systems for production of ceramic inlays, onlays, and veneers.

Dental ceramic technology is one of the fastest growing areas of dental materials research and development. During the past two decades numerous types of ceramics and processing methods have been introduced. Some of these materials can be formed into inlays, onlays, veneers, crowns, and FPDs, and several of the core ceramics can be resin-bonded micromechanically to tooth structure. The future of dental ceramics is bright because the increased demand for tooth-colored restorations will lead to an increased demand for ceramic-based and polymer-based restorations and the reduced use of amalgam and traditional cast metals.

CRITICAL QUESTION

Which four principal variables most strongly affect the fracture resistance of ceramic FPDs?

CLASSIFICATION OF DENTAL CERAMICS

Many different types of dental ceramics are available from dental laboratories. These include core ceramic, liner ceramic, margin ceramic, opaque dentin (also, body or gingival) ceramic, dentin ceramic, enamel (incisal) ceramic, **stain ceramic, glaze ceramic,** and addition ceramic. These products can be classified in several possible ways according to their: (1) use or indications (anterior, posterior, crowns, veneers, post and cores, FPDs, stain ceramic, and glaze ceramic); (2) composition (pure alumina, pure zirconia, silica glass, leucite-based glass-ceramic, and lithia-based glass-ceramic); (3) processing method (sintering, partial sintering and glass infiltration, CAD-CAM, and **copy-milling**); (4) firing temperature (low-fusing, medium-fusing, and high-fusing); (5) microstructure (glass, crystalline, and crystal-containing glass); (6) translucency (opaque, translucent, and transparent); (7) fracture resistance; or (8) abrasiveness. To allow a clinician to select the best material for a given clinical situation, this chapter describes the relative characteristics of dental ceramics as a function of one or more of these classifications.

The dentist and lab technician are faced with the complex challenge of deciding which ceramic should be used for each specific clinical situation. Although some ceramics are recommended for posterior 3-unit ceramic FPDs, the use of all-metal FPDs or metal-ceramic FPDs should first be considered because the latter prostheses will definitely have a much greater life expectancy relative to the fracture resistance of the prostheses. Only when a patient is highly resistant to accepting metallic components during the treatment planning discussions should all-ceramic FPDs be considered for posterior sites. The fracture resistance of posterior all-ceramic FPDs is based on (1) the strength and fracture toughness of the ceramic components, (2) the connector dimensions (minimum height of), (3) the connector shape (gingival embrasures must have large radii of curvature), and (4) the patient's biting force. The selection of ceramic for these prostheses is a very risky proposition since optimal conditions for their success are not yet known. For the few clinical studies that have been published, insufficient data have been reported on connector size and shape as a function of the patients' biting force capabilities.

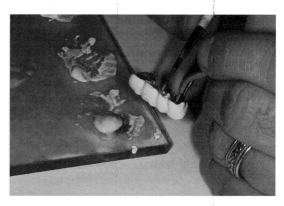

Fig. 21-2 Condensation of porcelain slurry on a metal framework for a four-unit fixed partial denture (FPD). See also color plate.

There are several categories of dental ceramics: conventional leucite-containing porcelain, leucite-enriched porcelain, ultralow-fusing porcelain that may contain leucite, glass-ceramic, specialized core ceramics (alumina, glass-infiltrated alumina, glass-infiltrated spinel, and glass-infiltrated zirconia), and **CAD-CAM ceramics.** Dental ceramics can be classified by type (feldspathic porcelain, leucite-reinforced porcelain, aluminous porcelain, alumina, glass-infiltrated alumina, glass-infiltrated spinel, glass-infiltrated zirconia and glass-ceramic), by use (denture teeth, metal-ceramics, veneers, inlays, crowns, anterior bridges, and posterior bridges), by processing method (sintering, casting, or machining), or by substructure material (cast metal, swaged metal, glass-ceramic, CAD-CAM porcelain, or sintered ceramic core). Methods of fabricating ceramic restorations include condensation and sintering (Fig. 21-2), pressure molding and sintering, casting and ceramming, slip-casting, sintering and glass infiltration, and milling by computer control. A classification of ceramic types by processing method is given in Table 21-3.

CRITICAL QUESTIONS

Which processing technique is most likely to cause damage to ceramic surfaces? What type of material is most likely to resist such damage?

CERAMIC PROCESSING METHODS

The single-unit crown may be a metal-ceramic crown (also called a *porcelain-fused-to-metal crown*), a traditional aluminous porcelain crown based on a core of aluminous porcelain, or the newer ceramic crowns based on a core of leucite-reinforced porcelain, injection- or pressure-molded leucite-based ceramic, glass-ceramic, sintered aluminous porcelain, sintered aluminum oxide, pressure-molded aluminum oxide, glass-infiltrated aluminum oxide, or glass-ceramic processed from cast glass. The types of restoration, with their variations, are discussed in detail in succeeding sections.

The processing stages of the ceramic core for production of ceramic prostheses are summarized in Table 21-3. These seven different processes represent the main procedures that were available in 2003. The quality of the final ceramic prosthesis is dependent on each stage of the fabrication process. Machining or grinding of the core structure is of particular importance since flaws or minute cracks can be introduced that can possibly be propagated to the point of fracture during subsequent

Table 21-3 Methods of Processing the Ceramic Core Form of a Ceramic Prosthesis

Initial forming method	Examples	Initial material form	Second processing method	Subsequent form	Subsequent process
Condensation	Aluminous porcelain (Vitadur-N, Hi-Ceram)	Powder and mixing liquid	Sintering of core ceramic	Dense core ceramic (less than 5 vol% porosity)	Application of veneering ceramic
Hot-pressing	IPS Empress2, OPC 3G, Finesse All Ceramic	High-quality ceramic ingot	Stain only or stain and glaze (inlays) or veneering ceramic	Stained/glazed inlay or veneered core	Stain and/or glaze for crowns and FPDs
Casting	Dicor	Glass ingot	Crystallization heat treatment (ceramming)	Glass-ceramic core containing a glass phase and tetrasilicic fluormica crystals	Application of shading porcelain
Slip-casting	In-Ceram Alumina, In-Ceram Spinell, In-Ceram Zirconia	Powder and mixing liquid	Partial sintering	Partially sintered core	Glass infiltration, trimming of excess glass, and application of veneering ceramic
Computer-aided machining/ milling (CAM)	Cerec Vitablocs (several types of core ceramics)	High-quality ceramic ingot	Margin repair (if necessary)	High-quality core possibly with repaired margin	Application of veneering ceramic
Computer-aided machining/ milling (CAM) of presintered form	Cercon and Lava	Partially sintered ceramic block	Final sintering of machined/ ground core and margin repair (if necessary)	Fully sintered core possibly with repaired margin	Application of veneering ceramic
Copy-milling	A variety of ceramic products	High-quality ceramic block	Margin repair (if necessary)	High-quality core possibly with repaired margin	Application of veneering ceramic
Milling of dry-pressed powder on enlarged die	Procera AllCeram	Dry pressed and machined alumina block	Sintering	High-quality core containing 99.9% alumina	Application of veneering ceramic

intraoral stressing cycles. The use of computer-aided manufacture (CAM) processes are most likely to induce such damage, although the ceramics with higher fracture toughness are less likely to exhibit such damage. It is possible that subsequent sintering or veneering procedures can reduce the potential for propagation of cracks in the prostheses while in service. However, insufficient data are available from clinical studies of ceramics.

The processing procedures for these ceramics are as follows. The feldspathic porcelain of traditional PFM restorations, some aluminous porcelains (Vitadur-N, Hi-Ceram), and pure alumina ceramic (Procera AllCeram) are condensed by vibration or dry-pressed (Procera) and sintered at high temperatures. **Pressable ceramics** (e.g., IPS Empress, IPS Empress2, Finesse All-Ceramic, OPC, and OPC-3G), when heated and subjected to hydrostatic pressure, flow into a mold and, after removal and divesting, are then veneered. Cast and cerammed crowns, such as the obsolete product Dicor, are made using the lost-wax technique. The molten glass is cast into a mold, heat-treated to form a glass-ceramic, and colored with shading porcelain and surface stains.

For **slip cast** ceramics (In-Ceram, In-Ceram Spinell, and In-Ceram Zirconia), a slurry of liquid and particles of alumina, magnesia-alumina silicate (spinel), or zirconia is placed on a dry refractory die that draws out the water from the slurry. The slip-cast deposit is sintered on this die, and then it is coated with a slurry of a glass-phase layer. During firing, the glass melts and infiltrates the porous ceramic core. Translucent porcelain veneers are then fired onto the core to provide the final contour and color.

For CAD-CAM processes, the ceramic block materials (Dicor MGC, Vita Cerec Mk I, and Vita Cerec Mk II) are shaped into inlays or crowns using a CAD-CAM system (Cerec). *CAM* refers to computer-aided milling or machining. This process is sometimes referred to as a *CAD-CIM process*, where *CIM* refers to computer-integrated machining or milling. These blocks can also be used in copy-milling devices (Celay) that mill or machine blocks into core shapes in a manner similar to that for cutting a key from a key blank, that is, by tracing over a master die of the shape to be produced out of the ceramic.

CRITICAL QUESTION

What is the potential benefit of the ultralow-fusing veneering ceramics (sintering temperature <850° C) over the traditional low-fusing porcelains (sintering temperatures of 850°–1100° C)?

METAL-CERAMIC PROSTHESES
Composition of Dental Porcelains

The composition of the noble and base metal alloys used in metal-ceramic restorations was discussed in Chapter 19. The reader is referred to the description of metal-ceramic restorations and the effects and purposes of the constituent metals.

The composition of the ceramic generally corresponds to that of the glasses in Table 21-1, except for an increased alkali content. The addition of greater quantities of soda, potash, and/or leucite is necessary to increase the thermal expansion to a level compatible with the metal coping. The opaque porcelains also contain relatively large amounts of metallic oxide opacifiers to conceal the underlying metal and to minimize the thickness of the opaque layer.

The high-contraction porcelains have a greater tendency to devitrify because of their alkali content. They should not be subjected to repeated firing, because this may increase the risk for cloudiness within the porcelain, as well as changes in the thermal contraction behavior. Thus it is obvious that a proper matching of the properties of the alloy and porcelain is imperative to success. Criteria and test methods for determining metal–porcelain compatibility have been suggested. Testing methods are focused on the measurement of coefficients of thermal expansion and contraction, thermal shock resistance, and the strength of the bond, which are discussed later.

Conventional dental porcelain is a vitreous ceramic based on a silica (SiO_2) network and potash feldspar ($K_2O \cdot Al_2O_3 \cdot 6SiO_2$) or soda feldspar ($Na_2O \cdot Al_2O_3 \cdot 6SiO_2$) or both. Pigments, opacifiers, and glasses are added to control the fusion temperature, sintering temperature, thermal contraction coefficient, and solubility. The feldspars used for dental porcelains are relatively pure and colorless. Thus pigments must be added to produce the hues of natural teeth or the color appearance of tooth-colored restorative materials that may exist in adjacent teeth.

Silica (SiO_2) can exist in four different forms: crystalline quartz, crystalline cristobalite, crystalline tridymite, and noncrystalline fused silica. Fused silica is a material whose high-melting temperature is attributed to the three-dimensional network of covalent bonds between silica tetrahedra, which are the basic structural units of the glass network. Fluxes (low-fusing glasses) are often included to reduce the temperature required to sinter the porcelain powder particles together at low enough temperatures so that the alloy to which it is fired does not melt or sustain sag (flexural creep) deformation.

Glass Modifiers

The sintering temperature of crystalline silica is too high for use in veneering aesthetic layers bonded to metal substrates. At such temperatures the alloys would melt. In addition, the thermal contraction coefficient of crystalline silica is too low for these alloys. Bonds between the silica tetrahedra can be broken by the addition of alkali metal ions such as sodium, potassium, and calcium. These ions are associated with the oxygen atoms at the corners of the tetrahedra and interrupt the oxygen-silicon bonds. As a result, the three-dimensional silica network contains many linear chains of silica tetrahedra that are able to move more easily at lower temperatures than the atoms that are locked into the three-dimensional structure of silica tetrahedra. This ease of movement is responsible for the increased fluidity (decreased viscosity), lower softening temperature, and increased thermal expansion conferred by glass modifiers. Too high a modifier concentration, however, reduces the chemical durability (resistance to attack by water, acids, and alkalis) of the glass. In addition, if too many tetrahedra are disrupted, the glass may crystallize (devitrify) during porcelain firing operations. Hence, a balance between a suitable melting range and good chemical durability must be maintained.

Manufacturers employ glass modifiers to produce dental porcelains with different firing temperatures. Dental porcelains are classified according to their firing temperatures. A typical classification is as follows:

High fusing	1300° C (2372° F)
Medium fusing	1101°–1300° C (2013°–2072° F)
Low fusing	850°–1100° C (1562°–2012° F)
Ultra-low fusing	<850° C (1562° F)

The medium-fusing and high-fusing types are used for the production of denture teeth. The low-fusing and ultralow-fusing porcelains are used for crown and bridge construction. Some of the ultralow-fusing porcelains are used for titanium and titanium alloys because of their low contraction coefficients that closely match those of these metals and because the low firing temperatures reduce the risk for growth of the metal oxide. However, some of these ultralow-fusing porcelains contain enough leucite to raise their thermal contraction coefficients as high as those of conventional low-fusing porcelains. The potential advantages of ultralow-fusing veneering ceramics are the reduction in sintering times, decrease in sag deformation of FPD frameworks, less thermal degradation of ceramic firing ovens, and less wear of opposing enamel surfaces.

Because commercial dental laboratories do not fabricate denture teeth for complete dentures or removable partial dentures, it has become more common to classify crown and bridge porcelains as high-fusing (850–1100° C) and low-fusing (<850° C). However, this change in classification has not been universally adopted. Thus, to avoid confusion, the sintering temperature range should be identified (at least initially) in discussions between dentists and dental technicians so that the less-abrasive benefit claimed for ultralow-fusing ceramics can be easily differentiated from the potentially more abrasive low-fusing porcelains that were used exclusively between the 1960s and 1990s.

Because it ensures adequate chemical durability, self-glazing of porcelain is preferred to an add-on glaze. A thin external layer of glassy material is formed during a self-glaze firing procedure at a temperature and time that cause localized softening of the glass phase and settling of crystalline particles within the surface region. The add-on glaze slurry material that is applied to the porcelain surface for an applied glaze procedure contains more glass modifiers and thus has a lower firing temperature. However, a higher proportion of glass modifiers tends to reduce the resistance of the applied glazes to leaching by oral fluids.

Another important glass modifier is water, although it is not an intentional addition to dental porcelain. The hydronium ion, H_3O^+, can replace sodium or other metal ions in a ceramic that contains glass modifiers. This fact accounts for the phenomenon of "slow crack growth" of ceramics that are exposed to tensile stresses and moist environments. It also may account for the occasional long-term failure of porcelain restorations after several years of service.

Feldspathic Porcelains

Potassium and sodium feldspar are naturally occurring minerals composed primarily of potash (K_2O) and soda (Na_2O), respectively. They also contain alumina (Al_2O_3), and silica (SiO_2) components. Feldspars are used in the preparation of many dental porcelains designed for metal-ceramic crowns and many other dental glasses and ceramics. When potassium feldspar is mixed with various metal oxides and fired to high temperatures, it can form leucite and a glass phase that will soften and flow slightly. The softening of this glass phase during porcelain firing allows the porcelain powder particles to coalesce together. For dental porcelains, the process by which the particles coalesce is called *liquid-phase sintering*, a process controlled by diffusion between particles at a temperature sufficiently high to form a dense solid. The driving force for sintering is the decrease in energy caused by a reduction in surface area. As explained in the key terms section, three dental products (In-Ceram Alumina, Spinell, and Zirconia) are slightly sintered to produce interconnected pore channels that are necessary for subsequent glass infiltration.

Another important property of feldspar is its tendency to form the crystalline mineral leucite when melted. Leucite is a potassium-aluminum-silicate mineral with a large coefficient of thermal expansion (20 to 25 ppm/° C) compared with feldspar glasses (which have coefficients of thermal expansion less than 10 ppm/° C). When feldspar is heated at temperatures between 1150° C and 1530° C, it undergoes incongruent melting to form crystals of leucite in a liquid glass. Incongruent melting is the process by which one material melts to form a liquid plus a different crystalline material. This tendency of feldspar to form leucite during incongruent melting is used to advantage in the manufacture of porcelains for metal bonding. Further information is provided in the sintering of porcelain section.

Many dental glasses do not contain leucite as a raw material. Since feldspar is not essential as a precursor to the formation of leucite, as described earlier, these glasses are modified with additions of leucite to control their thermal contraction coefficients.

Feldspathic porcelains contain a variety of oxide components, including SiO_2 (52–62 wt%), Al_2O_3 (11–16 wt%), K_2O (9–11 wt%), Na_2O (5–7 wt%), and certain additives, including Li_2O and B_2O_3. These ceramics are called *porcelains* because they contain a glass matrix and one or more crystal phases. They cannot be classified as *glass-ceramics* because crystal formation does not occur through controlled nucleation and crystal formation and growth. There are four types of veneering ceramics. These include (1) low-fusing ceramics (feldspar-based porcelain and nepheline syenite-based porcelain); (2) ultra low-fusing ceramics (porcelains and glasses); (3) stains; and (4) glazes (self-glaze and add-on glaze). The particle type and size of crystal particles, if present, will greatly influence the potential abrasiveness of the ceramic prosthesis. A listing of many of the veneering ceramics used for metal-ceramic prostheses is given in Table 21-4.

Table 21-4   Veneering Ceramics for Metal-Ceramic Prostheses

Veneering ceramic	Indications	Manufacturer
Synspar	Most alloys	Pentron
Pencraft Plus	Most alloys	Pentron
Finesse Low Fusing	Most Alloys	Dentsply Ceramco
Ceramco II	Most Alloys	Dentsply Ceramco
Ceramco II Silver	Silver-containing alloys	Dentsply Ceramco
Ceramco 3	Most Alloys	Dentsply Ceramco
Duceragold (hydrothermal)	Degunorm Type IV gold alloy for metal-ceramics	Dentsply Ceramco/Degussa
Duceram Plus	Most alloys	Dentsply Ceramco/Degussa
Duceram LFC	Most alloys	Dentsply Ceramco/Degussa
Excelsior	Most alloys	Dentsply Ceramco/Ney
IPS d.SIGN	Most alloys	Ivoclar Vivadent Inc.
IPS Classic V	Most alloys	Ivoclar Vivadent Inc.
Finesse Low-Fusing	Crown	Dentsply Ceramco
Vita Response	Degunorm (Degussa) and Mainbond A (Heraeus), Type IV gold alloys for metal-ceramics	Vident
Vita VMK 95	Most alloys	Vident
Vita Omega	Most alloys	Vident
Vita Omega 900 (Ultralow-fusing)	Most alloys	Vident

Modified from Kappert HF, and Krah MK, Keramiken—eine Übersicht, Quintessenz Zahntech 27(6):668-704, 2001.

Table 21-5	Thermal Expansion Coefficients of Some Low-Fusing and Ultralow-Fusing Ceramics
Low-fusing ceramics	**Thermal expansion coefficient**
Duceragold	15.8 ppm/° C (25°–500° C)
Duceram	14.2 ppm/° C (25°–600° C)
Duceram Plus	14.2 ppm/° C (25°–600° C)
Duceram LFC	12.2 ppm/° C (25°–500° C)
Finesse	11.8 ppm/° C (25°–500° C)[*]
Duceratin	8.6 ppm/° C (25°–500° C)
AllCeram	7.3 ppm/° C (25°–600° C)

*Data provided by Dentsply Ceramco, Inc.

The thermal expansion coefficients of some ultralow-fusing ceramics (sintering temperatures below 850° C) and low-fusing ceramics are listed in Table 21-5. These ultralow-fusing ceramics represent an exciting new family of ceramic core and veneering materials because of their microstructural features. They contain either a well-distributed dispersion of small crystal particles or few or no crystals, depending on the whether the ceramic is to be used as a veneer or glaze. Initial results of wear studies are promising in several cases relative to reduced enamel wear caused by these ceramics. These results are summarized in a later section of this chapter (see Wear of Enamel by Ceramic Products and Other Restorative Materials).

Other Additives

Other metallic oxides can be introduced, as indicated in Table 21-1. Boric oxide (B_2O_3) behaves as a glass modifier; that is, it decreases viscosity, lowers the softening temperature, and forms its own glass network. Because boric oxide forms a separate lattice interspersed with the silica lattice, it still interrupts the more rigid silica network and lowers the softening point of the glass. Alumina is not considered a true glass former by itself because of the dimensions of the ion and the oxygen/aluminum ratio. Nevertheless, it can take part in the glass network to alter the softening point and viscosity.

Pigmenting oxides are added to obtain the various shades needed to simulate natural teeth. These coloring pigments are produced by fusing metallic oxides together with fine glass and feldspar and then regrinding to a powder. These powders are blended with the unpigmented powdered frit to provide the proper hue and chroma. Examples of metallic oxides and their respective color contributions to porcelain include iron or nickel oxide (brown), copper oxide (green), titanium oxide (yellowish brown), manganese oxide (lavender), and cobalt oxide (blue). Opacity may be achieved by the addition of cerium oxide, zirconium oxide, titanium oxide, or tin oxide.

Aesthetic Potential of Metal-Ceramic Crowns Versus All-Ceramic Crowns

Although metal-ceramic prostheses account for about 70% of all fixed restorations, a metal-ceramic (MC) crown is not the best aesthetic choice for restoring a single maxillary anterior tooth. A ceramic crown offers a greater potential for success in matching the appearance of the adjacent natural tooth, but ceramic crowns are more susceptible to fracture, especially in posterior sites. A dark line at the facial margin of a MC crown occasionally associated with a metal collar or metal margin is of great concern when gingival recession occurs. This effect can be minimized by using a ceramic margin or by using a very thin knife-edge margin of metal coated with opaque **shoulder porcelain.** The technician should polish and glaze this margin to avoid a rough surface at the margin. The use of MC crowns with butt-joint margins or with very thin knife-edge metal margins on the facial surface are successful procedures for improving the aesthetics.

Porcelain Condensation

Porcelain for ceramic and metal-ceramic prostheses, as well as for other applications, is supplied as a fine powder that is designed to be mixed with water or another vehicle and condensed into the desired form (see Fig. 21-2). The powder particles are of a particular size distribution to produce the most densely packed porcelain when they are properly condensed. If the particles are of the same size, the density of packing would not be nearly as high. Thorough condensation is also crucial in obtaining dense packing of the powder particles. Dense packing of the powder particles provides two benefits: lower firing shrinkage and less porosity in the fired porcelain. This packing, or *condensation*, may be achieved by various methods, including vibration, spatulation, and brush techniques.

The first method uses mild vibration to pack the wet powder densely on the underlying framework. The excess water is blotted or wiped away with a clean tissue or fine brush, and condensation occurs toward the blotted or brushed area. In the second method, a small spatula is used to apply and smooth the wet porcelain. The smoothing action brings the excess water to the surface, where it is removed. The third method employs the addition of dry porcelain powder to the surface to absorb the water. The dry powder is placed by a brush to the side opposite from an increment of wet porcelain. As the water is drawn toward the dry powder, the wet particles are pulled together. Whichever method is used, it is important to remember that the surface tension of the water is the driving force for condensation, and the porcelain must never be allowed to dry out until condensation is complete.

Sintering of Porcelain

The thermochemical reactions between the porcelain powder components are virtually completed during the original manufacturing process. Therefore the purpose of firing is simply to sinter the particles of powder together properly to form the prosthesis. Some chemical reactions occur during prolonged firing times or multiple firings. Of particular importance are the observed changes in the leucite content of the porcelains designed for fabrication of metal-ceramic restorations. Leucite is a high-expansion (and high-contraction) crystal phase whose volume fraction in the glass matrix can greatly affect the thermal contraction coefficient of the porcelain. Changes in the leucite content can cause the development of a thermal contraction coefficient mismatch between the porcelain and the metal, which can produce tensile stresses during cooling that are sufficient to cause crack formation in the porcelain.

The condensed porcelain mass is placed in front of or below the muffle of a preheated furnace at approximately 650° C (1200° F) for low-fusing porcelain. This preheating procedure permits the remaining water vapor to dissipate. Placement of the condensed mass directly into even a moderately warm furnace results in a rapid production of steam, thereby introducing voids or fracturing large sections of the veneer. After preheating for approximately 5 min, the porcelain is placed into the furnace, and the firing cycle is initiated.

The size of the powder particles influences not only the degree of condensation of the porcelain but also the soundness or apparent density of the final product. At the initial firing temperature, the voids are occupied by the atmosphere of the furnace. As sintering of the particles begins, the porcelain particles bond at their points of contact. As the temperature is raised, the sintered glass gradually flows to fill up the air spaces. However, air becomes trapped in the form of voids because the fused mass is too viscous to allow all the air to escape. An aid in the reduction of porosity in dental porcelain is *vacuum firing*.

Vacuum firing reduces porosity in the following way. When the porcelain is placed in the furnace, the powder particles are packed together with air channels around them. As the air pressure inside the furnace muffle is reduced to about one-tenth of atmospheric pressure by the vacuum pump, the air around the particles is also reduced to this pressure. As the temperature rises, the particles sinter together, and closed voids are formed within the porcelain mass. The air inside these closed voids is isolated from the furnace atmosphere. At a temperature about 55° C (99° F) below the upper firing temperature, the vacuum is released and the pressure inside the furnace increases by a factor of 10, from 0.1 to 1 atm. Because the pressure is increased by a factor of 10, the voids are compressed to one-tenth of their original size, and the total volume of porosity is accordingly reduced. Not all the air can be evacuated from the furnace. Therefore a few bubbles are present in vacuum-sintered porcelains, but they are markedly smaller than the ones obtained by air-firing. A finished metal-ceramic multiple unit bridge is shown in Figure 21-3.

Overglazing and Shading Ceramics

As shown in Table 21-2, **natural glazed** (autoglazed or self-glazed), medium-fusing feldspathic porcelain is much stronger than ground, rough, nonglazed porcelain. If the glaze is removed by grinding, the transverse strength may be 40 to 46% less than that of the porcelain with the glaze layer intact. The glaze is effective in reducing crack propagation within the outer surface because the surface flaws may be bridged and the surface will be under a state of compressive stress. However, the results from one study indicate that porcelains with highly polished surfaces (1-μm abrasive paste) have comparable strength to that of specimens that were polished and glazed (Fairhurst et al, 1992). This observation is of clinical importance because after the porcelain prosthesis is cemented in the mouth, it is common practice for the dentist to adjust the occlusion by grinding the surface of the porcelain with a diamond bur. Unfortunately, this procedure weakens the porcelain markedly if the glaze is removed and the surface is left in a rough condition.

If the porcelain surface is rough, a natural glaze treatment is recommended since the fracture resistance of the surface is greater than that of unglazed porcelains. Porcelains for metal-ceramic and ceramic prostheses, porcelain veneers, or denture teeth may be characterized with stains and glazes to provide a more lifelike appearance. The fusing temperatures of glazes are reduced by the addition of glass modifiers that lower the chemical durability of glazes somewhat. Stains are simply tinted glazes and are subject to the same chemical durability problems. However, most of the currently available glazes have adequate durability if they are as thick as 50 μm or more.

One method for ensuring that the applied characterizing stains will be permanent is to use them internally. Internal staining and characterization can produce a lifelike result, particularly when simulated enamel craze lines and other features are built into the porcelain rather than merely applied to the surface. The disadvantage of internal staining and characterization is that the porcelain must be stripped away completely if the color or characterization is unsuitable.

It is logical to assume that fine polishing of a roughened surface followed by glazing produces smoother surfaces than polishing alone, sandblasting followed by glazing, or diamond grinding followed by glazing. A highly polished and glazed surface is smoother than the surfaces of glazed specimens that have been sandblasted or roughened with a diamond followed by glazing.

Cooling of Metal-Ceramic Prostheses

The proper cooling of a porcelain prosthesis from its firing temperature to room temperature is the subject of considerable controversy. The catastrophic fracture of glass that has been subjected to sudden changes in temperature is a familiar experience. The cooling of dental porcelain is a complex matter, particularly when the porcelain is fused to a metallic substrate. Multiple firings of a metal-ceramic restoration can cause the coefficient of thermal contraction of the porcelain to increase and can actually make it *more* likely to crack because of tensile stress development.

The chief limitation to the use of an all-porcelain crown in fixed prosthodontics is its lack of tensile strength. A method for minimizing this disadvantage is to fuse the porcelain directly to a metal coping that fits the prepared tooth. Such a metal-ceramic prosthesis is shown schematically in Figure 21-1. The metal on the facial side is approximately 0.3 to 0.5 mm thick. It is veneered with opaque porcelain approximately 0.3 mm in thickness. The **body porcelain** is about 1 mm thick.

If a stronger material is used as an inner core of a ceramic crown, cracks can develop only when the stronger material is deformed or broken, assuming that the veneering porcelain is firmly bonded to the stronger substrate. With proper design and physical properties of the porcelain and metal, the porcelain is reinforced so that brittle fracture can be avoided or at least minimized when these crowns are restricted to anterior teeth. Although most metal-ceramic prostheses involve cast metal copings, several novel noncast approaches (sintering, machining, swaging, and burnishing) to coping fabrication have been developed in recent years.

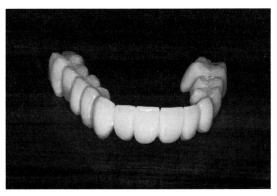

Fig. 21-3   A 13-unit metal-ceramic FPD. See also color plate.

Creep or Sag Resistance

Unfortunately, high-temperature creep or sag of some high noble and noble alloys occurs when the temperature approaches 980° C (1800° F). The creep can be reduced if the metal has the proper composition so that a dispersion strengthening effect occurs at the high temperature. When such a gold alloy is heated to 980° C or higher, a second phase is precipitated that can harden or strengthen the alloy. Such creep has been reduced in some of the commercial alloys, but it apparently cannot be eliminated. The solidus temperature (the lower end of the melting range) of base metal alloys, such as nickel-chromium, is higher than that of gold alloys; hence, base metal alloys are less susceptible to sag than are gold-based alloys.

However, the newer ultralow-fusing veneering ceramics that were introduced in the early 1990s are fired at lower temperatures (sintering temperatures below 850° C) than traditional low-fusing porcelains. For alloys with solidus temperatures of 1000° C or higher, creep (sag) deformation should be negligible. A schematic illustration of sag deformation is shown in Figure 19-1.

Copings for Metal-Ceramic Prostheses

Four types of process for producing a metal coping for metal-ceramic prostheses are available: (1) electrodeposition of gold or other metal on a duplicate die, (2) burnishing and heat-treating metal foils on a die, (3) CAD-CAM processing of a metal ingot, and (4) casting of a pure metal (CP Ti) or an alloy (high noble, noble, or predominantly base metal) through the lost-wax process. This discussion focuses primarily on the third option since it is the most widely used process.

The traditional development of the metal-ceramic prosthesis was the result of advances in the formulation of both alloys and porcelains. To bond a ceramic veneer to cast alloy copings, a ceramic must have a fusion temperature well above its sintering temperature and, it also must have a coefficient of thermal contraction that is closely matched to that of the alloys. A metal oxide is necessary to promote chemical bonding of the ceramic veneer to the metal substrate. Foil copings may or may not require a metal oxide or a bonding agent to ensure retention of the veneering ceramic. The use of one type of foil coping is discussed in the following section.

The gold alloys developed for porcelain bonding have higher melting ranges than typical gold alloys for cast metal prostheses; the higher melting ranges are necessary to prevent sag, creep, or melting of the coping during porcelain firing. These gold alloys contain small amounts (about 1%) of base metals such as iron, indium, and tin, as discussed in Chapter 19. The base metals form a surface oxide layer during the so-called "degassing" treatment, and this surface oxide is responsible for development of a bond with porcelain. This porcelain-metal bond is primarily chemical in nature and is capable of forming even when the metal surface is smooth and little opportunity exists for mechanical interlocking.

The alloys and porcelains used for the construction of such restorations have a number of rather stringent requirements. For example, if undesirable residual tensile stresses in the porcelain are to be avoided, both the metal and the ceramic must have thermal contraction profiles on cooling that are closely matched or with the metal exhibiting a slightly higher contraction. If the contraction differences are large, stresses may occur that weaken both the porcelain and the bond. For example, a difference in the coefficients of thermal contraction of 1.7 ppm/° C can produce a shear stress of 280 MPa (39,800 psi) in porcelain next to the gold-porcelain interface when the porcelain is cooled from 954° C (1750° F) to room temperature. Because the shear resistance to failure is far less than 280 MPa, these thermal stresses could cause spontaneous bond failure.

High tensile stresses are known to develop in porcelain veneers from a contraction coefficient mismatch between alloy and porcelain. The tensile stresses induced within the porcelain by occlusal forces would, of course, be added to residual thermal tensile stresses. However, when the metal and its porcelain veneer exhibit similar contraction curves and an average contraction coefficient difference of 0.5 ppm/° C or less (between the porcelain's glass transition temperature and room temperature), fracture is unlikely to occur except in cases of extreme stress concentration or extremely high intraoral forces. These metal-ceramic combinations are known as *thermally compatible systems.* Many prostheses made from metal and porcelain materials having contraction coefficient differences between 0.5 and 1.0 ppm/° C are known to survive for many years. These results are explainable by survival probability analyses that assume that the maximum biting forces on anterior crowns rarely exceed 890 N (200 lb) and the maximum force on posterior crowns rarely exceeds 2224 N (500 lb). In fact, the *Guinness Book of Records (1993)* cites the maximum clenching force ever recorded for posterior teeth as 4337 N (975 lb) sustained for 2 seconds. The second highest bite force ever recorded was 2447 N (550 lb). Most patients generate typical bite forces of 400 to 800 N (90 to 180 lb) between molar teeth and much lower forces between premolars and between anterior teeth. Thus a rather small number of patients have bite force capabilities that are likely to cause fracture of metal-ceramic crowns or bridges even when residual thermal incompatibility stresses are present. As a general rule, lower forces are generated by younger children versus older children, female patients versus male patients, a more closed bite versus a raised bite table, occlusion between natural teeth and denture teeth compared with the force generated between natural teeth against natural teeth.

Another equally important property of metal-ceramic systems is that the alloy should have a high proportional limit and, particularly, a high modulus of elasticity. Alloys with a high modulus of elasticity also share a greater proportion of stress compared with the adjacent porcelain. The metal framework must not melt during porcelain firing and also must resist high-temperature "sag" deformation. Sag or flexural creep can occur only at high temperatures. It does not occur at oral temperatures.

The **metal-ceramic prosthesis** is generally fabricated by a dental technician. The casting procedures are similar to those described for the casting of inlays and crowns. Because of the high melting temperature of the alloys, a phosphate-bonded investment must be used.

The casting should be carefully cleaned to ensure a strong bond to the porcelain. For example, an alloy such as Olympia (Heraeus Kulzer), a gold-palladium, silver-free alloy, is heated in the porcelain furnace to a temperature of 1038° C (1900° F) to burn off any remaining impurities and to form a thin oxide layer. In many alloy systems, this so-called degassing treatment does not actually degas the interior structure of the alloy, but it does produce an oxide layer on the alloy surface that is essential for the formation of the porcelain-metal bond.

The need for a clean metal surface cannot be overemphasized. The surface may be cleansed adequately by finishing with clean ceramic-bonded stones or sintered diamonds, which are used exclusively for finishing. Final sandblasting with high-purity alumina abrasive ensures that the porcelain is bonded to a clean and mechanically retentive surface.

Opaque porcelain is condensed with a thickness of approximately 0.3 mm and is then fired to its maturing temperature. Translucent porcelain is then applied, and the tooth form is built. Porcelain powder is applied by the condensation methods previously described. The unit is again fired. Several cycles of porcelain application and firing may be necessary to complete the prosthesis. A final glaze is then obtained.

Metal-Ceramic Crowns Based on Burnished Foil Copings

Captek (Precious Chemicals Company Inc.) is a technology that is based on the principle of capillary attraction to produce a gold composite metal. The Captek P and G metals can produce thin metal copings for single crowns or frameworks for metal-ceramic fixed partial dentures (FPDs) with a maximum span length of 18 mm (that allows space for up to two pontics). Captek is an acronym for "capillary casting technology." The finished metal coping may be described as a composite material consisting of a gold matrix reinforced with small particles of a Pt-Pd-Au alloy. The inner and outer surfaces contain approximately 97% Au. The grain size of the foil is 15 to 20 μm.

Malleable Captek metal strips are burnished on a refractory die to fabricate the metal coping of a metal-ceramic crown without the use of a melting and casting process. Examples of Captek metal-ceramic crowns are shown in Figure 21-4. The procedural steps are described below.

Starting with a master model of the prepared tooth or teeth, a Captek refractory die is produced. The Capsil relief liquid is sprayed onto the stone die(s) to reduce surface tension, allowing Capsil impression material or Capvest refractory die material to flow freely and to reduce bubbles and imperfections. After die spacer is applied to the master die, undercuts are blocked out. The master die is placed in the proper size-duplication flask, and Capsil silicone material is poured into the flask around the master die(s). The impression creates a mold into which refractory material (Capvest) is poured to create refractory dies. The master die is removed from the hardened silicone, and an accurate high-temperature refractory is poured into the new silicone mold.

The refractory die is heat-treated, the margins are marked with a red pencil, and an adhesive (Captek Adhesive) is applied to the die. The adhesive aids the adhesion of Captek material to the die and also enhances capillary attraction.

The next step requires the application of Captek P, a highly malleable gold, platinum, and palladium alloy. This internal reinforcing skeleton provides a three dimensional network of capillaries that will be eventually filled by Captek G

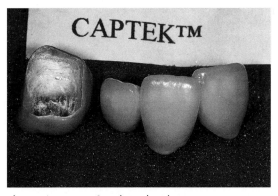

Fig. 21-4 Captek metal-ceramic crowns. See also color plate.

material forming a composite high gold metal alloy. This layer is burnished on the die, and after the margins are trimmed, it is sintered in a porcelain furnace on the recommended Captek thermal processing cycle.

This capillary structure is next infused with molten gold that is supplied by the Captek P material. The Captek P is pressed in place using uniform firm pressure so it conforms to the shape of the die. Excessive pressure or pulling of the material will cause it to tear or break. After trimming away any excess material, any voids are filled with trimmings of Captek P segments.

The crown and/or bridge units are now ready for firing. The pieces are heated at a rate of 55° to 80° C/minute to the recommended firing temperature. Next, Captek G strips are applied. The Captek G metal strip contains 97.5 wt% gold and 2.5 wt% silver. The copings and/or bridge components are fired again in the furnace according to the recommended Captek firing cycle. After processing, Captek G forms a high gold metal alloy composite through capillary attraction. The capillary action is used as the joining method of the hard particles and the resilient particles of metal present in the final coping. The gold melts, yet the Captek P structure remains stable. The Captek P reacts like a metal sponge and draws liquid gold completely into it. The Captek composite metal coping is now complete and ready for refractory die removal. The coping is divested, and the margins are finished. For the production of FPDs (bridges), Captek pontics are used. These are specially designed pontics that are precast using a metal-ceramic alloy and plated with pure gold.

The copings and/or pontics are coated with a mixture of a powder and liquid (Capbond), which will provide a thin covering of gold material to enhance areas of Captek P that have been ground during adjustment. The Capbond will also provide a gold color that is identical to that of areas that have not been ground.

Capcon liquid and powder are applied to areas between pontics and abutments, as well as pontic surface areas. The powder contains an alloy of gold, platinum, and palladium to provide the same base material structure as Captek P. Capcon absorbs, through capillary attraction, the Capfil material in the same way that Captek G is absorbed into Captek P, producing a gold connecting area that enhances the color of the pontic surface. Capcon is also used to enhance the buccal or labial pontic areas of Captek preformed pontics.

The units are veneered with two thin layers of opaque porcelain and other veneering porcelain layers. Before the opaque layer is applied, the finished Captek coping has a thickness of approximately 0.25 mm. Thus this technique provides a much thinner coping thickness than traditional cast metals (0.5 mm) and will provide additional space for veneering porcelain. The marginal adaptation is dependent on the skill of the technician in trimming the burnished materials. Unlike traditional cast metals that provide atomic bonding to opaque porcelain through an external oxide layer, Captek metal achieves bonding through a combination of surface interlocking and residual stresses produced by slight differences in thermal expansion coefficients. Although Captek metal is indicated for crowns and FPDs, no long-term clinical data are available to determine the survivability of Captek ceramic prostheses.

Bonding Porcelain to Metal

The primary requirement for the success of a metal-ceramic prosthesis is the development of a durable bond between the porcelain and the alloy. Once such a bond is achieved, there is an opportunity to introduce stresses in the prosthesis during the porcelain firing procedures. An unfavorable stress distribution during the cooling process can result in cracking of the porcelain, and delayed fracture can also occur. Thus, for a successful metal-ceramic prosthesis to be realized, both a strong interface bond and **thermal compatibility** are required.

Theories of metal-ceramic bonding have historically fallen into two groups: (1) mechanical interlocking between porcelain and metal and (2) chemical bonding across the metal-porcelain interface. Although chemical bonding is generally regarded to be responsible for metal-porcelain adherence, evidence exists that, for a few systems, mechanical interlocking may provide the principal bond. The oxidation behavior of these alloys largely determines their potential for bonding with porcelain. Research into the nature of metal-porcelain adherence has indicated that those alloys that form adherent oxides during the degassing cycle also form a good bond to porcelain, whereas those alloys with poorly adherent oxides form poor bonds. Some palladium-silver alloys form no external oxide at all but rather oxidize internally. It is for these alloys that mechanical bonding is needed.

A variety of tests have been advocated for measuring the bond strength. None can be regarded as an exact measure of the adhesion of porcelain to metal except in cases in which the metal-porcelain couple is matched thermally so that porcelain adjacent to the interface is essentially stress-free. This is a situation virtually impossible to attain because the metal exhibits a linear contraction behavior as a function of temperature and the porcelain exhibits a nonlinear contraction plot.

Clinical fractures of metal-ceramic restorations, although rare, still occur, especially when a new alloy or porcelain is being used or when a new coping technology has been adopted. As is generally true for all dental materials, there is a *learning curve* associated with the initial use of new products. When fractures occur, it is a good idea to make a vinyl polysiloxane impression of the fracture site for future fractographic analysis. All information on the crown or bridge should be recorded, including the visual appearance of the fracture site. Although there are an infinite number of fracture paths that may occur, three types are of particular importance in diagnosing the cause of fracture. Shown in Figure 21-5 are fracture paths that have occurred primarily at three sites: (1) along the interfacial region between opaque porcelain (*P*) and the interaction zone (*I*) between opaque porcelain and the metal substrate *(top)*; (2) within the interaction zone *(center)*; and (3) along the interfacial region between the metal and the interaction zone *(bottom)*. For conventional metal-ceramic crowns made from cast copings, the interaction zone is usually synonymous with the metal oxide layer.

For copings made using atypical methods such as the technologies associated with the Captek system, and electroforming processes, bonding to porcelain is achieved either through a combination of mechanical interlocking and residual stresses that occur because of a metal-ceramic contraction mismatch or through the application of a bonding agent. To characterize the principal site of fracture, magnification of 3 to 100 times is required because a thin layer of retained porcelain may not be visible without magnification. Each of the three principal fracture paths in Figure 21-5 may be caused by excessive stress development, a material deficiency, or a processing deficiency.

Bonding of Porcelain to Metal Using Electrodeposited Substrates

Ceramic bonding to metals in certain cases requires the electrodeposition of metal coatings and heating to form suitable metal oxides. Deposition of a layer of pure gold onto the cast metal and a subsequent short "flashing" deposition of tin have been shown to improve the wetting of porcelain onto the metal and to reduce the amount of porosity at the metal-porcelain interface. In addition, the

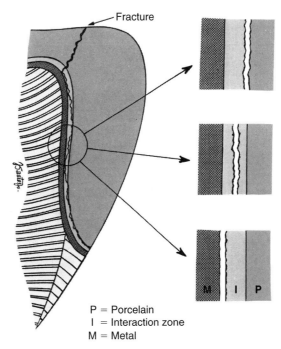

P = Porcelain
I = Interaction zone
M = Metal

Fig. 21-5   Cross-section of three principal types of interfacial zone fracture. See also color plate.

electrodeposited layer acts as a barrier between the metal casting and the porcelain to inhibit diffusion of atoms from the metal into the porcelain, within the normal limits of porcelain firing cycles.

A light color of the oxide film enhances the vitality of the porcelain when compared with the dark oxides that require heavy opaque layers to mask dark unaesthetic oxides. Because the activated surface can be controlled from golden, reddish-brown to gray, an additional dimension is available for color control of the porcelain.

Alloys and metals such as cobalt-chromium, stainless steel, palladium-silver, high- and low-gold–content alloys, and titanium all have been successfully electroplated and tin-coated to achieve satisfactory ceramic bonding. Various proprietary agents are also available that are intended for application to the metal surface before condensation of the opaque porcelain layer. These are applied as a thin liquid to the metal surface and are fired in a manner similar to that of opaque porcelain.

The function of these agents is twofold: (1) they are intended to improve metal-ceramic bonding by limiting the build-up of an oxide layer on the base metal surface during firing, and (2) they can improve aesthetics by helping to block the color of the dark metal oxide.

Benefits and Drawbacks of Metal-Ceramics

The properly made crown is stronger and more durable than the ordinary aluminous porcelain crown. However, a long-span bridge of this type may be subject to bending strains, and the porcelain may crack or fracture because of its low ductility. These difficulties can be partly overcome with proper prosthesis design, as discussed earlier. Proper occlusal relationships are also particularly important for this type of prosthesis.

The most outstanding advantages of metal-ceramic prostheses are the permanent aesthetic quality of the properly designed reinforced ceramic unit and their resistance to fracture. Unlike similar acrylic resin veneered structures, almost no wear of the porcelain occurs by abrasion and there is no staining along the interface between the veneer and the metal. Furthermore, as shown in a clinical study, the fracture rate of metal-ceramic crowns and bridges is as low as 2.3% after 7.5 years (Coornaert et al, 1984).

A slight advantage of metal-ceramic prostheses over ceramic prostheses is that less tooth structure needs to be removed to provide the proper bulk for the crown, especially if metal only is used on occlusal and lingual surfaces. As previously noted, high rigidity of the structure is needed to prevent fracture of the porcelain. Very little flexibility can be sustained by dental porcelains because of their moderately high modulus of elasticity (e.g., 69 GPa compared with values of 99.3 GPa for a Type IV gold alloy, 22.4 GPa for amalgam, and 16.6 GPa for a resin-based composite) and their relatively low tensile strength. As a result, only limited elastic deformation of the porcelain approximately (less than 0.1% strain) can be tolerated before fracture occurs. It follows, therefore, that a sufficient bulk of metal is necessary to provide the proper rigidity. The minimal metal coping thickness necessary in the occlusal region is approximately 0.3 mm. The shape of the crown cannot be conspicuously out of line with the anatomic form of adjacent teeth. Therefore the bulk of the natural tooth may need to be sacrificed to provide adequate space to ensure adequate fracture resistance and aesthetics.

The aesthetic capability of metal-ceramic restorations and their superb survivability are sufficient to overcome the drawbacks of metal-ceramic systems. For these reasons, metal-ceramics represent the most widely used prosthesis system used in fixed prosthodontics today.

CERAMIC PROSTHESES
Aluminous Porcelain Crowns

Another method of bonding porcelain to metal makes use of tin oxide coatings on platinum foil. The objective of this technique is to improve the aesthetics by a replacement of the thicker metal coping with a thin platinum foil, thus allowing more room for porcelain. The method consists of bonding aluminous porcelain to platinum foil copings. Attachment of the porcelain is secured by electroplating the platinum foil with a thin layer of tin and then oxidizing it in a furnace to provide a continuous film of tin oxide for porcelain bonding. The rationale is that the bonded foil will act as an inner skin on the fit surface to reduce subsurface porosity and formation of microcracks in the porcelain, thereby increasing the fracture resistance of crowns and bridges. The clinical performance of these crowns has been excellent for anterior teeth, but approximately 15% of these crowns fractured within 7 years after they were cemented to molar teeth with a glass ionomer cement.

Based on a 1994 survey, metal-ceramic crowns and bridges were used for approximately 90% of all fixed restorations. However, recent developments in ceramic products with improved fracture resistance and excellent aesthetic capability have led to a significant increase in the use of all-ceramic products. Ceramic crowns and bridges have been in widespread use since the beginning of the twentieth century. The ceramics employed in the conventional ceramic crown were high-fusing feldspathic porcelains. The relatively low strength of this type of porcelain prompted McLean and Hughes (1965) to develop an alumina-reinforced porcelain core material for the fabrication of ceramic crowns.

The alumina-reinforced crowns are generally regarded as providing slightly better aesthetics for anterior teeth than are the metal-ceramic crowns that employ a metal coping. However, the strength of the core porcelain used for alumina-reinforced crowns is inadequate to warrant the use of these prostheses for posterior teeth. In fact McLean reported a fracture rate of molar aluminous porcelain crowns of approximately 15% after 5 years.

Castable and Machinable Glass-Ceramics (Dicor and Dicor MGC)

When used for posterior crowns, ceramic crowns are most susceptible to fracture. Shown in Figure 21-6 (see also the color plate) is the stress distribution computed by finite element analysis in a 0.5-mm–thick molar Dicor crown loaded on the occlusal surface, just within the marginal ridge area. The maximum tensile stress is located within the internal surface directly below the point of applied force and just above the 50-μm–thick layer of resin cement (see the *arrow* in Fig. 21-6). This site represents the critical flaw responsible for crack initiation under an applied intraoral force. The location of initial crack formation was consistent with the location of maximum tensile stress predicted by the finite element calculations as shown in Figure 21-6. An SEM image of a fractured clinical crown of Dicor glass-ceramic is shown in Figure 21-7. The site of crack initiation (*arrow*) is the inner surface of the crown. A cross-sectional illustration of an anterior Dicor glass-ceramic crown is shown in Figure 21-8. Because of the smaller forces exerted on anterior crowns, the risk for fracture of anterior crowns is significantly less than that for posterior crowns.

The first commercially available **castable ceramic** material for dental use, Dicor, was developed by Corning Glass Works and marketed by Dentsply International. Dicor is a castable glass that is formed into an inlay, facial veneer, or full-crown restoration by a lost-wax casting process similar to that employed for metals. After the glass casting core or coping is recovered, the glass is sandblasted to remove residual casting investment and the sprues are gently cut away. The glass is then covered by a protective "embedment" material and subjected to a heat treatment that causes microscopic platelike crystals of crystalline material (mica) to grow within the glass matrix. This crystal nucleation and crystal growth process is called *ceramming*. Once

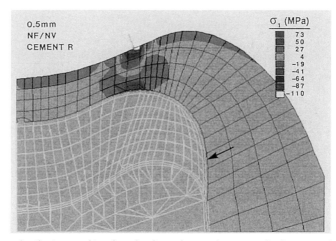

Fig. 21-6 Stress distribution resulting from loading (close to the marginal ridge area) of the occlusal surface of a finite element model of a Dicor glass-ceramic crown with an occlusal thickness of 0.5 mm. The maximum principal tensile stress is located directly below the point of occlusal loading within the internal surface of the crown adjacent to the 50-μm–thick layer of resin cement **(arrow)**. See also color plate.

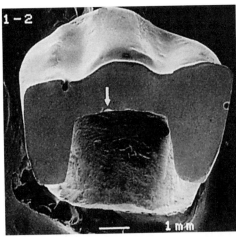

Fig. 21-7   Scanning electron microscopic image of a fractured Dicor glass-ceramic crown with a tetrasilicic fluormica-based core. The **arrow** indicates the site of the critical flaw responsible for crack initiation under intraoral loading. (From Thompson et al: Fracture surface characterization of clinically failed all-ceramic crowns. J Dent Res 73(12):1824-1832, 1994.)

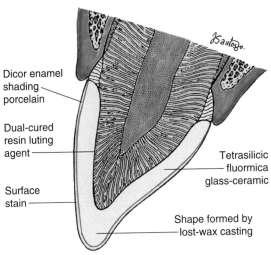

Fig. 21-8   Cross-section of cemented Dicor glass-ceramic crown. See also color plate.

the glass has been cerammed, it is fit on the prepared dies, ground as necessary, and then coated with veneering porcelain (as shown in Fig. 21-8) to match the shape and appearance of adjacent teeth. Dicor glass-ceramic is capable of producing surprisingly good aesthetics, perhaps because of the "chameleon" effect, where part of the color of the restoration is picked up from the adjacent teeth as well as from the tinted cements used for luting the restorations.

Dicor glass-ceramic contains about 55 vol% of tetrasilicic fluormica crystals. The ceramming process results in increased strength and toughness, increased resistance to abrasion, thermal shock resistance, chemical durability, and decreased translucency. Dicor MGC is a higher quality product that is crystallized by the manufacturer and provided as CAD-CAM blanks or ingots. The CAD-CAM ceramic Dicor MGC contains 70 vol% of tetrasilicic fluormica platelets, which are approximately 2 μm in diameter. The mechanical properties of Dicor MGC are similar to those of Dicor glass-ceramic, although it has less translucency (contrast ratio of 0.41–0.44 versus 0.56, respectively).

Dicor has recently been discontinued presumably because of low tensile strength and the need to color the prosthesis on the exterior region rather than within the core region, which would more closely resemble a natural tooth. Although Dicor is no longer sold, the principles for selection are useful when products of similar mechanical and physical properties are being considered. The advantages of Dicor glass-ceramic were ease of fabrication, improved aesthetics, minimal processing shrinkage, good marginal fit, moderately high flexural strength, low thermal expansion equal to that of tooth structure, and minimal abrasiveness to tooth enamel.

The disadvantages of Dicor glass-ceramic were its limited use in low-stress areas and its inability to be colored internally. As designed, it was colored with a thin outer layer of shading porcelain and surface stain to achieve acceptable aesthetics. However, Dicor MGC ingots have been supplied in light and dark shades, making it possible for technicians to build depth of color into the fabrication process.

Although both of the Dicor products were based on a glass-ceramic core that was minimally abrasive to opposing tooth enamel, the required shading or veneering porcelains were more abrasive. Aesthetically, Dicor crowns were more lifelike than metal-ceramic crowns, which often exhibit a metal collar, a gray shadow subgingivally, or poor translucency. The life expectancy of Dicor crowns in high-stress areas is not as good as that of PFM crowns. Two veneering materials were used to improve the color of Dicor crowns: Dicor Plus, which consisted a pigmented feldspathic porcelain veneer, and Willi's Glass, a veneer of Vitadur N aluminous porcelain.

Tooth preparation for glass-ceramic of this type is the same as that required for metal-ceramic prostheses except that, for first and second molars a reduction of 2 mm is recommended. Occlusal surfaces and incisal edges must be reduced a minimum of 1.5 mm. Axial surfaces should be reduced a minimum of 1.0 mm. The preparation should be either a shoulder with a rounded gingivoaxial line angle or a heavy chamfer.

Pressable Glass-Ceramics

A *glass-ceramic* is a material that is formed into the desired shape as a glass, then subjected to a heat treatment to induce partial devitrification (i.e., loss of glassy structure by crystallization of the glass). The crystalline particles, needles, or plates formed during this ceramming process serve to interrupt the propagation of cracks in the material when an intraoral force is applied, thereby causing increased strength and toughness. The use of glass-ceramics in dentistry was first proposed by MacCulloch in 1968. He used a continuous glass-molding process to produce denture teeth. He also suggested that it should be possible to fabricate crowns and inlays by centrifugal casting of molten glass.

Pressure molding is used to make small, intricate objects. This method uses a piston to force a heated ceramic ingot through a heated tube into a mold, where the ceramic form cools and hardens to the shape of the mold. When the object has solidified, the refractory mold (investment) is broken apart and the ceramic piece is removed. It is then debrided and either stained and glazed (certain inlays) or veneered with one or more layers of a thermally compatible ceramic.

IPS Empress is a glass-ceramic provided as core ingots that are heated and pressed until the ingot flows into a mold. It contains a higher concentration of leucite crystals that increase the resistance to crack propagation (fracture). The hot-pressing process occurs over a 45-min period at a high temperature to produce the ceramic substructure. This crown form can be either stained and glazed or built up using a conventional layering technique.

The advantages of this ceramic are its lack of metal, a translucent ceramic core, a moderately high flexural strength (similar to that of Optimal Pressable Ceramic), excellent fit, and excellent aesthetics. The disadvantages are its potential to fracture in posterior areas and the need to use a resin cement to bond the crown micromechanically to tooth structure.

IPS Empress and IPS Empress2 are typical products representative of several other leucite-reinforced and lithia disilicate–reinforced glass-ceramics, respectively. Some properties of IPS Empress and IPS Empress2 glass-ceramic core materials are listed in Table 21-6. IPS Empress is a leucite-containing glass-ceramic that contains about 35 vol% of leucite ($KAlSi_2O_6$) crystals, which increases the resistance to crack propagation (fracture). The veneering ceramic also contains leucite crystals in a glass matrix. After hot pressing, divesting, and separation of the ceramic units the sprue segments, they are veneered with porcelain containing leucite crystals in a glass matrix.

A cross-sectional illustration of an IPS Empress crown is illustrated in Figure 21-9. The IPS Empress2 is similar except that the core consists of lithia disilicate crystals in a glass matrix and the veneering ceramic contains apatite crystals. The very small

Table 21-6	Properties of Two Pressable Glass-Ceramics		
Property		**IPS Empress**	**IPS Empress2**
Flexural strength (MPa)		112 ± 10	400 ± 40
Fracture toughness (MPa·m$^{1/2}$)		1.3 ± 0.1	3.3 ± 0.3
Thermal expansion coefficient (ppm/° C)		15.0 ± 0.25	10.6 ± 0.25
Chemical durability (µg/cm^2)		100-200	50
Pressing temperature (° C)		1180	920
Veneering temperature (° C)		910	800

Modified from Höland W, and Beall G (eds): Glass-ceramic technology. Westerville, OH, The American Ceramic Society, 2002.

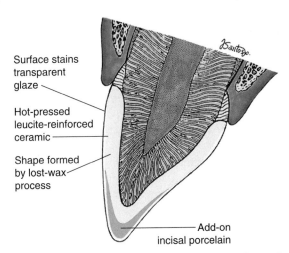

Fig. 21-9   Cross-section of cemented IPS Empress ceramic crown with a leucite-based ceramic core.

apatite crystals cause light scattering in a way that resembles the scattering by the structure and components of tooth enamel. The coefficient of expansion of the apatite glass-ceramic veneering ceramic is 9.7 ppm/° C, which is similar to that of IPS Empress2 core ceramic (10.6 ppm/° C). Obviously, this veneering ceramic should not be used with the IPS Empress core ceramic that has a much higher expansion coefficient (15.0 ppm/° C).

The core microstructure of IPS Empress2 glass ceramic is quite different from that of IPS Empress, as evidenced by the 70 vol% of elongated lithia disilicate crystals in IPS Empress2. The primary crystal particles in IPS Empress2 are 0.5 to 4 μm in length. A smaller concentration of lithium orthophosphate crystals ($Li_2Si_2O_5$) approximately 0.1 to 0.3 μm in diameter has also been reported (Höland et al, 2000). The microstructural difference between IPS Empress and IPS Empress2 results in a slight decrease in translucency for IPS Empress2 (0.55) (British Standard BS 5612: 1978) compared with that of IPS Empress (0.58) (Höland et al, 2000). As is the case for most pressable glass-ceramics, the advantages of IPS Empress and IPS Empress2 glass-ceramic core materials are their potential for accurate fit, excellent translucency and overall aesthetics, and a metal-free structure. Disadvantages are their low to moderately high flexural strength and fracture toughness. These properties limit their use to conservative designs in low to moderate stress environments. Shown in Figures 21-10, 21-11, and 21-12 are three-unit glass-ceramic FPDs made from a lithia-disilicate–based core material. The FPD shown in Figure 21-12 was made without a veneering ceramic to enhance the fracture resistance. A summary of important properties is presented in Table 21-7 for a variety of dental ceramics. A list of pressable ceramics and their veneering ceramics is summarized in Table 21-8.

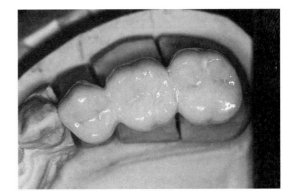

Fig. 21-10 Highly glazed surface on a three-unit FPD produced with a lithia disilicate-based core ceramic. See also color plate.

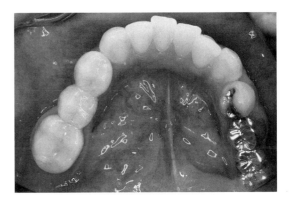

Fig. 21-11 A three-unit ceramic FPD (tooth numbers 19–21; FDI tooth numbers 34–36) produced with a lithia disilicate–based core ceramic. See also color plate.

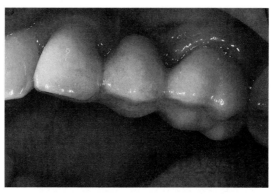

Fig. 21-12   A three-unit ceramic anterior-posterior FPD produced with a lithia disilicate–core ceramic. To increase the fracture resistance, no veneering ceramic was used in this case. Note the relatively large connector size (4 mm in height) that is necessary to reduce the risk for fracture in posterior areas. See also color plate.

OPC and OPC 3G are two pressable ceramics that are similar in nature to IPS Empress and IPS Empress2, respectively. OPC is a leucite-containing ceramic and OPC 3G contains lithia disilicate crystals. The ultralow-fusing temperature of the veneering porcelain suggests a low level of wear of opposing enamel. However, insufficient clinical data are available to support this hypothesis.

In-Ceram Alumina, In-Ceram Spinell, and In-Ceram Zirconia

In-Ceram is supplied as one of three core ceramics: (1) *In-Ceram Spinell*, (2) *In-Ceram Alumina*, and (3) *In-Ceram Zirconia*. A slurry of one of these materials is slip-cast on a porous refractory die and heated in a furnace to produce a partially sintered coping or framework. The partially sintered core is infiltrated with glass at 1100° C for 4 hr to eliminate porosity and to strengthen the slip-cast core. The initial sintering process for the alumina core produces a minimal shrinkage because the temperature and time are sufficient only to cause bonding between particles and to produce a desired level of sintering. Thus the marginal adaptation and fit of this core material should be adequate because little shrinkage occurs. The flexural strength (modulus of rupture) values of the glass-infiltrated core materials are approximately 350 MPa for In-Ceram Spinell (ICS), 500 MPa for In-Ceram Alumina (ICA), and 700 MPa for In-Ceram Zirconia (ICZ) compared with strengths of 100 to 400 MPa for Dicor, Optec Pressable Ceramic, IPS Empress, and IPS Empress2. Despite the relatively high strength of these materials, failures can still occur in single crowns as well as FPDs.

Because of the variation in strength, the primary indications for these core ceramics vary as shown in Table 21-9. For example, ICS is indicated for use as anterior single-unit inlays, onlays, crowns, and veneers. ICA is indicated for anterior and posterior crowns and anterior three-unit FPDs. Because of its high level of opacity, ICZ is not recommended for anterior prostheses. However, because of its extremely high strength and fracture toughness, it can be used for posterior crowns and posterior FPDs. As suggested in Chapter 4, it is essential that the gingival embrasure areas of ceramic FPD connectors be designed with a large radius of curvature to minimize the stress-raiser effect in areas of moderate to high tensile stress. The connectors also should be sufficiently thick to minimize stresses during loading. For Empress and Empress 2 ceramics used in molar areas, the connector height should be at least 4 mm.

Table 21-7 Comparative Characteristics of Dental Ceramic Products

Processing method	Sintered	Cast/cerammed	Presintered, milled, and postsintered	Enlarged die/sintered	Hot-Pressed	Sintered and glass infiltrated	CAD/CAM
Type of Construction	Metal-Ceramic	Ceramic	Ceramic	Ceramic	Ceramic	Ceramic	Ceramic
Indications	Anterior and posterior crowns and FPDs	Anterior and posterior crowns	Anterior and posterior crowns and FPDs	Anterior and posterior crowns	Leucite reinforced: anterior and posterior crowns Lithia disilicate reinforced: also indicated for premolar FPDs	Spinell core: anterior crowns Alumina core: anterior and posterior crowns and anterior 3-unit FPDs Zirconia core: posterior crowns and posterior FPDs	Anterior and posterior crowns and FPDs
Margin Quality	Poor margins	Good margins	Fair to good margins	Fair to good margins	Good to excellent margins	Fair to good margins	Fair to good margins
Appearance	Opaque	Translucent	Opaque	Opaque	Slightly translucent	Opaque	Slightly translucent to translucent
Relative Strength	Weak	Weak	Very strong	Strong	Moderately strong	Moderately to very strong	Moderately strong
Relative Toughness	Low	Low	Very high	High	Moderately high	Moderately high to high	Low to high
Acid Etchable	Etchable	Etchable	No	No	Etchable	Not indicated	Etchable
Abrasiveness of Core Ceramic	Moderately abrasive	Minimally abrasive	Highly abrasive	Highly abrasive	Moderately abrasive	Highly abrasive	Minimally to highly abrasive

Continued

Table 21-7   Comparative Characteristics of Dental Ceramic Products—cont'd

Processing method	Sintered	Cast/cerammed	Presintered, milled, and postsintered	Enlarged die/sintered	Hot-Pressed	Sintered and glass infiltrated	CAD/CAM
Ease of Cutting/Removal	Easy	Easy	Difficult	Difficult	Easy	Difficult	Easy to difficult
Treatment Time	Two visits	Two visits	Two visits	Two visits	Two visits	Two visits	One visit
Major Drawbacks	Weak and unsuitable as a core for full ceramic crowns or FPDs	No products are currently available	Tends to appear too opaque if tooth reduction is inadequate; not etchable	Tends to appear too opaque if tooth reduction is inadequate; not etchable	Leucite-reinforced type not indicated for FPDs; lithia disilicate–reinforced type limited to crowns and 3-unit FPDs extending to 2nd premolar; requires large connector size	All, but spinel type tend to look too opaque if tooth reduction is inadequate	Requires a uniform light-reflecting powder deposit to ensure adequate image quality

Table 21-8	Pressable Core Ceramics and Associated Veneering Ceramics for All-Ceramic Prostheses		
Core ceramic	**Veneering ceramic**	**Indications**	**Manufacturer**
Authentic	Authentic	Veneer/inlay/onlay/anterior crown	Ceramay
Carrara Press Core	Carrara Vincent	Veneer/inlay/onlay/anterior crown	Elephant
Carrara Press Inlay	Carrara Vincent	Inlay	Elephant
Cergo	Duceragold	Veneer/inlay/onlay/anterior crown	Dentsply Ceramco/Degussa
Cerpress	Sensation SL	Veneer/inlay/onlay/anterior and posterior crown	Dentagold
Cerapress	Creation LF	Veneer/inlay/onlay/anterior crown	Girrbach
IPS Empress	Empress	Veneer/inlay/onlay/anterior crown	Ivoclar Vivadent
IPS Empress2	Empress2, Eris	Veneer/inlay/onlay/anterior and posterior crown/anterior FPD	Ivoclar Vivadent
Evopress	Evolution	Veneer/inlay/onlay/anterior crown	Wegold
Finesse All Ceramic	Finesse	Veneer/inlay/onlay/anterior crown	Dentsply Ceramco
Fortress Pressable	—	—	Mirage
Imagine h.e. Press	Imagine h.e.	Veneer/inlay/onlay/anterior crown	Wieland
Magic Coating Caps Schicht-Pressing	Magic Ceram 2	Veneer/inlay/onlay/anterior crown	D.T.S. Denta TechnoStore
Magic Easy Press Colorier-Pressing	—	Veneer/inlay/onlay/anterior crown	D.T.S. Denta-TechnoStore
Nuance Presskeramik	Nuance 750	Veneer/inlay/onlay/anterior crown	Schutz Dental Group
Optec OPC Low Wear	Optec OPC Low wear	Veneer/inlay/onlay/anterior and posterior crown	Pentron
Optec OPC 3G	Optec OPC 3G Porcelain	Veneer/inlay/onlay/crown/anterior FPD	Pentron
Trendpress	Trendkeramik LFC	Veneer/inlay/onlay/anterior crown	Binder Dental
PLATINApress	Platina M	Veneer/inlay/onlay/anterior crown	Heimerle+Meule
Vision Aesthetic	Vision Aesthetic	Veneer/inlay/onlay/anterior crown	Wohlwend
VitaPress	Vita Omega 900	Veneer/inlay/onlay	Vident

Modified from Kappert HF, and Krah MK, Keramiken—eine Übersicht, Quintessenz Zahntech 27(6):668-704, 2001.

Until In-Ceram was introduced, aluminous porcelain had not been used successfully to produce FPDs because of low flexural strength and high sintering shrinkage. Thus the principal indications for aluminous porcelain crowns were the restoration of maxillary anterior crowns when aesthetics was important and their use in patients with allergies to metals. Its advantages and disadvantages are summarized in the following.

A schematic drawing of an In-Ceram crown is shown in Figure 21-13. The same diagram can be used to illustrate crowns made with In-Ceram Spinell (ICS) and In-Ceram Zirconia (ICZ), which will be discussed below. The three In-Ceram ceramics are glass-infiltrated core materials used for single anterior crowns (all three products), posterior crowns (In-Ceram Alumina and In-Ceram Zirconia), anterior three-unit FPDs (In-Ceram Alumina), and three-unit posterior bridges (In-Ceram Zirconia).

The most translucent of the three ceramics, *In-Ceram Spinell*, was introduced as an alternative to In-Ceram Alumina. This ceramic has a lower flexural strength, but its increased translucency provides improved aesthetics in clinical situations in which the adjacent teeth or restorations are quite translucent. The core of ICS is $MgAl_2O_4$ and that for ICZ is a mixture of Al_2O_3 and ZrO_2. These core ceramics are also infiltrated with glass, and they are fabricated in a manner similar to that for ICA, although the firing temperatures and times may be different.

The final ICA core consists of 70 wt% alumina infiltrated with 30 wt% sodium lanthanum glass. The final ICS core consists of glass-infiltrated magnesium spinel $(MgAl_2O_4)$. ICZ contains approximately 30 wt% zirconia and 70 wt% alumina. The power-liquid slurry is slip cast onto a porous die that absorbs water from the slurry, thereby densifying the agglomeration of particles onto the die. Steps for fabricating In-Ceram prostheses are as follows: (1) prepare teeth with an occlusal

Table 21-9	Core Ceramics That Are Reinforced with $MgAl_2O_4$, Al_2O_3, Al_2O_3-ZrO_2, and ZrO_2			
Ceramic block	**Ceramic type**	**Ceramic veneer**	**Indications**	**Manufacturer**
In-Ceram Spinell	MgO-Al_2O_3 ceramic	Vitadur Alpha (aluminous porcelain)	Anterior crowns	Vident
In-Ceram Alumina	Al_2O_3 ceramic	Vitadur Alpha (aluminous porcelain)	Anterior and posterior crowns and anterior FPDs	Vident
In-Ceram Zirconia	Al_2O_3-ZrO_2 ceramic	Vitadur Alpha (aluminous porcelain)	Posterior crowns and posterior FPDs	Vident
Cercon Base	ZrO_2, sintered	Cercon Ceram S	Crowns and FPDs	Dentsply Ceramco
Procera AllCeram	Dry pressed and sintered Al_2O_3	AllCeram	Crowns and FPDs	Nobel Biocare

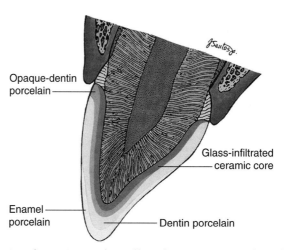

Fig. 21-13 Cross-section of an In-Ceram (glass-infiltrated core) crown. See also color plate.

reduction of 1.5 to 2.0 mm and a heavy circumferential chamfer (1.2 mm), (2) make an impression and pour two dies, (3) apply Al_2O_3 on a porous duplicate die, (4) heat at 120° C for 2 hours to dry Al_2O_3, (5) sinter the coping for 10 hours at 1120° C, (6) apply a sodium lanthanum glass slurry mixture on the coping, (7) fire for 4 hours at 1120° C to allow infiltration of glass, (8) trim excess glass from the coping with diamond burs, (9) build up the core with dentin and enamel porcelain, (10) fire in the oven, grind in the anatomy and occlusion, finish, and glaze.

The advantages of ICA include a moderately high flexural strength and fracture toughness, a metal-free structure, and an ability to be used successfully with conventional luting agents (Type I cements). The collective advantages of the three glass-infiltrated core materials are their lack of metal, relatively high flexural strength and toughness, and ability to be successfully cemented using any cement.

In spite of its high flexural strength (429 MPa), the Weibull modulus of ICA is quite low (5.7), which is indicative of a large scatter in the distribution of strength values relative to the probability of fracture (Tinschert et al, 2000). Its marginal adaptation may not be as good as that achieved with other ceramic products. In one study the mean marginal discrepancies were 83 μm for Procera AllCeram, 63 μm for IPS Empress, and 161 μm for In-Ceram Alumina. Other drawbacks of ICA include its relatively high degree of opacity, inability to be etched, technique sensitivity, and the relatively great amount of skilled labor required. These disadvantages apply also to In-Ceram Zirconia. Compared with ICM, the opacities of ICA and ICZ core ceramics are much greater.

Although these newer core ceramics have excellent fracture resistance, improper design of the connector area of a FPD can significantly reduce the fracture resistance and clinical survivability of the prosthesis. Shown in Figure 21-14 is the stress distribution in a three-unit FPD, which shows relatively high principal tensile stress (*red area*) at the tissue side of the interproximal connector when an occlusal load of 250 N is applied to the occlusal surface of the pontic.

In summary, In-Ceram Spinell (ICS) is a glass-infiltrated core ceramic that offers greater translucency for crowns than either the ICA or ICZ core ceramics. However,

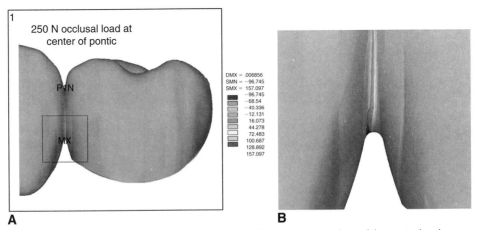

Fig. 21-14 Maximum principal tensile stress based on finite element analysis of the gingival embrasure area of the connector in a model of a three-unit fixed partial denture subjected to an occlusal load of 250 N. See also color plate. (Modified from Oh W, Götzen N, and Anusavice KJ: Influence of connector design on fracture probability of ceramic fixed-partial dentures. J Dent Res 81(9):623-627, 2002.)

ICS has lower strength and toughness compared with ICA and ICZ. Thus the use of ICS is limited to anterior inlays, onlays, veneers, and anterior crowns. Although ICZ is the strongest and toughest of the three core ceramics, its use is limited to posterior crowns and FPDs because of its high level of core opacity. ICZ is a much stronger and tougher material and has greater opacity than ICA.

Procera AllCeram

The Procera AllCeram crown is composed of densely sintered, high-purity aluminum oxide core combined with a compatible AllCeram veneering porcelain. This ceramic material contains 99.9% alumina, and its hardness is one of the highest among the ceramics used in dentistry. Procera AllCeram can be used for anterior and posterior crowns, veneers, onlays, and inlays.

A unique feature of the Procera system is the ability of the Procera Scanner to scan the surface of the prepared tooth and transmit the data to the milling unit to produce an enlarged die through a CAD-CAM process. The core ceramic form is dry pressed onto the die, and the core ceramic is then sintered and veneered. Thus the usual 15%–20% shrinkage of the core ceramic during sintering will be compensated by constructing an oversized ceramic pattern, which will shrink during sintering to the desired size to accurately fit the prepared tooth.

CAD-CAM Ceramics

As shown in the ceramic classification chart in Table 21-3, all-ceramic cores can be produced by processes of condensation and sintering, casting and ceramming, hot-pressing and sintering, sintering and glass infiltration, and CAD-CAM processing. For the Cerec CAD-CAM system the internal surface of inlays, onlays, or crowns is ground with diamond disks or other instruments to the dimensions obtained from a scanned image of the preparation. For some systems, the external surface must be ground manually, although some recent CAD-CAM systems are capable of forming the external surface as well.

Shown in Figure 21-15 is a milling operation within a Cerec CAD-CAM unit (Siemens Aktiengesellschaft, Bensheim, Germany). The ceramic block is being ground by a diamond-coated disk whose translational movements are guided

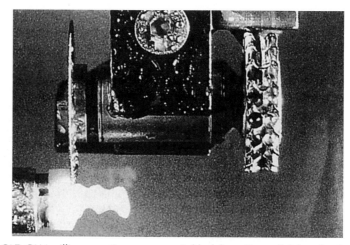

Fig. 21-15 CAD-CAM milling operation on a ceramic block by a diamond disk at the Cerec CAM station.

by computer-controlled input. A Cerec CAD-CAM ceramic block is shown in Figure 21-16 before milling, at an intermediate milling stage, and after completion of the milling operation for an inlay. These ceramics are supplied as small blocks that can be ground into inlays and veneers in a computer-driven CAD-CAM system. Vitablocs MK II are feldspathic porcelains that are used in the same way as is Dicor MGC (machinable glass-ceramic). The disadvantages of CAD-CAM restorations include the need for costly equipment, the lack of computer-controlled processing support for occlusal adjustment, and the technique-sensitive nature of surface imaging required for the prepared teeth. Advantages include negligible porosity levels in the CAD-CAM core ceramics, the freedom from making an impression, reduced assistant time associated with impression procedures, the need for only a single patient appointment (with the Cerec system), and good patient acceptance. A list of CAD-CAM and copy-milled ceramics is given in Table 21-10.

An advantage of CAD-CAM ceramics is that one can select a core ceramic either for strength and fracture resistance, for low abrasiveness, or for translucency. For example, the extensive wear of opposing enamel that occurs when it is opposed by a feldspathic porcelain surface in the absence of posterior occlusion (Fig. 21-17) can be minimized by selecting a core ceramic that is minimally abrasive to enamel.

Cercon and Lava Zirconia Core Ceramics

The Cercon Zirconia system (Dentsply Ceramco, Burlington, NJ) consists of the following procedures for production of zirconia-based prostheses. After preparing the teeth (2.0 mm incisal or occlusal reduction and 1.5 mm axial reduction), an impression is made and sent to the laboratory, where it is poured with a model material. A wax pattern approximately 0.8 mm in thickness is made for each coping or the crown areas of the framework of a FPD. The wax pattern is anchored on the holding appliance on the left side of the scanning and milling unit (Cercon Brain). A presintered zirconia blank is attached to the right side of the Brain unit. The blank has an attached barcode, which contains the enlargement factor and other milling parameters for computer control of the milling procedure After the unit is activated, the pattern is scanned and the blank is rough-milled and fine-milled on occlusal

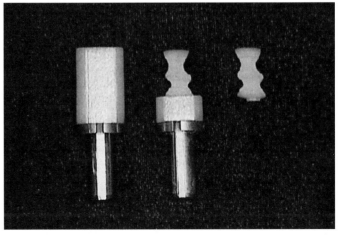

Fig. 21-16 Cerec CAD-CAM ceramic block before milling (**left**), at an intermediate stage of milling (**center**), and after removal of the inlay from the mounting stub (**right**).

Table 21-10	CAD-CAM and Copy-Milled Ceramics Used for All-Ceramic Prostheses			
Ceramic block	**Ceramic type**	**Ceramic veneer**	**Indications**	**Manufacturer**
CerAdapt	Highly sintered Al_2O_3	AllCeram	Implant superstructure	Nobel Biocare
Cercon Base	Presintered ZrO_2; postsintered after milling	Cercon Ceram S	Crowns and FPDs	Dentsply Ceramco
DC-Kristall	Leucite-based	Triceram	Crowns	DCS Dental AG/Esprident
DC-Zirkon	Presintered ZrO_2; hot isostatic postcompaction	Vitadur D Triceram	Crowns and FPDs	DCS Dental AG/Vita/Esprident
Denzir	Presintered ZrO_2; hot isostatic postcompaction	Empress2	Crowns and FPDs	Decim, Ivoclar
LAVA Frame	ZrO_2; presintered and postsintered	LAVA Ceram	Crowns and FPDs	3M ESPE
ProCad	Leucite-based	Maltechnik	Veneers, inlays, onlays, and crowns	Ivoclar
Procera AllCeram	Al_2O_3; presintered and postsintered	AllCeram	Crowns and FPDs	Nobel Biocare
Synthoceram	Al_2O_3 reinforced; pressed and postsintered	Sintagon	Crowns	Elephant
VitaBlocs Mark II	Feldspathic porcelain block	Maltechnik	Veneers, inlays, onlays, and crowns	Vident
VitaBlocs Alumina	Sintered Al_2O_3: followed by glass infiltration	Vitadur Alpha	Crowns and FPDs	Vident
VitaBlocs Spinell	Sintered $MgO-Al_2O_3$ spinel followed by glass infiltration	Vitadur Alpha	Crowns	Vident
VitaBlocs Zirconia	Sintered Al_2O_3/ZrO_2 followed by glass infiltration	Vitadur Alpha	Crowns and FPDs	Vident
Zircagon	ZrO_2; presintered and postsintered	Zircagon	Crowns	Elephant

Modified from Kappert HF, and Krah MK, Keramiken—eine Übersicht, Quintessenz Zahntech 27(6):668-704, 2001.

and gingival aspects in an enlarged size (Fig. 21-18) to compensate for the 20% shrinkage that will occur during subsequent sintering at 1350° C. The processing times for milling are approximately 35 min for a crown and 80 min for a four-unit fixed FPD. The milled prosthesis is removed from the unit, and the remaining extraneous extensions are removed. The zirconia coping or framework is then placed in

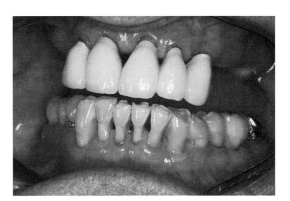

Fig. 21-17 Excessive wear of mandibular teeth caused by abrasion by opposing porcelain surfaces. (Courtesy of Dr. Henry Young.)

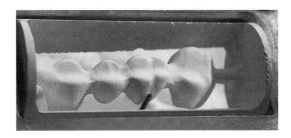

Fig. 21-18 Cercon zirconia core ceramic during initial milling of the "green state" ceramic. See also color plate. (Courtesy of Dentsply Ceramco, Burlington, NJ.)

the Cercon furnace (Fig. 21-19) and fired at 1350° C for approximately 6 hours to fully sinter the yttria-stabilized zirconia core coping or framework. The sintering shrinkage is achieved uniformly and linearly in three-dimensional space by the integrated process of scanning, enlarging the pattern design, controlled milling, and sintering.

After any subsequent trimming with a water-cooled, high-speed diamond bur (Fig. 21-20), the finished ceramic core framework (Fig. 21-21) is then veneered with a veneering ceramic (Cercon Ceram S) and stain ceramic (Fig. 21-22).

All-ceramic prostheses represent the most aesthetically pleasing, but also the most fracture-prone prostheses. However, with adequate tooth reduction, an excellent quality impression, a skilled technician, and a ceramic with reasonably high flexure strength ($\geq$250 MPa) and fracture toughness ($\geq$2.5 MPa·m$^{1/2}$), reasonably high success rates can be achieved. The material that has the greatest potential fracture toughness (9 MPa·m$^{1/2}$) and flexural strength (>900 MPa) is pure tetragonal-stabilized zirconia (ZrO_2). Tinschert et al (2001b) reported that the fracture resistance of three-unit ceramic FPDs (1278 N) made of Cercon zirconia core ceramic (Dentsply Ceramco) was more than twice as great as the values reported for In-Ceram Alumina (514 N) and Empress2 (621 N). Shown in Figure 21-23 is a comparison of the force required to fracture three-unit FPDs cemented to dies with zinc phosphate cement. The zirconia product (Cercon) would be expected to exhibit less fracture resistance in this case, but clinical data are needed to confirm this hypothesis.

To ensure maximum survival times, adequate occlusal tooth reduction is essential for posterior teeth. Optimal clinical performance of some ceramic products require a minimal occlusal reduction of 2 mm for molar tooth preparations. If the ceramic will be supported by a material with a high elastic modulus such as a ceramic or metal post or an amalgam build-up, less occlusal reduction (1.5 mm) may be possible without compromising the survivability of the crowns. For patients exhibiting extreme bruxism, either metal or metal-ceramic prostheses should be used.

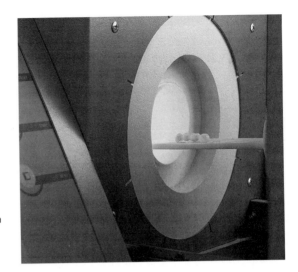

Fig. 21-19 Cercon FPD being placed in the furnace. See also color plate. (Courtesy of Dentsply Ceramco, Burlington, NJ.)

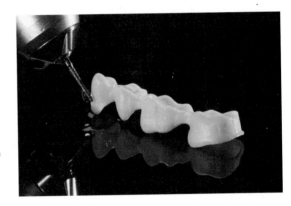

Fig. 21-20 Trimming of Cercon zirconia core ceramic. See also color plate. (Courtesy of Dentsply Ceramco, Burlington, NJ.)

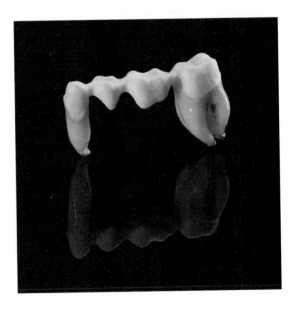

Fig. 21-21 Finished core ceramic framework made with Cercon core placed on teeth. See also color plate. (Courtesy of Dentsply Ceramco, Burlington, NJ.)

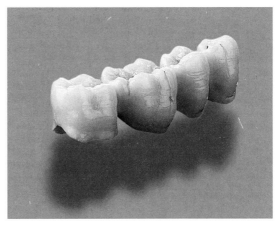

Fig. 21-22 Final Cercon FPD with veneering ceramic and stain characterization. See also color plate. (Courtesy of Dentsply Ceramco, Burlington, NJ.)

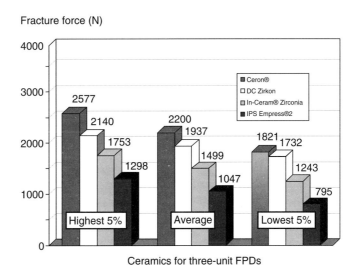

Fig. 21-23 Force required to fracture three-unit ceramic fixed partial dentures. (From Tinschert et al: Fracture resistance of lithium disilicate-, alumina-, and zirconia-based three-unit fixed partial dentures: A laboratory study. Int J Prosthodont 14(3)231-238, 2001 b.)

CRITICAL QUESTION

What occurs at the tips of cracks during the development of tensile stress to prevent crack growth in yttria stabilized zirconia?

METHODS OF STRENGTHENING CERAMICS
Minimize the Effect of Stress Raisers

Why do dental ceramic prostheses fail to exhibit the strengths that we would expect from the high bond forces between atoms? The answer is that numerous minute scratches and other defects are present on the surfaces of these materials. These surface flaws behave as sharp notches whose tips may be as narrow as the spacing between several atoms in the material. These stress concentration areas at the tip of each surface flaw can increase the localized stress to the theoretical strength of the material even though a relatively low average stress exists throughout the bulk of the structure. When the induced mechanical stress exceeds the actual strength of the material, the bonds at the notch tip break, forming a crack. This stress concentration phenomenon explains how materials fail at stresses far below their theoretical strength.

Stress raisers are discontinuities in ceramic and metal-ceramic structures and in other brittle materials that cause a stress concentration in these areas. The design of ceramic dental restorations should also avoid stress raisers in the ceramic. Abrupt changes in shape or thickness in the ceramic contour can act as stress raisers and make the restoration more prone to failure. Thus the incisal line angles on an anterior tooth prepared for a ceramic crown should be well rounded.

In ceramic crowns, several conditions can cause stress concentration. Creases or folds of the platinum foil or gold foil substrate that become embedded in the porcelain leave notches that act as stress raisers. Sharp line angles in the preparation also create areas of stress concentration in the restoration. Large changes in porcelain thickness, a factor also determined by the tooth preparation, can create areas of stress concentration.

A small particle of porcelain along the internal porcelain margin of a crown also induces locally high tensile stresses. A stray particle that is fused within the inner surface of a shoulder porcelain margin of a metal-ceramic crown can cause localized tensile stress concentrations in porcelain when an occlusal force is applied to the crown.

Even though a metal-ceramic restoration is generally stronger than most ceramic crowns of the same size and shape, care must be taken to avoid subjecting the porcelain in a PFM to loading that produces large localized stresses. If the occlusion is not adjusted properly on a porcelain surface, contact points rather than contact areas will greatly increase the localized stresses in the porcelain surface as well as within the internal surface of the crown.

Fracture mechanics is a science that allows scientists to analyze the influence of flaw/stress interactions on the probability of crack propagation through an elastic, brittle solid. The principles of linear elastic fracture mechanics were developed in the 1950s by Irwin (1957). This pioneering research on fracture phenomena was based on earlier investigations by Griffith (1921) and Orowan (1944, 1949, 1955). Irwin found that when a brittle material was subjected to tensile stresses, specific crack shapes in certain locations were associated with greatly increased stress levels. He also recognized the importance of determining the fracture toughness of these materials as a measure of their ability to resist fracture. The fracture toughness (K_{IC}) of a material represents the resistance of a material to rapid crack propagation. In contrast, the strength of a material depends primarily on the size of the initiating crack that is present. The strength of dental ceramics and other restorative materials is controlled by the size of the cracks or defects that are introduced during processing, production and handling. In this chapter a description is given of the processing methods used to produce ceramic prostheses and the potential of these methods to introduce flaws or cracks that may limit their clinical survival.

The brittle fracture behavior of ceramics and their low tensile strengths compared with those predicted from bonds between atoms can be understood by considering stress concentrations around surface flaws. As ceramics tend to have no mechanism for plastically deforming without fracture as do metals, cracks may propagate through a ceramic material at low average stress levels. As a result, ceramics and glasses have tensile strengths that are much lower than their compressive strengths. In the oral environment, tensile stresses are usually created by bending forces, and the maximum tensile stress created by the bending forces occurs at the surface of a prosthesis. It is for this reason that surface flaws are of particular importance in determining the strength of ceramics.

As the crack propagates through the material, the stress concentration is maintained at the crack tip unless the crack moves completely through the material or until it meets another crack, a pore, or a crystalline particle, which reduces the localized stress. The removal of surface flaws or the reduction of their size and number can produce a very large increase in strength. Reducing the depth of surface flaws in the surface of a ceramic is one of the reasons that polishing and glazing of dental porcelain is so important. The fracture resistance of ceramic prostheses can be increased through one or more of the following six options: (1) select stronger and tougher ceramics; (2) develop residual compressive stresses within the surface of the material by thermal tempering, (3) develop residual compressive stress within interfacial regions of weaker, less tough ceramic layers by properly matching thermal expansion coefficients, (4) reduce the tensile stress in the ceramic by appropriate selection of stiffer supporting materials, (5) minimize the number of porcelain firing cycles, (6) design the ceramic FPD prosthesis with greater bulk and broader radii of curvature to minimize the magnitude of tensile stresses and stress concentrations during function, and (7) adhesively bond ceramic crowns to tooth structure.

CRITICAL QUESTION

How can residual thermally-induced stress in a veneering ceramic weaken or strengthen a metal-ceramic or ceramic-ceramic prosthesis? Hint: Figure 19-4, A and B, should be used to explain your answer.

Develop Residual Compressive Stresses

One method of strengthening glasses and ceramics is the introduction of residual compressive stresses within the veneering ceramic. Consider three layers of porcelain: the outer two of the same composition and thermal contraction coefficient and the middle layer of a different composition and a higher thermal contraction coefficient. Suppose that the layers are bonded together and the bonded structure is allowed to cool to room temperature. The inner layer has a higher coefficient of thermal contraction and thus contracts more as it cools. Hence, on cooling to room temperature, the inner layer produces compressive stresses in the outer layers as previously described for thermal tempering. This three-layer laminate technique is used by Corning Glass Works to manufacture dinnerware.

A similar condition can develop in a veneering porcelain bonding to an alloy coping used for metal-ceramic crowns and FPDs and adjacent ceramic layers in all-ceramic prostheses. The metal and porcelain should be selected with a slight mismatch in their thermal contraction coefficients (the metal thermal contraction coefficient being slightly larger) so that the metal contracts slightly more than the porcelain on cooling from the firing temperature to room temperature. This mismatch leaves the porcelain in residual compression and provides additional strength for the prosthesis. Examples of how residual tensile stresses can weaken a metal-ceramic crown or FPD and how residual compressive stresses can increase fracture resistance are shown in Figure 19-4.

The same principle applies to ceramic prostheses in which the thermal contraction coefficient of the core ceramic is slightly greater than that of the veneering ceramic (such as opaceous dentin or body/gingival porcelain).

The fabrication of metal-ceramic and all-ceramic prostheses usually involves processing at high temperature, and the process of cooling to room temperature affords the opportunity to take advantage of mismatches in coefficients of thermal contraction of adjacent materials in the ceramic structure. Ideally, the porcelain should sustain slight compression in the final restoration. This objective is accomplished by selecting an alloy that contracts slightly more than the porcelain on cooling to room temperature.

A further, yet fundamentally different, method of strengthening glasses and ceramics is to reinforce them with a dispersed phase of a different material that is capable of hindering a crack from propagating through the material. There are two different types of dispersions used to interrupt crack propagation. One type relies on the toughness of the particle to absorb energy from the crack and deplete its driving force for propagation. The other relies on a crystal structural change under stress to absorb energy from the crack. These methods of strengthening are described below.

Minimize the Number of Firing Cycles

The purpose of porcelain firing procedures is to densely sinter the particles of powder together and to produce a relatively smooth, glassy layer (glaze) on the surface. In some cases, a stain layer is applied for shade adjustment or for characterization such as stain lines or fine cracks. Several chemical reactions occur over time at porcelain firing temperatures and of particular importance are increases in the concentration of crystalline leucite in the porcelains designed for fabrication of metal-ceramic restorations. Leucite, $K_2O\cdot Al_2O_3\cdot 4SiO_2$, is a high-expansion crystal phase, which can greatly affect the thermal contraction coefficient of the porcelain. Changes in the leucite content caused by multiple firings can alter the thermal contraction coefficient of the porcelain. Some porcelains undergo an increase in leucite crystals after multiple firings that will increase their thermal expansion coefficients. If the expansion coefficient increases above the value for the metal, the expansion mismatch between the porcelain and the metal can produce stresses during cooling that are sufficient to cause immediate or delayed crack formation in the porcelain.

Minimize Tensile Stress Through Optimal Design of Ceramic Prostheses

Tougher and stronger ceramics can sustain higher tensile stresses before cracks develop in areas of tensile stress. Conventional feldspathic porcelains should not be used as the core of ceramic crowns, especially in posterior areas, because occlusal forces can easily subject them to tensile stresses that exceed the tensile strength of the core ceramic. Of major concern are tensile stresses that are concentrated within the inner surface of posterior ceramic crowns. Sharp line angles in the preparation also will create areas of stress concentration in the restoration, primarily where a tensile component of bending stress develops. A small particle of ceramic along the internal porcelain margin of a crown will also induce locally high tensile stresses. Thus the ceramic surface that will be cemented to the prepared tooth or foundation material should be examined carefully when it is delivered from the laboratory. Furthermore, when grinding of this surface is required for adjustment of fit, one should use the finest grit abrasive that will accomplish the task.

Because the forces on anterior teeth are relatively small, the low to moderate tensile stresses produced can be supported by ceramic crowns more safely. However, if there is a great amount of vertical overlap (overbite) with only a moderate amount of horizontal overlap (overjet), high tensile stresses can be produced. Metal-ceramic crowns use a metal coping as the foundation of the restoration to which the porcelain is fused. The stiff, metal coping minimizes flexure of the porcelain structure of the crown that is associated with tensile stresses.

Most dental restorations containing ceramics should be designed in such a way as to overcome their weaknesses, that is, their relatively low tensile strength, their brittleness, and their susceptibility to flaws in the presence of surface flaws. The design should avoid exposure of the ceramic to high tensile stresses. It should also avoid stress concentration at sharp angles or marked changes in thickness. One way to reduce tensile stresses on the cemented surface in the occlusal region of ceramic inlays or crowns is to use the maximum occlusal thickness possible. However, within practical limits of tooth reduction, this thickness is typically 2.0 mm.

Aluminous porcelain crowns are contraindicated for restoring posterior teeth because occlusal forces can induce tensile stresses, which are often concentrated near the internal surface of the crown. Metal-ceramic crowns use a metal coping as the foundation of the restoration to which the porcelain is fused. In an attempt to overcome these stresses, the strong, stiff, yet ductile metal coping minimizes flexure of the porcelain structure of the crown that is associated with tensile stresses. Both the bonded platinum foil aluminous porcelain crown technique and the swaged gold alloy foil technique are also based on this same concept.

The tensile stresses in a ceramic FPD can be reduced by using a greater connector height and by broadening the radius of curvature of the gingival embrasure portion of the interproximal connector. However, a connector height greater than 4 mm makes the anatomic form in the buccal area of a posterior FPD too bulky and unaesthetic.

Ion Exchange

The technique of ion exchange is one of the more sophisticated and effective methods of introducing residual compressive stresses into the surface of a ceramic. The ion-exchange process is sometimes called *chemical tempering* (Anusavice et al, 1992) and can involve the sodium ion since sodium is a common constituent of a variety of glasses and has a relatively small ionic diameter. If a sodium-containing glass article is placed in a bath of molten potassium nitrate, potassium ions in the bath exchange places with some of the sodium ions in the surface of the glass article and remain in place after cooling. Since the potassium ion is about 35% larger than the sodium ion, the squeezing of the potassium ion into the place formerly occupied by the sodium ion creates very large residual compressive stresses.

The product GC Tuf-Coat (GC Corp., Tokyo, Japan) was a potassium-rich slurry that could be easily applied to a ceramic surface and, when heated to 450° C for 30 min (in any standard porcelain furnace), caused a sufficient exchange between the potassium ions in the slurry and the sodium ions in the ceramic. Increases of 100% or more in flexural strength have been achieved with several porcelain products that contained a significant concentration of small sodium ions. However, the depth of the compression zone is less than 100 μm (Anusavice et al, 1994). Therefore this strengthening effect could be lost if the porcelain or glass-ceramic surface is ground, worn, or eroded by long-term exposure to certain inorganic acids.

Thermal Tempering

Perhaps the most common method for strengthening glass is by thermal tempering. Thermal tempering creates residual surface compressive stresses by rapidly cooling (quenching) the surface of the object while it is hot and in the softened (molten) state. This rapid cooling produces a skin of rigid glass surrounding a soft (molten) core. As the molten core solidifies, it tends to shrink, but the outer skin remains rigid. The pull of the solidifying molten core, as it shrinks, creates residual tensile stresses in the core and residual compressive stresses within the outer surface.

Thermal tempering is used to strengthen glass for uses such as automobile windows and windshields, sliding glass doors, and diving masks. Often, the rapid cooling of the outer skin is accomplished by jets of air directed at the molten glass surface. If one observes the rear window of an automobile through polarized sunglasses, it is usually possible to discern a regular pattern of spots over the entire window. This pattern of spots corresponds to the arrangement of the air jets employed by the manufacturer in the tempering process. For dental applications, it is more effective to quench hot glass-phase ceramics in silicone oil or other special liquids rather than using air jets that may not uniformly cool the surface. This thermal tempering treatment induces a protective region of compressive stress within the surface (DeHoff and Anusavice, 1992).

Dispersion Strengthening

A further, yet fundamentally different, method of strengthening glasses and ceramics is to reinforce them with a dispersed phase of a different material that is capable of hindering a crack from propagating through the material. This process is referred to as *dispersion strengthening*. Almost all of the newer higher-strength ceramics derive their improved fracture resistance from the crack-blocking ability of the crystalline particles. Dental ceramics containing primarily a glass phase can be strengthened by increasing the crystal content of leucite ($K_2O \cdot Al_2O_3 \cdot 4SiO_2$), lithia disilicate ($Li_2O \cdot 2SiO_2$), alumina ($Al_2O_3$), magnesia-alumina spinel ($MgO \cdot Al_2O_3$), zirconia (ZrO_2), and other types of crystals. Some crystal phase additions are not as effective as others in toughening the ceramics. Toughening depends on the crystal type, its size, its volume fraction, the interparticle spacing, and its relative thermal expansion coefficient relative to the glass matrix. For example, the fracture toughness (K_{IC}) of soda-lime-silica glass is 0.75 MPa·m$^{1/2}$. If one disperses approximately 34 vol% of leucite crystals in the glass (IPS Empress), K_{IC} increases only to 1.3 MPa·m$^{1/2}$. If one disperses 70 vol% of tetrasilicic fluormica crystals in the glass (Dicor MGC glass-ceramic), the toughness increases only to 1.5 MPa·m$^{1/2}$. However, by dispersing 70 vol% of lithia disilicate crystals in the glass matrix (IPS Empress2), K_{IC} increases to 3.3 MPa·m$^{1/2}$ (Höland and Beall, 2002).

When a tough, crystalline material such as alumina (Al_2O_3) is added to a glass, the glass is toughened and strengthened because the crack cannot pass through the alumina particles as easily as it can pass through the glass matrix. This technique has found application in dentistry in the development of aluminous porcelains (Al_2O_3 particles in a glassy porcelain matrix) for porcelain jacket crowns. Most dental ceramics that have a glassy matrix utilize reinforcement of the glass by a dispersed crystalline substance.

Tinschert et al (2001b) evaluated the mean strength and standard deviation values for several ceramics. The mean strength values were as follows: (MPa ± SD) were: Cerec Mark II, 86.3 ± 4.3; Dicor, 70.3 ± 12.2; In-Ceram Alumina, 429.3 ± 87.2; IPS Empress, 83.9 ± 11.3; Vitadur Alpha Core, 131.0 ± 9.5; Vitadur Alpha Dentin, 60.7 ± 6.8; Vita VMK 68, 82.7 ± 10.0; and Zirconia-TZP, 913.0 ± 50.2. There was no statistically significant difference among the flexure strength of Cerec Mark II, Dicor, IPS Empress, Vitadur Alpha Dentin, and Vita VMK 68 ceramics (P >0.05). The highest Weibull moduli were associated with Cerec Mark II and Zirconia-TZP ceramics (23.6 and 18.4). Dicor glass-ceramic and In-Ceram Alumina had the lowest values of Weibull modulus (m) (5.5 and 5.7), whereas intermediate values were observed for IPS Empress, Vita VMK 68, Vitadur Alpha Dentin, and Vitadur Alpha Core ceramics (8.6, 8.9, 10.0, and 13.0, respectively).

Except for In-Ceram Alumina, Vitadur Alpha, and Zirconia-TZP core ceramics, the investigated ceramic materials fabricated under the condition of a dental laboratory were not stronger or more structurally reliable than Vita VMK 68 veneering porcelain. Only Cerec Mark II and Zirconia-TZP specimens, which were prepared from an industrially optimized ceramic material, exhibited m values greater than 18. Hence, we conclude that industrially prepared ceramics are more structurally reliable materials for dental applications, although CAD-CAM procedures may induce surface and subsurface flaws that may offset this benefit.

CRITICAL QUESTION

What is the difference between dispersion strengthening and transformation toughening?

Transformation Toughening

When small, tough crystals are homogeneously distributed in a glass, the ceramic structure is toughened and strengthened because cracks cannot penetrate the fine particles as easily as they can penetrate the glass. Dental ceramics are strengthened and toughened by a variety of dispersed crystalline phases including alumina (Vitadur Alpha, Procera AllCeram, In-Ceram alumina), leucite (Optec HSP, IPS Empress, OPC), tetrasilicic fluormica (Dicor, Dicor MGC), lithia disilicate (OPC 3G, IPS Empress2), and magnesia-alumina spinel (In-Ceram Spinell). In contrast, dental ceramics based primarily on zirconia crystals (Cercon and Lava) undergo transformation toughening that involves a transformation of ZrO_2 from a tetragonal crystal phase to a monoclinic phase at the tips of cracks that are in regions of tensile stress. The unit cells for tetragonal and monoclinic lattices are shown in Figure 2-14, *C* and *E*, respectively.

When pure ZrO_2 is heated to a temperature between 1470° and 2010° C and it is cooled, its crystal structure begins to change from a tetragonal to a monoclinic phase at approximately 1150° C. During cooling to room temperature, a volume increase of several percentage points occurs when it transforms from the tetragonal to monoclinic crystal structure. This polymorphic transformation can be prevented with certain additives such as 3 mol% yttrium oxide (yttria or Y_2O_3). This material is designated as $ZrO_2 \cdot TZP$ (tetragonal zirconia polycrystals). The volume increase in this case is constrained if the zirconia crystals are sufficiently small and the microstructure is strong enough to resist the resulting stresses. This material is extremely strong (flexural strength of approximately 900 MPa) and tough (fracture toughness, KIC, of approximately 9 MPa·m$^{1/2}$).

The toughening mechanism of crack shielding results from the controlled transformation of the metastable tetragonal phase to the stable monoclinic phase. Several types of crack shielding processes are possible, including microcracking, ductile zone formation, and transformation zone formation. By controlling the composition, particle size, and the temperature versus time cycle, zirconia can be densified by sintering at a high temperature and the tetragonal structure can be maintained as individual grains or precipitates as it is cooled to room temperature. The tetragonal phase is not stable at room temperature, and it can transform to the monoclinic phase with a corresponding volume increase under certain conditions. When sufficient stress develops in the tetragonal structure and a crack in the area begins to propagate, the metastable tetragonal crystals (grains) or precipitates next to the crack tip can transform to the stable monoclinic form. In this process a

3 vol% expansion of the ZrO_2 crystals or precipitates occurs that places the crack under a state of compressive stress and crack progression is arrested. For this crack to advance further, additional tensile stress would be required. Because of this strengthening and toughening mechanism, the yttria-stabilized zirconia ceramic is sometimes referred to as *ceramic steel*.

CRITICAL QUESTION

What factors affect the wear of enamel by ceramics, and what procedures can be performed by a lab technician or a dentist to minimize these effects?

ABRASIVENESS OF DENTAL CERAMICS

A review of the factors and material characteristics that cause excessive wear of enamel by ceramic prostheses is extremely important to optimize the performance of ceramic-based prostheses. Ceramics are generally considered the most biocompatible, durable, and aesthetic materials available for rehabilitation of teeth, occlusal function, and facial appearance. Currently available products exhibit variable mechanical properties (hardness, flexure strength, fracture toughness, and elastic modulus), physical properties (index of refraction, color parameters, translucency, chemical durability, and thermally compatible expansion coefficients for the core and veneering ceramics), and ability to be bonded to tooth structures and other substrates. In spite of their overall excellence in meeting the ideal requirements of a prosthetic material, dental ceramics have one major drawback. These materials can cause catastrophic wear of opposing tooth structure under certain conditions. The most extreme damage occurs when a roughened surface contacts tooth enamel or dentin under high occlusal forces, which may occur because of bruxing, premature occlusal contacts, and/or inadequate occlusal adjustments. When cuspid-guided disclusion is ensured, the wear of opposing enamel and dentin will be greatly reduced. In addition, if the occluding ceramic surface area is periodically refinished after occlusal adjustment or frequent exposure to carbonated beverages and/or acidulated phosphate fluoride, the abrasive wear of opposing tooth structure is further reduced.

Abrasive wear mechanisms for dental restorative materials and tooth enamel include (1) adhesion (metals and composites), in which localized bonding of two surfaces occurs, resulting in pullout and transfer of matter from one surface to the other, and (2) microfracture (ceramics and enamel), which results from gouging, asperities, impact, and contact stresses that cause cracks or localized fracture. For ceramic and enamel, two-phase brittle structures are involved. The ceramic consists of a glass matrix that contains variable levels and sizes of crystals. Tooth enamel consists of a small volume fraction of organic phase matrix and a high volume fraction of hydroxyapatite crystals. The wear of either material depends on the ease with which cracks can propagate through the structure. If microscopic cracks are forced to pass around the crystal particles rather than through them, the material will usually be more fracture- and abrasion-resistant unless residual stresses enhance the propagation of the cracks through the glass phase, the particles are less fracture-resistant than the glass matrix, or excessive voids or other defects exist along the pathway. The relative strengthening effect is dependent on several factors, including the strength of the glass and crystal phases, the size and spacing of crystalline particles, the interfacial bond strength of the crystal-glass interphase region, and the type and magnitude of residual stresses in the structure. These factors are beyond the control of the dentist, although the dentist and laboratory technician can select ceramics that are highly fracture-resistant.

The microfracture mechanism is the dominant mechanism responsible for surface breakdown of ceramics and the subsequent damage that a roughened ceramic surface can cause to tooth enamel surfaces. Enamel is also susceptible to this kind of microfracture through four specific mechanisms: (1) asperities extending from the ceramic surface that produce high localized stresses and microfracture; (2) gouging that results from high stresses and large hardness differences between two surfaces or particles extending from these surfaces; (3) impact or erosion that occurs through the action of abrasive particles carried in a flowing liquid such as saliva; and (4) contact stress microfracture that increases localized tensile stress and also enhances the damage caused by asperities, gouging, and impact or erosion. Because of microfracture mechanisms, it may be necessary to polish the ceramic surface periodically to reduce the height of asperities and to minimize enamel wear rates. Of major concern is the potential catastrophic damage that can be incurred by enamel in contact with polycrystalline asperities having high fracture toughness (K_{Ic}) values such as alumina (3.5-4.0 MPa·m$^{1/2}$), magnesium-stabilized zirconia (9-12 MPa·m$^{1/2}$), yttrium-stabilized zirconia (6-9 MPa·m$^{1/2}$), or cerium-stabilized zirconia (10-16 MPa·m$^{1/2}$). In contrast, glass has a fracture toughness of only 0.75 MPa·m$^{1/2}$ and should cause less gouging, contact stress, and impact damage within contacting enamel surfaces.

The abrasiveness of ceramics against enamel is affected by numerous factors and properties of the crystal phase particles and the glass matrix (if present). These include hardness, tensile strength, fracture toughness, fatigue resistance, particle-glass bonding, particle-glass interface integrity, chemical durability, exposure frequency to corrosive chemical agents (acidulated phosphate fluoride, carbonated beverages), abrasiveness of foods, residual stress, subsurface quality (voids or other imperfections), magnitude and orientation of applied forces, chewing and bruxing frequency, contacting area, lubrication by saliva, and wear frequency. Thus it is understandable why the hardness of the ceramic is not a good predictor of the potential wear of enamel surfaces by a ceramic. However, the larger the hardness difference between two sliding surfaces, the greater is the degree of gouging.

Wear of Ceramics Compared with Other Materials

To minimize enamel abrasion by a contacting ceramic structure, we should use a ceramic that exhibits uniform surface microfracture at the same rate as tooth enamel under the same conditions of loading, antagonist structure, food substance abrasiveness, applied forces, and degree of lubrication. The breakdown of the ceramic surface should be uniform so that asperities such as large crystalline inclusions do not project out from the surface.

These asperities produce high stress concentration areas within the opposing enamel surface that lead to gouging, troughing, and greater localized microfracture of the enamel structure. If such nonuniform surface wear of ceramics occurs during oral function, the only solutions available to reduce enamel wear are to reduce the occlusal load by occlusal adjustment or to polish the ceramic surface periodically to reduce stress concentrations and the height of these asperities.

Some of the new ultralow-fusing ceramics have a wide range of thermal expansion coefficients as listed in Table 21-5. These are approximate values estimated for several low-fusing ceramic products produced by the Ducera company: Duceragold (780° C) and Duceram LFC (Dentsply Ceramco) were introduced between 1991 and 1992. Duceram LFC is classified as a hydrothermal ceramic that was claimed to develop a hydrothermal layer approximately 1 µm thick in vivo and 3 µm thick in vitro. In theory, this property allows a protective layer to seal microscopic surface cracks. Its veneer is a low-fusing ceramic that minimizes shrinkage of the core ceramic during subsequent firings. Duceram LFC and Duceragold do not contain large leucite crystals and thereby retain a stable thermal expansion coefficient over several firings. The opalescence and fluorescence are also easier to achieve than for conventional low-fusing feldspathic porcelains because of the ability to maintain very small crystal particles (400–500 nm). Because of its high expansion coefficient, Duceragold is intended as a veneer for high-expansion alloys such as Degunorm, which exhibits an intense yellow hue and, potentially, superb PFM aesthetics.

Duceratin and AllCeram, ultralow-expansion, low-fusing porcelains, were subsequently developed as veneering ceramics for titanium metals and Procera AllCeram (Nobel Biocare, Göteborg, Sweden) core ceramics, respectively. TiCeram is another ultralow-fusing ceramic and has a firing temperature of approximately 740° C. The initial veneering porcelain for Procera AllCeram was Vitadur N (Vita Zahnfabrik, Bad Säckingen, Germany), a large-particle aluminous porcelain. Currently, AllCeram porcelain (Degussa Dental) is used. Finesse, an ultralow-fusing ceramic (~760° C) that contains larger leucite crystals, was introduced by Dentsply Ceramco, Inc. (E. Windsor, NJ). Vita Omega 900 (Vita Zahnfabrik) is another ultralow-fusing ceramic. For CAD-CAM processing, Dicor MGC glass-ceramic (Caulk/Dentsply, Milford, DE), Vita Mk I ceramic (Vita Zahnfabrik), and Vita Mk II ceramic (Vita Zahnfabrik) blocks are available, which also offer a small-particle distribution of crystals that may reduce wear of opposing enamel surfaces.

It is not known what effect, if any, thermal mismatch differences will produce on the surface quality of these ceramics. Microcracking can lead to surface flaws, loss of surface material, and increased wear of enamel. However, this effect should only occur when a gross mismatch occurs between a core ceramic and its veneering ceramic.

Based on a study of abrasion by a 500-g slurry of glass (Derand and Vereby, 1999), 100 g alumina (100 µm), and 120 g water, the mean wear depths (in microns) after a specified time period for several ceramics and tooth enamel were as follows: enamel (24.3), Finesse (20.3), Vitadur Alpha (16.3), Procera (14.8), Dentsply Ceramco II (13.6), Vita Omega (13.1), Ti-Ceram (12.1), IPS Empress (11.8), Duceragold (11.5), and Creation (10.8). The enamel wear was significantly greater than that of all ceramics tested. The wear depth of Vitadur Alpha was significantly greater than that for IPS Empress, Duceragold, and Creation ceramics. It is clear that the relative wear rate of enamel by a highly abrasive medium is greater than that of most porcelains.

Wear of Enamel by Ceramic Products and Other Restorative Materials

Another factor that can increase wear of ceramics against enamel is the nonuniform distribution or clustering of crystals. IPS Empress after hot-pressing at 1180° C exhibits clusters of relatively large (5–10 µm) leucite crystals ($KAlSi_2O_6$) with cracks between the crystal agglomerates. This noninterlocking arrangement of leucite crystals also occurs in the veneering ceramic after it is sintered at 910° C. In contrast, IPS Empress2 core ceramic exhibits a uniform dispersion of smaller lithia disilicate ($LiSi_2O_4$) crystals after hot pressing at 920° C and veneering at 800° C.

One should expect greater wear of enamel by IPS Empress compared with IPS Empress2. IPS Empress ceramic contains 35 ± 5 vol% of leucite crystals that are formed in a noninterlocking particle cluster pattern (Höland et al, 2000). The core microstructure of IPS Empress2 is quite different from that of IPS Empress, evidenced by elongated lithia disilicate crystals 0.5 to 4 μm in length and a smaller concentration of lithium orthophosphate crystals ($Li_2Si_2O_5$) approximately 0.1 to 0.3 μm in diameter (Höland et al, 2000).

Studies of ultralow-fusing ceramics have generally revealed significantly lower enamel wear rates than those produced by conventional low-fusing porcelains. However, the results of a recent study suggest that one of these ceramics, Duceram LFC, caused significantly more enamel wear (0.197 mm^3) than Creation porcelain (0.135 mm^3) or Vitadur Alpha porcelain (0.153 mm^3), presumably because of the higher void volume within the surface layer of Duceram (Magne et al, 1999). In this study, the combined enamel/ceramic wear rates were significantly greater for Duceram LFC (0.363 mm^3) and Vitadur Alpha (0.333 mm^3) compared with that for Creation porcelain (0.260 mm^3). Veneering ceramics contain either large crystalline filler particles or a glass structure with no crystals or very small crystals.

Similarly, the results from another in vitro study (Al-Hiyasat et al, 1999) of enamel wear (after 25,000 simulated chewing cycles) by ceramics using a corn meal slurry (three-body condition) revealed greater relative wear depth in enamel by Duceram LFC (0.74 mm) and Vitadur Alpha (0.80 mm) compared with Vita Cerec Mk II (0.48 mm). The explanation given for the higher wear rate of enamel by Duceram LFC was the presence of porosities within the surface of the ceramic. This result for Duceram LFC is in contrast with two-body wear data (al-Hiyasat et al, 1998a) that indicated significantly less enamel wear by Duceram LFC [also Vita Mk II (0.65 mm) and a gold alloy (0.09 mm)] in distilled water without an abrasive food medium (0.54 mm after 25,000 simulated chewing cycles) compared with Vitadur Alpha porcelain (0.93 mm) and Vita Omega porcelain (0.96 mm). The wear rate of enamel by gold alloy was significantly less than by the four ceramics.

One would expect the latter types of ceramics to cause minimal wear of enamel. Metzler et al (1999) reported that the relative enamel loss was less for two lower-fusing ceramics, Finesse (0.56) and Vita Omega 900 (0.60), compared with Dentsply Ceramco II porcelain (0.85), a large-particle leucite-based porcelain.

Krejci et al (1994) reported significantly lower estimated 5-year enamel wear rates for amalgam (50 μm) and a new Cerec CAD-CAM ceramic (95 μm), Vita Cerec Mk II V7K, compared with the original Vita Cerec Mk I ceramic (225 μm). In comparison, the wear of enamel by enamel was 107 μm. Hacker et al (1996) found considerably lower enamel wear rates for a gold-palladium alloy (9 μm) compared with AllCeram veneer ceramic (60 μm) and Dentsply Ceramco porcelain (230 μm).

Jagger et al (1995) reported the following wear depths of dentin after exposure to wear by restorative materials: amalgam (0 μm), microfilled composite (7 μm), gold alloy (16.7 μm), conventional composite (31.7 μm), and Vitadur N aluminous porcelain (100 μm). These results indicate that direct filling materials are less abrasive to dentin than aluminous porcelain. This result is not surprising. What is of importance is the significant potential benefit of amalgam and microfilled composite as the least abrasive restorative materials for situations in which dentin is exposed.

Al-Hiyasat et al (1998b) investigated the effect of a carbonated beverage (Coca Cola) on the wear of human enamel and three dental ceramics: Vitadur Alpha (feldspathic porcelain), Duceram LFC (ultralow-fusing porcelain), and Vita Mark II, a machinable ceramic. Tooth and ceramic specimens were tested in a wear machine under a load of 40 N, at 80 cycles per minute, for a total of 25,000 cycles. The test was performed in distilled water or with intermittent exposure to a carbonated beverage (Coca Cola). When tested in water, Alpha porcelain caused significantly more enamel wear and also exhibited greater wear than Duceram LFC and Vita Mark II. However, after exposure to the carbonated beverage, the enamel wear produced by

Duceram LFC did not differ significantly from that produced by Alpha porcelain. Vita Mark II produced the least amount of enamel wear. Exposure to the carbonated beverage significantly increased the enamel wear. The wear of Duceram LFC and Vita Mark II increased with exposure to the carbonated beverage. It was concluded that exposure to the carbonated beverage accelerated the enamel wear produced by Duceram LFC and Vita Mark II ceramics. Overall, Vita Mark II was the most resistant to wear and also significantly less abrasive than Vitadur Alpha porcelain.

Reducing Abrasiveness of Ceramics by Polishing and Glazing

In theory, the smoothest surface should cause the least wear damage to opposing surfaces. Depending on the initial surface roughness of the ceramic surface, glazing the surface may not adequately decrease the surface roughness since the glassy layer may be of insufficient thickness to fill in scratches and grooves within the ground surface. Thus, under certain conditions, polishing or polishing followed by glazing may be required.

Jagger and Harrison (1994) reported that the amount of enamel wear produced by both glazed (28.8 μm) and unglazed Vitadur N aluminous porcelain (29 μm) was similar; however, the wear produced by polished porcelain (12 μm) was substantially less. Polished or glazed porcelain caused significantly less wear than unglazed porcelain. Polishing was accomplished with 3M Soflex disks and Shofu rubber points.

After 25,000 cycles of abrasion testing of various porcelain surfaces on human enamel in vitro, Al-Hiyasat et al (1997) reported no significant difference between the enamel wear of glazed and polished groups, but wear produced by the unglazed groups was significantly higher (P <0.05). Sixty pairs of tooth-porcelain specimens were tested under load in distilled water with and without intermittent exposure to a carbonated beverage. Wear of enamel and Vitadur Alpha porcelain specimens was determined after 5,000, 15,000, and 25,000 cycles. Exposure to carbonated Coca Cola and Schweppes beverages significantly increased the amount of enamel wear produced by all porcelain surfaces (P <0.001). The finish of the porcelain surface did not influence its wear resistance under these conditions.

Guidelines for Minimizing Excessive Wear of Enamel by Dental Ceramics

To minimize the wear of enamel by dental ceramics, the following steps should be taken: (1) ensure cuspid-guided disclusion; (2) eliminate occlusal prematurities; (3) use metal in functional bruxing areas; (4) if occlusion in ceramic, use ultralow-fusing ceramics (5) polish functional ceramic surfaces; (6) repolish ceramic surfaces periodically; and (7) readjust occlusion periodically if needed.

Some ultralow-fusing ceramics are less abrasive than traditional low-fusing ceramics, but few clinical studies have been reported on any of these materials to validate the in vitro findings. Caution should be exercised in selecting these new ceramics for use since they exhibit widely variable expansion coefficients and may not be thermally compatible with certain ceramic core materials or metal substrates. Malocclusion is likely the major wear-causing factor that must be avoided to achieve acceptable wear performance with any ceramic product.

Polishing is preferred over glazing as a procedure to reduce abrasion damage of enamel. Ceramic surfaces should be refinished periodically after acid exposure, especially acidulated phosphate fluoride. The Shofu porcelain polishing kit followed with diamond paste or SofLex disks (3M) without a diamond paste follow-up are useful as effective finishing products.

Ceramic and opposing surfaces should be examined periodically for evidence of excessive wear. Occlusal adjustment and polishing of the ceramic surfaces should be performed to reduce the risk for further surface degradation. Noble metal surfaces are especially indicated for individuals who exhibit evidence of severe bruxing since the wear rates of gold alloys are very low compared with the wear damage caused by either traditional ceramics or recent lower-fusing ceramics.

A rough ceramic surface that is in hyperocclusion with opposing enamel is very likely to cause great abrasive wear of tooth surfaces. To minimize the risk of such wear damage to tooth enamel or other surfaces, the smoothest possible ceramic surface should be produced. This can be accomplished by (1) polishing only, (2) polishing followed by glazing, or (3) glazing only. The second choice is preferred. Glazing is recommended whenever possible before cementation of a prosthesis. If this is not possible, polishing alone is acceptable. However, glazing of a very rough ceramic surface may not sufficiently reduce the surface roughness to minimize wear damage. It is clear that a glazed rough surface is better than a rough, nonglazed surface because the more-abrasive crystalline particles tend to be covered by the less-abrasive glass phase.

It is not always possible to polish a ceramic surface in the clinic. Because of the heat generated during the polishing of ceramic-based prostheses that require extensive polishing, the temperature increase of pulpal tissue may lead to irreversible pulpitis. This is especially true when the tooth has been greatly reduced in size and the pulp chamber is within 0.5 mm of the external surface of the prepared tooth.

There are several clear indications for polishing ceramic surfaces. Polishing of ceramic prostheses should be performed when they cannot be autoglazed. Polishing of ceramic restorations that have functional occlusal pathways or subgingival extensions will ensure optimal smoothness. All CAD-CAM inlays or other ceramic prostheses that will not receive veneering ceramic should also be polished.

Intraoral instrumentation can produce a smoother surface than an autoglazing procedure. Highly polished porcelain may also be naturally glazed or overglazed without significantly increasing the surface roughness. Increased time or cycles of glazing will decrease surface roughness.

Polishing instruments should be selected according to type of ceramic, type of restoration, and level of smoothness desired. If the crown was ground with a 100 μm grit diamond, the first polishing abrasive should be 75 μm or less. If the abrasive is too fine, more time will be needed to polish the surface.

Hulterstrom and Bergman (1993) found that two of the best polishing systems are Sof-Lex disks (3M Dental) and Shofu Porcelain Laminate Polishing Kit followed by diamond paste. For the Sof-Lex disks, one should start with a disk that is the most effective at removing the initial grinding patterns. If the abrasive grit size on the disk is too small, it will take too long to decrease the roughness. If the grit size is too large (e.g., extra-coarse or coarse), the surface will become rougher. Also, if the polishing procedure is performed in the mouth, care should be taken to avoid heat build-up. Sof-Lex disks are made to be used in a wet environment, so water coolant should be used whenever possible.

The Shofu kit contains a series of rubber point abrasives and rubber wheels. The shank of the rubber tips is color-coded to distinguish the abrasive grit characteristic. The diamond paste is expressed from a tube or removed from a jar and applied to the ceramic surface using either a Robinson Wheel brush or a felt wheel. This paste is more amenable to use for extraoral polishing of dental ceramics.

CLINICAL PERFORMANCE OF CERAMIC PROSTHESES

As stated earlier, the survival of metal-ceramic crowns and fixed partial bridges is as high as 97.7% after 7.5 years (Coornaert et al, 1984). This represents the standard against which ceramic prostheses should be judged. This section is focused on several relevant studies that are at least three years in duration.

Few published reports on the long-term clinical performance of ceramic prostheses are available, and of those that exist, the dimensions of the crowns usually have not been reported. McLean reported in the results of a comprehensive analysis of the clinical performance of porcelain jacket crowns constructed with an aluminous-core that has an inner layer of a 25 μm–thick platinum foil electroplated with a 0.2–μm thick layer of tin, which was subsequently oxidized. Although the theory of this approach was that bonding of core porcelain to the plated and oxidized tin film on platinum foil would eliminate open surface defects from which tensile failure may originate, McLean indicated that the cumulative failure rates after five years for these crowns were 2.1% for incisor crowns and 1.3% for canines. The failure rates for premolar and molar crowns after 5 years were unacceptably high (8% and 15%, respectively) and suggest that extreme caution should be exercised before using aluminous porcelain crowns or onlays for posterior teeth on a routine basis.

A reduced failure rate of 1.3% was reported for 143 anterior and 254 posterior Dicor crowns, which were luted with a resin cement (Dicor Light-Activated Cement, Dentsply). A possible explanation of this improvement is that resin cement may fill in macroscopic flaws and may prevent water access to the ceramic surface. Microcracks that are present within the internal surface of a crown can be blunted during the etching procedure before bonding. This blunting process reduces the stress concentration at the crack tips. If any voids are trapped within the interface between the crown and cement in the occlusal area, occlusal loads above this site can generate tensile stresses in the ceramic that may cause crack formation or fracture.

Malament and Socransky (1999) reported survival probabilities for acid-etched Dicor and nonetched Dicor restorations of 76% and 50%, respectively, at 14 years (P <0.001). Nonetched Dicor crowns exhibited a 2.2 times greater risk for failure than acid-etched, resin-bonded restorations (P <0.01). The survival probability of acid-etched, resin-bonded crowns was 76% after 14 years compared with 50% for the nonetched crowns. Ceramic crown survival was greatest for incisor teeth and decreased progressively to a maximum failure level for second molar crowns. All lateral incisor crowns survived during the 14-year study. Survival of acid-etched Dicor crowns for subjects 33 to 52 years of age was 62% at 14 years compared with 82% for those 52 years of age and older.

Tooth preparation for these ceramic crowns is virtually the same as that required for PFM restorations. Occlusal surfaces and incisal edges must be reduced about 2.0 mm. Axial surfaces should be reduced at least 1.0 mm circumferentially. The preparation should be either a shoulder with a rounded gingivoaxial line angle or a 120° chamfer (deep chamfer).

Odén et al (1998) reported a 5.2% fracture rate for Procera AllCeram crowns after 5 years. Of the 97 crowns that were placed, 3.1% fractured through the core and veneering ceramic and 2.1% fractured only though the veneer. Odman and Andersson (2001) reported survival rates for Procera crowns of 97.7% after 5 years and 93.5% after 10 years. The marginal integrity was judged to be acceptable to excellent in 92% of the cases. Gingival bleeding occurred adjacent to 35% of the teeth with crowns and 27% of the contralateral teeth. Boening et al (2000) reported a median maximal gap width of 80 to 180 μm for anterior teeth restored with Procera AllCeram crowns and 115 to 245 μm for posterior crowns.

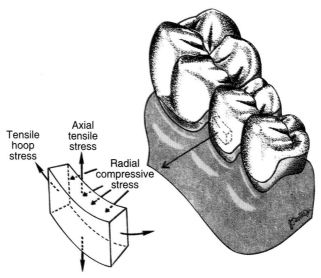

20 Residual stress in the porcelain veneer of a metal-ceramic crown for a case in which the coefficient of thermal contraction for the porcelain is greater than that for the metal.

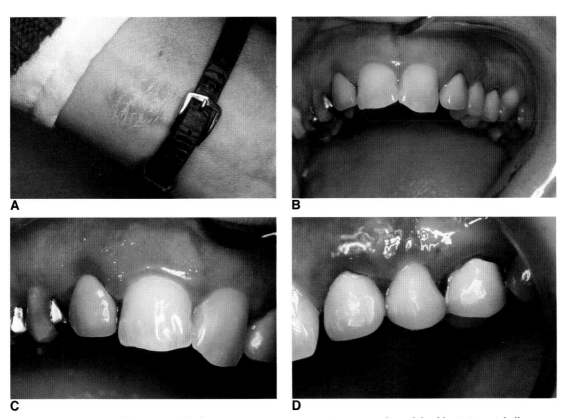

21 Allergy to nickel alloy. **A,** Eczematous type reaction to metal watch buckle. **B,** Potential allergy to nickel-based alloys used for metal-ceramic crowns on FPD (**B** and **C**) and single crown (**D**).

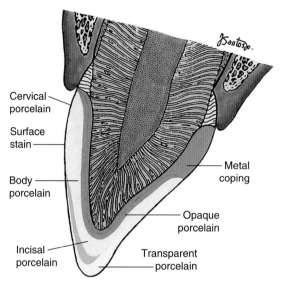

22 Cross-section of a metal-ceramic crown.

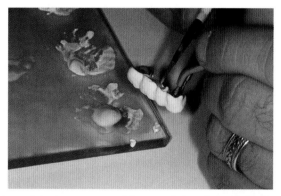

23 Condensation of porcelain slurry on a metal framework for a four-unit fixed partial denture (FPD).

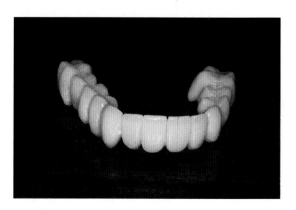

24 A 13-unit metal-ceramic FPD.

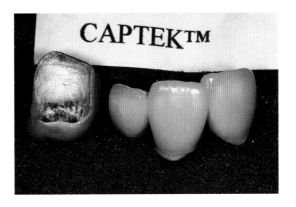

25 Captek™ metal-ceramic crowns.

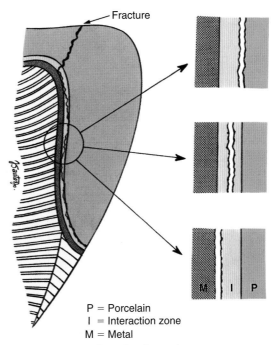

P = Porcelain
I = Interaction zone
M = Metal

26 Cross-section of three principal types of interfacial zone fracture.

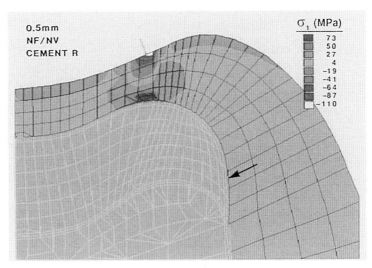

27 Stress distribution resulting from loading (close to the marginal ridge area) of the occlusal surface of a finite element model of a Dicor glass-ceramic crown with an occlusal thickness of 0.5 mm. The maximum principal tensile stress is located directly below the point of occlusal loading within the internal surface of the crown adjacent to the 50-μm–thick layer of resin cement **(arrow)**.

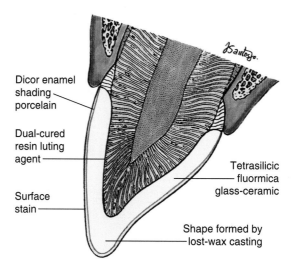

28 Cross-section of cemented Dicor glass-ceramic crown.

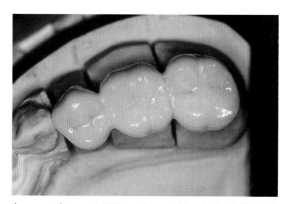

29 Highly glazed surface on a three-unit FPD produced with a lithia disilicate-based core ceramic.

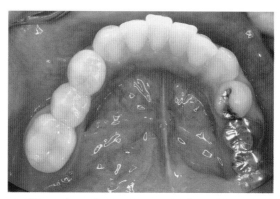

30 A three-unit ceramic FPD (tooth numbers 19–21; FDI tooth numbers 34–36) produced with a lithia disilicate–based core ceramic.

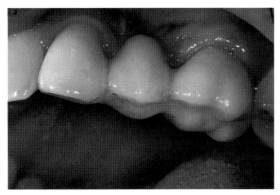

31 A three-unit ceramic anterior-posterior FPD produced with a lithia disilicate–core ceramic. To increase the fracture resistance, no veneering ceramic was used in this case. Note the relatively large connector size (4 mm in height) that is necessary to reduce the risk for fracture in posterior areas.

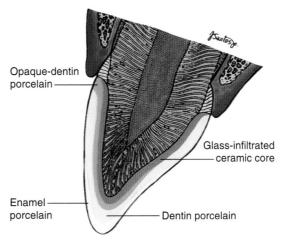

Opaque-dentin porcelain

Glass-infiltrated ceramic core

Enamel porcelain

Dentin porcelain

32 Cross-section of an In-Ceram (glass-infiltrated core) crown.

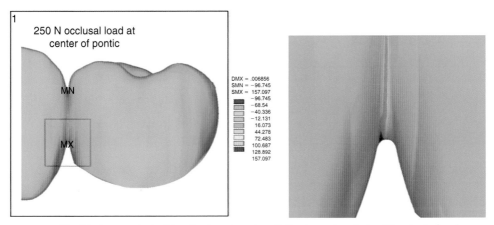

250 N occlusal load at center of pontic

MN

MX

DMX = .006856
SMN = −96.745
SMX = 157.097
−96.745
−68.54
−40.336
−12.131
16.073
44.278
72.483
100.687
128.892
157.097

33 Maximum principal tensile stress based on finite element analysis of the gingival embrasure area of the connector in a model of a three-unit fixed partial denture subjected to an occlusal load of 250 N. (Modified from Oh W, Götzen N, and Anusavice KJ: Influence of connector design on fracture probability of ceramic fixed-partial dentures. J Dent Res 81(9):623-627, 2002.)

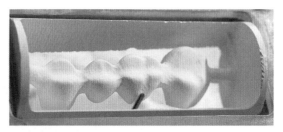

34 Cercon zirconia core ceramic during initial milling of the "green state" ceramic. (Courtesy of Dentsply Ceramco, Burlington, NJ.)

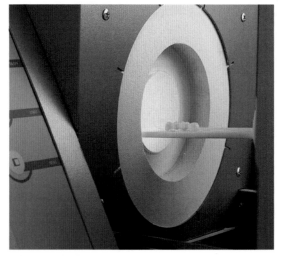

35 Cercon FPD being placed in the furnace. (Courtesy of Dentsply Ceramco, Burlington, NJ.)

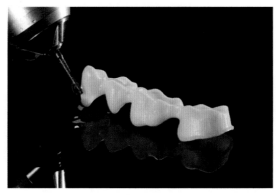

36 Trimming of Cercon zirconia core ceramic. (Courtesy of Dentsply Ceramco, Burlington, NJ.)

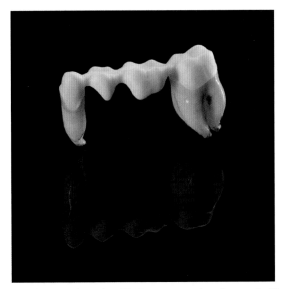

37 Finished core ceramic framework made with Cercon core placed on teeth. (Courtesy of Dentsply Ceramco, Burlington, NJ.)

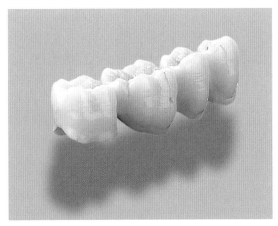

38 Final Cercon FPD with veneering ceramic and stain characterization. (Courtesy of Dentsply Ceramco, Burlington, NJ.)

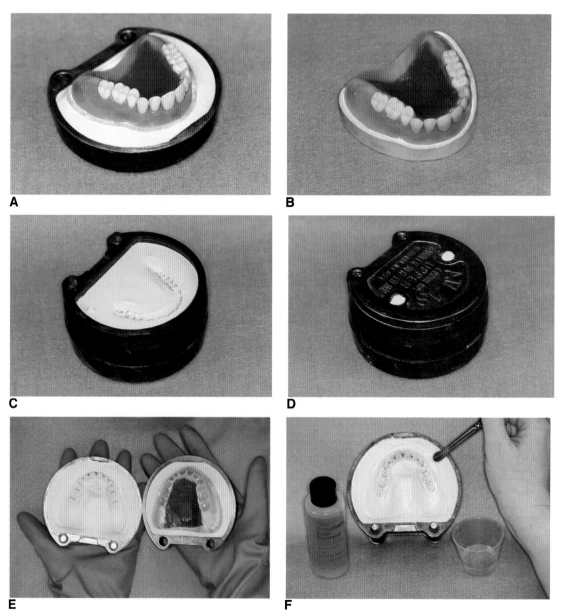

39 Steps in mold preparation (compression molding technique). **A,** Completed tooth arrangement prepared for flasking process. **B,** Master cast embedded in properly contoured dental stone. **C,** Occlusal and incisal surfaces of the prosthetic teeth are exposed to facilitate subsequent denture recovery. **D,** Fully flasked maxillary complete denture. **E,** Separation of flask segments during wax elimination process. **F,** Placement of alginate-based separating medium.

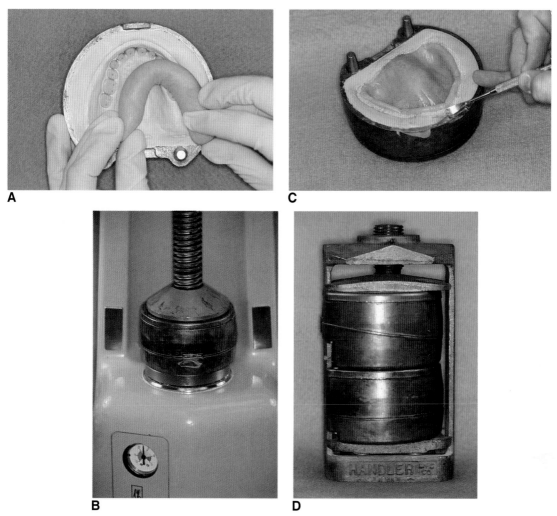

40 Steps in resin packing (compression molding technique). **A,** Properly mixed resin is bent into a horseshoe shape and placed into the mold cavity. **B,** The flask assembly is placed into a flask press, and pressure is applied. **C,** Excess material is carefully removed from the flask. **D,** The flask is transferred to a flask carrier, which maintains pressure on the assembly during processing.

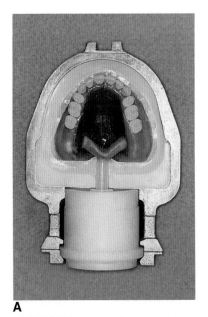

A

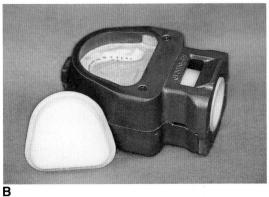

B

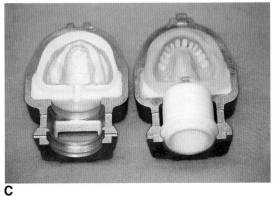

C

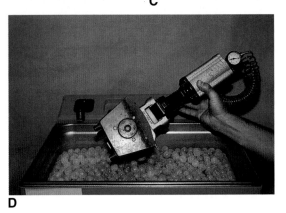

D

41 Steps in mold preparation (injection molding technique). **A,** Placement of sprues for introduction of resin. **B,** Occlusal and incisal surfaces of the prosthetic teeth are exposed to facilitate denture recovery. **C,** Separation of flask segments during wax elimination process. **D,** Injection of resin and placement of assembly into water bath.

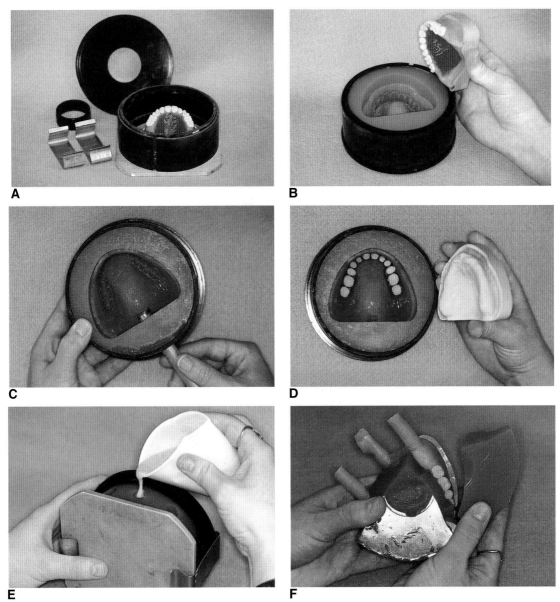

42 Steps in mold preparation (Fluid resin technique). **A,** Completed tooth arrangement positioned in a fluid resin flask. **B,** Removal of tooth arrangement from reversible hydrocolloid investment.
C, Preparation of sprues and vents for the introduction of resin. **D,** Repositioning of the prosthetic teeth and master cast. **E,** Introduction of pour-type resin. **F,** Recovery of the completed prosthesis.

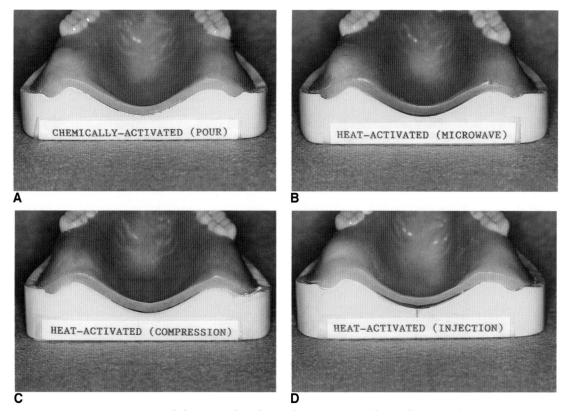

43 Dimensional changes resulting from polymerization. **A,** Chemically activated resin, pour technique. **B,** Microwave resin, compression molding. **C,** Conventional heat-activated resin, compression molding. **D,** Heat-activated resin, injection molding.

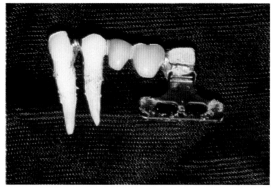

44 Failed blade implant prosthesis that was also attached to natural teeth. (Courtesy of Dr. Mickey Calverley.)

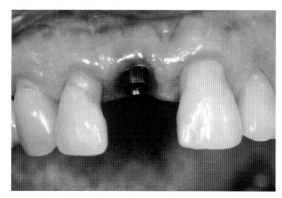

45 Endosteal implants are placed directly into bone, and they mimic root forms for proper placement and location in bone.

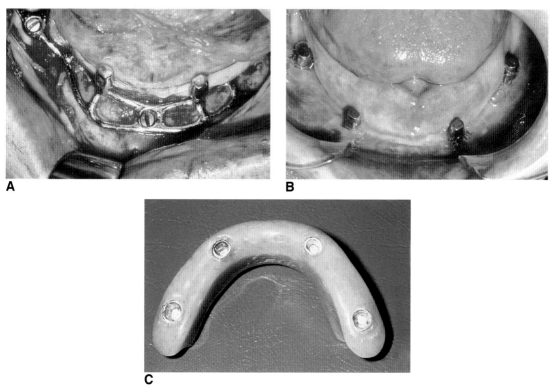

A

B

C

46 A, Subperiosteal implant positioned beneath the periosteum. Impression making often requires a difficult surgical technique. **B,** Superstructure for subperiosteal implant allowing for attachment of prosthesis. **C,** Denture restoration for subperiosteal implant. (Courtesy of Dr. Joseph Cain and Dr. Richard Seals.)

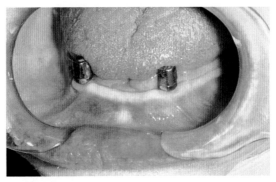

47 Transmucosal abutment for transosteal implant allowing for placement of denture restoration. (Courtesy of Dr. Joseph Cain and Dr. Richard Seals.)

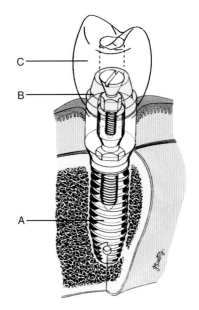

48 Diagram of implant components. **A,** The implant fixture (endosteal root form). **B,** Transmucosal abutment that serves as the attachment between fixture and the actual prosthesis. **C,** The actual prosthesis that can either be cemented, screwed, or swaged.

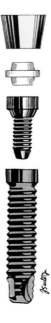

49 Intramobile element that is believed to act as an internal shock absorber.

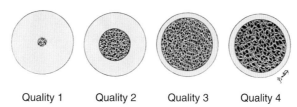

Quality 1   Quality 2   Quality 3   Quality 4

50 Four types of bone ranging from homogenous compact bone to low-density trabecular bone.

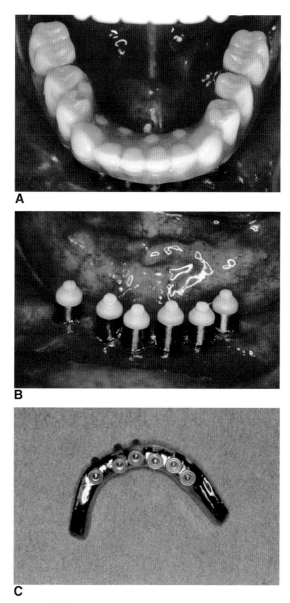

51 **A,** The original Branemark hybrid prosthesis designed to accommodate severely atrophic mandibles. **B,** The hybrid prosthesis usually requires 4 to 6 implants. **C,** Corresponding superstructure that is screwed onto the implants.

Von Steyern et al (2001) reported that 10% (2 of 20) of In-Ceram FPDs had fractured during a 5-year period. Both occurred in the connector area. Although not stated, it is assumed that the material used as the core ceramic was In-Ceram alumina.

Clinicians have experienced fractures of crowns during initial seating because of overextended marginal areas, undetected or incompletely removed ceramic particles on the internal surface, distortion of impressions or trays, undercut areas on the tooth that were not properly blocked out, and inadequate occlusal or connector thickness under hyperocclusion conditions

A light seating force combined with internal inspection and correction of these irregularities is indicated as a routine procedure. For cementation, a resin cement is indicated for the weaker products such as Dicor, OPC, OPC-3G, Finesse All-Ceramic, IPS Empress, IPS Empress2, and In-Ceram Spinell. All but the last product can be etched to create micromechanical retention areas on the internal surface. A dual-curing or self-curing cement is recommended. A vibratory instrument or a light tapping procedure will ensure complete seating since some of these cements are quite viscous or behave in a thixotropic manner (increased flow under vibratory or light tapping action). The cement excess should be removed completely immediately after seating. After polymerization, residual resin can be removed with abrasive disks, stones, or burs. For any ceramic crown, large voids in the cement must be minimized since the tensile stresses in the adjacent ceramic crown will be increased under occlusal forces.

PORCELAIN DENTURE TEETH

The manufacture of denture teeth constitutes virtually the sole current use for high-fusing or medium-fusing dental porcelains. Denture teeth are made by packing two or more porcelains of differing translucencies for each tooth into metal molds. They are fired on large trays in high-temperature ovens. Porcelain teeth are designed to be retained on the denture base by mechanical interlocking. The anterior teeth are made with projecting metal pins that become surrounded with the denture base resin during processing, whereas the posterior teeth are molded with diatoric spaces into which the denture base resin may flow.

Either porcelain denture teeth or acrylic resin denture teeth can be employed in the fabrication of complete and partial dentures. Porcelain teeth are generally considered to be more aesthetic than acrylic teeth. They are also much more resistant to wear, although the development of new polymers has improved the wear resistance of acrylic teeth. Porcelain teeth also have the advantage of being the only type of denture teeth that allow the denture to be rebased (replacement of all the acrylic denture base).

The disadvantages of porcelain teeth are their brittleness and the clicking sound produced on contact with the opposing teeth. Porcelain teeth also require a greater interridge distance because they cannot be ground as thin in the ridge lap area as acrylic teeth without destroying the diatoric channels that provide their only means of retention to the denture base.

FACTORS AFFECTING THE COLOR OF CERAMICS

The principal reason for the choice of porcelain as a restorative material is its aesthetic quality in matching the adjacent tooth structure in translucence, color, and chroma. Color phenomena and terminology are discussed in Chapter 3. Perfect color matching is extremely difficult, if not impossible. The structure of the tooth influences its color. Dentin is more opaque than enamel and reflects light. Enamel is a crystalline layer over the dentin and is composed of tiny prisms or rods cemented together by an organic substance. The indices of refraction of the rods and the cementing substance are different. As a result, a light ray is scattered by reflection and refraction to produce a translucent effect, and a sensation of depth as the scattered light ray reaches the eye. As the light ray strikes the tooth surface, part of it is reflected, and the remainder penetrates the enamel and is scattered. Any light reaching the dentin is either absorbed or reflected to be again scattered within the enamel. If dentin is not present, as in the tip of an incisor, some of the light ray may be transmitted and absorbed in the oral cavity. As a result, this area may appear to be more translucent than that toward the gingival area. Thus, because the law of energy conservation must apply, the following relationship shows the four energy components that are derived from the energy (E) of the incident light:

$$E_{incident} = E_{scattered} + E_{reflected} + E_{absorbed} + E_{transmitted} + E_{fluoresced}$$

Although some of the absorbed light may be converted into heat, some may be transmitted back to the eye as fluorescent energy. When the ultraviolet rays of daylight or of nightclub lighting contact teeth or restorations, some of the radiant energy is converted into light of one or more colors, for example, red, orange, and yellow.

Light rays can also be dispersed, giving a color or shade that varies in different teeth. The dispersion can vary with the wavelength of the light. Therefore the appearance of the teeth may vary according to whether they are viewed in direct sunlight, reflected daylight, tungsten light, or fluorescent light. This phenomenon is called *metamerism*. It is impossible to imitate such an optical system perfectly. The dentist and/or laboratory technician can, however, reproduce the aesthetic characteristics sufficiently so that the difference is conspicuous only to the trained eye.

Dental porcelains are pigmented by the inclusion of oxides to provide desired shades, as discussed earlier. Specimens of each shade (collectively called a *shade guide*, as shown in Chapter 3) are provided for the dentist, who in turn attempts to match the tooth color as nearly as possible. Shade guides made of solid porcelain are used most often by dentists to describe a desired appearance of a natural tooth or ceramic prosthesis. However, there are several deficiencies of shade guides. Shade guide tabs are much thicker than the thickness of ceramic used for dental crowns or veneers, and they are more translucent than teeth and ceramic crowns that are backed by a nontranslucent dentin substructure. Much of the incident light is transmitted through a tab. In contrast, most of the incident light on a crown is reflected back except at the incisal edge and at inciso-proximal areas. Furthermore, the necks of shade tabs are made from a deeper hue, that is, higher chroma, and this region tends to distract the observer's ability to match the gingival third of the tab. To avoid this situation, some clinicians grind away the neck area of a set of shade tabs (see Fig. 3–7).

The production of color sensation with a pigment is a physically different phenomenon from that obtained by optical reflection, refraction, and dispersion. The color of a pigment is determined by selective absorption and selective reflection. For example, if white light is reflected from a red surface, all the light with a wavelength different from that of red is absorbed and only the red light is reflected. It follows, then, that if a red hue is present in a ceramic crown, but the red wavelength is not present in the light beam, the tooth will appear as a different shade. If the tooth or restoration surface is rough, most of the light will be scattered and little will penetrate the structure. In some instances, almost no color can be seen.

CHEMICAL ATTACK OF GLASS-PHASE CERAMICS BY ACIDULATED PHOSPHATE FLUORIDE

Topical fluorides are routinely used for caries control. The effect of such agents on the surface of ceramic restorations has been studied. Acidulated phosphate fluoride (APF), one of the most commonly used fluoride gels, is known to etch glass, typically by selective leaching of sodium ions, thereby disrupting the silica network. When glazed feldspathic porcelain is contacted by 1.23% APF or by 8% stannous fluoride, a surface roughness is produced within 4 min. As can be seen in Figure 21-24, a 30-min exposure to 1.23% APF gel appears to preferentially attack the glass phase (areas with white precipitate particles) of a gingival (body) porcelain. When the exposure time is increased to 300 min, a generalized severe degradation of the porcelain surface has occurred (Fig. 21-25). Obviously, this roughness could lead to staining, plaque accumulation, and further breakdown of the structure. However, other fluoride agents, such as 0.4% stannous fluoride and 2% sodium fluoride, have no significant effect on a ceramic surface. Dentists should be aware of

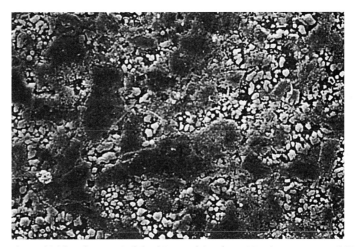

Fig. 21-24 Surface of feldspathic gingival (body) porcelain after a 30-min exposure to 1.23% acidulated phosphate fluoride.

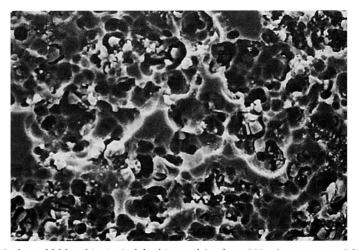

Fig. 21-25 Surface of feldspathic gingival (body) porcelain after a 300-min exposure to 1.23% acidulated phosphate fluoride.

these long-term clinical effects of fluorides on ceramic and composite restorations (because of their glass filler particles) and avoid the use of APF gels when composites and ceramics are present. APF gels should not be used on glazed porcelain surfaces. If such a gel is used, the surface of the restoration should be protected with petroleum jelly, cocoa butter, or wax.

CRITERIA FOR SELECTION AND USE OF DENTAL CERAMICS

Before a decision is made to use an all-ceramic crown, six criteria should be considered to minimize the risks for poor aesthetics, clinical failures, remakes, and possible lawsuits among dentist, patient, technician, and manufacturer.

1. The dentist should not use all-ceramic crowns for patients with evidence of extreme bruxism, clenching, or malocclusion. In this case, metal-ceramic or all-metal prostheses should be used.

2. The experience of the laboratory technician should be extensive to ensure a success rate of at least 98% over a 3-year period. This is the success rate for metal-ceramic crowns and bridges after 7.5 years. Only technicians who demonstrate meticulous attention to detail should be selected. Technicians with high ethical standards are reluctant to accept impressions with unreadable or incomplete margins.

3. The dentist should judge whether previous aesthetic success with metal-ceramic prostheses combined with the aesthetic demands of the specific patient would yield more predictable outcomes and longevity than an all-ceramic crown. A metal-ceramic crown made from metal-ceramic systems with which one had previous clinical success is preferred over a ceramic crown when the patient has an average or less-than-average appreciation of aesthetics.

4. Use all-ceramic crowns when adjacent anterior teeth exhibit a high degree of translucency. Because of their relatively translucent core materials, Optimal Pressable Ceramic, OPC 3G, IPS Empress, IPS Empress2, and Finesse All-Ceramic systems are useful for matching adjacent tooth shades for young patients and others who may exhibit a high degree of translucency. Use the toughest ceramic core materials (Table 21-11) in posterior areas when limited space or high stress conditions exist.

5. Patients must accept the described benefits, risks, and alternatives to the proposed treatment, and they must give their consent for the treatment to be performed. This means that informed consent must be obtained from the patient, preferably in writing. As one gains experience and success with these prostheses, this precaution will be of secondary importance. Initially, however, the patient should be informed of the higher success rates of metal-ceramic crowns over longer periods of time, especially when used for posterior applications. In addition, the cost differential between the ceramic crowns and metal-ceramic crowns should be considered. The initial cost and the expenses associated with remakes for the ceramic crowns will be higher than those associated with metal-ceramic crowns. The patient should again be informed of the relative cost of these restorations and their consent obtained for the proposed material of choice.

6. The skill of the dentist is of paramount importance in producing perfect impressions derived from smooth preparations free of undercuts with continuous, well-defined margins and with adequate tooth reduction. If this performance cannot be consistently maintained without a significant increase in preparation time compared with preparations for metal-ceramic prostheses, the use of the ceramic crowns is contraindicated. As stated in criterion 2, a reputable technician should not accept impressions with incomplete or unreadable margins.

Table 21-11	Flexure Strength and Fracture Toughness of Some Ceramics and a Gold Alloy		
Material	Type	Flexure strength (MPa)	Fracture toughness (MPa·m$^{1/2}$)
Feldspathic porcelain	Veneering ceramic	55–87	0.9–1.5
Glass-ceramic reinforced with tetrasilicic fluormica	Core ceramic	90–124	1.2–1.3
Aluminous porcelain	Core ceramic	139–160	2.0–2.9
Glass-ceramic reinforced with leucite	Core ceramic	73–182	1.0–2.0
Glass-ceramic reinforced with lithia disilicate	Core ceramic	215–350	3.4
Glass-infiltrated spinel	Core ceramic	150–350	2.7
Glass-infiltrated alumina	Core ceramic	256–500	4.4–4.8
Glass-infiltrated alumina-zirconia	Core ceramic	700	6.8
Alumina	Core ceramic	420–670	3.8–4.5
Zirconia (yttria stabilized)	Core ceramic	900–1345	9.0
Gold alloy	Metal-ceramic alloy	350–600	~20

Although an all-ceramic crown exhibits superb aesthetics, ceramic FPDs are not usually as aesthetic because the connectors must be sufficiently thick to minimize the risk for fracture. Some ceramic crowns will not be aesthetic if the tooth preparations are inadequate, particularly when insufficient tooth structure has been removed. Not all patients will benefit from the placement of all-ceramic crowns or FPDs. Some individuals exhibit certain characteristics that would allow only a metal or metal-ceramic FPD to be used. For example, if an individual bruxes frequently and with great force, an all-ceramic FPD would not be likely to survive. Patients with short crown heights should not be treated with ceramic FPDs because inadequate connector height will increase the risk for connector fracture. A ceramic FPD should not be placed in patients who have a long span across the pontic site, since the higher stresses under function could lead to premature fracture. These conditions should be kept in mind when planning crown and bridge cases. Ceramics are appropriate when aesthetics is a primary concern, when PFM aesthetics is unacceptable, and when a history of metal hypersensitivity exists. Contraindications for all-ceramic prostheses include severe bruxism, extensive wear of tooth structure or restorations, excessive bite force capability, and a previous history of all-ceramic inlay or crown fractures.

Recent alumina-core ceramics are stronger and tougher (see Table 21-11), and they have very opaque cores (In-Ceram Alumina, In-Ceram Zirconia, Procera AllCeram, Cercon, and Lava) that are veneered with layers of more translucent ceramics. Other products (e.g., OPC, OPC-3G, IPS Empress, IPS Empress2, and Finesse All Ceramic) are less tough, but they have more translucent cores.

The success rate of etched and bonded porcelain veneers has been well established since the concept of acid etching of porcelain was established in 1981. In general, ceramic veneers are not as aesthetic as full ceramic crowns.

ACKNOWLEDGMENT

The author gratefully acknowledges the constructive comments provided by Mr. Ben Lee, a senior dental laboratory technician at the University of Florida.

SELECTED READINGS

Adair PJ, and Grossman D: The castable ceramic crown. Int J Periodontics Restorative Dent 4(2):32-46, 1984.

Anusavice KJ, DeHoff PH, Hojjatie B, and Gray A: Influence of tempering and contraction mismatch on crack development in ceramic surfaces. J Dent Res 68:1182-1187, 1989.

Anusavice KJ, and Hojjatie B: Effect of thermal tempering on strength and crack propagation of feldspathic porcelain. J Dent Res 70:1009-1013, 1991.

A study that showed a 158% increase in biaxial flexure strength of a porcelain subjected to thermal tempering.

Anusavice KJ, Hojjatie B, and Chang T-C: Effect of grinding and fluoride-gel exposure on strength of ion-exchanged porcelain. J Dent Res 73(8):1444-1449, 1994.

A study that demonstrated the weakening of an ion-exchanged porcelain by grinding to a depth of 100 μm or more.

Anusavice KJ, DeHoff PH, Hojjatie B, and Gray A: Influence of tempering and contraction mismatch on crack development in ceramic surfaces. J Dent Res 68:1182, 1989.

A study of the application of thermal tempering to strengthen dental porcelain.

Anusavice KJ, Shen C, Vermost B, and Chow B: Strengthening of porcelain by ion exchange subsequent to thermal tempering. Dent Mater 8:149, 1992.

The influence of ion exchange and tempering on strengthening of porcelain.

Anusavice KJ, and Tsai YL: Stress distribution in ceramic crown forms as a function of thickness, elastic modulus, and supporting substrate. In: Proceedings of Sixteenth Southern Biomedical Engineering Conference, Bumgardner JD, and Puckett AD (eds). Biloxi, MS, 264-267, 1997.

A finite element study that revealed a decrease in the maximum principal tensile stress under an occlusal load of 200 N from 343 to 101 MPa when the occlusal thickness of a ceramic crown increased from 0.5 mm to 1.5 mm. In addition, the maximum principal stress near the ceramic-cement interface decreased progressively as the elastic modulus of the substrate material increased from 4.5 to 18.6 GPa.

Binns DB: Some physical properties of two-phase crystal-glass solids. In: Stewart GH (ed): Science of Ceramics, Vol 1. London, Academic Press, 1962, p 315.

A classic paper on the reinforcement of glasses with crystalline particles.

Boening KW, Wolf BH, Schmidt AE, Kastner K, and Walter MH: Clinical fit of Procera AllCeram crowns. J Prosthet Dent 84:419-424, 2000.

An in vivo study of median and maximum marginal discrepancies of anterior and posterior ceramic crowns.

Chai J, Takahashi Y, Sulaiman F, Chong K, and Lautenschlager EP: Probability of fracture of all-ceramic crowns. Int J Prosthodont 13:420-424, 2000.

An in vitro study that found no significant differences in the fracture probabilities of In-Ceram Alumina, In-Ceram Alumina (Cerec processed), IPS Empress, and Procera AllCeram crowns.

Coornaert J, Adriaens P, and De Boever: Long-term clinical study of porcelain-fused-to-gold restorations. J Prosthet Dent 51(3):338-342, 1984.

A 7.5-year study that demonstrated an excellent survival level of 97.7% for metal-ceramic crowns and FPDs.

DeHoff PH, and Anusavice KJ: Analysis of tempering stresses in bilayered porcelain discs. J Dent Res 71(5):1139-1144, 1992.

This study demonstrated the feasibility of controlled air blasting of a porcelain surface to induce surface compression.

Dorsch P: Thermal compatibility of materials for porcelain-fused-to-metal (PFM) restorations. Ceramic Forum International/Ber Dt Keram Ges 59:1, 1982.

This article presents a review of the factors that affect porcelain-metal compatibility.

Duret F, Blouin J-L, and Duret B: CAD-CAM in dentistry. J Am Dent Assoc 117:715, 1988.

A clinician-oriented description of the computer-aided design and machining of a ceramic restoration.

Erpenstein H, Borchard R, and Kerschbaum T: Long-term clinical results of galvano-ceramic and glass-ceramic individual crowns. J Prosthet Dent 83:530-534, 2000.

A 7-year clinical study that revealed survival levels for anterior and posterior Dicor crowns, respectively, of 82.7% and 70.0% compared with 92.0% and 96.5%, respectively, for Auvo-Galvano crowns.

Esquivel-Upshaw JF, and Anusavice KJ: Ceramic design concepts based on stress distribution analysis. Compend Contin Educ Dent 21:649-652, 654; quiz 656, 2000.

A review of design concepts based on finite element analyses of stresses in ceramic crowns.

Fairhurst C W, Anusavice K J, Hashinger D T, Ringle R D, and Twiggs S W: Thermal expansion of dental alloys and porcelains. J Biomed Mater Res 14:435, 1980.

Thermal expansion data are provided for a number of alloys and porcelains, and the changes in porcelain thermal expansion that can be caused by multiple firings are described.

Fairhurst C W, Lockwood PE, Ringle RD, and Thompson WO: The effect of glaze on porcelain strength. Dent Mater 8(3):203-207, 1992.

Griffith AA: The phenomenon of rupture and flow in solids. Phil Trans Roy Soc Lond A221:163-198, 1921.

A classical article that led to the foundation of the science of fracture mechanics.

Höland W, and Beall G (eds): Glass-Ceramic Technology, The American Ceramic Society, Westerville, OH, 2002.

An excellent reference on glass-ceramic composition, processing, microstructure, and properties.

Höland W, Schweiger M, Frank M, and Rheinberger V: A comparison of the microstructure and properties of the IPS Empress 2 and the IPS Empress glass-ceramics. J Biomed Mater Res 53(4):297-303, 2000.

The authors of this report analyzed the microstructures and properties of glass-ceramics of the IPS Empress2 and IPS Empress systems by scanning electron microscopy. The flexural strength of the pressed glass-ceramic (core material) was improved by a factor of more than 3 for IPS Empress2 (lithium disilicate glass-ceramic) in comparison with IPS Empress (leucite glass-ceramic). The K_{IC} value was 3.3 ± 0.3 MPa for IPS Empress2 and 1.3 ± 0.1 MPa for IPS Empress. The authors suggest that IPS Empress2 can be used to fabricate three-unit bridges up to the second premolar.

Hulterstrom AK, and Bergman M: Polishing systems for dental ceramics. Acta Odontol Scand 51(4) 229-34, 1993.

Two products were superior in their polishing effectiveness compared with several other porcelain polishing systems.

Irwin GR: Analysis of stresses and strains near the end of a crack traversing a plate. J Appl Mech 24:361-364, 1957.

Another key contribution to the field of fracture mechanics.

Jones DE: Effects of topical fluoride preparations on glazed porcelain surfaces. J Prosthet Dent 53:483, 1985.

Kappert HF, and Krah MK: Keramiken—eine Übersicht, Quintessenz Zahntech 27(6):668-704, 2001.

An excellent overview of ceramic products in use at the end of the 20th century.

Kelly JR, Nishimura I, and Campbell SD: Ceramics in dentistry: Historical roots and current perspectives. J Prosthet Dent 75:18-32, 1996.

A historical review of ceramic use in dentistry.

Land C: Porcelain dental arts. Dental Cosmos 45:615-620, 1903.

A historical article describing one of the first ceramic crowns made in dentistry.

MacCulloch WT: Advances in dental ceramics. Br Dent J 124:361, 1968.

This paper represents the first description of the use of glass ceramics for dental applications.

Mackert JR Jr, Butts MB, and Fairhurst CW: The effect of the leucite transformation on dental porcelain expansion. Dent Mater 2:32, 1986.

Analysis of the influence of mineral leucite in regulating the expansion of dental porcelain.

Mackert JR Jr, Butts MB, Morena R, and Fairhurst CW: Phase changes in a leucite-containing dental porcelain frit. J Am Ceram Soc 69:C-69, 1986.

A study of the susceptibility of dental porcelains to phase changes during heat treatment is described.

Mackert JR Jr, Ringle RD, Parry EE, et al: The relationship between oxide adherence and porcelain-metal bonding. J Dent Res 67(2):474-478, 1988.

Evidence that the quality of the porcelain bond is dependent on the adherence of the oxide formed during the degassing treatment of the alloy is documented.

Malament KA, and Socransky SS: Survival of Dicor glass-ceramic dental restorations over 14 years: Part I. Survival of Dicor complete coverage restorations and effect of internal surface acid etching, tooth position, gender, and age. J Prosthet Dent 81(1):23-32, 1999.

A long-term clinical study that demonstrated greater fracture rates of posterior Dicor crowns, maxillary crowns, in male patients, and in patients between the ages of 33 and 52 years.

McCabe JF, and Carrick TE: A statistical approach to the mechanical testing of dental materials. Dent Mater 2:139-142, 1986.

A useful review of Weibull statistical parameters.

McLaren EA, and Sorensen JA: High-strength alumina crowns and fixed partial dentures generated by copy-milling technology. Quint Dent Technol 18:310, 1995.

A technique article on the Celay system that is used for copy-milling of In-Ceram cores for all-ceramic restorations.

McLean JW: The Science and Art of Dental Ceramics, Vol 1. Chicago, Quintessence, 1979; and McLean JW: The Science and Art of Dental Ceramics, Vol 2. Chicago, Quintessence, 1980.

Classic overview of dental ceramics that covered the entire state of the art in the field up to that time.

McLean JW (ed): Proceedings of the First International Symposium on Ceramics. Chicago, Quintessence, 1983.

A collection of papers from the First International Symposium on Ceramics, containing valuable insights and information on all aspects of dental ceramics.

McLean JW, and Hughes TH: The reinforcement of dental porcelain with ceramic oxides. Br Dent J 119:251, 1965.

A description of the development of alumina-reinforced porcelain, which is the ceramic used as the core of porcelain jacket crowns.

McLean JW, Hughes TH: The reinforcement of dental porcelain with ceramic oxides. Brit Dent J 119:251-267, 1965.

Proceedings of a symposium that stimulated a great interest in the development of new ceramics.

Mecholsky JJ Jr: Fracture mechanics principles. Dent Mater 11(2):111-112, 1995.

A useful review of the principles of the fracture behavior of brittle materials.

Morena R, Lockwood PE, Evans AL, and Fairhurst CW: Toughening of dental porcelain by tetragonal ZrO_2 additions. J Am Ceram Soc 69:C75, 1986.

The use of partially stabilized zirconia to increase the toughness of dental porcelains is explored via a process termed transformation toughening.

Naleway CA: Laboratory methods of assessing fluoride dentifrices and other topical fluoride agents. In: Wei SH (ed): Clinical Uses of Fluorides. Philadelphia, Lea & Febiger, 1985, p 147.

A group of publications showing the deleterious effects of topical fluorides on the surface of glazed porcelain.

Nassau K (ed): The fifteen causes of color. In: The Physics and Chemistry of Color. New York, John Wiley & Sons, 1983, pp 1–454.

An excellent review of the principles of color and color perception.

Odén A, Andersson M, Krystek-Ondracek I, and Magnusson D: Five-year evaluation of Procera AllCeram Crowns. J Prosthet Dent 80:450-456, 1998.

Odman P, and Andersson B: Procera AllCeram crowns followed for 5 to 10.5 years: A prospective clinical study. Int J Prosthodont 2001; 14:504-509.

Clinical survival rates of 97.7% and 93.5%, respectively, were reported for Procera AllCeram crowns. Margin integrity was found to be acceptable to excellent in 92% of the crowns, although gingival bleeding was greater for teeth with Procera AllCeram crowns (35%) compared with unrestored contralateral teeth (27%).

Orowan E: The fatigue of glass under stress. Nature 154:341-343, 1944.

Orowan E: Fracture and strength of solids. Rep Prog Phys 12:185, 1949.

Orowan E: Energy criteria of fracture. Weld J Res Suppl 20:157s, 1955.

Ozcan M, and Niedermeier W: Clinical study on the reasons for and location of failures of metal-ceramic restorations and survival of repairs. Int J Prosthodont 15:299-302, 2002.

An vivo study that showed a survival level of repaired metal-ceramic crowns with previous porcelain fractures of 89% after 3 years.

Sulaiman F, Chai J, Jameson LM, and Wozniak WT: A comparison of the marginal fit of In-Ceram, IPS Empress, and Procera crowns. Int J Prosthodont 1997; 10:478-84.

An in vitro study that reported maximum marginal discrepancies of 161 μm for In-Ceram crowns compared with 83 μm and 63 μm for Procera AllCeram and IPS Empress crowns, respectively.

Thompson JY, Anusavice KJ, Naman A, and Morris HF: Fracture surface characterization of clinically failed all-ceramic crowns. J Dent Res 73(12):1824-1832, 1994.

A fractographic analysis of fractured clinical crowns of Dicor glass-ceramic crowns and Cerestore crowns (magnesia-alumina spinel core) revealed that fractures initiated within the inner surface of all Dicor crowns and along the porcelain/core interface of 78% of the Cerestore crowns.

Tinschert J, Zwez D, Marx R, and Anusavice KJ: Structural reliability of alumina-, feldspar-, leucite-, mica- and zirconia-based ceramics. J Dent 28(7):529-535, 2000.

Tinschert J, Natt G, Mautsch W, Augthun M, and Spiekerman H: Fracture resistance of lithium disilicate-, alumina-, and zirconia-based three-unit fixed partial dentures: A laboratory study. Int J Prosthodont 14(3):231-238, 2001b.

Tinschert J, Natt G, Mautsch W, Spiekermann H, and Anusavice KJ: Marginal fit of alumina- and zirconia-based fixed partial dentures produced by a CAD/CAM system. Oper Dent 26(4):367-374, 2001a.

Traini T: Electroforming technology for ceramo-metal restorations. Quint Dent Technol 18:21, 1995.

A technique article that describes a method for electroforming metal copings for metal-ceramic restorations and the method of preparing the metal for bonding to porcelain.

Vergano PJ, Hill DC, and Uhlmann DR: Thermal expansion of feldspar glasses. J Am Ceram Soc 50:59, 1967.

A classic paper on thermal expansion of feldspar glasses. It is one of the first reports to demonstrate the influence of the high-expanding leucite phase on the thermal expansion of feldspar glasses.

Von Steyern PV, Jönsson O, and Nilner K: Five-year evaluation of posterior all-ceramic three-unit (In-Ceram) FPDs. Int J Prosthodont 14:379-384, 2001.

Vrijhoef MMA, Spanauf AJ, Renggli HH, et al: Electroformed gold crowns and bridges. Gold Bull 17:13, 1983.

Gold electroforming technology is presented with data on the mechanical properties as influenced by the conditions of the electrodeposition bath.

Weinstein M, Katz S, and Weinstein AB: Fused porcelain-to-metal teeth. US Patent No. 3,052,982, September 11, 1962.

This patent represents one of the major advances in ceramics used for metal-ceramic restorations.

Weinstein M, and Weinstein AB: Porcelain-covered metal-reinforced teeth. US Patent No. 3,052,983, September 11, 1962.

These two patents of Weinstein et al describe the development of high-expanding porcelains suitable for fusing with dental alloys. The materials developed by Weinstein and colleagues form the basis for all modern metal-ceramic restorations.

Wen MY, Mueller HJ, Chai J, and Wozniak WT: Comparative mechanical property characterization of three all-ceramic core materials. Int J Prosthodont 12:534-541, 1999.

A study of the fracture toughness and flexural strength of three core ceramics and a comparison of these properties with other dental ceramics.

SELECTED READINGS ON WEAR ASSOCIATED WITH DENTAL CERAMICS

al-Hiyasat AS, Saunders WP, Sharkey SW, Smith GM, and Gilmour WH: The abrasive effect of glazed, unglazed, and polished porcelain on the wear of human enamel, and the influence of carbonated soft drinks on the rate of wear. Int J Prosthodont 10(3):269-82, 1997.

al-Hiyasat AS, Saunders WP, Sharkey SW, Smith GM, and Gilmour WH: Investigation of human enamel wear against four dental ceramics and gold. J Dent 26(5-6): 487-95, 1998a.

al-Hiyasat AS, Saunders WP, Sharkey SW, and Smith GM: The effect of a carbonated beverage on the wear of human enamel and dental ceramics. J Prosthodont 7(1):2-12, 1998b.

al-Hiyasat AS, Saunders WP, and Smith G: Three-body wear associated with three ceramics and enamel. J Prosthet Dent 82(4):476-481, 1999.

DeLong R, Sasik C, Pintado MR, and Douglas WH: The wear of enamel when opposed by ceramic systems. Dent Mater 5(4):266-271, 1989.

Delong R, Pintado MR, and Douglas WH: The wear of enamel opposing shaded ceramic restorative materials: an in vitro study. J Prosthet Dent 68(1):42-48, 1992.

Derand P, and Vereby P: Wear of low-fusing porcelains. J Prosthet Dent 81:460-463, 1999.

Ekfeldt A, and Oilo G: Occlusal contact wear of prosthodontic materials. Acta Odontol Scand 46:159-169, 1988.

Fisher RM, Moore BK, Swartz ML, and Dykema RW: The effects of enamel wear on the metal-porcelain interface. J Prosthet Dent 50(5):627-631, 1983.

Hacker CH, Wagner WC, and Razzoog ME: An in vitro investigation of the wear of enamel on porcelain and gold in saliva. J Prosthet Dent 75(1):14-17, 1996.

Jacobi R, Shillingburg HT, and Duncanson MG: A comparison of the abrasiveness of six ceramic surfaces and gold. J Prosthet Dent 66:303-309, 1991.

Jagger DC, and Harrison A: An in vitro investigation into the wear effects of unglazed, glazed, and polished porcelain on human enamel. J Prosthet Dent 72(3):320-323, 1994.

Jagger DC, and Harrison A: An in vitro investigation into the wear effects of selected restorative materials on dentine. J Oral Rehabil 22(5):349-354, 1995.

Krejci I, Lutz F, Reimer M, and Heinzmann JL: Wear of ceramic inlays, their enamel antagonists, and luting cements. J Prosthet Dent 69(4):425-430, 1993.

Krejci I, Lutz F, and Reimer M: Wear of CAD/CAM ceramic inlays: restorations, opposing cusps, and luting cements. Quintessence Int 25(3):199-207, 1994.

Magne P, Oh WS, Pintado MR, DeLong R: Wear of enamel and veneering ceramics after laboratory and chairside finishing procedures. J Prosthet Dent 82(6):669-679, 1999.

Mahalick JA, Knap FJ, Weiter EJ: Occlusal wear in prosthodontics. J Am Dent Assoc 82:154-159, 1971.

Metzler KT, Woody RD, Miller AW III, Miller BH: *In vitro* investigation of the wear of human enamel by dental porcelain. J Prosthet Dent 81(3):356-364, 1999.

Monasky GE, Taylor DF: Studies on the wear of porcelain, enamel, and gold. J Prosthet Dent 25(3):299-306, 1971.

Oh W-S, Delong R, Anusavice KJ: Factors affecting enamel and ceramic wear: A literature review, J Prosthet Dent 87(4): 451-459, 2002.

Palmer DS, Barco MT, Pelleu GB, Jr., McKinney JE: Wear of human enamel against a commercial castable ceramic restorative material. J Prosthet Dent 65(2):192-195, 1991.

Ramp MH, Suzuki S, Cox CF, Lacefield WR, Koth DL: Evaluation of wear: enamel opposing three ceramic materials and a gold alloy. J Prosthet Dent 77(5):523-530, 1997.

Ratledge DK, Smith BG, and Wilson RF: The effect of restorative materials on the wear of human enamel. J Prosthet Dent 72(2):194-203, 1994.

Richardson DW: Time, Temperature, Environmental Effects on Properties. In: Richardson DW, (ed): Modern Ceramic Engineering. New York, Marcel Dekker, Inc, p 358, 1992.

Seghi RR, Rosenstiel SF, and Bauer P: Abrasion of human enamel by different dental ceramics in vitro. *J Dent Res* 70(3):221-225, 1991.

22

Denture Base Resins

Rodney D. Phoenix

KEY TERMS

Inhibitor—Chemical component that prevents or inhibits undesirable polymerization of the monomeric liquid during storage.

Liner—The polymeric material used to replace the tissue-contacting surface of an existing denture.

Long-term soft liner—Heat-activated polymeric material that is more durable than chemically activated liners.

Rebasing—Process of replacing an entire denture base on an existing complete or partial denture.

Relining—Process of replacing the tissue-contacting surface of an existing denture.

Soft denture liner—Polymeric material placed on the tissue-contacting surface of a denture base to absorb some of the energy produced by masticatory impact and to act as a type of "shock absorber" between the occlusal surfaces of a denture and the underlying oral tissues.

Short-term soft liner (tissue conditioner)—Chemically activated polymeric material that tends to degrade more rapidly than heat-activated resins.

The *Glossary of Prosthodontic Terms* defines a complete denture as a removable dental prosthesis that replaces the entire dentition and associated structures of the maxilla or mandible. Such a prosthesis is composed of artificial teeth attached to a denture base. In turn, the denture base derives its support through contact with the underlying oral tissues, teeth, or implants.

Although individual denture bases may be formed from metals or metal alloys, the majority of denture bases are fabricated using common polymers. Such polymers are chosen based on availability, dimensional stability, handling characteristics, color, and compatibility with oral tissues.

A discussion of commonly used denture base polymers is presented in this chapter. Considerable attention is given to individual processing systems and polymerization techniques. In addition, methods for improving the fit and dimensional stability of resin-based prostheses are provided.

General Technique

Several processing techniques are available for the fabrication of denture bases. Each technique requires the fabrication of an accurate impression of the associated arch. Using this impression, a dental cast is generated. In turn, a resin record base is fabricated on the cast. Wax is added to the record base, and the teeth are positioned in the wax.

A denture flask is chosen, and the completed tooth arrangement is encased in a suitable investing medium. Subsequently, the denture flask is opened, and the wax is eliminated. After a thorough cleansing of the mold, a resin denture base material is introduced into the mold cavity. Subsequently, the denture base resin is polymerized. Following polymerization, the denture is recovered and prepared for insertion.

Acrylic Resins

Since the mid-1940s, the majority of denture bases have been fabricated using poly(methyl methacrylate) resins. Such resins are resilient plastics formed by joining multiple methyl methacrylate molecules or *"mers."* The chemical basis for this reaction is described in Chapter 7.

Pure poly(methyl methacrylate) is a colorless, transparent solid. To facilitate its use in dental applications, the polymer may be tinted to provide almost any shade and degree of translucency. Its color and optical properties remain stable under normal intraoral conditions, and its physical properties have proven adequate for dental applications.

One decided advantage of poly(methyl methacrylate) as a denture base material is the relative ease with which it can be processed. Poly(methyl methacrylate) denture base material usually is supplied as a powder-liquid system. The liquid contains nonpolymerized methyl methacrylate. The powder contains prepolymerized poly(methyl methacrylate) resin in the form of small beads. When the liquid and powder are mixed in the proper proportions, a workable mass is formed. Subsequently, the material is introduced into a mold cavity of the desired shape and polymerized. Upon completion of the polymerization process, the resultant prosthesis is retrieved and prepared for delivery to the dentist and patient.

HEAT-ACTIVATED DENTURE BASE RESINS

Heat-activated materials are used in the fabrication of nearly all denture bases. The thermal energy required for polymerization of such materials may be provided using a water bath or microwave oven. Emphasis will be placed on heat-activated systems because of the prevalence of these resins.

Composition

As previously noted, most poly(methyl methacrylate) resin systems include powder and liquid components (Fig. 22-1). The powder consists of prepolymerized spheres of poly(methyl methacrylate) and a small amount of *benzoyl peroxide*. The benzoyl peroxide is responsible for starting the polymerization process and is termed the

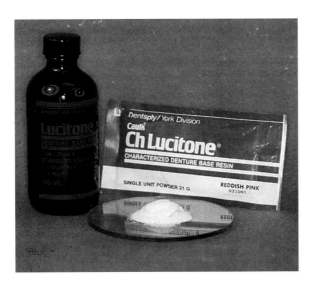

Fig. 22-1 A representative heat-activated resin. The majority of heat-activated resins are supplied as powder-liquid systems.

initiator. The liquid is predominantly nonpolymerized methyl methacrylate with small amounts of hydroquinone. *Hydroquinone* is added as an **inhibitor** and it prevents undesirable polymerization or *"setting"* of the liquid during storage.

A cross-linking agent also may be added to the liquid. *Glycol dimethacrylate* commonly is used as a *cross-linking agent* in poly(methyl methacrylate) denture base resins. Glycol dimethacrylate is chemically and structurally similar to methyl methacrylate and therefore may be incorporated into growing polymer chains (Fig. 22-2). It is important to note that although methyl methacrylate possesses one carbon—carbon double bond per molecule, glycol dimethacrylate possesses two double bonds per molecule. As a result, an individual molecule of glycol dimethacrylate

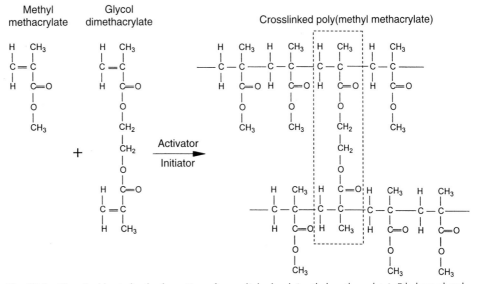

Fig. 22-2 Chemical basis for the formation of cross-linked poly(methyl methacrylate). Ethylene glycol dimethacrylate is incorporated into poly(methyl methacrylate) chains and may "bridge" or "interconnect" such chains.

may serve as a "bridge" or "cross-member" that unites two polymer chains. If sufficient glycol dimethacrylate is included in the mixture, several interconnections may be formed. A polymer formed in this manner yields a netlike structure that provides increased resistance to deformation. Cross-linking agents are incorporated into the liquid component at a concentration of 1% to 2% by volume.

Storage

Manufacturers of heat-activated resin systems generally recommend specific temperature and time limits for storage. Strict observance of such recommendations is essential. If recommendations are not followed, components may undergo changes that can affect working properties of these resins, as well as the chemical and physical properties of processed denture bases.

COMPRESSION MOLDING TECHNIQUE

As a rule, heat-activated denture base resins are shaped via compression molding. Therefore the compression molding technique will be described in detail.

Preparation of the Mold

Before mold preparation, prosthetic teeth must be selected and arranged in a manner that will fulfill both aesthetic and functional requirements. This necessitates absolute accuracy in impression making, cast generation, record base fabrication, articulator mounting, tooth arrangement, and wax contouring. When these objectives have been accomplished, the completed tooth arrangement is sealed to the master cast.

At this stage, the master cast and completed tooth arrangement are removed from the dental articulator (Fig. 22-3, A). The master cast is coated with a thin layer of separator to prevent adherence of dental stone during the flasking process. The lower portion of a denture flask is filled with freshly mixed dental stone, and the master cast is placed into this mixture. The dental stone is contoured to facilitate wax elimination, packing, and deflasking procedures (Fig. 22-3, B). Upon reaching its initial set, the stone is coated with an appropriate separator.

The upper portion of the selected denture flask is then positioned atop the lower portion of the flask. A surface-tension-reducing agent is applied to exposed wax surfaces, and a second mix of dental stone is prepared. The dental stone is poured into the denture flask. Care is taken to ensure that the investing stone achieves intimate contact with all external surfaces. The investing stone is added until all surfaces of the tooth arrangement and denture base are completely covered. Incisal and occlusal surfaces are minimally exposed to facilitate subsequent deflasking procedures (Fig. 22-3, C). The stone is permitted to set and is coated with separator.

At this point, an additional increment of dental stone is mixed, and the remainder of the flask is filled. The lid of the flask is gently tapped into place, and the stone is allowed to set (Fig. 22-3, D).

Upon completion of the setting process, the record base and wax must be removed from the mold. To accomplish this, the denture flask is immersed in boiling water for 4 min. The flask is then removed from the water, and the appropriate segments are separated. The record base and softened wax remain in the lower portion of the denture flask, while the prosthetic teeth remain firmly embedded in the investing stone of the remaining segment (Fig. 22-3, E). The record base and softened wax are carefully removed from the surface of the mold. Residual wax is

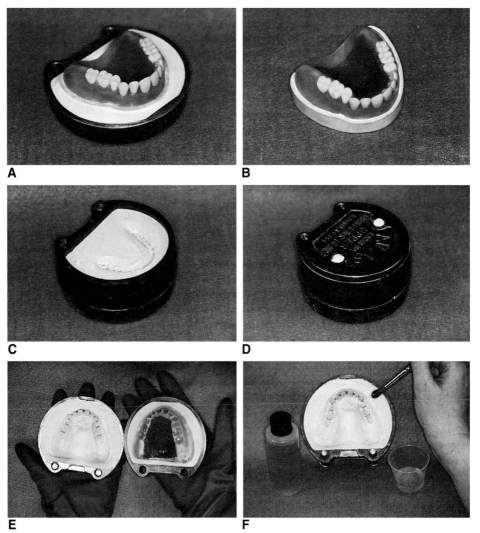

Fig. 22-3 Steps in mold preparation (compression molding technique). **A,** Completed tooth arrangement prepared for flasking process. **B,** Master cast embedded in properly contoured dental stone. **C,** Occlusal and incisal surfaces of the prosthetic teeth are exposed to facilitate subsequent denture recovery. **D,** Fully flasked maxillary complete denture. **E,** Separation of flask segments during wax elimination process. **F,** Placement of alginate-based separating medium. See also color plates.

removed from the mold cavity using wax solvent. The mold cavity subsequently is cleaned with a mild detergent solution and rinsed with boiling water.

Selection and Application of a Separating Medium

The next step in denture base fabrication involves the application of an appropriate separating medium onto the walls of the mold cavity. This medium must prevent direct contact between the denture base resin and the mold surface. Failure to place an appropriate separating medium may lead to two major difficulties: (1) If water is permitted to diffuse from the mold surface into the denture base resin, it may affect the polymerization rate as well as the optical and physical properties of the resultant denture base. (2) If dissolved polymer or free monomer is permitted to soak into the mold surface, portions of the investing medium may become fused to the denture base. These difficulties often produce compromises in the physical and aesthetic properties of processed denture bases. Hence the importance of selecting an appropriate separating medium should not be overlooked.

One of the first widely accepted methods for protecting denture base materials was to line molds with thin sheets of tin foil. Unfortunately, placement of tin foil sheets was time- and labor-intensive. Therefore practical substitutes were sought. A variety of paint-on separating media were introduced during subsequent years. These materials included cellulose lacquers, as well as solutions containing alginate compounds, soaps, and starches. Because these separating media were used in lieu of tin foil liners, they were termed *tin foil substitutes*.

Currently, the most popular separating agents are water-soluble alginate solutions. When applied to dental stone surfaces, these solutions produce thin, relatively insoluble calcium alginate films. These films prevent direct contact of denture base resins and the surrounding dental stone. Therefore undesirable interactions between denture base resins and dental stones are eliminated. It is important to note that the physical properties of denture base resins polymerized against calcium alginate films are not significantly different from those of resins polymerized against tin foil liners.

Placement of an alginate-based separating medium is relatively uncomplicated. A small amount of separator is dispensed into a disposable container. Then a fine brush is used to spread the separating medium onto the exposed surfaces of a warm, clean stone mold (Fig. 22-3, *F*). The separating medium is carefully guided into interdental regions. Separator should not be permitted to contact exposed portions of acrylic resin teeth, since its presence interferes with chemical bonding between acrylic resin teeth and denture base resins. The mold is inspected to ensure that a thin, even coating of separating medium is evident on all stone surfaces. Subsequently, the mold sections are oriented to prevent "pooling" of separator, and the solution is permitted to dry.

Polymer-to-Monomer Ratio

A proper polymer-to-monomer ratio is of considerable importance in the fabrication of well-fitting denture bases with desirable physical properties. Unfortunately, most discussions of polymer-to-monomer ratio are vague and provide little practical information for dental personnel. Furthermore, these discussions do not address relationships between molecular events and gross handling characteristics of denture base resins. The following paragraphs are intended to provide such information in an understandable manner.

The polymerization of denture base resins results in volumetric and linear shrinkage. This is understandable when one considers the molecular events that occur during the polymerization process.

Envision two methyl methacrylate molecules. Each molecule possesses an electrical field that repels nearby molecules. Consequently, the distance between molecules is significantly greater than the length of a representative carbon-to-carbon bond. When the methyl methacrylate molecules are chemically bonded, a new carbon-to-carbon linkage is formed. This produces a net decrease in the space occupied by the components.

Research indicates that the polymerization of methyl methacrylate to form poly(methyl methacrylate) yields a 21% decrease in the volume of material. As might be expected, a volumetric shrinkage of 21% would create significant difficulties in denture base fabrication and clinical use. To minimize dimensional changes, resin manufacturers prepolymerize a significant fraction of the denture base material. This may be thought of as "preshrinking" the selected resin fraction. At this point, the prepolymerized material is mixed with compatible monomer, and the resultant mass is then polymerized.

As previously noted, the majority of denture base resin systems are composed of powder and liquid components. The *powder* consists of prepolymerized poly(methyl methacrylate) beads, commonly referred to as *polymer*. The *liquid* contains nonpolymerized methyl methacrylate, and therefore is termed the *monomer*. When the powder and liquid components are mixed in the proper proportions, a doughlike mass results. The accepted polymer-to-monomer ratio is 3:1 by volume. This provides sufficient monomer to thoroughly wet the polymer particles, but this ratio does not contribute excess monomer that would lead to increased polymerization shrinkage. Using a 3:1 ratio, the volumetric shrinkage may be limited to approximately 6% (0.5% linear shrinkage).

Polymer-Monomer Interaction

When monomer and polymer are mixed in the proper proportions, a workable mass is produced. Upon standing, the resultant mass passes through five distinct stages. These stages may be described as (1) *sandy*, (2) *stringy*, (3) *doughlike*, (4) *rubbery* or *elastic*, and (5) *stiff*.

During the *sandy* stage, little or no interaction occurs on a molecular level. Polymer beads remain unaltered, and the consistency of the mixture may be described as "coarse" or "grainy." Later, the mixture enters a *stringy* stage. During this stage, the monomer attacks the surfaces of individual polymer beads. Some polymer chains are dispersed in the liquid monomer. These polymer chains uncoil, thereby increasing the viscosity of the mix. This stage is characterized by "stringiness" or "stickiness" when the material is touched or drawn apart.

Subsequently, the mass enters a *doughlike* stage. On a molecular level, an increased number of polymer chains enter solution. Hence a sea of monomer and dissolved polymer is formed. It is important to note that a large quantity of undissolved polymer also remains. Clinically, the mass behaves as a pliable dough. It is no longer tacky and does not adhere to the surfaces of the mixing vessel or spatula. The physical and chemical characteristics exhibited during the latter phases of this stage are ideal for compression molding. Hence the material should be inserted into the mold cavity during the latter phases of the doughlike stage.

Following the doughlike stage, the mixture enters a *rubbery* or *elastic* stage. Monomer is dissipated by evaporation and by further penetration into remaining polymer beads. In clinical use, the mass rebounds when compressed or stretched. Because the mass no longer flows freely to assume the shape of its container, it cannot be molded by conventional compression techniques.

Upon standing for an extended period, the mixture becomes *stiff*. This may be attributed to the evaporation of free monomer. From a clinical standpoint, the mixture appears very dry, and is resistant to mechanical deformation.

Dough-Forming Time

The time required for the resin mixture to reach a doughlike stage is termed the *dough-forming time*. American National Standards Institute/American Dental Association (ANSI/ADA) Specification No. 12 for denture base resins requires that this consistency be attained in less than 40 min from the start of the mixing process. In clinical use, the majority of resins reach a doughlike consistency in less than 10 min.

Working Time

Working time may be defined as the time that a denture base material remains in the doughlike stage. This period is critical to the compression molding process. ANSI/ADA Specification No. 12 requires the dough to remain moldable for at least 5 min.

The ambient temperature affects working time. Hence the working time of a denture resin may be extended via refrigeration. A significant drawback associated with this technique is that moisture may condense on the resin when it is removed from the refrigerator. The presence of moisture may degrade the physical and aesthetic properties of a processed resin. Moisture contamination may be avoided by storing the resin in an airtight container. Following removal from the refrigerator, the container should not be opened until it reaches room temperature.

Packing

The placement and adaptation of denture base resin within the mold cavity is termed *packing*. This process represents one of the most critical steps in denture base fabrication. It is essential that the mold cavity be properly filled at the time of polymerization. The placement of too much material, that is, "overpacking," leads to a denture base that exhibits excessive thickness and resultant malpositioning of prosthetic teeth. Conversely, the use of too little material, that is, "underpacking," leads to noticeable denture base porosity. To minimize the likelihood of overpacking or underpacking, the mold cavity is packed in several steps.

As previously stated, the packing process should be performed while the denture base resin is in a doughlike state. The resin is removed from its mixing container and rolled into a ropelike form. Subsequently, the resin form is bent into a horseshoe shape and placed into the portion of the flask that houses the prosthetic teeth (Fig. 22-4, *A*). A polyethylene sheet is placed over the resin, and the flask is reassembled.

The flask assembly is placed into a specially designed press, and pressure is applied incrementally (Fig. 22-4, *B*). Slow application of pressure permits the resin dough to flow evenly throughout the mold space. Excess material is displaced eccentrically. The application of pressure is continued until the denture flask is firmly closed. The major flask portions subsequently are separated, and the polyethylene packing sheet is removed from the surface of the resin with a rapid, continuous tug.

Excess resin will be found on the relatively flat areas surrounding the mold cavity. This excess resin is called *flash*. Using a gently rounded instrument, the flash is carefully teased away from the body of resin that occupies the mold cavity (Fig. 22-4, *C*). Care is taken not to chip the stone surfaces of the mold. Pieces of stone that have become dislodged must be removed so that they are not incorporated into the processed denture base.

A fresh polyethylene sheet is placed between the major portions of the flask, and the flask assembly is once again placed in the press. Another trial closure is made. In most instances, the flask can be closed entirely during the second trial closure. Care should be taken not to apply excessive force to effect closure. Trial closures are repeated until no flash is observed.

When flash is no longer apparent, definitive closure of the mold may be accomplished. During the final closure process, no polyethylene sheet is interposed between the major mold sections. The mold sections are properly oriented and placed in the flask press. Again, pressure is incrementally applied. The flask is then transferred to a flask carrier (Fig. 22-4, *D*), which maintains pressure on the flask assembly during denture base processing. A cross-sectional representation of the denture flask and its contents are presented in Figure 22-5.

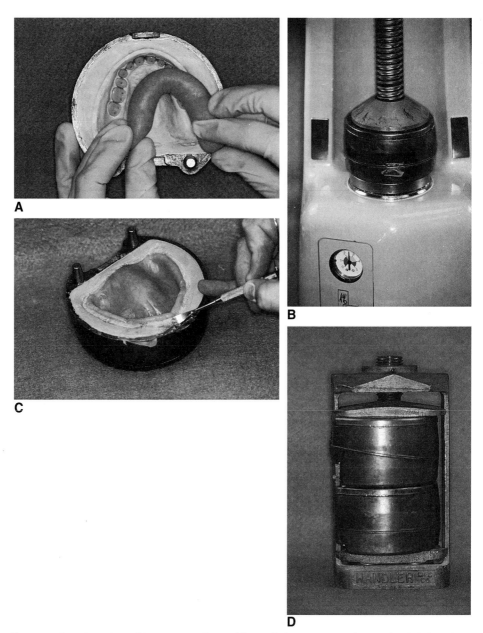

Fig. 22-4 Steps in resin packing (compression molding technique). **A,** Properly mixed resin is bent into a horseshoe shape and placed into the mold cavity. **B,** The flask assembly is placed into a flask press, and pressure is applied. **C,** Excess material is carefully removed from the flask. **D,** The flask is transferred to a flask carrier, which maintains pressure on the assembly during processing. See also color plate.

Injection Molding Technique

In addition to compression molding techniques, denture bases also may be fabricated via injection molding using a specially designed flask. One half of the flask is filled with freshly mixed dental stone, and the master cast is settled into the stone. The dental stone is appropriately contoured and permitted to set. Subsequently, sprues are attached to the wax denture base (Fig. 22-6, *A*). The remaining portion of the flask is positioned, and the investment process is completed (Fig. 22-6, *B*). Wax elimination is performed as previously described (Fig. 22-6, *C*), and the flask is

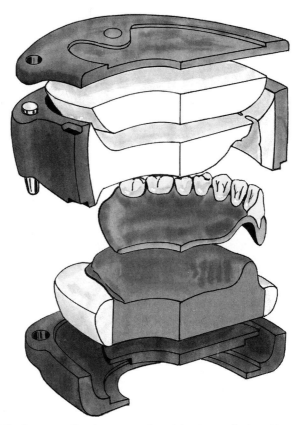

Fig. 22-5   A cross-sectional representation of the denture flask and its contents.

reassembled. Afterward, the flask is placed into a carrier that maintains pressure on the assembly during resin introduction and processing. Upon completion of these steps, resin is injected into the mold cavity (Fig. 22-6, *D*).

When a powder-liquid mixture is used, the resin is mixed and introduced into a room-temperature mold while at room temperature. The flask is then placed into the water bath for polymerization of the denture base resin (see Fig. 22-6, *D*). As the material polymerizes, additional resin is introduced into the mold cavity. This process offsets the effects of polymerization shrinkage. Upon completion, the denture is recovered, adjusted, finished, and polished.

Currently, there is some debate regarding the comparative accuracy of denture bases fabricated by compression molding and those fabricated by injection molding. Available data and clinical information indicate denture bases fabricated by injection molding may provide slightly improved clinical accuracy.

Polymerization Procedure

As previously noted, denture base resins generally contain benzoyl peroxide. When heated above 60° C, molecules of benzoyl peroxide decompose to yield electrically neutral species containing unpaired electrons. These species are termed *free radicals*. Each free radical rapidly reacts with an available monomer molecule to initiate chain-growth polymerization. Since the reaction product also possesses an unpaired electron, it remains chemically active. Consequently, additional monomer molecules become attached to individual polymer chains. This process occurs very

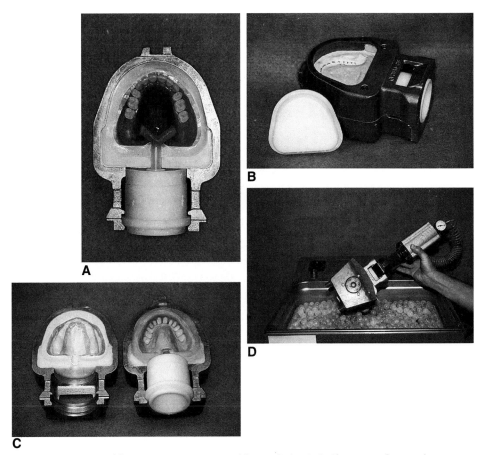

Fig. 22-6 Steps in mold preparation (injection molding technique). **A,** Placement of sprues for introduction of resin. **B,** Occlusal and incisal surfaces of the prosthetic teeth are exposed to facilitate denture recovery. **C,** Separation of flask segments during wax elimination process. **D,** Injection of resin and placement of assembly into water bath. See also color plate.

rapidly, and terminates by either (1) coupling of two growing chains (i.e., combination) or (2) transfer of a single hydrogen ion from one chain to another.

In the system under discussion, heat is required to cause decomposition of benzoyl peroxide molecules. Therefore *heat* is termed the *activator*. Decomposition of benzoyl peroxide molecules yields free radicals that are responsible for the initiation of chain growth. Hence *benzoyl peroxide* is termed the *initiator*.

During denture base fabrication, heat is applied to the resin by immersing a denture flask and flask carrier in a water bath. Subsequently, the water is heated to a prescribed temperature and maintained at that temperature for a period suggested by the manufacturer.

Temperature Rise

The polymerization of denture base resins is exothermic, and the amount of heat evolved may affect the properties of the processed denture bases. Representative temperature changes occurring in water, investing stone, and resin are illustrated in Figure 22-7.

As shown in Figure 22-7, the temperature profile of the investing stone (denoted as "plaster") closely parallels the heating curve for the water. The temperature of the

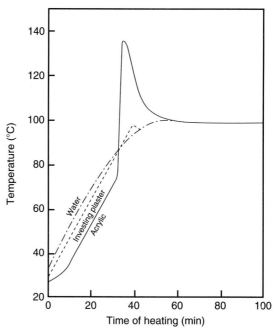

Fig. 22-7 Temperature-time heating curves for the water bath, investing plaster, and acrylic resin during the polymerization of a 25.4-mm cube of denture resin. (Modified from Tuckfield WJ, Worner HK, and Guerin BD: Acrylic resins in dentistry. Aust Dent J 47:119-121, 1943. Reproduced with permission from the Australian Dental Journal.)

denture base resin lags somewhat during the initial stages of the heating process. This may be attributed to the fact that the resin occupies a position in the center of the mold and, therefore, heat penetration takes longer.

As the denture base resin attains a temperature slightly above 70° C, the temperature of the resin begins to increase rapidly. In turn, the decomposition rate of benzoyl peroxide is significantly increased. This sequence of events leads to an increased rate of polymerization, and an accompanying increase in the exothermic heat of reaction. Because resin and dental stone are relatively poor thermal conductors, the heat of reaction cannot be dissipated. Therefore the temperature of the resin rises well above the temperatures of the investing stone and surrounding water. It should be noted that the temperature of the resin also exceeds the boiling point of the monomer (100.8° C). As will be discussed, this temperature increase produces significant effects on the physical characteristics of the processed resin.

Internal Porosity

As we have seen, the polymerization process is exothermic. If the temperature of the resin exceeds the boiling point of unreacted monomer and/or low molecular weight polymer(s), these components may boil.

Clinically, boiling yields porosity within the completed denture base. Such porosity usually will *not* be seen at the surface of the denture base. The heat generated as a result of polymerization is conducted away from the surface of the resin and into the surrounding dental stone. Consequently, heat is dissipated, and the surface temperature of the resin does not reach the boiling point of the monomer.

Because resin is an extremely poor thermal conductor, heat generated in a thick segment of resin cannot be dissipated. As a result, the peak temperature of this resin may rise well above the boiling point of monomer. This causes boiling of unreacted monomer and produces porosity within the processed denture base.

CRITICAL QUESTIONS

What causes porosity in denture bases? How can these defects be minimized?

Polymerization Cycle

The heating process used to control polymerization is termed the *polymerization cycle* or *curing cycle*. Ideally, this process should be well controlled to avoid the effects of uncontrolled temperature rise, such as the boiling of the monomer, or denture base porosity.

As might be expected, the curing cycle presented in Figure 22-7 is unsatisfactory because of the marked temperature increase during the early stages of polymerization. Fortunately, this process may be controlled by heating the resin more slowly during the polymerization cycle.

The relationship between the rate of heating and temperature rise within the denture base resin is illustrated in Figure 22-8. The polymerization cycle represented by curve C probably would yield porosity in thick portions of the denture, since the temperature of the resin exceeds the boiling point of the monomer (100.8° C). On the other hand, the polymerization cycle represented by curve A probably would result in the presence of unreacted monomer, since the resin temperature fails to reach the boiling temperature of the monomer (100.8° C). Thus it is logical to assume that an optimum polymerization cycle lies somewhere between curves A and C.

Research has led to the development of guidelines for polymerization of denture base resins. The resultant polymerization cycles have been quite successful for denture bases of various sizes, shapes, and thicknesses.

One technique involves processing the denture base resin in a constant-temperature water bath at 74° C (165° F) for 8 hr or longer, with no terminal boiling treatment. A second technique is consists of processing in a 74° C water bath for 8 hr and then increasing the temperature to 100° C for 1 hr. A third technique involves processing the resin at 74° C for approximately 2 hr and increasing the temperature of the water bath to 100° C and processing for 1 hr.

Following completion of the chosen polymerization cycle, the denture flask should be cooled slowly to room temperature. Rapid cooling may result in warping of the denture base because of differences in thermal contraction of resin and investing

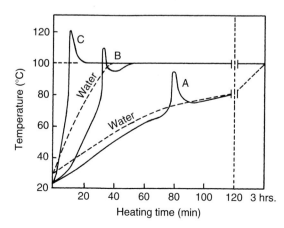

Fig. 22-8 Temperature changes in acrylic resin when subjected to various curing schedules. (Modified from Tuckfield WJ, Worner HK, and Guerin BD: Acrylic resins in dentistry. Aust Dent J 47:119-121, 1943. Reproduced with permission from the Australian Dental Journal.)

stone. Slow, uniform cooling of these materials minimizes potential difficulties. Hence the flask should be removed from the water bath and bench cooled for 30 min. Subsequently, the flask should be immersed in cool tap water for 15 min. The denture base may then be deflasked and prepared for delivery. To decrease the probability of unfavorable dimensional changes, the denture should be stored in water until it is delivered to the patient.

Polymerization Via Microwave Energy

Poly(methyl methacrylate) resin also may be polymerized using microwave energy. This technique employs a specially formulated resin and a nonmetallic flask (Fig. 22-9). A conventional microwave oven is used to supply the thermal energy required for polymerization.

The major advantage of this technique is the speed with which polymerization may be accomplished. Available information indicates the physical properties of microwave resins are comparable to those of conventional resins. Furthermore, the fit of denture bases polymerized using microwave energy are comparable to those processed via conventional techniques.

CRITICAL QUESTION

What are the main benefits and drawbacks of denture base resins cured by a chemical-activation process compared with those that are heat-cured?

CHEMICALLY ACTIVATED DENTURE BASE RESINS

As discussed, heat and microwave energy may be used to induce denture base polymerization. The application of thermal energy leads to decomposition of benzoyl peroxide, and the production of free radicals. The free radicals formed as a result of this process initiate polymerization.

Chemical activators also may be used to induce denture base polymerization. Chemical activation does not require the application of thermal energy, and therefore may be completed at room temperature. As a result, chemically activated resins often are referred to as *cold-curing*, *self-curing*, or *autopolymerizing* resins.

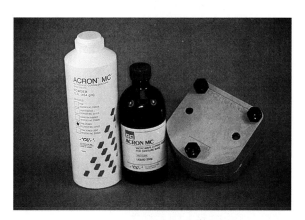

Fig. 22-9 A representative microwave resin and nonmetallic microwave flask.

In most instances, chemical activation is accomplished through the addition of a tertiary amine, such as dimethyl-*para*-toluidine, to the denture base liquid (i.e., monomer). Upon mixing powder and liquid components, the tertiary amine causes decomposition of benzoyl peroxide. Consequently, free radicals are produced and polymerization is initiated. Polymerization progresses in a manner similar to that described for heat-activated systems.

It should be noted that the fundamental difference between heat-activated resins and chemically activated resins is the method by which benzoyl peroxide is divided to yield free radicals. All other factors in this process (e.g., initiator and reactants) remain the same.

As might be expected, denture bases fabricated using chemically activated resins and heat-activated resins are quite similar. Nonetheless, chemically activated resins exhibit certain advantages and disadvantages worthy of discussion.

As a general rule, the degree of polymerization achieved using chemically activated resins is not as complete as that achieved using heat-activated systems. This indicates there is a greater amount of unreacted monomer in denture bases fabricated via chemical activation. This unreacted monomer creates two major difficulties. First, it acts as a plasticizer that results in decreased transverse strength of the denture resin. Second, the residual monomer serves as a potential tissue irritant, thereby compromising the biocompatibility of the denture base.

From a physical standpoint, chemically activated resins display slightly less shrinkage than their heat-activated counterparts. This imparts greater dimensional accuracy to chemically activated resins.

The color stability of chemically activated resins generally is inferior to the color stability of heat-activated resins. This property is related to the presence of tertiary amines within the chemically activated resins. Such amines are susceptible to oxidation and accompanying color changes that affect the appearance of the resin. Discoloration of these resins may be minimized via the addition of stabilizing agents that prevent such oxidation.

Technical Considerations

Chemically activated denture base resins are most often molded using compression techniques. Therefore mold preparation and resin packing are essentially the same as those described for heat-activated denture resins.

Polymer and monomer are supplied in the form of a powder and a liquid, respectively. These components are mixed according to manufacturer's directions and permitted to attain a doughlike consistency. The working time for chemically activated resins is shorter than for heat-activated materials. Therefore special attention must be paid to the consistency of the material and rate of polymerization.

A lengthy initiation period is desirable, since this provides adequate time for trial closures. One method for prolonging the initiation period is to decrease the temperature of the resin mass. This may be accomplished by refrigerating the liquid component and/or mixing vessel before the mixing process. When the powder and liquid are mixed, the rate of polymerization process decreases. As a result, the resin mass remains in a doughy stage for an extended period, and the working time is increased.

Mold preparation and resin packing are accomplished in the same manner described for heat-activated resins. In cases of chemically activated resins with minimal working times, it is doubtful that more than two trial closures can be made. Therefore extreme care must be taken to ensure that a proper amount of resin is employed and a minimal number of trial closures are needed.

Processing Considerations

Following final closure of the denture flask, pressure must be maintained throughout the polymerization process. The time required for polymerization will vary with the material chosen.

Initial hardening of the resin generally will occur within 30 min of final flask closure. However, it is doubtful that polymerization will be complete at this point. To ensure sufficient polymerization, the flask should be held under pressure for a minimum of 3 hr.

As previously noted, the polymerization of chemically activated resins is never as complete as the polymerization of heat-activated materials. Resins polymerized via chemical activation generally display 3% to 5% free monomer, whereas heat-activated resins exhibit 0.2% to 0.5% free monomer. Therefore it is important that the polymerization of chemically activated resins be as complete as possible. Failure to achieve a high degree of polymerization will predispose the denture base to dimensional instability and may lead to soft tissue irritation.

Fluid Resin Technique

The *fluid resin technique* employs a pourable, chemically activated resin for the fabrication of denture bases. The resin is supplied in the form of powder and liquid components. When mixed in the proper proportions, these components yield a low viscosity resin. Subsequently, this resin is poured into a mold cavity, subjected to increased atmospheric pressure, and allowed to polymerize. Laboratory aspects of the fluid resin technique are described in the following paragraphs.

Tooth arrangement is accomplished using accepted prosthodontic principles. The completed tooth arrangement is then sealed to the underlying cast and placed in a specially designed flask (Fig. 22-10, *A*). The flask is filled with a reversible hydrocolloid investment medium, and the assembly is cooled. Following gelation of the hydrocolloid, the cast with the attached tooth arrangement is removed from the flask (Fig. 22-10, *B*). At this stage, sprues and vents are cut from the external surface of the flask to the mold cavity (Fig. 22-10, *C*).

Wax is eliminated from the cast using hot water. The prosthetic teeth are retrieved and carefully seated in their respective positions within the hydrocolloid investing medium. Subsequently, the cast is returned to its position within the mold (Fig. 22-10, *D*).

The resin is mixed according to manufacturer's directions and poured into the mold via the sprue channels (Fig. 22-10, *E*). The flask is then placed in a pressurized chamber (i.e., pressure pot) at room temperature and the resin is permitted to polymerize. According to available information, only 30 to 45 min are required for polymerization. Nevertheless, a longer period is suggested.

Following completion of the polymerization process, the denture is retrieved from the flask (Fig. 22-10, *F*), and the sprues are removed. The denture/cast assembly is returned to the articulator for correction of processing changes. Subsequently, the denture base is finished and polished. After finishing and polishing, the denture should be stored in water to prevent dehydration and warping.

Advantages claimed for the fluid resin technique include (1) improved adaptation to underlying soft tissues, (2) decreased probability of damage to prosthetic teeth and denture bases during deflasking, (3) reduced material costs, (4) and simplification of the flasking, deflasking, and finishing procedures.

Potential disadvantages of the fluid resin technique include (1) noticeable shifting of prosthetic teeth during processing, (2) air entrapment within the denture base

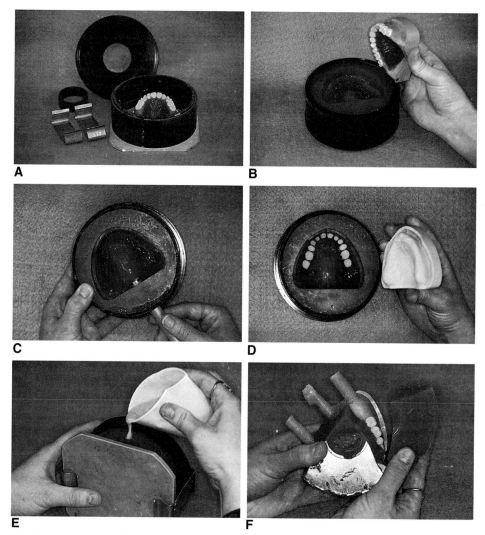

Fig. 22-10 Steps in mold preparation (fluid resin technique). **A,** Completed tooth arrangement positioned in a fluid resin flask. **B,** Removal of tooth arrangement from reversible hydrocolloid investment. **C,** Preparation of sprues and vents for the introduction of resin. **D,** Repositioning of the prosthetic teeth and master cast. **E,** Introduction of pour-type resin. **F,** Recovery of the completed prosthesis. See also color plate.

material, (3) poor bonding between the denture base material and acrylic resin teeth, and (4) technique sensitivity.

In general, denture bases fabricated in this manner exhibit physical properties that are somewhat inferior to those of conventional heat-processed resins. Nonetheless, clinically acceptable dentures can be obtained using fluid resins.

LIGHT-ACTIVATED DENTURE BASE RESINS

A visible light-activated denture base resin has been available to the dental community for several years. This material has been described as a composite having a matrix of urethane dimethacrylate, microfine silica, and high molecular weight acrylic resin monomers. Acrylic resin beads are included as organic filler. *Visible light* is the *activator*, whereas *camphorquinone* serves as the *initiator* for polymerization.

The single-component denture base resin is supplied in sheet and rope forms and is packed in light-proof pouches to prevent inadvertent polymerization (Fig. 22-11, *A*).

As might be expected, denture base fabrication using a light-activated resin is significantly different from the techniques described in previous sections. Opaque investing media prevent the passage of light; therefore light-activated resins cannot be flasked in a conventional manner. Instead, teeth are arranged, and the denture base is molded on an accurate cast (Fig. 22-11, *B*). Subsequently, the denture base is exposed to a high-intensity visible light source for an appropriate period (Fig. 22-11, *C*). Following polymerization, the denture is removed from the cast, finished, and polished in a conventional manner.

PHYSICAL PROPERTIES OF DENTURE BASE RESINS

The physical properties of denture base resins are critical to the fit and function of removable dental prostheses. Characteristics of interest include polymerization shrinkage, porosity, water absorption, solubility, processing stresses, and crazing. These characteristics are addressed in the following sections.

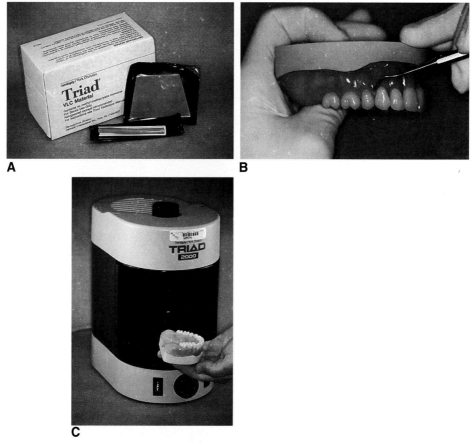

Fig. 22-11   Steps in denture fabrication (light-activated denture base resins). **A,** Representative light-activated denture base resin. Sheet and rope forms are supplied in light-proof pouches to prevent inadvertent polymerization. **B,** Teeth are arranged and the denture base sculpted using light-activated resin. **C,** The denture base is placed into a light chamber and polymerized according to manufacturer's recommendations.

Polymerization Shrinkage

When methyl methacrylate monomer is polymerized to form poly(methyl methacrylate), the density of the mass changes from 0.94 g/cm^3 to 1.19 g/cm^3. This change in density results in a volumetric shrinkage of 21%. When a conventional heat-activated resin is mixed at the suggested powder-to-liquid ratio, about one-third of the mass is liquid. The remainder of the mass is pre-polymerized poly(methyl methacrylate). Consequently, the volumetric shrinkage exhibited by the polymerized mass should be approximately 7%. This figure is in agreement with values observed in laboratory and clinical investigations.

There are several possible reasons why materials exhibiting such high volumetric shrinkages can be used to produce clinically satisfactory denture bases. It appears the shrinkage exhibited by these materials is distributed uniformly to all surfaces. Hence the adaptation of denture bases to underlying soft tissues is not significantly affected, provided the materials are manipulated properly.

In addition to volumetric shrinkage, one also must consider the effects of linear shrinkage. Linear shrinkage causes significant effects upon denture base adaptation and cuspal interdigitation.

By convention, linear shrinkage values are determined by measuring the distance between two predetermined reference points in the second molar regions of a completed tooth arrangement. Following polymerization of the denture base resin and removal of the prosthesis from the master cast, the distance between these reference points is measured once again. The difference between pre- and postpolymerization measurements is recorded as linear shrinkage. The greater the linear shrinkage, the greater is the discrepancy observed in the initial fit of a denture.

CRITICAL QUESTION

Why is the relatively high volumetric shrinkage of a denture base resin not usually considered as a significant clinical problem?

Based on a projected volumetric shrinkage of 7%, an acrylic resin denture base should exhibit a linear shrinkage of approximately 2%. In reality, the observed linear shrinkage generally observed is less than 1% (Table 22-1).

Examination of the polymerization process indicates thermal shrinkage of resin is primarily responsible for the linear shrinkage phenomenon in heat-activated systems. During the initial stages of the cooling process, the resin remains relatively

Table 22-1 Polymerization Shrinkage of Maxillary Denture Bases	
Material	**Linear shrinkage (%)**
High-impact acrylic resin	0.12
Vinyl acrylic resin	0.33
Conventional acrylic resin	0.43
Pour-type acrylic resin	0.48
Rapid heat-cured acrylic resin	0.97

Adapted from Stafford GD, Bates JF, Huggett R, and Handley RW: A review of the properties of some denture base polymers. J Dent 8: 292, 1960.

soft. Therefore the pressure maintained on the flask assembly causes the resin to contract at approximately the same rate as the surrounding dental stone.

As cooling proceeds, the soft resin approaches its *glass transition temperature*. The glass transition temperature is a thermal range in which the polymerized resin passes from a soft, rubbery state to a rigid, glassy state. Hence, cooling the denture base resin beyond the glass transition temperature yields a rigid mass. In turn, this rigid mass contracts at a rate different from that of surrounding dental stone. The shrinkage occurring below the glass transition temperature is thermal in nature and varies according to the composition of the resin.

To illustrate the effect of thermal shrinkage, consider the following example. The glass transition temperature for poly(methyl methacrylate) is approximately 105° C. Room temperature is 20° C. The generally accepted value for linear coefficient of thermal expansion, α, for poly(methyl methacrylate) is 81 ppm/° C. Therefore, as the denture base resin cools from the glass transition temperature to room temperature, it undergoes a linear shrinkage that may be expressed as:

$$\text{Linear Shrinkage} = \alpha \Delta T = (81 \text{ ppm/}° \text{ C})(105° \text{ C} - 20° \text{ C})(100\%) = 0.69\% \qquad (1)$$

This value is in agreement with linear shrinkages of 0.12% to 0.97% reported for various commercial denture resins (see Table 22-1).

Complete dentures constructed using chemically activated resins generally display better adaptation than those constructed using heat-activated resins. This phenomenon may be attributed to the negligible thermal shrinkage displayed by chemically activated resins. Processing shrinkage has been measured as 0.26% for a representative chemically activated resin, compared with 0.53% for a representative heat-activated resin.

Given the preceding information regarding polymerization shrinkage and denture base adaptation, chemically activated resins appear to provide significant advantages over heat-activated resins. However, there are several other factors that affect the overall dimensional characteristics of processed denture bases including the type of investing medium selected, method of resin introduction, and the temperature used to activate the polymerization process.

On completion of the polymerization process, individual denture bases and master casts are retrieved and returned to their respective articulator(s). At this stage, dimensional changes are assessed with respect to proposed vertical dimension of occlusion.

Fluid resin techniques used in conjunction with hydrocolloid investing media generally yield decreases in vertical dimension. Conversely, dentures processed using heat-activated or chemically activated resins in conjunction with compression-molding techniques usually display increases in overall vertical dimension. Minimal increases in vertical dimension are considered desirable, since they permit a return to the proposed occlusal vertical dimension through occlusal grinding procedures. Dimensional changes occurring in denture bases fabricated from various resins are illustrated in Figure 22-12.

CRITICAL QUESTIONS

What are the causes of porosity when using fluid resin denture fabrication techniques? How can this problem be minimized?

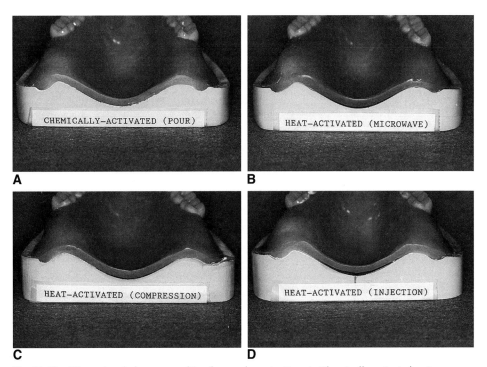

Fig. 22-12 Dimensional changes resulting from polymerization. **A,** Chemically activated resin, pour technique. **B,** Microwave resin, compression molding. **C,** Conventional heat-activated resin, compression molding. **D,** Heat-activated resin, injection molding. See also color plate.

Porosity

The presence of surface and subsurface voids may compromise the physical, aesthetic, and hygienic properties of a processed denture base. It has been noted that porosity is likely to develop in thicker portions of a denture base. Such porosity results from the vaporization of unreacted monomer and low molecular weight polymers, when the temperature of a resin reaches or surpasses the boiling points of these species. Nonetheless, this type of porosity may not occur equally throughout affected resin segments.

To facilitate an understanding of this concept, consider the specimens in Figures 22-13, *A* (no porosity) and 22-13, *B* (localized subsurface porosity). Specimens B and C were flasked in such a manner that the section displaying porosity was nearer the center of the investment mass, whereas the nonporous section was nearer the surface of the metal flask. As might be expected, the metal of the flask conducted heat away from the periphery with sufficient rapidity to prevent a substantial temperature rise. Consequently, the low–molecular-weight species did not boil, and porosity did not develop. In contrast, resin specimens occupying central positions in the mold were surrounded by larger amounts of dental stone. Because this material is a poor thermal conductor, heat was not readily dissipated, low–molecular-weight species were vaporized, and noticeable porosity was produced.

Porosity also may result from inadequate mixing of powder and liquid components. If this occurs, some regions of the resin mass will contain more monomer than others. During polymerization these regions shrink more than adjacent regions, and the localized shrinkage tends to produce voids (Fig. 22-13, *D*).

The occurrence of such porosity can be minimized by ensuring the greatest possible homogeneity of the resin. Hence, the use of proper polymer-to-monomer ratios and well-controlled mixing procedures is essential. Furthermore, because the

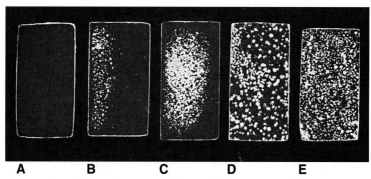

Fig. 22-13   Heat-activated denture base resin exhibiting different types and degrees of porosity.
A, Properly polymerized; no porosity. **B** and **C,** Rapid heating, relatively small subsurface voids.
D, Insufficient mixing of monomer and polymer; large voids resulting from localized polymerization
shrinkage. **E,** Insufficient pressure during polymerization; relatively large, irregular voids. (From
Tuckfield WJ, Worner HK, and Guerin BD: Acrylic resins in dentistry. Aust Dent J, March, 1943.)

material is more homogeneous in the doughlike stage, it is wise to delay packing
until this consistency has been reached. In evaluating the information presented in
Figure 22-13, it should be recognized that such porosities can occur in surface and
subsurface locations. Porosities resulting from rapid temperature elevation can be
much larger than those presented in Figure 22-13, *B* and *C*.

A third type of porosity may be caused by inadequate pressure or insufficient
material in the mold during polymerization (Fig. 22-13, *E*). Voids resulting from
these inadequacies are not spherical; they assume irregular shapes. These voids may
be so abundant that the resultant resin appears significantly lighter and more
opaque than its intended color.

A final type of porosity is most often associated with fluid resins. Such porosity
appears to be caused by air inclusions incorporated during mixing and pouring procedures. If these inclusions are not removed, sizable voids may be produced in the
resultant denture bases. Careful mixing, spruing, and venting seem to help reduce
the incidence of air inclusions.

Water Absorption

Poly(methyl methacrylate) absorbs relatively small amounts of water when placed
in an aqueous environment. This water exerts significant effects on the mechanical
and dimensional properties of the polymer.

Although absorption is facilitated by the polarity of poly(methyl methacrylate)
molecules, a diffusion mechanism is primarily responsible for the ingress of water.
Diffusion is the migration of one substance through a space, or within a second substance. In this instance, water molecules penetrate the poly(methyl methacrylate)
mass, and occupy positions between polymer chains. Consequently, the affected
polymer chains are forced apart. The introduction of water molecules within the
polymerized mass produces two important effects. First, it causes a slight expansion
of the polymerized mass. Second, water molecules interfere with the entanglement
of polymer chains, and thereby act as plasticizers.

Poly(methyl methacrylate) exhibits a water sorption value of 0.69 mg/cm^2.
Although this amount of water may seem inconsequential, it produces significant
effects in polymerized resins. It has been estimated that for each 1% increase in
weight produced by water absorption, acrylic resin expands 0.23% linearly.
Laboratory trials indicate the linear expansion caused by water absorption is approx-

imately equal to the thermal shrinkage encountered as a result of the polymerization process. Hence, these processes very nearly offset one another.

As previously noted, water molecules also may interfere with entanglement of polymer chains, and thereby change the physical characteristics of the resultant polymer. When this occurs, polymer chains generally become more mobile. This permits the relaxation of stresses incurred during polymerization. As stresses are relieved, polymerized resins may undergo changes in shape. Fortunately, these changes are relatively minor and do not exert significant effects on the fit or function of the processed bases.

Because the presence of water adversely affects the physical and dimensional properties of denture base resins, diffusion coefficients also warrant consideration. The diffusion coefficient (D) of water in representative heat-activated denture acrylic resin is 0.011×10^{-6} cm^2/s at 37° C. For a representative chemically activated resin, the diffusion coefficient is 0.023×10^{-6} cm^2/s. Since the diffusion coefficients of water in representative denture resins are relatively low, the time required for a denture base to reach saturation can be considerable. This depends on the thickness of the resin, as well as the storage conditions. A typical denture base may require a period of 17 days to become fully saturated with water.

Results of laboratory investigations indicate there are very slight differences in the dimensions of heat-activated and chemically activated denture bases following prolonged storage in water. Compression molded, heat-activated denture bases are slightly undersize when measured from second molar to second molar. Conversely, compression-molded, chemically activated denture bases are slightly oversize when measured in the same region. The clinical significance of this difference appears negligible.

ANSI/ADA Specification No. 12 identifies guidelines regarding the testing and acceptance of denture base resins. To test water absorption, a disk of material with specified dimensions is prepared and dried to a constant weight. This weight is recorded as a baseline value. The disk is then soaked in distilled water for seven days. Again, the disk is weighed, and this value is compared with the baseline value. According to the specification, the weight gain following immersion must not be greater than 0.8 mg/cm^2. Additional information regarding ANSI/ADA Specification No. 12 is presented in subsequent sections.

Solubility

Although denture base resins are soluble in a variety of solvents, they are virtually insoluble in the fluids commonly encountered in the oral cavity. ANSI/ADA Specification No. 12 prescribes a testing regimen for the measurement of resin solubility. This procedure is a continuation of the water sorption test described in the preceding section. Following the required water immersion, the test disk is permitted to dry and is reweighed. This value is compared with the baseline value to determine weight loss. According to the specification, weight loss must not be greater than 0.04 mg/cm^2 from the specimen surface. Such a loss is negligible from a clinical standpoint.

CRITICAL QUESTIONS

What are the causes of processing stresses? What are the clinical implications of these stresses, if any?

Processing Stresses

Whenever a natural dimensional change is inhibited, the affected material contains stresses. If stresses are relaxed, a resultant distortion of the material may occur. This principle has important ramifications in the fabrication of denture bases, since stresses are always induced during processing.

For purposes of this discussion, consider the events that occur during denture base polymerization. As previously stated, a moderate amount of shrinkage occurs as individual monomers are linked to form polymer chains. During this process, it is possible that friction between the mold walls and soft resin may inhibit normal shrinkage of these chains. As a result, the polymer chains are stretched, and the resin sustains tensile stresses.

Stresses also are produced as the result of thermal shrinkage. As a polymerized resin is cooled below its glass transition temperature, the resin becomes relatively rigid. Further cooling yields thermal shrinkage. The clinician must remember that a denture base resin generally is encased in a rigid investing medium such as dental stone, during this process. Since denture base resins and dental stones contract at markedly different rates, a contraction differential is established. This disparity in contraction rates also yields stresses within the resin. Additional factors that may contribute to processing stresses include improper mixing and handling of the resin, and poorly controlled heating and cooling of the flask assembly.

The release of stresses yields dimensional changes that are cumulative in nature. Fortunately, these dimensional changes are quite small. Total dimensional changes occurring as a result of processing and water sorption are in the range of 0.1 to 0.2 mm (as measured from second molar to second molar). Therefore it is doubtful such changes would be noticed by a patient.

Crazing

Although dimensional changes may occur during relaxation of processing stresses, these changes generally do not cause clinical difficulties. In contrast, stress relaxation may produce small surface flaws that can adversely affect the aesthetic and physical properties of a denture. The production of such flaws, or microcracks, is termed *crazing*.

In a clinical setting, crazing is evidenced by small linear cracks that appear to originate at a denture's surface. Crazing in a transparent resin imparts a "hazy" or "foggy" appearance. In a tinted resin, crazing imparts a whitish appearance. In addition, surface cracks predispose a denture resin to fracture.

From a physical standpoint, crazing may result from stress application or partial dissolution of a resin, for example, attack by a solvent. Tensile stresses are most often responsible for crazing in denture base applications. It is believed that crazing is produced by mechanical separation of individual polymer chains that occurs on application of tensile stresses.

Crazing generally begins at the surface of a resin and is oriented at right angles to tensile forces. Microcracks formed in this manner subsequently progress internally. An example of crazing is presented in Figure 22-14.

As noted, crazing also may be produced as a result of solvent action. Microcracks produced in this manner are oriented more randomly than those depicted in Figure 22-14. Solvent-induced crazing generally results from prolonged contact with liquids such as ethyl alcohol. The development of improved acrylic resin teeth and cross-linked denture base resins has resulted in a decreased incidence of denture base crazing.

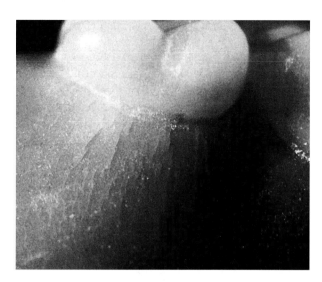

Fig. 22-14 Crazing around porcelain teeth.

CRITICAL QUESTIONS

What variables reduce the strength of acrylic dentures? What processing method is most likely to produce denture bases with lower fracture resistance?

Strength

The strength of an individual denture base resin is dependent on many factors. These factors include composition of the resin, processing technique, and conditions presented by the oral environment.

To provide acceptable physical properties, denture base resins must meet or exceed the standards presented in ANSI/ADA Specification No. 12. A transverse test is used to evaluate the relationship between applied load and resultant deflection in a resin specimen of prescribed dimensions. Typical load-deflection results are presented in Figure 22-15.

Inspection of Figure 22-15 reveals a curvature to each component of the deflection load plot. Since no straight-line portion is evident, one may assume that plastic deformation (i.e., irreversible deformation) occurs during the loading process. Some elastic deformation (i.e., recoverable deformation) also occurs. From a clinical standpoint, this means that load application produces stresses within a resin and a change in the overall shape of the denture base. When the load is released, stresses within the resin are relaxed and the denture base begins to return to its original shape. Nevertheless, plastic deformation prevents complete recovery and some permanent deformation will exist.

Perhaps the most important determinant of resin strength is the degree of polymerization exhibited by the material. As the degree of polymerization increases, the strength of the resin also increases. In this regard, the polymerization cycle employed with a heat activated resin is extremely important. Figure 22-16 reveals the effects that processing cycles exert upon load-deflection properties. Note that increased duration of the polymerization cycle appears to yield improved physical properties.

In comparison with heat-activated resins, the chemically activated resins generally display lower degrees of polymerization. As a result, chemically activated resins

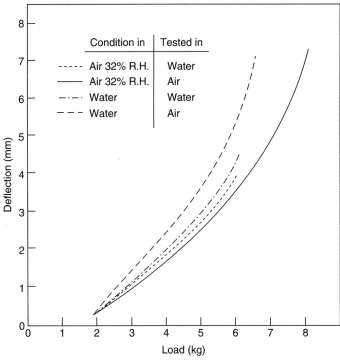

Fig. 22-15   Transverse load-deflection curve for a typical denture base resin, showing the influences of different conditioning procedures and testing environments. All specimens were conditioned for 3 days as indicated before testing. (From Swaney AC, Paffenbarger GC, Caul HJ, and Sweeney WT: American Dental Association Specification No. 12 for denture base resin, ed. 2, J Am Dent Assoc 46(1):54-66, January, 1953. Reprinted by permission of ADA Publishing, a Division of ADA Business Enterprises, Inc.)

exhibit increased levels of residual monomer and decreased strength and stiffness. Despite these characteristics, heat- and chemically activated resins display similar elastic moduli.

Creep

Denture resins display *viscoelastic behavior*. In other words, these materials act as rubbery solids that recover elastic deformation over time once the stresses induced in the resin have been eliminated. When a denture base resin is subjected to a sustained load, the material exhibits an initial deflection or deformation. If this load is not removed, additional plastic deformation may occur over time. This additional deformation is termed *creep*.

The rate at which this progressive deformation occurs is termed the *creep rate*. This rate may be elevated by increases in temperature, applied load, residual monomer, and the presence of plasticizers. Although creep rates for heat-activated and chemically activated resins are very similar at low stresses, (e.g., 9 MPa) creep rates for chemically activated resins increase more rapidly as stresses are raised.

Miscellaneous Properties

The Charpy impact strength for a heat-activated denture resin may range from 0.98 to 1.27 joules, whereas that for a chemically activated resin is somewhat lower (0.78 joules). Values for high-impact resins such as Lucitone 199, can be twice as high as

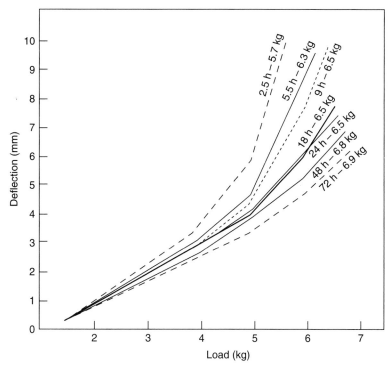

Fig. 22-16 Transverse stress-strain curves for samples of poly(methyl methacrylate) polymerized for different periods at 71° C (160° F). Processing times and fracture loads are noted on individual curves. (From Harman IM: Effects of time and temperature on polymerization of a methacrylate resin denture base, J Am Dent Assoc 38(2):188-203, February, 1949. Reprinted by permission of ADA Publishing, a Division of ADA Business Enterprises, Inc.)

the values reported for conventional poly(methyl methacrylate) resins. The clinician should recognize that these figures are useful only for comparisons of products, since the energy absorbed by an individual specimen is dependent on specimen size and geometry, distance between specimen supports, and the presence or absence of notching.

The Knoop hardness values for heat-activated resins may be as high as 20, whereas chemically activated resins generally display Knoop hardness values of 16 to 18.

CRITICAL QUESTION

What is the optimal technique for repairing a fractured acrylic denture base?

MISCELLANEOUS RESINS AND TECHNIQUES
Repair Resins

Despite the favorable physical characteristics of denture base resins, denture bases sometimes fracture. In most instances, these fractures may be repaired using compatible resins. Repair resins may be light-, heat-, or chemically activated.

To accurately accomplish repair of a fractured prosthesis, the clinician must realign and lute components together using an adherent wax or modeling plastic. When this has been accomplished, a repair cast is generated using dental stone. The denture is then removed from the cast, and the luting medium is eliminated. Subsequently, the fracture surfaces are trimmed to provide sufficient room for repair material. The cast is coated with separating medium to prevent adherence of repair resin, and the denture base sections are repositioned and affixed to the cast.

At this point, a repair material is chosen. Chemically activated resins generally are preferred over heat- and light-activated resins, despite the fact that chemically activated resins display lower transverse strengths. The principal advantage of chemically activated resins is that they may be polymerized at room temperature. Heat- and light-activated repair materials must be placed in water baths and light chambers, respectively. Heat generated by water baths and light chambers often causes stress release and distortion of previously polymerized denture base segments.

The following sequence is employed to accomplish denture base repair using a chemically activated resin. A small amount of monomer is painted onto prepared surfaces of the denture base to facilitate bonding of the repair material. Increments of monomer and polymer are added to the repair area using a small sable-hair brush or suitable substitute. A slight excess of material is placed at the repair site to account for polymerization shrinkage. Subsequently, the assembly is placed in a pressure chamber and allowed to polymerize. The repair site is then shaped, finished, and polished using conventional techniques.

The minimum requirements for chemically activated resins used in repair applications are identified in ANSI/ADA Specification No. 13.

CRITICAL QUESTION

Why are denture reliner materials considered temporary-use products?

Relining Resin Denture Bases

Because soft tissue contours change during denture service, it is sometimes necessary to alter tissue surfaces of prostheses to ensure proper fit and function. In some instances, this may be achieved by selective grinding procedures. In other instances, tissue surfaces must be replaced by **relining** or **rebasing** existing dentures.

Relining involves replacement of the tissue surface of an existing denture, whereas rebasing involves replacement of the entire denture base. In both instances, an impression of the soft tissues is obtained using the existing denture as an impression tray. A stone cast is generated in the impression, and the resultant assembly is invested in a denture flask. Subsequently, the flask is opened and prepared for the introduction of resin.

If the denture is to be relined, the impression material is removed from the denture. The tissue surface is cleaned to enhance bonding between the existing resin and the reline material. Following this sequence, an appropriate resin is introduced and shaped using a compression molding technique.

For relining, a low polymerization temperature is desirable to minimize distortion of the remaining denture base. Hence, a chemically activated resin usually is chosen. The selected material is mixed according to manufacturer's recommendations, placed into the mold, compressed, and permitted to polymerize. In turn, the denture is recovered, finished, and polished.

If a chemically activated resin is selected for relining the existing denture, a specialized mounting assembly (i.e., reline fixture) may be used in lieu of flasking. This assembly maintains the correct vertical and horizontal relationships between the cast and the denture, while eliminating the need to encase the remaining denture base in dental stone. This facilitates recovery of the denture at the end of the relining process.

Several manufacturers offer chemically activated resins for relining dentures intraorally. Unfortunately, many of these materials generate sufficient heat to injure oral tissues. To receive ADA approval, materials must comply with ANSI/ADA Specification No. 17, which places limits on the rate of temperature rise and maximum acceptable temperature.

Relining also may be accomplished using resins that are activated by heat, light, or microwave energy. In all of these instances, significant heat may be generated, and distortion of the existing denture base is more likely.

Some materials are manufactured for repair as well as relining purposes. The practitioner should be extremely cautious in using such products. Some of these materials comply with ANSI/ADA Specification No. 13 for repairs but fail to meet temperature requirements set forth in ANSI/ADA Specification No. 17. Other materials comply with specification No. 17 but fail to meet the requirements of specification No. 13. Such materials often discolor, harbor microorganisms, and separate from underlying denture bases.

Similar materials are marketed for home use. Unfortunately, the majority of patients do not possess adequate knowledge to manipulate these materials correctly. As a result, the use of such products may result in irreparable damage to the oral tissues. Consequently, the purchase and use of such products should be discouraged.

Rebasing Resin Dentures

The steps required in denture rebasing are very similar to those described for relining. An accurate impression of the soft tissues is obtained using the existing denture as a custom tray. Subsequently, a stone cast is fabricated in the impression. The cast and denture are mounted in a device designed to maintain the correct vertical and horizontal relationships between the stone cast and surfaces of the prosthetic teeth. The resultant assembly provides indices for the occlusal surfaces of the prosthetic teeth. After these indices have been established, the denture is removed and the teeth are separated from the existing denture base. The teeth are repositioned in their respective indices and held in their original relationships to the cast while they are waxed to a new baseplate.

At this point, the denture base is waxed to the desired form. The completed tooth arrangement is sealed to the cast, and the assembly is invested as previously described. Following elimination of the wax and removal of the baseplate, resin is introduced into the mold cavity. The material subsequently is processed. After processing, the denture is recovered, finished, and polished. Consequently, the prosthesis consists of a new denture base in conjunction with teeth from the patient's previous denture.

CRITICAL QUESTION

Under what conditions might soft denture liners be used rather than rebasing an acrylic denture base?

Short-Term and Long-Term Soft Denture Liners

The purpose of a **soft denture liner** is to absorb some of the energy produced by masticatory impact. Hence a soft liner serves as a "shock absorber" between the occlusal surfaces of a denture and the underlying oral tissues. The most commonly used **liners** are *plasticized acrylic resins*. These resins may be heat-activated or chemically activated, and are based on familiar chemistries.

Chemically activated soft liners generally employ poly(methyl methacrylate) or poly(ethyl methacrylate) as principal structural components. These polymers are supplied in powder form, and subsequently are mixed with liquids containing 60% to 80% of a plasticizer. The *plasticizer* usually is a large molecular species such as *dibutyl phthalate*. The distribution of large plasticizer molecules minimizes entanglement of polymer chains, thereby permitting individual chains to "slip" past one another. This slipping motion permits rapid changes in the shape of the soft liner and provides a cushioning effect for the underlying tissues. It is important to note that the liquids used in such applications do not contain acrylic monomers. Consequently, the resultant liners are considered **short-term soft liners**, or **tissue conditioners**.

Unlike chemically activated soft liners, heat-activated materials generally are more durable and may be considered **long-term soft liners**. Nonetheless, these materials degrade over time and should not be considered permanent.

A number of heat-activated soft liners are supplied as powder-liquid systems. The powders are composed of acrylic resin polymers and copolymers, whereas the liquids consist of appropriate acrylic monomers and plasticizers. When mixed, these materials form pliable resins exhibiting glass transition temperatures (T_g) below mouth temperature.

Although plasticizers impart flexibility, they also present certain difficulties. Plasticizers are not bound within the resin mass and therefore may be "leached out" of soft liners. As this occurs, soft liners become progressively more rigid. Consequently, it is advantageous to use liners that are less prone to leaching phenomena.

As poly(methyl methacrylate) is replaced by higher methacrylates (e.g., ethyl, n-propyl, and n-butyl), the T_g becomes progressively lower. As a result, less plasticizer is required and the effects of leaching can be minimized.

Vinyl resins also have been used in soft liner applications. Unfortunately, plasticized poly(vinyl chloride) and poly(vinyl acetate) are subject to leaching and harden during sustained use.

Perhaps the most successful materials for soft liner applications have been the silicone rubbers. These materials are not dependent on leachable plasticizers; therefore they retain their elastic properties for prolonged periods. Unfortunately, silicone rubbers may lose adhesion to underlying denture bases.

Silicone rubbers may be chemically activated or heat-activated. Chemically activated silicones are supplied as two-component systems that polymerize via condensation reactions. Hence, these materials are quite similar to condensation silicone impression materials.

Placement of chemically activated soft liners is relatively uncomplicated. Relief is provided to permit an acceptable thickness of the chosen material. Adhesive is then applied to the surface of the denture base to facilitate bonding of the hard and soft resins. The resilient material is mixed, applied to the denture base via compression molding, and permitted to polymerize. Subsequently, the denture is recovered, finished, and polished.

Heat-activated silicones are one-component systems supplied as pastes or gels. These materials are applied and contoured using compression molding techniques.

Heat-activated silicones may be applied to polymerized resin bases, or they may be polymerized in conjunction with freshly mixed resins.

To promote adhesion between silicone soft liners and rigid denture base materials, rubber-poly(methyl methacrylate) cements often are used. These cements serve as chemical intermediates that bond to both soft liners and denture resins.

At least one silicone liner does not require an adhesive when it is cured together with an acrylic denture base material. This material actually is a silicone copolymer that contains components capable of bonding with acrylic resins.

Laboratory procedures for heat-activated silicones are similar to those described for chemically activated materials. Bases are invested, and mold spaces are prepared as required. Relief is provided to permit an acceptable thickness of the chosen material(s). Packing, compression molding, and processing are performed in accordance with manufacturer's recommendations. The denture is then recovered, finished, and polished.

Other polymers that have been used as soft liners include polyurethane and polyphosphazine. All of the described liners display certain shortcomings. For instance, silicone liners are poorly adherent to denture base resins. Silicone liners also undergo significant volume changes with the gain and loss of water. Many soft liners bond well to denture bases but become progressively more rigid as plasticizers leach from liner materials. Hardening rates for these liners are associated with the initial plasticizer content. As the plasticizer content is increased, the probability for leaching also is increased. Hence materials with a high initial plasticizer content tend to harden rather rapidly.

Soft liners also exert significant effects on associated denture bases. As the thickness of a soft liner is increased, the thickness of the accompanying denture base must be decreased, and this results in decreased denture base strength. Furthermore, materials used in conjunction with soft liners (e.g., adhesives and monomers) may cause partial dissolution of the accompanying denture bases. The resultant decrease in base strength may result in fracture during clinical service.

Perhaps the greatest difficulty associated with long- and short-term soft liners is that these materials cannot be cleaned effectively. As a result, patients often report disagreeable tastes and odors related to these materials. Research indicates the liners themselves do not support mycotic growth, but such growth is supported by debris that accumulates in the pores of these materials. The most common fungal growth associated with soft liners is *Candida albicans*.

Several regimens have been used in attempts to improve the hygienic characteristics of soft liners. Unfortunately, these regimens have met with limited success. Both oxygenating and hypochlorite-type denture cleansers have been employed. These agents can cause significant damage to soft liners, especially the silicone materials.

Mechanical cleaning of soft liners may lead to damage, but such debridement often is necessary. If mechanical cleaning is undertaken, a soft brush should be used in conjunction with a mild detergent solution or nonabrasive dentifrice.

In attempts to address potential problems, antimycotic agents have been incorporated into soft liners. Although this approach appears promising, the duration of antimycotic activity is questionable. Hence additional research is needed.

Based on the preceding information, it appears that none of the existing soft liners may be considered entirely satisfactory. Few of the materials remain soft indefinitely, although some harden more slowly than others. In addition, existing materials accumulate stains and are difficult to clean. For these reasons, available materials should be considered temporary and not permanent clinical agents.

Resin Impression Trays and Tray Materials

Resin trays are often used in dental impression procedures. Unlike stock trays, resin impression trays are fabricated to fit the arches of individual patients. As a result, resin impression trays are often called *custom trays*.

The steps in custom tray fabrication may be described as follows: A preliminary impression is made using a stock tray and an appropriate impression material. In turn, a gypsum cast is generated. A suitable spacer is placed on the stone cast to provide the desired relief. Subsequently, a separating medium is painted onto exposed cast surfaces.

A resin dough is formed by mixing an inorganically filled polymer and the appropriate monomer. In most instances, the material of choice is a chemically activated poly(methyl methacrylate) resin. The dough is rolled into a sheet approximately 2 mm thick, adapted to the diagnostic cast, and allowed to polymerize.

It should be noted that a resin impression tray may undergo noticeable dimensional changes for 24 hr following fabrication and therefore should not be used during this period. At the end of the prescribed period, the fit of the tray is evaluated intraorally, and necessary modifications are made. Subsequently, the spacer is removed and a master impression is made using an appropriate elastomeric impression material.

In recent years, light-activated urethane dimethacrylate resins also have been used in tray fabrication. These resins are supplied in sheet and gel forms. Sheet forms are preferred for custom tray fabrication because of their favorable handling characteristics.

Tray fabrication procedures for urethane dimethacrylate resins are similar to those described in the previous paragraphs. To facilitate tray fabrication, a diagnostic cast is made and one or more layers of wax relief are placed. A separating medium is applied to exposed cast surfaces, and a tray is fashioned using urethane dimethacrylate sheet material. The cast and tray are placed in a light chamber, and the resin is polymerized.

Trays fabricated using urethane dimethacrylate resins are dimensionally stable during post-polymerization stages. Nonetheless, these materials are brittle and produce fine particles during grinding procedures.

Denture Cleansers

Patients use a wide variety of agents for cleaning artificial dentures. In approximate order of preference, these include the following: dentifrices, proprietary denture cleansers, mild detergents, household cleansers, bleaches, and vinegar. Both immersion and brushing techniques are used with these materials.

The most common commercial denture cleansers are based upon or require immersion techniques. These cleansers are marketed in powder and tablet forms. Immersion agents contain alkaline compounds, detergents, sodium perborate, and flavoring agents. When dissolved in water, sodium perborate decomposes to form an alkaline peroxide solution. This peroxide solution subsequently releases oxygen that loosens debris via mechanical means.

Household bleaches (hypochlorites) also are used in denture cleaning applications. Dilute bleach solutions may be used to remove certain types of stains. Concentrated solutions should be avoided, because prolonged use may affect denture coloration. Bleaches also may discolor soft relining materials, particularly the silicones.

Bleaches and bleach solutions should not be used for cleaning metal prostheses, such as removable partial denture frameworks. Such solutions produce significant darkening of base metals and may irreparably damage the serviceability of affected prostheses.

The effects of abrasive agents on acrylic resin surfaces also have been investigated. Toothbrushes alone exert little effect on resin surfaces. Toothbrushes in conjunction with most commercial dentifrices, mild detergents, and soaps do not appear to be harmful. Conversely, household cleansers, such as kitchen and bathroom abrasives, are definitely contraindicated. Prolonged use of such cleansers may cause noticeable wear of resin surfaces and may adversely affect the function and aesthetics of these prostheses. As a result, each patient should be educated regarding the care and cleaning of resin prostheses.

Infection Control Procedures

Care should be taken to prevent cross-contamination between patients and dental personnel, including those personnel in the dental laboratory. New appliances should be disinfected before leaving the dental laboratory. Existing prostheses should be disinfected before entering the laboratory and after completion of laboratory procedures. All materials used for finishing and polishing procedures should be handled according to established infection control guidelines. Items such as rag wheels should be autoclaved, and materials such as pumice should be used according to unit-dose recommendations.

CRITICAL QUESTION

Which components of denture resins are most likely to cause an allergic reaction?

Allergic Reactions

Possible toxic or allergic reactions to poly(methyl methacrylate) have long been postulated. Theoretically, such reactions could occur following contact with the polymer, residual monomer, benzoyl peroxide, hydroquinone, pigments, or a reaction product between some component of the denture base and its environment.

Clinical experience indicates that true allergic reactions to acrylic resins seldom occur in the oral cavity. Residual monomer is the component most often cited as an irritant. It should be recognized that the residual monomer content of a properly processed denture is less than 1%. Furthermore, surface monomer is completely eliminated following storage in water for 17 hr.

Based on the preceding information, reactions to residual monomer should occur shortly after prosthesis delivery. However, the majority of patients reporting denture sore mouth have worn the offending prostheses for months or even years. Clinical evaluation of these cases indicates tissue irritation generally is related to nonhygienic conditions or trauma caused by poorly fitting denture bases.

Repeated or prolonged contact with monomer also may result in contact dermatitis. This condition is most commonly experienced by personnel involved in the manipulation of denture resins. Because of this possibility, dental personnel should refrain from handling such materials with ungloved hands. The high concentration of monomer in freshly mixed resins may produce local irritation and serious sensitization of the fingers.

Finally, it should be noted that inhalation of monomer vapor may be detrimental. Therefore the use of monomer should be restricted to well-ventilated areas.

Toxicology

There is no evidence that commonly used dental resins produce systemic toxic effects in humans. As previously noted, the amount of residual monomer in processed poly(methyl methacrylate) is extremely low. To enter the circulatory system, residual monomer must pass through the oral mucosa and underlying tissues. These structures function as barriers that significantly diminish the volume of monomer reaching the bloodstream.

Residual monomer that does reach the bloodstream is rapidly hydrolyzed to methacrylic acid and excreted. It is estimated that the half-life of methyl methacrylate in circulating blood is 20 to 40 min. (See Chapter 8 for more information on biocompatibility of dental materials.)

CRITICAL QUESTIONS

What precautions should be taken when using porcelain teeth in a denture? What are the clinically relevant differences between porcelain teeth and acrylic resin teeth?

RESIN TEETH FOR PROSTHETIC APPLICATIONS

The majority of preformed artificial teeth sold in the United States are made of acrylic or vinyl-acrylic resins. As might be expected, the majority of resin teeth are based on poly(methyl methacrylate) compositions.

Poly(methyl methacrylate) resins used in the fabrication of prosthetic teeth are very similar to those used in denture base construction. Nevertheless, the degree of cross-linking within prosthetic teeth is somewhat greater than that within polymerized denture bases. This increase is achieved by elevating the amount of cross-linking agent in the denture base liquid. The resultant polymer displays enhanced stability and improved clinical properties.

Cervical portions of prosthetic teeth often exhibit reduced cross-linking. This feature facilitates chemical bonding with denture base resins. Additional enhancement of chemical bonding may be achieved by removing the glossy "ridge-lap" surfaces of resin teeth.

Chemical bonding between resin teeth and heat-activated denture base materials has proven extremely effective. Nonetheless, bond failures may occur if ridge-lap surfaces are contaminated by residual wax or misplaced separating media. The stone molds must be flushed with hot water and exposed cervical portions of prosthetic teeth must be thoroughly cleaned with mild detergent solutions. Separating media must be applied to stone mold surfaces but should not be permitted to extend onto the exposed surfaces of resin teeth. As a final measure, ridge-lap surfaces should be wetted with monomer immediately before resin introduction. Adherence to these guidelines facilitates effective chemical interaction and enhanced bonding.

The use of mechanical retention has been the primary means for securing resin teeth to chemically activated denture base materials. It should be noted that chemical bonding also may be used in joining these resins. To accomplish this, a mixture of equal volumes methylene chloride and chemically activated methyl methacrylate monomer is applied to the necks of preformed resin teeth for approximately 5 min. Excess solution is then removed. This treatment produces softening of the resin and facilitates chemical bonding during denture base polymerization. Resultant bond strengths are similar to those obtained between resin teeth and heat-activated denture base resins.

Despite the current emphasis on resin teeth, prosthetic teeth also may be fabricated using dental porcelains. Hence a comparison of resin and porcelain teeth is provided for completeness.

Resin teeth display greater impact resistance and ductility than porcelain teeth. As a result, resin teeth are less likely to chip or fracture on impact, such as when a denture is dropped. Furthermore, resin teeth are easier to adjust and display greater resistance to thermal shock. In comparison, porcelain teeth display better dimensional stability and increased wear resistance. Unfortunately, porcelain teeth often cause significant wear of opposing enamel and gold surfaces, especially when contacting surfaces have been roughened. As a result, porcelain teeth should not oppose such surfaces, and if they are used, they should be polished periodically to reduce abrasive damage.

As a final note, resin teeth are capable of chemical bonding with commonly used denture base resins. Porcelain teeth do not form chemical bonds with denture resins and must be retained by other means, for example, mechanical undercuts and silanization.

CRITICAL QUESTION

What are the benefits and drawbacks of materials used in the construction of maxillofacial prostheses?

MATERIALS FOR MAXILLOFACIAL PROSTHETICS

For centuries, prostheses have been used to mask maxillofacial defects. The ancient Egyptians and Chinese used waxes and resins to reconstruct missing portions of the craniofacial complex. By the 16th century, the French surgeon Ambroise Paré described a variety of simple prostheses used for the cosmetic and functional replacement of maxillofacial structures. During subsequent years, restorative techniques and materials improved slowly. Casualties in World Wars I and II established a great need for maxillofacial prosthetics, and the dental profession assumed a major role in reconstruction and rehabilitation processes.

Despite improvements in surgical and restorative techniques, the materials used in maxillofacial prosthetics are far from ideal. An ideal material should be inexpensive, biocompatible, strong, and stable. In addition, the material should be skinlike in color and texture. Maxillofacial materials must exhibit resistance to tearing, and should be able to withstand moderate thermal and chemical challenges. Currently, no material fulfills all of these requirements. A brief summary of maxillofacial materials is included in the following paragraphs.

Latexes

Latexes are soft, inexpensive materials that may be used to create lifelike prostheses. Unfortunately, these materials are weak, degenerate rapidly, and exhibit color instability. Consequently, latexes are infrequently used in the fabrication of maxillofacial prostheses.

One synthetic latex is a tripolymer of butyl acrylate, methyl methacrylate, and methyl methacrylamide. Superior to natural latex, this material is nearly transparent. Colorants are sprayed onto the reverse or tissue side of the prosthesis, thereby providing enhanced translucency and improved blending. Despite these advantages, technical processes are lengthy and resultant prostheses last only a few months. As a result, synthetic latexes have limited applications.

Vinyl Plastisols

Plasticized vinyl resins sometimes are used in maxillofacial applications. Plastisols are thick liquids composed of small vinyl particles dispersed in a plasticizer. Colorants are added to these materials to match individual skin tones. Subsequently, vinyl plastisols are heated to impart desired physical characteristics. Unfortunately, vinyl plastisols harden with age as a result of plasticizer migration. Ultraviolet light also has an adverse effect on these materials. For these reasons, the use of vinyl plastisols is limited.

Silicone Rubbers

Although silicones were introduced in the mid-1940s, only in recent years have they been used in maxillofacial applications. Both heat-vulcanizing and room temperature–vulcanizing silicones are in use today, and both exhibit advantages and disadvantages.

Room temperature–vulcanizing silicones are supplied as single-paste systems that are colored by the addition of dyed rayon fibers, dry earth pigments, and/or oil paints. Prostheses can be polymerized in artificial stone molds, but more durable molds can be made from epoxy resins or metals. These silicones are not as strong as the heat-vulcanized silicones, and they are generally monochromatic.

Heat-vulcanizing silicones are supplied as semisolid or puttylike materials that require milling, packing under pressure, and a 30-min heat application cycle at 180° C. Pigments are milled into these materials. As a result, intrinsic color can be achieved. Heat-vulcanizing silicones display better strength and color stability than room temperature–vulcanizing silicones.

The major disadvantage of heat-vulcanizing silicones is the requirement for a milling machine and a press. Furthermore, a metal mold normally is used, and fabrication of the mold is a lengthy procedure. A stone mold within a denture flask may be used, but this increases the risk for damage to the material during deflasking.

Polyurethane Polymers

Polyurethane is the most recent addition to materials used in maxillofacial prosthetics. Fabrication of a polyurethane prosthesis requires accurate proportioning of three components. The material is placed in a stone or metal mold and allowed to polymerize at room temperature. Although a polyurethane prosthesis has a natural feel and appearance, it is susceptible to rapid deterioration.

Additional information may be found in texts that deal with the fabrication of maxillofacial prostheses.

SELECTED READINGS

Bates JF, Stanford GD, Huggett R, and Handley RW: Current status of pour-type denture base resins. J Dent 5:177, 1977.

The mechanical properties of pour-type denture resins were somewhat lower than those of conventional heat-cured resins, and they were more sensitive to laboratory variables.

Caswell CW and Norling BK: Comparative study of the bond strengths of three abrasion-resistant plastic denture teeth bonded to a cross-linked and a grafted, cross-linked denture base material. J Prosthet Dent 55:701, 1986.

Testing bond strength of denture base resin to resin teeth revealed that 83% of fractures occurred within the teeth. Thus the tensile strength of the tooth is as critical a factor as is the bond strength.

Chaing BKP: Polymers in the service of prosthetic dentistry. J Dent 12:203, 1984.

A comprehensive discussion of polymers used in prosthodontics and a citation of pertinent literature on materials such as denture polymers, soft liners, tissue conditioners, and impression materials.

Chalian VA: Evaluation and comparison of physical properties of materials used in maxillofacial prosthetics. Thesis, Indiana University School of Dentistry, Indianapolis, 1976.

A complete review of the materials used in maxillofacial prostheses, their comparative properties, and characteristics.

Clancy JMS and Boyer DB: Comparative bond strengths of light-cured, heat-cured, and autopolymerizing denture resins to denture teeth. J Prosthet Dent 61:457, 1989.

Tensile bond strength of heat-cured, autopolymerizing, and light-cured resins to two types of plastic teeth were measured.

Devlin H and Watts DC: Acrylic "Allergy"? Br Dent J 157:272, 1984.

A review of the possible mechanisms of acrylic allergy.

The Glossary of Prosthodontic Terms, 7th ed, GPT-7, The Academy of Prosthodontics Foundation, Mosby, St. Louis, 1999.

Heath JR, Davenport JC, and Jones PA: The abrasion of acrylic resin by cleaning pastes. J Oral Rehabil 10:159, 1983.

A number of abrasive pastes were evaluated for wear on denture resin; the clinical relevance is discussed.

Levin B, Sanders JL, and Reitz PV: The use of microwave energy for processing acrylic resins. J Prosthet Dent 61:381, 1989.

A description of the techniques and equipment for microwave processing.

McCabe JF and Wilson HJ: The use of differential scanning calorimetry for the evaluation of dental materials. Part II. Denture base materials. J Oral Rehabil 7:235, 1980.

Results of this investigation indicate that the Tg for self-polymerizing resins is considerably lower than the Tg for heat-cured resins.

Monsenego P, Baszkin A, deLourdes Costa J, and Lejoyeaus J: Complete denture retention, wettability studies on various acrylic resin denture base materials. J Prosthet Dent 62:308, 1989.

Hydrophilic properties of denture resins were studied. Authors cautiously suggest that air-particle-abraded, heat-polymerized resin provided the best surface for denture retention.

Nyquist G: Study of denture sore mouth. An investigation of traumatic, allergic, and toxic lesions of the oral mucosa arising from the use of full dentures. Acta Odontol Scand 10:154, 1952.

Probably the most comprehensive survey of reported allergic reactions to acrylic resins. The incidence of a true allergy is extremely small.

Sanders JL, Levin B, and Reitz PV: Porosity in denture acrylic resins cured by microwave energy. Quint Int 18:453, 1987.

Microwave polymerization is an effective way of processing acrylic resins. Resultant denture bases appear extremely dense.

Shlosberg SR, Goodacre CJ, Munoz CA, et al: Microwave energy polymerization of poly(methyl methacrylate) denture base resin. Int J Prosthodont 2:453, 1989.

Transverse strength and hardness were comparable with microwave and traditional polymerization techniques. Significant porosity was produced when conventional resins were polymerized using microwave energy.

Smith DC, and Baines MED: Residual methyl methacrylate in the denture base and its relation to denture sore mouth. Br Dent J 98:55, 1955.

Free monomer in a properly polymerized denture leaches out within 17 hr, suggesting that this component is not a likely cause for tissue irritation.

Takamata T, Setcos JC, Phillips RW, and Boone ME: Adaptation of acrylic resin dentures influenced by the activation mode of polymerization. J Am Dent Assoc 118:271, 1989.

Five resins and four processing techniques were evaluated. The two best-fitting groups were prepared from an autopolymerizing resin and the microwave-activated resin.

Takamata T, and Setcos JC: Resin denture bases: Review of accuracy and methods of polymerization. Int J Prosthodont 2:555, 1989.

A review of the literature as related to modifications in denture base resins, including pourable, microwave, and light-activated systems.

Tan H-K, Brudvik JS, Nicholls JI, and Smith DE: Adaptation of a visible light-cured denture base material. J Prosthet Dent 61:326, 1989.

Various methods were used to adapt light-polymerizing resin sheets to casts. Vacuum forming produced the best adaptation.

Tulacha GJ and Moser JB: Evaluation of viscoelastic behavior of a light-cured denture resin. J Prosthet Dent 61:695, 1989.

The viscoelastic properties of a light-polymerizing reline resin (Triad) were compared with those of a rubber base impression material and a prototype light-polymerizing resin paste.

Vermilyea SG, Powers JM, and Koran A: The rheological properties of fluid denture base resins. J Dent Res 57:227, 1978.

The rheological properties of six fluid resins were determined. Materials displayed initial non-Newtonian behavior and increased viscosity over time.

23
Dental Implants

Josephine Esquivel-Upshaw

OUTLINE

History of Dental Implants

Classification of Implants

Implant Components

Clinical Success of Dental Implants

Implant Materials

Selecting an Implant Material

Biocompatibility of Implants

Biomechanics

Summary

KEY TERMS

Alloplastic—Related to implantation of an inert foreign body.

Ankylosis—A condition of joint or tooth immobility resulting from oral pathology, surgery, or direct contact with bone.

Anodization—An oxidation process in which a film is produced on the surface of a metal by electrolytic treatment at the anode.

Bioacceptance—Ability to be tolerated in a biological environment in spite of adverse effects.

Bioactive—Capable of promoting the formation of hydroxyapatite and bonding to bone.

Biocompatibility—Ability of a material to elicit an appropriate biological response in a given application in the body.

Biointegration—Process in which bone or other living tissue becomes integrated with an implanted material with no intervening space.

Endosteal implant—A device that is placed into the alveolar and/or basal bone of the mandible or maxilla, which transects only one cortical plate.

Epithelial implant—A device placed within the oral mucosa.

Implantation—Process of grafting or inserting a material such as an inert foreign body (alloplast) or tissue within the body.

Ion implantation—Process of altering the surface of a metal with desirable ionic species.

Osseointegration—Process in which living bony tissue forms to within 100 Å of the implant surface without any intervening fibrous connective tissue.

Osteoinductive—Ability to promote bone formation through a mechanism that induces the differentiation of osteoblasts.

Passivation—Process of transforming a chemically active surface of a metal to a less active surface.

Replantation—Reinsertion of a tooth back into its jaw socket soon after intentional extraction or accidental removal.

Subperiosteal implant—A dental device that is placed beneath the periosteum and overlies cortical bone.

Texturing—Process of increasing surface roughness of the area to which bone can bond.

Toxicity—Ability of a material to cause cell or tissue death.
Transosteal implant—A device that penetrates both cortical plates and the thickness of the alveolar bone.

HISTORY OF DENTAL IMPLANTS

The restoration of missing teeth is an important aspect of modern dentistry. As teeth are lost to decay or periodontal disease, there is a demand for replacement of aesthetics and/or function. Conventional methods of restoration include a removable complete denture, a removable partial denture, or a fixed prosthesis. Each method has its own indications and its share of advantages and disadvantages. Removable dentures have long been considered cumbersome because of the inconvenience of removing them one or more times per day. The stigma of removing one's teeth is a major drawback, especially for the younger generation. Also, these removable dentures are bulky, they complicate chewing, and they are often unaesthetic.

Fixed prostheses appear to be more natural and more convenient, but they involve preparation of adjacent teeth that could lead to a different set of problems, such as secondary decay or irreversible pulpitis. If the adjacent teeth are not restored, the decision to prepare them for a fixed prosthesis is quite difficult because two or more natural teeth must be surgically altered to provide retention for one or more artificial teeth.

For centuries, people have attempted to replace missing teeth using **implantation**. *Implantation* is defined as the insertion of any object or material, such as an **alloplastic** substance or other tissue, either partially or completely, into the body for therapeutic, diagnostic, prosthetic, or experimental purposes. Implantation should be differentiated from two other similar procedures: namely, **replantation** and **transplantation**. *Replantation* refers to the reinsertion of a tooth back into its jaw socket after accidental or intentional removal, whereas *transplantation* is the transfer of a body part from one site to another.

CRITICAL QUESTION

How did the concept of implantation evolve into one of the most widely used restorative techniques in dentistry?

The origins of dental implants began as early as the Greeks, Etruscans, and Egyptians. These civilizations employed different designs and materials ranging from jade and bone to metal. Some of the designs they used have evolved into the modern implants we see today.

Albucasis de Condue (936-1013) attempted to use ox bone to replace missing teeth and this treatment was the first documented placement of implants. This was followed through the centuries by a series of tooth transplants of either human or animal teeth. These transplants became a status symbol and quickly replaced other artificial alternatives for restoring missing teeth. Toward the 18th century, Pierre Fauchard and John Hunter further documented tooth transplantation with conditions for its success. They claimed that success was greater with anterior teeth or premolar replacement and in young people with healthy tooth sockets. Failure was believed to be the result of the incompatibility of the type of tooth used or the lack of conformity of the tooth to the socket.

The increased failure rates of transplants brought about interest in implantation of artificial roots. In 1809 Maggiolo fabricated gold roots that were fixed to pivot teeth by means of a spring. These gold implants were placed into fresh extraction sites although not truly submerged into bone. The crowns were placed after healing had occurred around the implant. Harris followed in 1887 with the implantation of a platinum post coated with lead. The post was shaped like a tooth root, and the lead was roughened for retention in the socket. Bonwell in 1895 used gold or iridium tubes implanted into bone to restore a single tooth or to support complete dentures. Payne, in 1898, implanted a silver capsule as a foundation for a porcelain crown that was cemented several weeks later. In 1905 Scholl demonstrated a porcelain corrugated root implant. The implant was successful for two years and was anchored to adjacent teeth and fillings through the use of pins.

In 1913 Greenfield introduced a hollow basket implant made from a meshwork of 24-gauge iridium-platinum wires soldered with 24-karat gold. This was used to support single implants, as well as fixed partial dentures using as many as eight implants.

Consistent failures with these artificial implant materials brought about a scientific approach to implant placement. More emphasis was placed on the tissue tolerance as well as the bone reaction toward metal implants. In 1937 Venable, Strock, and Beach analyzed the effects of metals on bone. They concluded that certain metals produce a galvanic reaction that leads to corrosion when they contact tissue fluids. They proposed the use of Vitallium, a material composed of cobalt, chromium, and molybdenum. This metal was considered to be inert, compatible with living tissue, and resistant to body fluids. Vitallium has been used in different forms of surgical appliances, such as skull plates and orthopedic screws, nails, and hip joints. The earliest successful documented case of Vitallium implants indicated survival times of 15 years or more.

Many other materials and designs followed, including the use of porcelain, high-density aluminum oxide (alumina), sapphire (alpha alumina), bioactive glass (Bioglass), and carbon. In 1947 Formiggini developed a single helix wire spiral implant made from tantalum or stainless steel. In 1948 Goldberg and Gershkoff reported the insertion of the first viable **subperiosteal implant.** In 1963 Linkow designed and introduced the hollow basket design with vents and screw threads. In 1952 Branemark developed a threaded implant design made of pure titanium that increased the popularity of implants to new levels. Unlike his predecessors, Branemark studied every aspect of implant design, including biological, mechanical, physiological, and functional phenomena relative to the success of the **endosteal implant.** The result is an implant system that was not marketed until 17 years of extensive clinical testing and study had been completed.

CLASSIFICATION OF IMPLANTS

Implants can be classified according to implant design, implant properties, or implant attachment mechanism. There are four types of implant designs that have evolved during centuries of development.

Implant Design

There are four types of implant designs that have evolved during centuries of development. The first and most commonly used type is the endosteal implant, which is a device that is placed into the alveolar and/or basal bone of the mandible or maxilla and transects only one cortical plate. These implants are formed in different shapes, such as cylindrical cones or thin plates, and can be used in all areas of the mouth. One example of an endosteal implant is the blade implant (Fig. 23-1), which was developed independently in 1967 by two groups led by Linkow and Roberts. Endosteal blade implants consist of thin plates embedded into bone; they are used for narrow spaces such as posterior edentulous areas.

Because of the predictable failure rates of blade implants, the associated excessive bone loss, and lack of documented long-term success, their application in modern

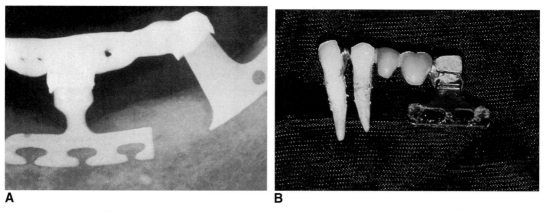

Fig. 23-1 **A,** Blade implants embedded in bone showing some bone loss. **B,** Failed blade implant prosthesis that was also attached to natural teeth. See also color plate. (Courtesy of Dr. Mickey Calverley.)

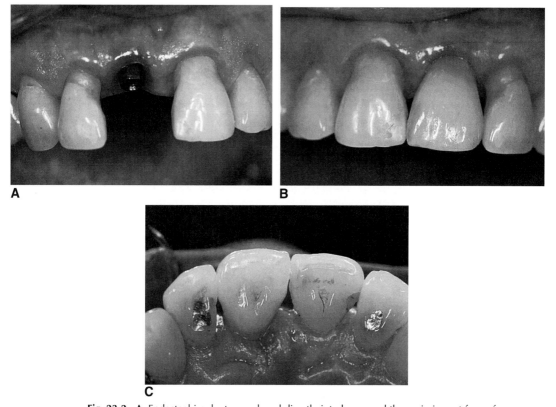

Fig. 23-2 **A,** Endosteal implants are placed directly into bone, and they mimic root forms for proper placement and location in bone. See also color plate. **B** and **C,** Restored anterior implant blending well with adjacent teeth.

implantology is minimal. Another example of an endosteal implant is the ramus frame implant, which is a horseshoe-shaped stainless steel device inserted into the mandible from one retromolar pad to the other, passing through the anterior symphysis area. As with the blade implants, there is no documentation of success or longevity, and failure is associated with great morbidity. The most popular endosteal implant is the root-form (Fig. 23-2), which was designed to mimic the shape of tooth

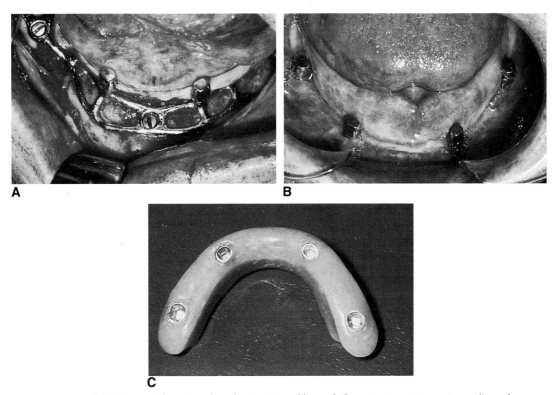

Fig. 23-3 **A,** Subperiosteal implant positioned beneath the periosteum. Impression making often requires a difficult surgical technique. **B,** Superstructure for subperiosteal implant allowing for attachment of prosthesis **C,** Denture prosthesis for subperiosteal implant. See also color plate. (Courtesy of Dr. Joseph Cain and Dr. Richard Seals.)

roots for directional load distribution, as well as for proper positioning in bone. In longitudinal studies, the root-form has the most documented success level of the endosteal implants, although several surgical stages may be needed for completion and the procedure is technically sensitive in the surgical and prosthetic stages.

The second implant design is the subperiosteal implant (Fig. 23-3), which employs an implant substructure and superstructure. The custom-cast frame is placed directly beneath the periosteum overlying the bony cortex. This implant was first developed by Dahl (1940) and refined by Berman (1951) who used a direct bone impression technique. It can be used to restore partially dentate or completely edentulous jaws and is used when there is inadequate bone for endosseous implants. Use of the subperiosteal implant has been limited because of numerous disadvantages, which include slow, but predictable rejection of the implant, difficult retrievability, and excessive bone loss associated with failure.

The **transosteal implant** (Fig. 23-4) combines the subperiosteal and endosteal components. This type of implant penetrates both cortical plates and passes through the full thickness of the alveolar bone. Use of the transosteal implant is restricted to the anterior area of the mandible and provides support for tissue-borne overdentures. The concept of transosseous implants was first conceived in Germany in the early 1930s. Small (1968) developed the mandibular staple implant, which was modified by Bosker (1982) with the transmandibular implant (TMI) made of gold alloy. Other names for transosteal implants include staple bone implant, mandibular staple implant, and transmandibular implant.

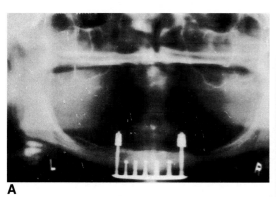 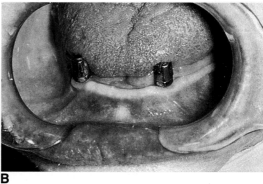

A   **B**

Fig. 23-4   A, Panoramic radiograph of a transosteal implant showing perforation of both cortical plates. Hence, the name *staple implant.* **B,** Transmucosal abutment for transosteal implant allowing for placement of denture restoration. See also color plate. (Courtesy of Dr. Joseph Cain and Dr. Richard Seals.)

The fourth implant design is the **epithelial implant,** which is inserted into the oral mucosa. This type is associated with a very simple surgical technique and requires that the mucosa be used as an attachment site for the metal inserts. There are several disadvantages associated with the epithelial implant, most notably painful healing and the requirement for continual wear, which probably explains why it is no longer used.

Implant Properties

Implant biomaterials can also be classified according to their composition and their physical, mechanical, chemical, and biological properties. These classifications often include ranked comparisons of properties such as elastic moduli, tensile strength, and ductility to determine optimal clinical applications (Table 23-1). These properties are used to aid in the design and the fabrication of the prosthesis. For example, the elastic modulus of the implant is inversely related to the strain transmitted across the implant-tissue interface. An implant with a comparable elastic modulus to bone should be selected to produce a more uniform stress distribution across the interface. Metals possess high strength and ductility, whereas the ceramics and carbons are brittle materials. Ductility is also important because it relates to the potential for permanent deformation of abutments or fixtures in areas of high tensile stress.

CRITICAL QUESTIONS

What is the preferred method of implant attachment? How has this affected the popularity of implant placement?

Attachment Mechanisms

Another way of classifying implants is through the nature of their attachment mechanisms. Periodontal fibers, which attach a tooth to the bone, consist of highly differentiated fibrous tissue. These fibers are replete with numerous cells and nerve endings that allow for shock absorption, sensory function, bone formation, and tooth movements. Although this is the most ideal form of attachment, there is no known implant material or system at present that can stimulate the growth of these fibers and mimic the function of a natural tooth.

| Table 23-1 | Mechanical Properties and Density of Metallic and Ceramic Implant Materials |

Material	Grade or Condition	Yield Strength (MPa)	Elongation (%)	Modulus of Elasticity (GPa)	Tensile Strength (MPa)	Density (g/cm³)
CP Titanium	1	170	24	102	240	4.5
	2	275	20	102	345	4.5
	3	380	18	102	450	4.5
	4	483	15	104	550	4.5
Ti-6Al-4V		860	10	113	930	4.4
Ti-6Al-4V ELI		795	10	113	860	4.4
Co-Cr-Mo	Cast	450	8	240	700	8.0
Stainless steel	Annealed	190	40	200	490	8.0
	Cold-worked	690	12	200	860	8.0
Aluminum oxide	Polycrystalline	400*(550) (flexure)	0.1	380	220	3.96
Zirconium oxide	Y_2O_3 (stabilized)	1200 (flexure)	0.1	200	350	6.0
Cortical bone		N/A	1	18	140	0.7
Dentin		N/A	0	18.3	52	2.2
Enamel		N/A	0	84	10	3.0

*ASTM Standard: Minimum Values

Historically, implant attachment through low-differentiated fibrous tissue was widely accepted as a measure of successful implant placement. However, it was later learned that this type of attachment is a manifestation of adverse reactions that later lead to implant failure. Such reactions include tissue rejection where an acute or chronic inflammatory response is accompanied by pain and eventual loss of the implant. Another manifestation is implant encapsulation by poorly differentiated fibers that have often been called a "pseudo-periodontium." Despite numerous claims by some that this constitutes implant success, clinical studies indicate that this type of attachment can eventually lead to an acute rejection or acute reaction, and progressive looseness will occur.

Osseointegration is characterized by the direct contact between bone and the surface of the loaded implant. This was initially described by Branemark as direct anchorage to bone and is now the primary attachment mechanism of commercial dental implants. This mode is described as the direct adaptation of bone to implants without any other intermediate interstitial tissue, and it is similar to a tooth **ankylosis** where no periodontal ligament exists. The strength of this contact increases over time, as opposed to the pseudoperiodontium described previously, which results eventually in loosening of the implant. Integration occurs initially through osteoconduction wherein bone-producing cells migrate alongside the implant surface through a connective tissue scaffolding formed adjacent to the implant surface. Attachment of this scaffold is highly dependent on the implant surface design. Bone apposition is encouraged through microscopic surface ridges. Osseointegration can also be achieved through the use of **bioactive** materials that stimulate the formation of bone along the surface of the implant. A second mechanism of osseointegration involves "de novo" bone formation wherein a mineralized interfacial matrix is deposited along the implant surface. Once again, the surface topography will determine the bond strength of bone to the implant surface.

CRITICAL QUESTION

What is the purpose of pretreating implant surfaces?

IMPLANT COMPONENTS

To understand the material characteristics and function of an implant, one must first be knowledgeable of its numerous parts. Although each implant system varies, the parts are basically consistent. The fixture (Fig. 23-5, *A*) is the implant component that actually engages bone. Depending on the implant system, the fixture can have different surfaces—threaded, grooved, perforated, plasma-sprayed, or coated. Each surface type is meant to serve a particular purpose—for example, increased surface area enhances osseointegration, or better cortex engagement ensures immediate and long-term bone anchorage. The coated or plasma-sprayed materials are used to enhance attachment to bone. These materials are discussed later in this chapter. The second component (Fig. 23-5, *B*) is the transmucosal abutment, which provides the connection between the implant fixture and the prosthesis that will be fabricated (Fig. 23-5, *C*). The abutment is usually connected to the fixture by means of a screw; it can also be cemented or swaged. Abutments can engage either an internal or external hexagon on the fixture that serves as an antirotation device, which is particularly important for single-unit restorations. The last part of an implant is the prosthesis. This can be attached to the abutments through the use of screws, cement, or precision attachments, such as those used for implant overdentures.

Placement and restoration of implants are usually performed in stages. The first stage involves the surgical part where the actual implant is placed into the bone. The implant is left alone for a period of four to six months depending on the bone quality and allowed to heal and become osseointegrated. A secondary surgery is required

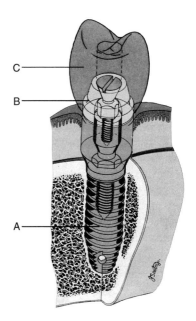

Fig. 23-5   Diagram of implant components. **A,** The implant fixture (endosteal root form). **B,** Transmucosal abutment that serves as the attachment between fixture and the actual prosthesis. **C,** The actual prosthesis that can either be cemented, screwed, or swaged. See also color plate.

in which the implant is uncovered and exposed through the oral environment with a healing cap placed to ensure proper healing of soft tissues around the site of the future abutment. The restorative phase then follows with placement of abutments and either a fixed partial denture or a removable denture. There are some implant systems that require only one surgical intervention, and the implant is immediately placed in contact with the oral environment. Some of these systems have even been advocated for immediate loading with reports of relative success.

CRITICAL QUESTIONS

When can an implant restoration be considered successful? What criteria are used to determine this success? What clinical situations can affect the success rate of dental implants?

CLINICAL SUCCESS OF DENTAL IMPLANTS

There have been several long-standing debates about what is considered successful in implant dentistry. It was originally believed that the encapsulation of an implant with a pseudoperiodontium was a successful implant until the fixture loosened itself out of the bone. The most frequently cited success criteria are those by Schnitman and Schulman (1979) and by Albrektsson et al (1986). Schnitman and Schulman proposed the following requirements:
  1. The mobility of an implant must be less than 1 mm when tested clinically.
  2. There must be no evidence of radiolucency.
  3. Bone loss should be less than one-third the height of the implants.
  4. There should be an absence of infection, damage to structures, or violation of body cavities. Inflammation present must be amenable to treatment.
  5. The success rate must be 75% or more after 5 years of functional service.
These requirements are differentiated from the criteria of Albrektsson et al (1986), which include the following conditions:
  1. The individual, unattached implant is immobile when tested clinically.
  2. The radiograph does not demonstrate any evidence of periapical radiolucency.
  3. Vertical bone loss should be less than 0.2 mm annually following the implant's first year of service.
  4. Individual implant performance must be characterized by an absence of signs and symptoms such as pain, infections, neuropathies, paresthesia, or violation of the mandibular canal.
  5. Success rates of 85% or more at the end of a 5-year observation period and 80% at the end of a 10-year period are the minimum criteria for success.
Smith and Zarb (1989) modified Albrektsson's criteria by stating that the patient's and dentist's satisfaction with the implant prosthesis should be the primary consideration and that aesthetic requirements should be met. Patient satisfaction and patient attitude toward the prosthesis have been included in some subsequent lists of criteria for success. Although these criteria have become more stringent in recent years, measurement of success in implant dentistry is still difficult to quantify. It is important that standardized criteria for success be established to enable proper evaluation and evolution of implant dentistry.

Clinical success is no longer a game of chance. With the progress achieved by Branemark in studying osseointegration, a more scientific approach to implant dentistry has emerged. Performing a risk assessment analysis of the patient and minimizing the risk factors involved can maximize clinical survival. Subject risks include factors such as cigarette smoking, osteopenia, osteoporosis, diabetes, patient debilitation, and polypharmacy. The presence of these conditions has been known to compromise the success of osseointegration. Studies have concluded that the success rates for patients with controlled diabetes are 85.5% and 85.7% for the maxilla and mandible, respectively, with an overall success rate of 85.7% after 6.5 years. This is somewhat lower than the success rate for noncompromised patients, which is reported to be above 95%. This increase in failure rate usually occurs during the first year of loading of a prosthesis.

The reasons for tooth loss and the presence of uncontrolled periodontal disease and infections have also been implicated in the success or failure of the implant. Peri-implantitis, which causes inflammation of the supportive tissues around the implants, has been linked to the same bacteria prevalent in periodontal disease. There are also more internal factors specific to the site of placement, including bone height, bone density, and the amount of attached mucosa. Minimal bone height indicates the need for shorter implants, which have a relatively poorer prognosis. In comparison, implant placement in dense bone as opposed to spongy bone has a higher success rate. Some studies have noted the success rate for implants to be 94.5% when placed in the edentulous mandible consisting of denser bone, but only 72.4% when placed in the maxilla with spongy bone. Movable tissue around an implant has also been implicated in inducing the onset of peri-implantitis, which can lower the prognosis. Surprisingly, even the choice of implant type or material plays a role in clinical success. For example, studies have shown that hydroxyapatite-coated implants have a higher failure rate than other implant materials. However there are certain indications for use of hydroxyapatite crystals; these are discussed later in this chapter.

In a recent statistical study, implant failure has also been associated with immediate loading of the implants as well as implant staging (two-stage versus one-stage). Other critical factors include implant proximity to natural teeth and other existing implants.

CRITICAL QUESTION

Why are ceramic implants not ideal for posterior sites?

IMPLANT MATERIALS

Today, implant materials are subjected to significant scientific scrutiny before they are used in vivo. The most commonly used implant materials are made from some form of metallic substance. Implants also differ in the nature of their surface coating. Some implants are not coated; others are coated with ceramic, carbon, or a polymer. Of the four types of implants, endosteal implants are the most commonly used for dental applications.

Metallic Implants

Metallic implants undergo one or more of several surface modifications to enable them to become suitable for implantation. These modifications are **passivation, anodization, ion implantation,** and **texturing.** Passivation refers to the enhancement of the oxide layer to prevent the release of metallic ions as a result of surface breakdown. Minimizing ion release also enhances the **biocompatibility** of these materials. Passivation treatments can be performed through immersion in 40% nitric acid or anodization where an electric current is passed through the metal.

The former method of treatment minimally increases the oxide layer thickness, whereas the latter treatment results in a thicker oxide layer, which is more beneficial in enhancing corrosion resistance.

Surface texturing increases the surface area of the implant by up to six times and enhances osseointegration by increasing the area to which bone can bond. This is accomplished through several methods, including plasma spraying with titanium, acid etching, and blasting with aluminum oxide or another ceramic material. It is important that the increased implant surfaces remain passive, because a greater surface area tends to encourage the release of metallic ions.

Another surface modification for the implant is ion implantation, which consists of bombarding the surface of the implant with high-energy ions up to a surface depth of 0.1 μm. This procedure is claimed to increase the corrosion resistance of the metal through the formation of a TiN surface layer.

The most popular implant material in use today is titanium. As a result of Branemark's extensive studies, titanium has become the gold standard in implant materials. Titanium exists in nature as a pure element with an atomic number of 22 in the periodic table. With an atomic weight of 47.9, titanium composes about 0.6% of the earth's crust and is a million times more abundant than gold. This metal exists as rutile (TiO^2) or ilmenite ($FeTiO_3$) and requires specific extraction methods to be recovered in its elemental state. The Kroll process involves reduction of $TiCl_4$ by magnesium, whereas the iodide process involves formation of titanium iodide through the reaction of raw titanium with iodine. The titanium iodide is later decomposed on a heated titanium wire.

Titanium has several favorable physical properties, which include a low specific gravity with a density of 4.5 g/cm^3, high heat resistance, and high strength comparable with that of stainless steel. Titanium is also very resistant to corrosion as a result of the passivating effect afforded by a thin layer of titanium oxide that is formed on its surface. It has the ability to form an oxide layer 10 Å in thickness within a millisecond and is generally self-healing. If left unchecked, this oxide layer can become 100-Å thick within a minute. Pure titanium has the ability to form several oxides, including TiO, TiO_2, and Ti_2O_3. Of these, TiO_2 is considered the most stable and is used more often under physiological conditions.

The most commonly used titanium products are pure Ti and titanium alloys, namely, Ti-6Al-4V and Ti-6Al-4V extra low interstitial (ELI). Titanium can be alloyed with different elements to modify its properties. Pure titanium can undergo a transformation from a hexagonal-close-packed alpha phase to a body-centered-cubic beta phase at 883° C. Alloying elements are added to stabilize either phase. Ti-6Al-4V is one of the more commonly used titanium alloys. Aluminum acts as an alpha stabilizer for the purpose of increasing strength and decreasing the mass. Vanadium, copper, and palladium are beta phase stabilizers, which are used to minimize the formation of $TiAl_3$ to approximately 6% or less to decrease its susceptibility to corrosion. With the exception of pure titanium, the modulus of elasticity of Ti-6Al-4V is closer to that of bone than any other widely used implant material. This ensures a more uniform distribution of stress, particularly along the bone-implant interface, as the bone and the implant flex similarly.

A combination of these phases enhances the alloy's strength. ELI contains low levels of oxygen dissolved in interstitial sites in the metal. Lower amounts of oxygen and iron improve the ductility of the ELI alloy. Newer titanium alloys have been developed, which include Ti-13Nb-13Zr and Ti-15Mo-2.8Nb. These alloys utilize other phase stabilizers instead of aluminum and vanadium, and they may exhibit a greater corrosion resistance.

Table 23-2	Composition of CP Titanium and Alloys (Weight Percent)							
Titanium	*N*	*C*	*H*	*Fe*	*O*	*Al*	*V*	*Ti*
CP grade I	0.03	0.08	0.015	0.20	0.18	—	—	balance
CP grade II	0.03	0.08	0.015	0.30	0.25	—	—	balance
CP grade III	0.05	0.08	0.015	0.30	0.35	—	—	balance
CP grade IV	0.05	0.08	0.015	0.50	0.40	—	—	balance
Ti-6Al-4V alloy	0.05	0.08	0.015	0.30	0.20	5.50-6.75	3.50-4.50	balance
Ti-6Al-4V (ELI alloy)	0.05	0.08	0.012	0.25	0.13	5.50-6.50	3.50-4.50	balance

ASTM standard: minimum values.

Commercially pure Ti comes in different grades, from CP grade I to CP grade IV. The compositions of these metals in weight percentage are given in Table 23-2. The strength of CPTi is less than that of Ti-6Al-4V alloy, although the modulus of elasticity values are comparable. The elastic modulus of Ti alloys (113 GPa) (see Table 23-1) is only slightly higher than that for the CP grade IV Ti (102 GPa). The yield strength values for ELI and Ti6Al4V alloys (795 MPa and 860 MPa, respectively) are 65% to 78% greater than that for CPTi. Ti alloys are able to maintain that fine balance between sufficient strength to resist fracture under occlusal forces and a lower modulus of elasticity for a more uniform stress distribution across the bone-implant interface.

Another alloy used for implantation is stainless steel. Used in the form of surgical austenitic steel, these metals have 18% chromium for corrosion resistance and 8% nickel to stabilize the austenitic structure. Stainless steel is most often used in the wrought and heat-treated state and possesses high strength and ductility. This metal is not widely used in implant dentistry despite its low cost and ease of fabrication because of the allergenic potential of nickel, as well as its susceptibility to crevice and pitting corrosion. Its corrosion products include iron, chromium, nickel, and molybdenum. These elements or their ions can accumulate in the tissues surrounding the implant and subsequently be transported to different parts of the body to produce a potentially unfavorable immune response. Surface treatments such as surface passivation and ion implantation are used to improve the corrosion resistance, although austenitic stainless steels are still prone to localized attack in long-term applications. The presence of a galvanic potential with the use of different metals is also an area of concern for the decreased corrosion resistance of stainless steel.

Cobalt-chromium-molybdenum alloys generally consist of 63% cobalt, 30% chromium, and 5% molybdenum with small amounts of carbon, manganese, and nickel. Molybdenum is a stabilizer; chromium provides the passivating effect to ensure corrosion resistance; and carbon serves as a hardener. Vitallium was introduced by Venable in the late 1930s and is part of the Co-Cr-Mo alloy family. It was initially shown to lack electrochemical activity and tissue reaction. Ticonium, a Ni-Cr-Mo-Be alloy, was also used as a dental implant material, although it showed less biocompatibility. In later studies, Vitallium was shown to evoke a chronic inflammation with no epithelial attachment and with fibrous encapsulation accompanied by mobility.

In an attempt to improve the alloy's performance, inert materials in the form of aluminum oxide ceramics were added to the surface. Aluminum oxide and zirconium oxide coated on Vitallium were found to have no effect on improving biological acceptability of the metal. Co-Cr-Mo alloys have a high elastic modulus and resistance to corrosion, although they have low ductility. Studies have shown that this low ductility is a result of the agglomeration of particles, which are rich in carbon, chromium, and molybdenum. Ductility can be improved through the reduction of the carbon content in the metal. In spite of titanium's excellent biocompatibility, Co-Cr-Mo alloys and stainless steel are still sometimes used for larger implants such as subperiosteal and transosteal implants because of their castability and lower cost.

Ceramic and Ceramic-Coated Implant Systems

There are several synthetic and biological materials that have been used in the –treatment of bone defects, ridge augmentation, and osteoporotic lesions. These materials are also used to coat metallic implants to produce an ionic ceramic surface, which is thermodynamically stable and hydrophilic, thereby producing a high-strength attachment to bone and the surrounding tissues. These ceramics can either be plasma-sprayed or coated onto the metal implant to produce a bioactive surface. The term *bioactive* refers to a variety of inorganic materials that can stimulate adhesion and bonding to bone. These materials are generally brittle and have a high elastic modulus and low tensile strength.

Ceramic implants can withstand only relatively low tensile stresses induced by occlusal loads, but they can tolerate quite high levels of compressive stress. Aluminum oxide (Al_2O_3) is used as the gold standard for ceramic implants because of its inertness with no evidence of ion release or immune reactions in vivo. Zirconia (ZrO_2) has also demonstrated a high degree of inertness, although alumina (Al_2O_3) has shown a higher surface wettability compared with those of metallic surface implants. These ceramic implants are not bioactive in that they do not promote the formation of bone. They have high strength, stiffness, and hardness and function well as subperiosteal or transosteal implants. Table 23-1 lists the mechanical properties of different metallic materials compared with ceramic implant materials.

Of the synthetic types of materials, calcium phosphates are the most successful for grafting and augmentation of bone. This performance is probably associated with the fact that vital bone is composed of 60% to 70% calcium phosphate. These materials are nonimmunogenic and are biocompatible with host tissues. The two most commonly used calcium phosphates are hydroxyapatite (HA), or $Ca_{10}(PO_4)_6(OH)_2$, and tricalcium phosphate (TCP), or $Ca_3(PO_4)_2$. Hydroxyapatite and tricalcium phosphate are used as bone graft materials in granular or block form to serve as a template for the formation of new bone. Because these materials are known to promote and achieve a direct bond of the implant to hard tissues, they are classified as bioactive. Both also promote vertically directed bone growth, as well as a stronger bond to bone. **Biointegration** is defined in the 7th edition of the *Glossary of Prosthodontic Terms* as "the benign acceptance of a foreign object by living tissue." More specifically, the biointegration of bone with an implanted material indicates the bond of bone to HA. HA, TCP, and other calcium phosphates are biocompatible as a result of the release of calcium and phosphate ions to the surrounding tissue. However, the attachment strength of the calcium phosphates is far below that of alumina and zirconia. Studies have revealed several differences in the tissue response to these materials following implantation. TCP is resorbed more rapidly than HA and results in a breakdown of material and replacement by mesenchymal cells with features resembling osteoprogenitor cells. It has also been shown that after 4 weeks of implantation, osteocytes accumulate adjacent to HA granules, indicating the possibility of osteogenesis with these implants.

Use of these calcium phosphates as coating materials for metallic implants is directly related to their crystallinity. The more crystalline the HA coating, the more resistant it is to clinical dissolution. A minimum of 50% crystalline HA is considered an optimal concentration in a coating for implants. Commercial implants coated with HA have ranged from 85% crystalline HA and 15% TCP to 97% crystalline HA. Dissolution of the ceramic coating occurs at a higher rate with a more amorphous HA structure. Heat treatment after the deposition process has been shown to improve the crystallinity of HA. The major advantage of these ceramic coatings is that they can stimulate the adaptation of bone, and they exhibit a more intimate bone-to-implant contact compared with a metallic surface. The amount of osseointegration was compared between metallic implants and ceramic-coated implants in numerous studies. These studies suggest that there is a greater bone-to-implant integration with the HA-coated implants, with values ranging from 17.1% for 7 days to 75.9% for 3 months for HA-coated implants versus 1.2% (7 days) to 45.7% (3 months) for titanium implants. However, a study by Gottlander and Albrektsson (1992) concluded that there was no significant difference between the ceramic-coated and the uncoated implants after 6 months of integration, which implies that early integration and resistance to torque failure of HA-coated implants over uncoated ones may be only of short-term duration.

The bioglasses (SiO_2-CaO-Na_2O-P_2O_5-MgO) are another form of bioactive ceramics. These materials are known to form a carbonated hydroxyapatite layer in vivo as a result of their calcium and phosphorus content. The formation of this layer is initiated by the migration of calcium, phosphate, silica, and sodium ions toward tissue as a result of external pH changes. A silica-rich gel layer forms on the surface as elements are released and lost. The silicon depletion initiates a migration of calcium and phosphate ions to the silica gel layer from both the bioglass surface and tissue fluids. This results in the formation of a calcium-phosphorus layer that stimulates osteoblasts to proliferate. These osteoblasts produce collagen fibrils that become incorporated into the calcium-phosphorus layer and are later anchored by the calcium-phosphorus crystals. This layer is 100 to 200 μm thick and has been shown to form a very strong bone-bioglass interface. Bioglasses are classified as bioactive materials, because they stimulate the formation of bone. These materials are more often used as grafting materials for ridge augmentation or bony defects than as coating materials for metallic implants because the interfacial bond strength of bioglasses with metal and other ceramic substrates is weak and is subject to dissolution in vivo. Despite their favorable **osteoinductive** ability, bioglasses are also very brittle, which makes them unsuitable for use as a stress-bearing implant materials.

CRITICAL QUESTION

How does an intramobile element affect the function of an implant?

Polymers

Polymeric implants in the form of polymethylmethacrylate and polytetrafluoroethylene were first used in the 1930s. These substances are made of simple and recurring structural units called monomers, which are connected by covalent bonds formed during the polymerization process to form a polymeric substance. They are generally complex molecules of high molecular weight, but they are much softer and more flexible with a lower modulus of elasticity than the other classes of biomaterials. The low mechanical strength of the polymers has precluded their use as implant materials because of their susceptibility for mechanical fracture during function. Also, physical properties of the polymers are greatly influenced by changes in temperature, environment, and composition, and as such, their sterilization can be accomplished only by gamma irradiation or exposure to ethylene oxide gas. Contamination of these polymers is another disadvantage, because electrostatic charges often attract dust and other impurities from the environment.

During the mid 1940s, methyl methacrylate was used for temporary acrylic implants to preserve the dissected space to receive a Co-Cr implant at a later time. The tissues did not show any evidence of irritation or destruction with the use of this material.

The use of polymers for osseointegrated implants is now confined to components. The IMZ implants are either titanium plasma-sprayed or HA-coated and incorporate a polyoxymethylene (POM) intramobile element (IME), which acts as an internal shock absorber. The IME is placed between the prosthesis and the implant body (Fig. 23-6) to initiate mobility, stress relief, and shock absorption capability to mimic that of the natural tooth. When incorporated into the IMZ implant, the IME initiates the biomechanical function of the natural tooth unit, periodontal ligament, and alveolar bone. The IME is designed to ensure a more uniform stress distribution along the bone-implant interface. Studies have demonstrated that this shock-absorbing element also helps in reducing occlusal loads.

Other Implant Materials

Carbon and a carbon compound (C and SiC) were introduced in the 1960s for use in implantology. Vitreous carbon, which elicits a very minimal response from host tissues, is one of the most biocompatible materials. Studies have confirmed that the morphology of the bone-implant interface is similar to that associated with an HA implant. Compared with metallic implants, carbon is inert under physiological conditions and has a modulus of elasticity equivalent to that of dentin and bone. Thus it deforms at a rate similar to those tissues, enabling adequate transmission of stress. However, because of its brittleness, carbon is susceptible to fracture under tensile stress, which is usually generated as a component of flexural stress. It also has a relatively low compressive strength. Thus a large surface area and geometry are

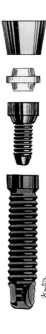

Fig. 23-6 Intramobile element that is believed to act as an internal shock absorber. See also color plate.

required to resist fracture. Carbon-based materials are also used for ceramic and metallic implant coatings.

CRITICAL QUESTION

With the abundance of implant materials to choose from, how does a clinician know which material to use for a particular situation?

SELECTING AN IMPLANT MATERIAL

Because of the abundance of different implant materials and implant systems, it is important to know the indications for use of these different materials. Perhaps the most important consideration is the strength of the implant material and the type of bone in which the implant will be placed. The other factors to consider are implant design, abutment choices and availability, surface finish, and biomechanical considerations.

The strength of an implant is often a consideration, depending on the area of placement of the implant. If the implants are located in a high load zone (e.g., in the posterior areas of the arch), the clinician might consider using a higher-strength material such as CP grade IV titanium or one of the titanium alloys. Some controversy exists as to which titanium metal to use, because some researchers believe that aluminum and vanadium can be toxic if released in sufficient quantities.

Other considerations for selection include a history of implant fracture in the placement area of interest, the use of narrower implants, and a history of occlusal or parafunctional habits. Anterior implants designated for use in narrow spaces have smaller diameters in the range of 3.25 mm. Conversely, single implants placed in posterior areas have larger diameters up to 5.0 mm. Table 23-3 shows some implant systems and the type of metal used by the manufacturers.

CRITICAL QUESTION

How do bone height and dental bone quality affect the survival time of implants?

As previously stated, the type of bone in which the implant will be placed is of critical importance. Bone quality has been classified into four types: Type I consists of mostly homogenous compact bone; Type II consists of a thick layer of compact

Table 23-3	Compositions of Current Implant Systems					
	CP Ti grade I	CP Ti grade II	CP Ti grade III	CP Ti grade IV	Ti-6Al-4V ELI alloy	Ti-6Al-4V alloy
3i	*	*	X			
BioHorizons				X		
Lifecore			X	X	X	
Nobel Biocare	X					
Paragon				X	X	
Steri-Oss			X	X		
Sulzer Calcitek						X

From McCracken M: Dental implant materials: Commercially pure titanium and titanium alloys. J Prosthodont 8:40-43, 1999.

bone surrounding a core of dense trabecular bone; Type III is a thin layer of cortical bone surrounding a core of dense trabecular bone; and Type IV is composed of a thin layer of cortical bone with a core of low-density trabecular bone (Fig. 23-7). Type IV bone is by far the worst possible bone environment for implant placement because of inadequate stability and poor bone quality.

There is much debate about when to use metal implants or ceramic-coated implants. As mentioned earlier, HA-coated implants stimulate bone growth and have been shown to have a greater bone-to-implant integration. However, there are also some studies showing that HA is a very unstable implant material and can prove detrimental to bone and tissues in the long term. Gottlander and Albrektsson (1991) examined the bone-to-implant contact area both at 6 weeks and 12 months for HA-coated and CPTi implants. They concluded that the bone-to-implant contact area at 6 weeks was 65% for HA and 59% for Ti. However at 12 months, Ti exhibited a 75% contact area versus 53% for HA. The bond for HA is formed from a very dynamic bone reaction to the material and is later maintained by a continuous ion exchange. Some contend that the bond of HA to bone is biologically unstable as a result of this exchange. As mentioned earlier, HA is also subject to dissolution, and high crystallinity must be maintained to minimize this occurrence. Unfortunately, some amount of amorphous substance must be present to complete the bond to metal, and this substance is susceptible to dissolution. The long-term stability of the HA-coated implants is still very controversial. Although the bond between HA and bone is considered to be strong, the mechanical stability of the interface between the coating and the metallic substrate can be unstable.

Some studies have shown that the survival rate of HA-coated implants is initially higher than that for titanium plasma-sprayed implants, but the survival rate significantly decreases after 4 years. Failures are caused by inflammation of the surrounding tissues with delamination and exfoliation. Some implants were retrieved before failure, and these revealed partial loss of the HA coating with flattening and thinning in some areas, as well as an increase in Cl and Mg ions. The implications of these factors relative to clinical implant failure are still unknown.

Another concern is the adherence of microorganisms to the HA surface. A study of failed titanium and HA-coated implants revealed a colonization of coccoid and rod-shaped bacteria on HA implants, possibly as a result of the bioreactivity of HA. The roughened surface of the HA implants can also contribute to plaque growth once the coating is exposed. This can lead to peri-implantitis, which decreases the chance of long-term survival.

In spite of all the disadvantages, hydroxyapatite still has some indications for implant applications. Studies reported on the biological response to both the coated and uncoated implants suggest that HA-coated implants were interfaced intimately with bone and that the mineralized matrix extended into the microporosity of the HA coating. Numerous osteocytes were found along the periphery of HA-coated implants, which indicates that HA-coated implants are a better option for poor bone quality areas such as the maxilla. In one study, Branemark-type titanium implants

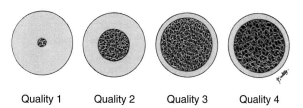

Fig. 23-7 Four types of bone ranging from homogenous compact bone to low-density trabecular bone. See also color plate.

were evaluated in Type IV bone and a survival rate of 63% was found for mandibular implants and 56% for maxillary implants. These values are lower than the survival rates of 90% or more when these implants were placed in Type I and II bone. Another study compared the survival rates of titanium screw-type implants and HA-coated cylinders in Type IV bone. At 36 months, Ti implants had a survival rate of 78.3%, compared with 98% for HA implants. At 48 months this survival rate fell to 74.7% for the metal implants. In a follow-up study, titanium screws exhibited a 91% 3-year survival rate and 89% for a 7-year period in Type IV maxillary bone. These rates can be compared with a survival level of 95% for HA implants during a 7-year period. All of these studies indicate that HA-coated implants have a greater survival rate in Type IV bone. Therefore the dentist should be inclined to use HA-coated implants for areas where poor or less than ideal bone is to be used for implant placement.

The bone height available for implant placement is also a factor for consideration of which type of implant to use. A five-year study revealed a 70% failure rate for titanium screws with only a height of 8 mm. The same height of HA-coated screws resulted in only a 4% failure. There was no significant difference in the failure rates between the two types of implants when the length of the screws was increased to 12 mm.

Another indication for HA-coated implants is their placement in fresh extraction sites. Immediate implant placement can sometimes be performed immediately after an extraction if there are time constraints and no existing pathological conditions, such as periodontal conditions or diseased bone states. Initial stability is difficult to obtain in some of these cases, and this leads to implant failure. A comparison of the survival rate of HA-coated implants, metallic implants, and hollow basket implants was made after 7 years of immediate implant placement. Survival rates of 95%, 90%, and 82% were found, respectively. The implant-bone interface contact area was also shown to be 61.8% for HA-coated implants and 29.2% for metallic implants after 28 days of placement. The initial stability afforded by the HA-coated implants makes them more suitable for placement in fresh extraction sites.

Further advances in the field of dental surgery have allowed placement of implants in areas in which bone is not normally present. Maxillary and nasal sinus lifts are commonplace in partially dentate individuals who require an implant. Bone grafts have enabled placement of a sinus lift in posterior areas where bone is deficient. Unfortunately, the quality of bone produced from these bone grafts is poor and an implant is required to establish a substantial implant-bone contact area. Most of these implant sites oppose fully dentate arches, which exert a higher amount of masticatory force. Thus initial stability, proper osseointegration, and high shear strength are important implant properties for these locations. Studies have revealed that HA-coated implants exhibited a push shear bond strength of 7.3 MPa versus a value of 1.2 MPa for titanium metallic implants after a period of 10 weeks. After 32 weeks HA-coated implants still had shear bond strength values that were five times greater than those for metallic surface implants.

Another study compared the torsional strength of commercially pure titanium, Ti-6Al-4V, and HA-coated implants. Values for a period of up to 4 months ranged from 74.0 Ncm to 186.0 Ncm (HA-coated implants). These torsion strength values reflect the failure resistance of the implant. Thus HA-coated implant surfaces can provide a greater implant-bone interface, higher shear bond strength, and higher torsional strength in areas that require a sinus lift procedure.

A recent meta-analysis review was conducted to compare the performance of coated and noncoated implants. The review suggests that the survival rates are similar for both coated and uncoated implants and that the HA-coating did not compromise the long-term survival of these implants. Indications to support the selection of HA-coated implants over titanium or metallic surfaced implants include (1) the need for greater bone-implant interface contact area, (2) the ability to place the implant in Type IV bone, (3) fresh extraction sites, and (4) newly grafted sites. It has also been shown that the advantages of HA-coated implants are mainly short-term in nature and are related to the initial stability of the implant, which most often determines its prerestorative success or failure.

CRITICAL QUESTION

Several types of biocompatibility test data may be useful for selection of an appropriate implant. What is the principal factor on which an implant material should be selected as suitable or unsuitable for osseointegration?

BIOCOMPATIBILITY OF IMPLANTS

The concept of biomaterial biocompatibility does not refer to total inertness, but rather the ability of a material to perform with an appropriate response in a specific application. Biocompatibility is affected by the intrinsic nature of the material, as well as its design and construction. Therefore the state of biocompatibility may be confined to a particular situation or function in the human body. The American Dental Association outlines some acceptance provisions for dental implants, including (1) evaluation of physical properties that ensure sufficient strength; (2) demonstration of ease of fabrication and sterilization potential without material degradation; (3) biocompatibility evaluation, including cytotoxicity testing; (4) freedom from defects; and (5) a minimum of two clinical trials, each with a minimum of 50 human subjects conducted for 3 years to earn provisional acceptance or 5 years to earn acceptance.

Other materials such as stainless steel and cobalt-chromium alloys are mainly used for construction of the superstructure in the restoration phase or as fixation screws. Concern exists over the potential electrolytic action and increased corrosion associated with the combination of contacting metals; another concern is the possible release of nickel and beryllium ions.

The primary interactions between an implant material and its host take place at the surface of the implant within a region of approximately the size of one water molecule ($\sim$0.1–1.0 nm). However, this does not mean that the implant-tissue interactions are isolated at this interface. Some studies have reported unusually high titanium levels in both the spleen and lungs of rabbits immediately following surgery, but these concentrations were well within normal limits. In humans, Ti levels are normally 50 ppm, but they can reach levels of up to 300 ppm in tissues surrounding titanium implants. Tissue discoloration at this level may be visible, but it is still well tolerated by the body. Kasemo and Lausmaa (1991) demonstrated the dissolution of corrosion products into the bioliquid and adjacent tissues. Thus the outermost atomic layers of an implant are critical regions associated with biochemical interactions of the implant-tissue interface. This should have a tremendous influence on a high degree of standardization and surface control in the production of implants.

Disintegrating particles of HA, which result from dissolution of the amorphous substance, are believed to be toxic to fibroblasts, especially when they are smaller than 5 μm. Direct interaction with the cells has resulted in irreversible cell membrane damage.

The response of bone to different implant materials is the principal factor on which an implant material is selected as suitable or unsuitable for osseointegration.

Reports have concluded that the percentage of bone volume in cortical bone around CPTi and HA implants were the same. However, when these implant materials were placed in bone marrow, a marked difference was reported. Titanium implants induced a steady increase in bone volume directly adjacent to the implant and surrounding it for up to 8 weeks. The volume of bone adjacent to the surface of HA implants increased to a maximum level at 4 weeks. This clearly emphasizes the need for more studies highlighting the effects of biomaterials to surrounding tissues as well as their effect on clinical effectiveness.

Reaction to polymers includes a chronic irritation of the surrounding connective tissue with a fibrous encapsulation. Polymers are also allergenic and have caused carcinogenic reactions in some studies. Other reactions include bone loss, gingival recession, and peri-implantitis. As such, polymers are no longer being used as implant materials.

CRITICAL QUESTION

How does a tooth-implant–supported prosthesis compare with an implant-supported prosthesis?

BIOMECHANICS

The attachment of bone to implants serves as the basis for the biomechanics analyses performed for dental implants. Close approximation of osseointegrated bone with the surface of an implant fixture permits the transfer of stresses with little relative displacement of the bone and implant. The stresses that are generated are highly affected by three main variables: (1) masticatory factors (frequency, bite force, and mandibular movements), (2) support for the prosthesis (implant-supported, implant-tissue–supported, implant-tooth–supported), and (3) the mechanical properties of the materials involved in the implant restoration (elastic modulus, ductility, fracture strength, etc.). One of the most important variables affecting the close apposition of bone to the implant surface is the relative movement, or "micro-motion." It has long been documented that movement shortly after implantation prevents the formation of bone and encourages the formation of fibrous connective tissue around the implant surface. This collagen-rich connective tissue is considered to be nonretentive and provides no support for the implant fixture. This is the reason that a delay of 4 to 6 months is recommended before loading after surgery. As mentioned previously, there has been some success reported with immediate loading of implants depending on bone quality and patient selection.

There are two main types of loading condition that can occur in an implant site. These are represented by axial forces and bending moments. A bending moment can best be demonstrated by visualizing a cantilever beam design in which the maximum bending moment that is located at the fixed base of support is calculated as force (perpendicular to the beam) times the length of the lever arm. These bending moments become highly significant, depending on the type and design of implant restoration that is planned.

Rangert (1989), Skalak (1983), and Brunski (1988) analyzed the theoretical effects of cantilever length, number of implants, the arrangement of implants, and prosthesis design. Their models were based on the initial Branemark hybrid prosthesis for the atrophic mandible (Fig. 23-8). This type of restoration usually involves four to six implant fixtures confined to the area between the mental foramina of the mandible with cantilevers extending from the most distal implant. These were

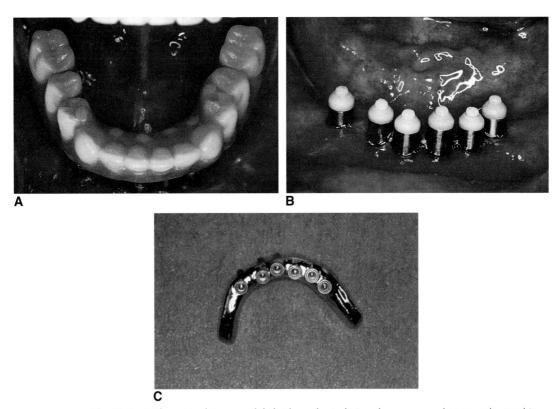

Fig. 23-8 **A,** The original Branemark hybrid prosthesis designed to accommodate severely atrophic mandibles. **B,** The hybrid prosthesis usually requires 4 to 6 implants. **C,** Corresponding superstructure that is screwed onto the implants. See also color plate.

restored with acrylic resin and denture teeth, which were attached to the implant metal superstructure through the use of chemical and mechanical bonding. The most significant aspect of these studies is the optimal ratio of the cantilever length to the interfixture distance.

When two or more implants are placed in a straight line, the bending moment will be distributed proportionately to all fixtures, provided that the prosthesis is sufficiently rigid. Placement of the implants in an offset manner has been suggested as a more favorable orientation because it is believed to increase the resistance to loading. However, recent studies have shown that tripodization of implants does not necessarily minimize stresses as much as the use of wider-diameter implants placed in a straight line. An increase in the anterior-posterior placement of implants is also recommended to minimize the angular loading of the implant components. The load is greatest at the most distal fixture when an anteriorly positioned cantilever prosthesis exists. Thus the distance between the most terminal abutment and the one directly adjacent to it should be increased to reduce the stress and strain induced within the most distal abutment.

Another important factor to consider is the fit of the prosthesis on the implant. An inaccurate fit will lead to a nonuniform distribution of load with the unit closest to the load bearing most of the forces. For well-integrated implant fixtures, the weakest link in the system becomes the gold or abutment screw, which is regarded as the safety feature in these restorations. All of the external tension is usually borne entirely by the gold screw if an inaccurate fit exists and a preload is applied to the screw connection. These screws are fairly retrievable and are easy to replace.

The ultimate tensile strength of the gold screw is approximately twice the stress induced by maximum occlusal force in the molar region.

The Branemark hybrid implant has been designed with variable cantilever distances based on the number of implants available in the prosthesis. Branemark recommended a maximum length of three premolars. Others have suggested a 20-mm distance with five to six implants for the restoration and a 15-mm distance if only four implants are to be used. Other recommendations include a 15- to 20-mm separation in the mandible and 10 mm in the maxilla because of poorer bone quality. Some guidelines include computing the anterior-posterior span of all the implants and allowing a distance of 1.5 times the cantilever width but limiting the maxilla to a maximum of 8 mm because of poor bone quality. Any cantilever length over 7 mm causes the largest increases in microstrain within both the framework and bone. Therefore for any length over 7 mm, ideal conditions should be ensured, or the decision to proceed under less ideal conditions should be approached with extreme caution.

Another area of debate is the attachment of implants to natural teeth. The consensus seems to be that attaching them to natural teeth should be avoided and that having lone-standing implants is a better restorative option. However, in cases in which it is absolutely necessary to include a natural tooth in the restoration (e.g., when a low maxillary sinus position is present), there is disagreement as to whether or not this lowers the prognosis of the entire restoration. The issue stems from the different nature of attachments to bone between the implant and the tooth. The implant is osseointegrated, meaning that it has a direct connection with bone. In essence, the fixture itself is ankylosed to bone. On the other hand, a tooth is attached to bone through the periodontal ligament, which provides sensory functions to the tooth and also cushions the masticatory load.

Bone formation or resorption is determined by the tension or compression within the periodontal ligament. A concern associated with attachment of an implant to a natural tooth is that the mobility of the tooth might minimize its load sharing ability and overload the implant or understimulate the tooth. Several devices, such as the IMZ intramobile element, have been developed to allow the implant to accommodate the movement of the periodontal ligament. In any event, studies will continue to elucidate the effects of implant and natural tooth attachment on the probability of success. The results from most of the previous studies suggest that the attachment of natural teeth to implants does not compromise the prognosis of the prosthesis. Because these studies also confirm the overall excellent success rates of implant-supported prostheses, it is still recommended that this be the first approach for treatment.

SUMMARY

The implant systems currently available are diverse. In 2002 there were at least 30 companies manufacturing 20 different implant systems. The implant materials range from commercially pure titanium to HA-coated devices. Manufacturers have developed individualized designs for their implants, and they are continually altering marketing strategies to highlight the features of each implant. Although most of the implant materials that have been described in this chapter are believed to be biocompatible, the precise bone-bonding mechanisms are not fully characterized on a molecular level. When the mechanisms that ensure implant **bioacceptance** and structural stabilization are fully understood, implant failures will become a rare occurrence, provided that they are used properly and placed in sites for which they are indicated.

SELECTED READINGS

Akagi K, Okamoto Y, Matsuura T, and Horibe T: Properties of test metal ceramic titanium alloys. J Prosthet Dent 68:462-467, 1992.

Akca K, and Iplikcioglu H: Finite element stress analysis of the influence of staggered versus straight placement of dental implants. Int J Oral Maxillofac Implants 16:722-730, 2001.

Albrektsson T, and Sennerby L: State of the art in oral implants. J Clin Periodontol 18:474-481, 1991.

Albrektsson T, and Zarb G, Worthington P, and Eriksson RA: The long-term efficacy of currently used dental implants: a review and proposed criteria of success. Int J Oral Maxillofac Implants 1:11-25, 1986.

ASTM F 67-00: Standard specification for unalloyed titanium, for surgical implant applications (UNS R 50250, UNS R 50400, UNS R 50550, UNS R 50700). In: Annual Book of ASTM Standards, Philadelphia, American Society for Testing and Materials, 2000.

ASTM F 136-98: Wrought titanium—6 aluminum—4 vanadium ELI (extra low interstitial) alloy (UNS R 56401) for surgical implant applications. In: Annual Book of ASTM Standards, Philadelphia, American Society for Testing Materials, 2000.

ASTM F 139-00: Standard specification for wrought 18 chromium-14 nickel—2.5 molybdenum stainless steel bar and wire for surgical implants (UNS S 31673). In: Annual Book of ASTM Standards, Philadelphia, American Society for Testing Materials, 2000.

Balkin B: Implant Dentistry: Historical overview with current perspective. J Dent Educ 1988; 52:683-695.

Baltag I, Watanabe K, Kusakari H, Taguchi N, et al: Long-term changes of hydroxyapatite-coated dental implants. J Biomed Mater Res 53:76-85, 2000.

Branemark PI, Zarb GA, and Albrektsson T: Tissue Integrated Prostheses: Osseointegration in Clinical Dentistry. Chicago, Quintessence Publishing Co, 1987.

Brunski JB: Biomechanics of oral implants: future research directions. J Dent Educ (special issue) 52:755-787, 1988.

Brunski JB, and Skalak R: Biomechanical Considerations in Advanced Osseointegration Surgery: Applications in the Maxillofacial Region. Worthington P, Branemark PI (eds): Carol Stream, IL, Quintessence, 1992, pp 15-40.

Chang YL, Lew D, Park JB, and Keller JC: Biomechanical and morphometric analysis of hydroxyapatite-coated implants with varying crystallinity. J Oral Maxillofac Surg 57:1096-1109, 1999.

Chuang SK, Wei LJ, Douglass CW, and Dodson TB: Risk factors for dental implant failure: a strategy for the analysis of clustered failure-time observations. J Dent Res 81:572-577, 2002.

Craig RG (ed): Restorative Dental Materials, 11th ed. St Louis, Mosby, 2001.

Davies JE: Mechanisms of endosseous integration. Int J Prosthodont 11:391-401, 1998.

Driskell TD: History of implants. Calif Dent Assoc J 15:16-25, 1987.

Fiorellini JP, Chen PK, Nevins M, and Nevins ML: A retrospective study of dental implants in diabetic patients. Int J Periodontics Restorative Dent 20:366-373, 2000.

Glossary of Prosthodontic Terms, 7th edition. GPT-7, Mosby, reprinted from J Prosthet Dent, 81(1):39-110, 1999.

Ichikawa T, Hanawa T, Ukai H, and Murakami K: Three-dimensional bone response to commercially pure titanium, hydroxyapatite, and calcium-ion-missing titanium in rabbits. Int J Oral Maxillofac Implants 15:231-238, 2000.

Kasemo B, and Lausmaa J: The Biomaterial-Tissue Interface and Its Analogues in Surface Science and Technology. In: Davis JE (ed): The Bone-Biomaterials Interface, 1st ed. Toronto, University of Toronto, 1991, pp 19-32.

Lacefield WR: Materials characteristics of uncoated/ceramic-coated implant materials. Adv Dent Res 13:21-26, 1999.

Lautenschlager EP, and Monaghan P: Titanium and titanium alloys as dental materials. Int Dent J 43:245-253, 1993.

Lee JJ, Rouhfar, and Beirne OR: Survival of hydroxyapatite-coated implants: A meta-analytic review. J Oral Maxillofac Surg 58:1372-1379, 2000.

Lindh T, Back T, Nystromm E, and Gunne J: Implant versus tooth-implant supported prostheses in the posterior maxilla: A 2-year report. Clin Oral Implants Res 12:441-449, 2001.

McCracken M: Dental implant materials: Commercially pure titanium and titanium alloys. J Prosthodont 8:40-43, 1999.

Meffert RM: Ceramic-coated implant systems. Adv Dent Res 13:170-172, 1999.

Misch CM, and Ismail YH: Finite element stress analysis of tooth-to-implant fixed partial denture designs. J Prosthodont 2:83-92, 1993.

Ogiso M, Yamashita Y, and Matsumoto T: Differences in microstructural characteristics of dense HA and HA coating. J Biomed Mater Res 41:296-303, 1998.

Parr GR, Gardner LK, and Toth RW: Titanium: The mystery metal of implant dentistry. Dental materials aspects. J Prosthet Dent 54:410-414, 1985.

Rangert B, Gunne J, and Sullivan DY: Mechanical aspects of a Branemark implant connected to a natural tooth: An in vitro study. Int J Oral Maxillofac Implants 6:177-186, 1991.

Rodriguez AM, Aquilino SA, Lund PS, Ryther JS, and Southard TE: Evaluation of strain at the terminal abutment site of a fixed mandibular implant prosthesis during cantilever loading. J Prosthodont 2:93-102, 1993.

Schnitman PA: Implant dentistry: Where are we now? J Am Dent Assoc 124:39-47, 1993.

Schnitman PA, and Shulman LB (eds): Dental Implants: Benefits and Risk, An NIH-Harvard consensus development conference. U.S. Dept. of Health and Human Services, 1979, p 1-135.

Skalak R: Biomechanical considerations in osseointegrated prostheses. J Prosthet Dent 49:843-849, 1983.

Smith D: Dental implants: Materials and design considerations. Int J Prosthodont 6:106-117, 1993.

Steflik DE, Corpe RS, Young TR, Sisk AL, and Parr GR: The biologic tissue responses to uncoated and coated implanted biomaterials. Adv Dent Res 13:27-33, 1999.

Tonetti MS: Determination of the success and failure of root-form osseointegrated dental implants. Adv Dent Res 13:173-180, 1999

Appendix
The FDA Modernization Act of 1997

The FDA Modernization Act of 1997 is major legislation that is designed to reform the regulation of food, medical products, and cosmetics. The coded initiatives include measures to modernize the regulation of biological products by bringing them in harmony with the regulations for drugs. The act (1) eliminates the need for establishment license application, batch certification, and monograph requirements for insulin and antibiotics; (2) streamlines the approval processes for drug and biological manufacturing changes; and (3) reduces the need for environmental assessment as part of a product application.

The act is designed to increase patient access to experimental drugs and medical devices and to accelerate review of important new medications. The law provides for an expanded database of clinical trials, which is accessible by patients. Results of such clinical trials will be included in the database when a sponsor consents to it.

The law allows dissemination of information by manufacturers about unapproved uses of drugs and medical devices. It allows a company to provide peer-reviewed journal articles about off-label indications of its products, provided that the company files, within a specified time, a supplemental application based on appropriate research to establish the safety and effectiveness of the unapproved use.

The act ensures an increased emphasis on resources covering medical devices that present the greatest risks to patients. The law exempts from premarket notification any Class I device that is not intended for a use that is of substantial importance in preventing impairment of human health, or that do not present a potential unreasonable risk of illness or injury. The law directs the FDA to focus its postmarket surveillance on higher-risk devices.

Although the act simplifies many regulatory obligations for manufacturers, it does not reduce the standards by which medical problems are introduced into the market place. The act preserves the general rule that requires at least two well-controlled studies to prove a product's safety and effectiveness. The acts specifies that the FDA may keep out of the market products whose manufacturing processes are so deficient that they could present a serious health hazard. The law also gives the agency authority to take appropriate action if the technology of a device suggests that it is likely to be used for a potentially harmful unlabeled use.

Index

Italicized page numbers indicate figures. Page numbers followed by t indicate tables; b, boxes.